# ENCYCLOPAEDIC DICTIONARY OF GENETICS AND ORGANIC EVOLUTION

# Encyclopaedic Dictionary of Genetics and Organic Evolution

**Vol. 1**
[A — F]

*Editor*
**Kiran Narang**

**ANMOL PUBLICATIONS PVT LTD**
**New Delhi-110 002**

ANMOL PUBLICATIONS PVT LTD
4374/4B, Ansari Road
Daryaganj, New Delhi-110 002

*Encyclopaedic Dictionary of Genetics and Organic Evolution*

First Edition 1995
**ISBN 81-7488-044-5 (Set)**

**PRINTED IN INDIA**

Published by J.L. Kumar for Anmol Publications Pvt. Ltd. and
Printed at Mehra Offset Press, Delhi.

# Preface

This encyclopaedic dictionary has been essentially a compilation and editing of the terms and concepts taken from genetics and organic evolution. Many words borrowed from more general usage have been endowed with very special meaning, sometimes not obvious to the uninitiated.

The entries have been represented in a clear and explanatory style to provide both straight forward definitions and invaluable background informations. This approach combined with an extensive cross referencing system enables the reader to place each entry into a broader scientific context. Many diagrams have been incorporated whenever the meaning of a term can be best conveyed by means of a diagram.

Every effort has been made to include certain entries which take into account of recent developments and trends in genetics and organic evolution.

The terms included in this encyclopaedic dictionary have been presented in brief analytical phrases thereby avoiding the more comprehensive type of treatment appropriate to large reference works. The extent of each entry has been determined by the need for definition of meaning, function and agricultural relevance. Also, certain entries have been added to take into account of recent developments and trends in agriculture.

This encyclopaedic dictionary will be of immense value to the students of genetics and organic evolution, botany, ecology, biology, microbiology, anthropology, biochemistry, archaeology, geography, geology, agriculture and environmental science.

**Editor**

Vol. 1

# A

*Å or A.* Abbrev. for Angstrom.

*A-.* Prefix. denoting not, without, away.

*A (Amino Acid) Site.* The location at which specific transfer RNA molecules become attached to ribosomes during the translation phase of protein synthesis.

*A24 Protein (Semihistone).* Protein complex resulting from the conjugation of ubiquitin to histone H2A. The amount of H2A histone that is in the form of A24 varies in different cells. Some evidence exists to suggest that chromatin which includes actively transcribed DNA sequences is enriched in A24 protein.

*A Band.* One of the bands visible in striated muscle. A bands are distinguished from 1 bands with which they alternate in striated muscle, the former being composed of myosin fibrils and the latter of actin, troponin and tropomyosin.

*A, B Antigens.* Human blood group substances composed of oligosaccharides and found attached to glycolipid in the plasma membrane of erythrocytes, or to soluble glycoproteins in tears, gastric juice and saliva. Their function is not known, but they are detected by means of 'naturally occurring antibodies' present in individuals lacking the corresponding antigen and which probably arise because similar oligosaccharides are present on cell membranes of enteric bacteria.

***Abiotic Factor.*** Any contribution to the environment that is of a non-living nature, e.g. climate.

***ABO Blood Group.*** A classification of blood based on natural variation in human blood types, identified and named by Karl Landsteiner (1868-1943) in 1901. There are four groups : A, B, AB and O, each classified by a particular combination of antigen(s) on the red blood cells and naturally occurring antibodies in the blood plasma. The relative frequency of the four ABO groups in the genetic polymorphism has been investigated in most human populations and differs widely between races.

Antigens and antibodies of the same type cause agglutination when mixed, resulting in difficulties in blood transfusion. Although possessing no A or B antigens, Group O individuals have an H-antigen which is a precursor to the A and B types. H, A and B antigens are found also in human body secretions such as saliva and semen, often a useful fact in forensic tests.

Inheritance of grouping is controlled by a single autosomal gene on chromosome 9 with three major alleles, A, B and O (sometimes written as $I^A$, $I^B$ and $I^O$). Four types of the A group are now known, making six multiple alleles at this locus.

***Abortive Transduction.*** Transduction of bacterial genes into a new host cell by a viral vector that is not followed by integration of the new genes into the genome of the recipient cell. The transduced genes may, however, persist for a time in the cell as a plasmid, conferring on the recipient bacterium new but transient genetic properties.

Abortive transduction is characterized by the presence of small (often microscopic) colonies on media selective for the donor phenotype. Only one cell in each of these colonies actually contains the exogenote, so the colonies grow non-exponentially. When minute colonies are absent from appropriate selective media then no part of the exogenote can compensate for the functional deficiency of the recipient endogenote and the mutations are therefore allelic. The presence of abortive transductants indicates genetic complementation between exogenote and endogenote; this can be interallelic (allelic complementation) or intergenic.

***Abscisic Acid.*** A plant hormone. It is called abscisin when found in ageing leaves and it is partly responsible for leaf abscission. It is also called dormin when in buds and seeds, and cause induction of dormancy. See Figure A.1.

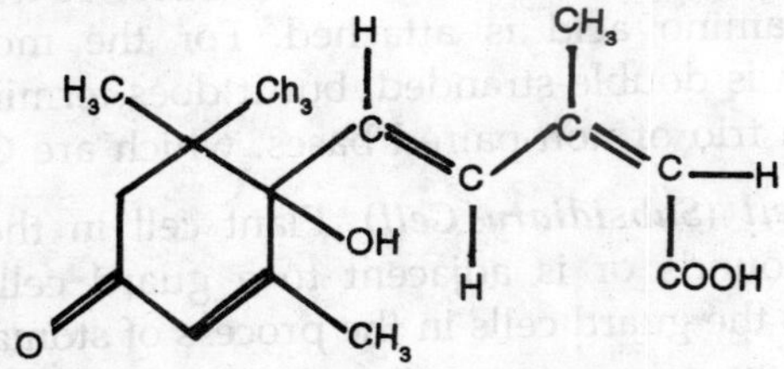


Figure A.1. Abscisic acid. Molecular structure.

***Abscission.*** The process by which plant organs are shed. The process occurs in the stalks of unfertilized flowers, ripe fruits and deciduous leaves in autumn, or in diseased leaves at any time. It is due to the formation of an abscission layer of thin-walled cells in the stalk base which rupture under strain, e.g. wind. A layer of cork forms beneath the abscission layer to seal the plant surface. Abscission is controlled by plant hormones present; a low concentration of auxin, high amounts of ethylene, and (in some plants) a high concentration of abscisic acid all stimulate production of the abscission layer. See Figure A.2.

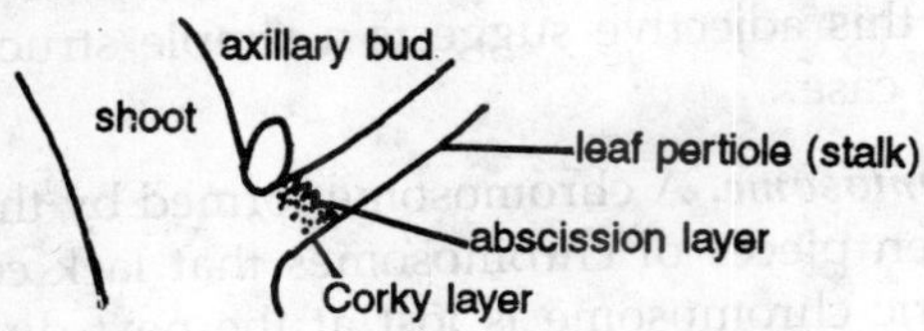


Figure A.2. Abscission. Abscission layer in a leaf stalk.

***Abyssal.*** Designating or inhabiting the deep waters of an ocean (approximately below 2000 metres), where conditions are cold, dark, and still.

***Absorptive Endocytosis.*** Uptake of material from the surrounding medium by means of active endocytosis through the plasma membrane of the cell.

***Acceptor Molecule.*** A molecule that has a high affinity for electrons, usually passing them on to another acceptor molecule in a series (called an electron transport system).

***Acceptor Splicing Site.*** Junction between the intron and the exon at the right-hand end of an intron.

***Acceptor Stem.*** Linear extension of a transfer RNA to which a specific amino acid is attached. For the most part the extension is double-stranded, but it does terminate at its 3' -end in a trio of non-paired bases, which are CCA.

***Accessory Cell (Subsidiary Cell).*** Plant cell in the epidermis that surrounds or is adjacent to a guard cell. Accessory cells help the guard cells in the process of stomatal opening and closing.

***Accessory Nuclei.*** Small nuclei found in the oocytes of some hymenopteran insects. They are derived from the main oocyte nucleus.

***Acclimatization or Acclimation.*** The process by which a range of adjustments occur in the body, e.g. in temperature control and respiration, when an organism is subjected to unusual environmental stresses.

***Acellular (of an organism).*** Having a body which is not composed of cells. Acellular organisms may have a complex structure differentiated into specialized areas and organelles. Such organisms are also described as unicellular, although this adjective suggests a simple structure, which is not the case.

***Acentric Chromosome.*** A chromosome formed by the joining of two broken pieces of chromosomes that lack centromeres; the acentric chromosome is lost at the next division.

***Acetabularia.*** A genus of marine algae. Individuals may reach a size of 30 mm and are acellular with a body consisting of three distinct areas : head, stalk and a base containing the single nucleus. Experiments by the German biologist Joachim Hammerling (b. 1901) using grafts between two species demonstrated that the nucleus alone is responsible for body morphology and produces a chemical substance which can control development. Such results can now be interpreted as indications of the role of DNA and messenger RNA.

***Aceto-Carmine.*** Dye consisting of 5 percent carmine solution in acetic acid; formerly used as a chromosome stain, but now largely replaced by aceto-orcein.

***Aceto-Orcein.*** Dye consisting of a solution of orcein in acetic acid. Squash preparations of chromosomes are often stained with aceto-orcein.

***Acetylcholine (ACh).*** A transmitter substance that is secreted at the ends of cholinergic nerve fibres on the arrival of a nerve impulse. ACh then passes the impulse across a synapse and immediately ACh has depolarized the postsynaptic membrane it is destroyed by the enzyme cholinesterase.

***Acetylcholinesterase.*** The enzyme present in the synaptic cleft that destroys acetylcholine.

***Acetylcoenzyme A (Acetyl-CoA).*** An organic compound important in the process of oxidation of energy-rich compounds to $CO_2$ and water. In the presence of oxygen the three-carbon pyruvic acid produced in glycolysis is broken down in the mitochondria to produce $CO_2$, two hydrogen

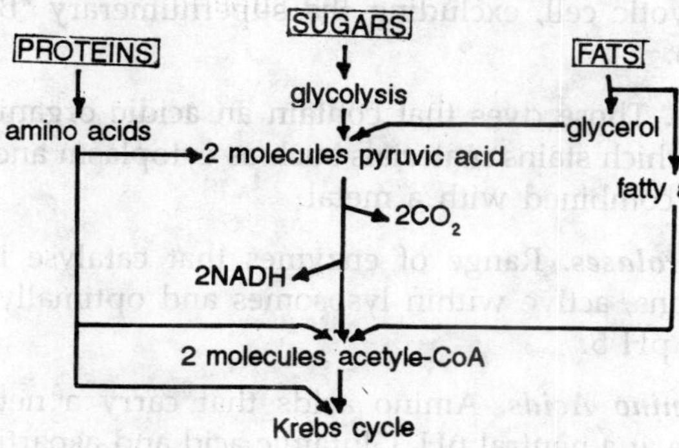


Figure A.3. Acetylcoenzyme A. Production of acetyl-CoA from food.

atoms (reducing NAD to $NADH_2$), and an active form of two-carbon acetic acid bonded to coenzyme A, called acetylcoenzyme A, Metabolism of fats and proteins also produces acetyl-CoA, either via pyruvic acid or directly. Thus acetyl-CoA is common to the metabolism of all major types of food, forming a step leading to the krebs cycle. See Figure A.3.

***Acetylmuramic Acid.*** Disaccharide found in linear polymers in peptidoglycan that occurs in the periplasm between the inner and outer membranes of gram-negative bacteria.

***Achiasmate.*** Designating a meiosis in which no chiasmata occur. In some species, such as Drosophila melanogaster, crossing-over is limited to one sex, and in these cases the heterogametic sex has achiasmate meiosis.

***Achondroplasia.*** The commonest form of human dwarfism. It results from abnormal cartilage development, producing numerous bone defects : stunted trunk, shortened and deformed limbs, and bulging skull. The condition is controlled by an autosomal dominant gene and thus affected children born to normal parents must result from a mutation in one or other parent. The majority (around 80%) of achondroplastics die in early childhood but those surviving are fertile, have the normal range of intelligence and can live more or less normal lives. The typical circus dwarf is achondroplastic.

**A *Chromosomes.*** The main chromosome complement of a eukaryotic cell, excluding the supernumerary *B chromosomes.

***Acid Dyes.*** Those dyes that contain an acidic organic component which stains materials such as cytoplasm and collagen when combined with a metal.

***Acid Hydrolases.*** Range of enzymes that catalyse hydrolytic reactions, active within lysosomes and optimally active at about pH 5.

***Acidic Amino Acids.*** Amino acids that carry a net negative charge at a neutral pH. Glutamic acid and aspartic acid are examples of such amino acids, possessing negatively charged side-chains at normal cellular pH.

***Acidic Dye.*** Dye (e.g. Acid Fuchsin) that specifically stains positively charged material since the dye carries a net negative charge.

***Acidic Protein.*** Protein that possesses a net negative charge at neutral pH because it is rich in acidic amino acids. Most proteins in eukaryotic cells are acidic, notable exceptions being the basic proteins — the histones. Some acidic proteins are believed to have important roles as gene-regulatory molecules.

***Acidophil or Acidophile or Acidophilic or Acidophilous.*** 1. (of a cell such as a leucocyte) having tissues that are easily stainable with acid dyes. 2. (of organisms, particularly microorganisms) preferring an acidic environment.

***Acid Phosphatase.*** Enzyme that splits the phosphate groups from a variety of substances and is optimally active at acid pH. It is an important constituent of lysosomes and was originally used as an assay to identify cell fractions rich in lysosomes. There is evidence that acid phosphatase is packaged in the golgi apparatus of the cell.

***Acinar Cell.*** Exocrine cell in the pancreas that secretes digestive enzymes and zymogens, including amylase, lipase, trypsinogen, chymotrypsinogen, DNase and RNase. Acinar cells have provided information about cellular secretion processes; for example, pulses of radiolabelled amino acids are given to the cells and the subsequent fate of the amino acids is traced by autoradiography.

***Acinus.*** Basic secretory unit of an exocrine gland. It has a sacular or tubular shape, the wall of which is typically cuboidal or columnar epithelial cells. Secretory product is released from the apical cell surfaces into the enclosed lumen form which it drains into a collecting duct. In a compound exocrine gland, the acini may resemble a bunch of grapes (acinus = grape) and drain into a complex, branched ductal system.

***Acquired Characters.*** Characteristics of an organism which, according to Lamarck become well developed through use or through environment influences during an organism's lifetime, and which are inherited by its progeny. However, no clear experimental evidence has yet been found to support the theory. Current opinion is that the environment does play a large part in evolution, though only through natural selection.

***Acridine.*** One of a class of organic dyes that can act as mutagens, causing deletions and additions of base pairs, especially in plasmids and other extrachromosomal DNA molecules. The flat acridine molecules intercalate between adjacent base pairs in DNA and cause unwinding of the helix. An example is proflavin (2,8-diaminoacridine).

***Acrocentric (of a chromosome).*** Having the centromere near one end, making one chromosome arm much longer than the other.

***Acromegaly.*** A chronic disease characterized by enlargement of the head, hands and feet. It is caused by over-secretion of growth hormones.

***Acropetal.*** 1. (of plant structures, e.g. leaves and flowers) produced one after another from the base of the stem to the apex. 2. (of substances, e.g. water) moving from the base of a plant to the apex.

***Acrosome.*** A membrane-bound sac derived from the golgi apparatus, located at the tip of the sperm. The acrosome plays an important role in fertilization. It contains enzymes that, when the sac ruptures upon contacting the egg, aid in penetration of the egg membrane so enabling transfer of the sperm nucleus to the egg cell. See Figure A.4.

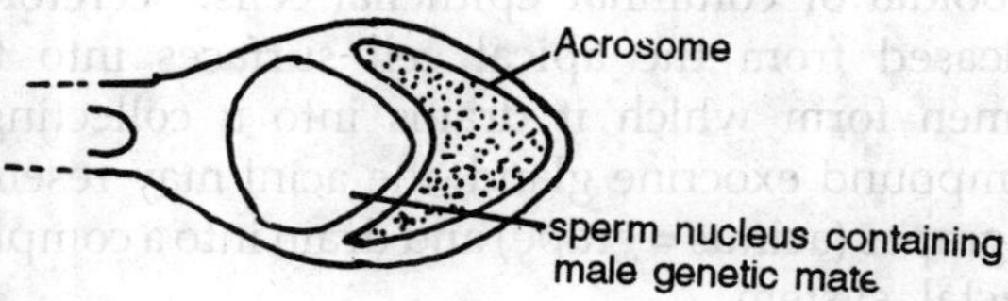


Figure A.4. Acrosome. Head of a typical mammalian sperm.

***Acrosome Reaction.*** Initial response of an egg cell to contact with a spermatozoon. The acrosome vesicle of the sperm, a package of hydrolytic enzymes, is released by exocytosis, digesting a path for the sperm through the zona pellucida of the egg and enabling it to reach the egg cell plasma membrane with which it fuses. In invertebrate sperm, the reaction also releases specific protein molecules which help to bind the sperm to the egg coat.

***Acrosyndesis.*** Pairing of homologous chromosomes at meiosis by means of their telomeric portions.

***Acrylamide.*** Monomer resin used, together with a crosslinking agent, in the formation of polyacrylamide gels for electrophoresis.

***ACTH (adrenocorticotrophic hormone, corticotrophin).*** A hormone produced by the anterior pituitary gland in response to stress that controls secretion of certain hormones (the corticosteroids) by the adrenal glands. It can be administered by injection to treat such disorders as rheumatic diseases and asthma, but it only relieves symptoms and is not a cure.

***Actimycin.*** Inhibitor of mitochondrial electron transport.

***Actin.*** Chief protein constituent of muscle and of other contractile systems (e.g. cilia and flagella). Actin molecules are filamentous proteins, consisting of two strings of globular units (G actin) wound round one another to form a rope-like structure (F actin). See Figure A.5.

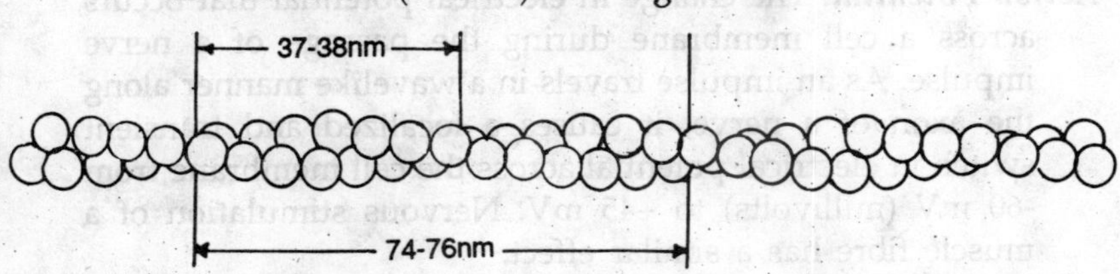


Figure A.5. Linkage of actin molecules to form a microfilament. Each spherical unit in the double spiral is an actin molecule.

***Actin Filament.*** Filamentous structure of F actin, consisting of two strands of globular molecules, each about 4 nm diameter, twisted into a helix with 13.5 molecules per turn. Such filaments have been identified as the chief components of thin filaments in striated muscle.

***Actin Genes.*** Genes coding for actin constitute an important gene family in animal cells. Up to 20 distinct coding sequences have been distinguished in mammals, but not all are necessarily transcribed. Although some actin sequences are linked, others are dispersed widely in the genome. Distinct actin genes are activated in mammalian cardiac and skeletal muscle. At least one pseudogene has been discovered in the actin gene family.

***Actinins.*** Accessory muscle proteins. found mainly in the Z disc of striated muscle; alpha-actinin ($M_r$ = 200 000); beta-actinin.

***Actinomycetes.*** Group of gram-positive bacteria capable of mycelial growth. This group include the genus Streptomyces.

***Actinomycin D.*** A substance that inhibits the transcription of RNA from DNA. When isolated from soil bacteria and used pharmaceutically it acts as an antibiotic.

***Actinosphaerium.*** A protozoan, known as the sun-animalcule, which is related to Amoeba.

***Actinozoa.*** A less usual term for the anthozoa.

***Action Potential.*** The change in electrical potential that occurs across a cell membrane during the passage of a nerve impulse. As an impulse travels in a wavelike manner along the axon of a nerve, it causes a localized and transient switch in electrical potential across the cell membrane from -60 mV (millivolts) to +45 mV. Nervous stimulation of a muscle fibre has a similar effect.

***Action Spectrum.*** A plot of the relative efficiencies of different wavelengths of radiation (usually light) in causing a reaction. The action spectrum for photosynthesis is shown in the diagram and corresponds closely with the absorption spectrum of the chlorophylls, indicating that the latter pigments are the primary light-trapping molecules in photosynthesis. See Figure A.6.

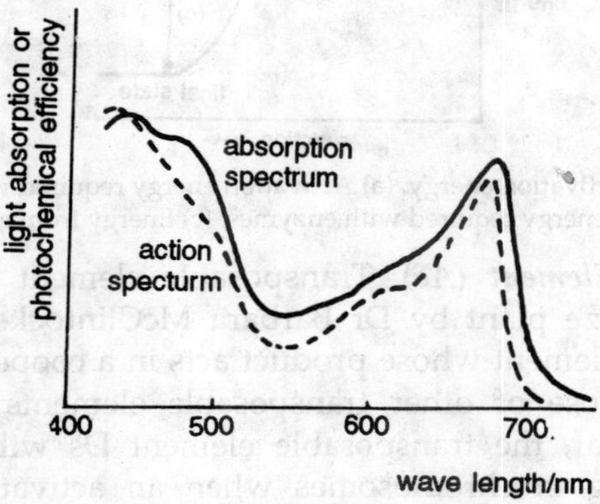


Figure A.6. Light absorption spectrum and action spectrum of photosynthesis for a green plant.

***Activated Macrophage.*** Macrophage which, following stimulation by lymphokines, is enlarged and highly active in phagocytosis.

***Activated Sludge.*** Any material used in sewage treatment, consisting mainly of bacteria and protozoans, that purifies the sewage and increases by multiplication during the process. Part of the new sludge is used in the continuing treatment of the sewage.

***Activation Energy.*** The energy required to initiate a reaction. Chemical bonds holding molecules together are difficult to break, requiring extra 'activation' energy to push the bonded atoms apart. This extra energy makes the bonds less stable so that the molecule releases not only the activation energy but also the energy unlocked when the chemical bonds break, forming an exergonic reaction.

Activation energy can be applied externally as heat, but this is inappropriate for living organisms. Instead, they rely on biological catalysis (Enzymes) which decrease the activation energy needed for the reaction to take place. See Figure A.7.

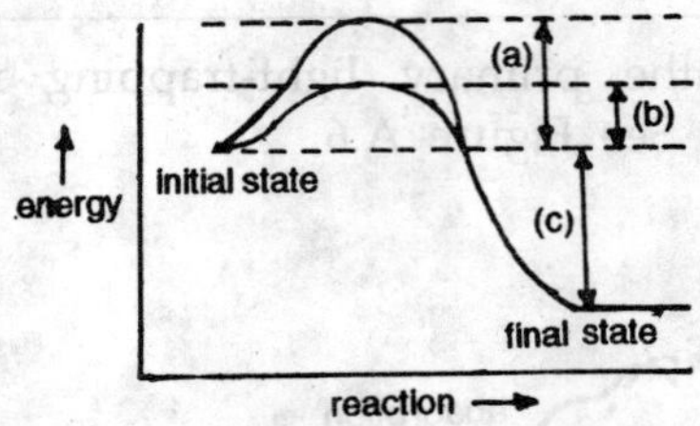


Figure A.7. Activation energy. (a) Activation energy required without enzymes. (b) Activation energy required with enzymes. (c) Energy from exergonic reaction.

***Activator Element (Ac).*** Transposable element discovered in the maize plant by Dr Barbara McClintock. It is a trans-acting element whose product acts in a cooperative fashion with those of other transposable elements in maize. In particular, the transposable element Ds will only induce breaking in chromosomes when an activator element is also present.

***Activator Molecule.*** Molecule that specifically activates or induces a biochemical reaction; most frequently applied to molecules that act as gene regulators.

***Active Centre.*** 1. The part of an enzyme molecule that interacts with and binds are substrate, forming an enzyme substrate. 2. The part of an antibody molecule that interacts with and binds the antigen, forming an antibody/antigen complex.

***Active Gene.*** Gene sequence that is being actively transcribed. Since the rates of transcription vary, the activity of a gene is not an 'all-or-nothing' phenomenon. Some genes, such as those coding for tRNA, are transcribed at a high rate throughout the life of the cell, and are said to be constitutive. Others, such as those coding for histones, are expressed in all cells but are active only at certain times during the cell cycle, and some (e.g. globin gene), are active only in blood-forming tissue during times when haemoglobin synthesis is required.

Active genes have certain biochemical characteristics, some of which may be partially responsible for the process of activation, others may follow from the fact of activation. The characteristics of most active genes are : (1) that they are in an open conformation in chromatin and therefore more easily digested by degradative enzymes such as Dnase I; (2) that they have highly acetylated histones associated with them; (3) that they are poorly methylated, if at all; (4) some active genes are also associated with histone that is enriched for A24 protein.

***Active Immunity.*** Development of an immune reaction by the host's immune system following injection of, or natural exposure to, an antigen oand often resulting in long-term protection should the antigen be a pathogen or some inocuous form of it.

***Active Ingredient.*** The chemically active part of a manufactured product such as an herbicide, the remainder being inert.

***Active Site.*** An area of enzyme surface which has a shape complementary to a particular substrate, enabling the enzyme and substrate to become temporarily bonded to form an enzyme-substrate complex. Such a lock-and-key mechanism explains the great specificity of enzymes for substrates and also why changes in enzyme three-dimensional shape (by pH, temperature) cause alterations to enzyme activity. See Figure A.8.

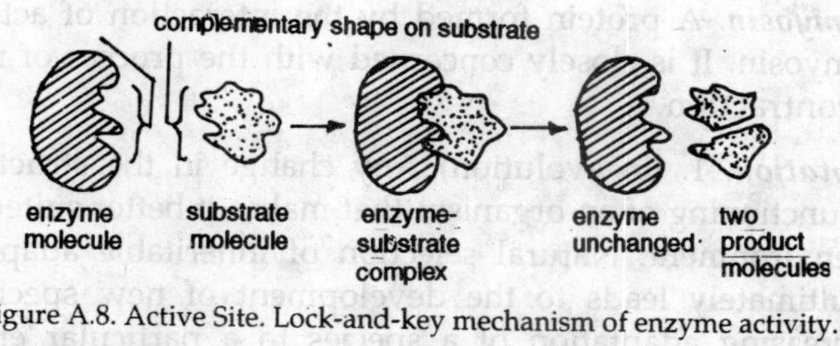


Figure A.8. Active Site. Lock-and-key mechanism of enzyme activity.

***Active Transport.*** The transport of molecules across a biological membrane against a concentration gradient (i.e. from a region of low concentration to one of high concentration). Active transport is mediated by a carrier (C), thought to be a protein or lipoprotein, which becomes saturated at high concentration levels. It also requires a source of energy, e.g. ATP (see Figure A.9(a)), and is usually unidirectional (unlike passive diffusion, which is reversible). Active transport is responsible for the entry of amino acids into cells and for the exclusion of sodium from neurones to produce a resting potential across the cell membrane.

Passive transport (i.e. without expenditure of energy) may occur reversibly by carrier-mediated systems. Two such systems are facilitated diffusion, which occurs along a concentration gradient (see Figure A.9(b)), for example in the transport of glucose into red blood cells; and exchange diffusion. in which molecules are exchanged between one side of the membrane and the other (see Figure A.9(c)), for example in the exchange of phosphate across the mitochondrial membrane.

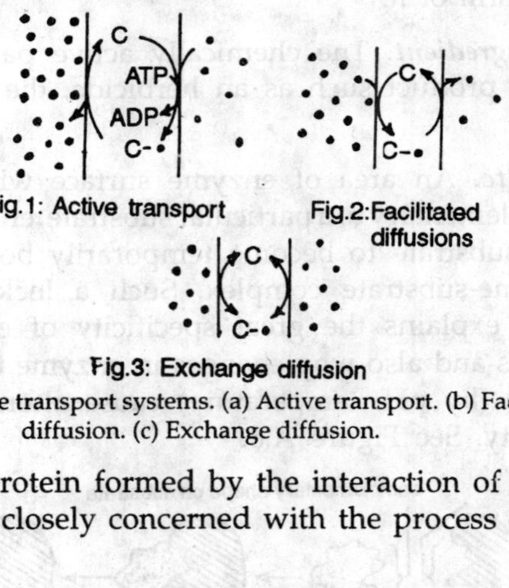


Figure. Membrane transport systems. (a) Active transport. (b) Facilitated diffusion. (c) Exchange diffusion.

***Actomyosin.*** A protein formed by the interaction of actin and myosin. It is closely concerned with the process of muscle contraction.

***Adaptation.*** 1. (in evolution) Any change in the structure or functioning of an organism that makes it better suited to its environment. Natural selection of inheritable adaptations ultimately leads to the development of new species. Increasing adaptation of a species to a particular environment tends to diminish its ability to adapt to any sudden change in that environment. 2. (in physiology) The alteration in the degree of sensitivity (either an increase or a decrease) of a sense organ to suit conditions more extreme than normally encountered. An example is the adjustment of the eye to vision in very bright or very dim light.

***Adaptation, Genetic.*** Any characteristic that improves the chances of an organism transmitting genes to the next generation (i.e. producing offspring). Such beneficial changes are genetically controlled and can be distinguished from alterations occurring within one generation which may not lead to genetic change. Adaptations can affect any level of organization, from cells to whole organisms, and their behaviour. Adaptions are favoured by the process of natural selection.

***Adaptation, Physiological.*** Change in the reaction that organisms show as a result of prolonged exposure to conditions that normally produce a different or more extensive reaction. For example, mountain sickness (headache, nausea, fatigue) in man passes off as he becomes acclimatized to high altitudes because of adjustments that occur in the respiratory and circulatory systems.

***Adaptive Enzyme.*** An enzyme that is produced by an organism, e.g. bacteria, only in the presence of its normal substrate or a closely similar substance. Such enzymes are not produced in circumstances to which the organism is not adapted.

***Adaptive Evolution.*** Process of evolution that makes a species or population more suited to its environmental niche.

***Adaptive Landscape.*** Topographical representation of two gene frequencies each plotted against average fitness.

***Adaptive Radiation.*** The evolutionary divergence of many forms of animals or plants from a single ancestral stock to fill many ecological niches. These forms can become new species or even, in time, new genera and families. For example, insects underwent adaptive radiation into types suited for flying, burrowing, aquatic life, parasitism, etc.; mammals, both placental and marsupial, evolved into carnivores, herbivores, burrowers, and aquatic, arboreal, and flying types. Flowering plants adapted to suit desert conditions, freshwater, marshland, and salt-marsh habitats, and into climbing, insectivorous, and parasitic modes of life.

***Adaptive Valve.*** Worth of a particular genotype in conferring an advantage, or increased fitness, on an organism in a particular environment.

***Adaptor.*** Short sequence of DNA used to splice together two longer DNA molecules, only one of which has cohesive ends.

***Addison's Disease.*** A disease caused by a deficiency of adreno-corticosteroid hormones (e.g. cortisone, aldosterone) produced by cells of the adrenal gland cortex. Named after Thomas Addison (1793-1860), the English physician who first described it. The major symptoms of the disease are lowered blood pressure, lowered blood-sugar levels, reduced kidney function, loss of weight, extreme muscular weakness, and a brownish pigmentation of the skin and mucous membranes.

***Additive Factors (Additive Genes).*** Series of non-ellelic gene sequences which each affect the same phenotypic character in a synergistic fashion.

***Additive Genes.*** Those in which more than one gene controls a character, with each allele making a definite and measurable contribution towards the character, there is no dominance between alleles of one gene and no epistasis between different loci. Many pigment systems are controlled by additive genes, producing a wide spread of variability.

***Additive Genetic Variation.*** Component of variation with respect to some quantitatively measurable character that behaves in heredity as if determined by gene differences of additive effect. Taken literally it implies the absence of dominance in allelic interactions and of epistasis in non-allelic (intergene) interactions, both of which generally occur to a greater or lesser extent. So the additive model is at best a statistical approximation, dependent on the particular array of mutational differences that happen to be present in the population under study. Additivity of effect is a property of particular combinations of particular alleles, not of genes as such. The same gene can often mutate either to alleles of minor and more or less additive effect (in comparison with the progenitor) or to alleles of major non-additive effect.

***Additive Recombination.*** Genetic recombination, which involves insertion of a new DNA sequence into an existing genome without any reciprocal loss of DNA. Such recombination may be achieved by devices such as insertion elements, which pair up with a short sequence in the DNA, initiate a local break in the DNA and then by a splicing procedure come to be included as a colinear addition to the original sequence.

***Adductor.*** 1. Also called a depressor. A muscle that pulls a structure or limb towards the main part of the body. An example is the adductor mandibulae, which closes the jaws in amphibians. 2. A muscle that pulls two structures together, e.g. the two valves of a shell.

***Adenine.*** One of four types of nitrogenous bases found in DNA, having the double-ring structure of a class known as purines (See Figure A.10).

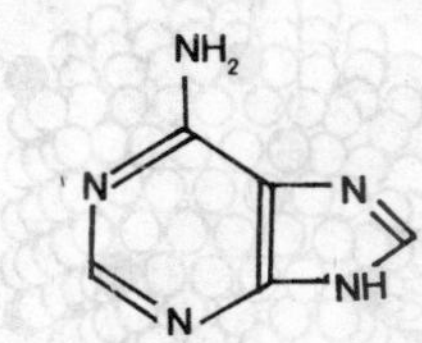


Figure A.10. Adenine. Molecular structure.

Adenine forms part of a DNA unit called a nucleotide and always forms complementary base pairing with a DNA pyrimidine base called thymine (see Figure A.11). When pairing with RNA during transcription, adenine is complementary to uracil. Adenine also occurs in RNA molecules, ATP and AMP.

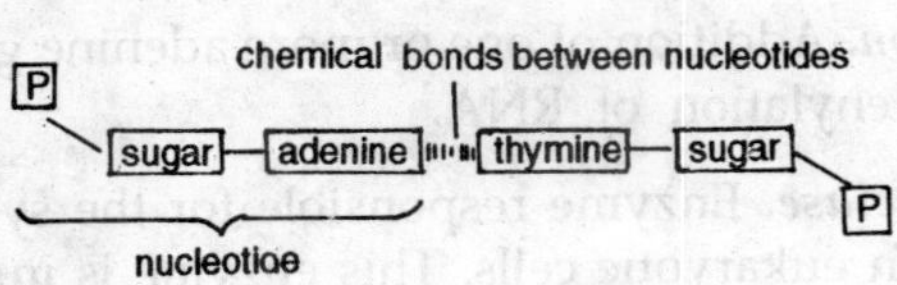


Figure A.11. Adenine. Complementary pairing. P = phosphate group.

***Adenine Deoxyriboside.*** Nucleoside formed by bonding of adenine with deoxyribose.

***Adenosine.*** Nucleoside formed by the bonding of adenine with ribose.

***Adenosine Phosphates.*** Compounds in which adenosine in combined with either one, two or three phosphoric acid groups. The various phosphates of adenosine—AMP, ADP and ATP—are easily converted from one to the other.

***Adenoviruses.*** Group of DNA viruses having double-stranded DNA as a genome enclosed within a capsid with icosahedral symmetry. Their genomes are small, with coding potential for only about 12 genes. Some adenoviruses cause acute respiratory diseases in man and other mammals. See Figure A.12.

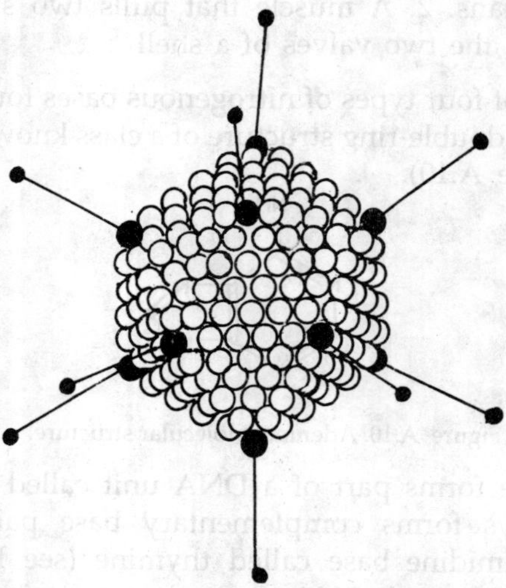

Figure A.12. Model of adenovirus particle based on electron microscopic observations.

***Adenylation.*** Addition of one or more adenine groups, as in the polyadenylation of RNA.

***Adenyl Cyclase.*** Enzyme responsible for the synthesis of cycle AMP in eukaryotic cells. This enzyme is involved in many cellular processes and particularly in the action of polypeptide hormones (e.g. insulin). When such hormones attach to the plasma membrane of a cell they stimulate adenyl cyclase to produce cyclic AMP. This is the initial step in the second messenger system, which enables these hormones to affect the gene expression of cells to which they bind.

***Adenylic Acid.*** Nucleotide found in RNA consisting of the purine base adenine, a pentose sugar and a phosphoric acid group.

***ADH (Antidiuretic Hormone).*** A hormone secreted by neurosecretory cells of the hypothalamus and released by the posterior lobe of the pituitary gland. ADH stimulates the resorption of water through the distal-convoluted tubule of the kidney nephron in mammals and thus limits the water content and the overall volume of urine.

***Adjuvant.*** A substance that is not itself antigenic but, when mixed with an antigen, enhances antibody production. Adjuvant not only helps to produce antibody against small amounts of antigen but also prolongs the period of antibody production. Adjuvants for therapeutic use must be easily metabolizable and ultimately eliminated. Although the exact mode of action of adjuvants is uncertain, they are known to promote the persistence of antigen and to cause an inflammatory response that leads to a local influx of antibody-forming cells.

***A DNA.*** Form of double helical DNA which, like the common B form, is a right-handed double helix of antiparallel strands, but differing slightly in helical pitch and base pair orientation from the B form. Only very localized regions of DNA occur as A-form molecules, but the A-form helix is the most stable configuration for double-stranded RNA.

***Adoptive Transfer.*** Transfer, from one organism to another, of an immunological potential by the transfer of immune competent cells.

***ADP (Adenosine Diphosphate).*** A molecule consisting of an adenosine unit into which are attached two phosphate groups, which are joined by a high-energy bond. ADP can be converted to ATP by the addition of inorganic phosphate and about 34 kJ energy. See Figure A.13.

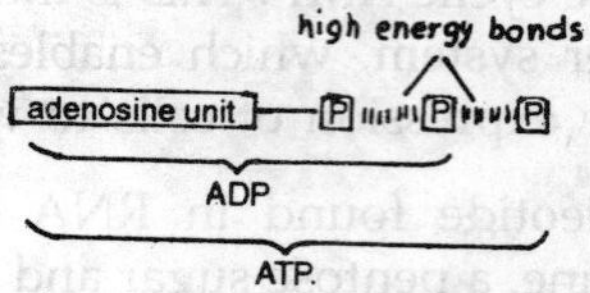


Figure A.13. ADP. General structure of ADP and ATP. P = phosphate group.

***Adrenal Cortical Hormones.*** Hormones secreted by the cortex of the adrenal glands. They are generally of three main types : (a) mineralocorticoids, e.g. aldosterone and deoxycorticosterone, which are concerned with salt and water balance; (b) Glucocorticoids, e.g. cortisone and hydrocortisone, which aid the formation of carbohydrates from fat and protein; and (c) sex hormones, particularly androgens in both male and female mammals.

***Adrenal Gland.*** An endocrine organ consisting of a medulla (central part) secreting adrenaline and noradrenaline and a cortex (outer zone) secreting adrenal cortical hormones. The two parts are closely associated in mammals, but are sometimes separated into distinct organs in other vertebrates, e.g. fish. The activity of the medulla is controlled by the sympathetic nervous system, and that of the cortex by adrenocorticotropic hormone secreted by the pituitary gland. In mammals there is a pair of adrenal glands situated anteriorly to the kidneys; other vertebrates have more than two adrenals.

***Adrenaline or Epinephrine.*** A hormone secreted by the medulla (central part) of the adrenal gland. It prepares the body for emergency action (fight-or-flight reaction); it increases the cardiac frequency, constricts the vessels supplying the skin and gut, increases the blood pressure, increases blood sugar, dilates the blood vessels of the muscles, heart and brain, widens the pupils, and causes hair erection. It is usually secreted with noradrenaline, whose effects are similar. Both hormones are also secreted by the adrenergic nerve endings of the sympathetic nervous system.

***Adrenergic (of nerve endings).*** Secreting adrenaline and nonadrenaline on the arrival of a nerve impulse. These substances then stimulate the effector nerve fibres in the sympathetic nervous system of many vertebrates in much the same way as acetylcholine acts as a transmitter substance in cholinergic nerve fibres.

***Adrenocorticotropic or Adrenocorticotrophic Hormone (ACTH) or Corticotrophin.*** A small, proteinaceous hormone secreted by the anterior lobe of the pituitary. It controls the secretion of other hormones of the cortex of the adrenal gland.

***Adrenogenital Syndrome.*** Disease in humans typified by hormonal inbalance and an accumulation of a testosterone-like compound, and therefore presenting as masculinization of affected females.

***Adsorption.*** The taking up of gas or liquid by a surface or interface. In physical adsorption, molecules are held by Van Der Waal's forces of attraction; in chemical adsorption there is exchange or sharing of electrons.

***Advanced.*** Non-primitive; descriptive of a character or evolutionary stage that is, relative to others, a late development, especially if complex and beneficial.

***Adventitious Embryony.*** Production of one sporophyte from another without any intervening gametophyte generation.

***Aerial Respiration.*** A process of gas exchange occurring in terrestrial and some aquatic organisms, by which oxygen is absorbed from the air and carbon dioxide released. Respiratory surfaces are usually internal (e.g. the mesophyll of leaves, the tracheae of insects, the lung books of spiders and scorpions, and the lungs of land vertebrates), although some respiratory organs are external, e.g. the skin of amphibia. All surfaces rely on a water layer for gas exchange and may also depend on a blood system for transport of gases to and from distant parts of the body.

***Aerobe.*** Any organism (typically a microorganism) that can survive only in the presence of oxygen required for aerobic respiration.

***Aerobic Respiration.*** A type of cellular respiration that requires oxygen. Glucose is broken down to release energy in a series of steps which can be grouped into three main stages :

Stage 1 : glucose is converted to pyruvic acid in a process called glycolysis which takes place in the cell cytoplasm. A stable glucose molecule is first energized by the addition of a phosphate group from two ATP molecules (Phosphorylation) and then broken down to two molecules of three-carbon phosphoglyceraldehyde (PGAL). Each PGAL molecule is oxidized by removal of two hydrogen atoms which are picked up by an NAD molecule. Since oxygen is present, NADH can undergo a mitochondrial shunt to enter an electron transport system (ETS). Four molecules of ATP are then synthesized in substrate-level phosphorylation over several steps, giving a net gain of two ATP molecules per molecule of glucose. Glycolysis is completed with the production of two molecules of three-carbon pyruvic acid (pyruvate).

Stage 2 : oxidation and decarboxylation of pyruvic acid in the mitochondria to form two molecules of two-carbon acetylcoenzyme A (acetyl-CoA). $CO_2$ is released in this process, together with two hydrogen atoms per pyruvic acid molecule, which are picked up by NAD and passed down an ETS located on the inner membranes of mitochondrial cristae. Three molecules of ATP are produced per NADH, with oxygen acting as the final acceptor of hydrogen, producing water.

Stage 3 : entry of acetyl-CoA into the krebs cycle (TCA cycle). Each molecule of acetyl-CoA can turn the cycle once. As each glucose molecule is broken down to two acetyl-CoA molecules, the cycle will turn twice per glucose molecule, yielding $2 \times 2$ molecules of $CO_2$ and $2 \times 8$ atoms of hydrogen. Six pairs of hydrogen atoms are picked up by NAD to produce 18 ($6 \times 3$) molecules of ATP via the ETS. The remaining two pairs of hydrogen atoms are accepted by fad molecules which move to the ETS to produce 4 ($2 \times 2$) molecules of ATP. One molecule of ATP is produced directly by substrate-level phosphorylation for each turn of the cycle. The three stages are summarized in Figure A.14.

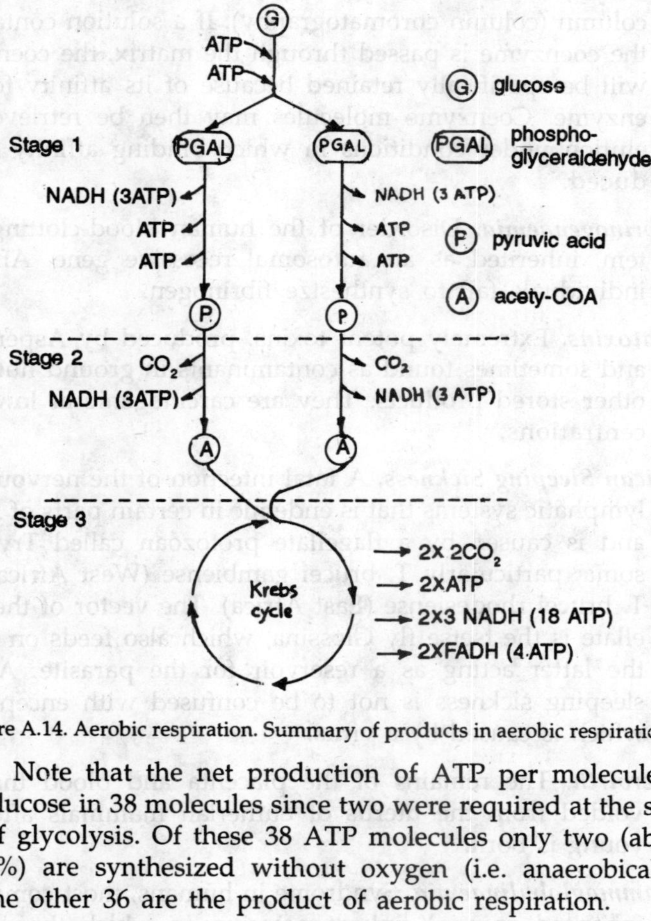


Figure A.14. Aerobic respiration. Summary of products in aerobic respiration.

Note that the net production of ATP per molecule of glucose in 38 molecules since two were required at the start of glycolysis. Of these 38 ATP molecules only two (about 5%) are synthesized without oxygen (i.e. anaerobically); the other 36 are the product of aerobic respiration.

Fats and proteins can also undergo aerobic respiration, entering the reactions at various stages.

***Aflatoxin.*** Any of four related toxic compounds produced by the mould Aspergillus flavus. Aflatoxins bind to DNA and prevent replication and transcription. They can cause acute liver damage and cancers; man may be poisoned by eating stored peanuts and cereals contaminated with the mould.

***Affinity Chromatography.*** A technique for isolating biological molecules that depends on the specific affinity of one molecule for another. For example, to isolate a coenzyme, enzyme molecules may be bound to an inert matrix in a column (column chromatography). If a solution containing the coenzyme is passed through the matrix, the coenzyme will be specifically retained because of its affinity for the enzyme. Coenzyme molecules may then be retrieved by elution under conditions in which binding affinity in reduced.

***Afibrinogenaemia.*** Disorder of the human blood-clotting system, inherited as an autosomal recessive gene. Affected individuals fail to synthesize fibrinogen.

***Aflatoxins.*** Extremely potent toxins, produced by Aspergillus and sometimes found as contaminants in ground nuts and other stored products. They are carcinogenic at low concentrations.

***African Sleeping Sickness.*** A fatal infection of the nervous and lymphatic systems that is endemic in certain parts of Africa and is caused by a flagellate protozoan called Trypanosoma, particularly T. brucei gambiense (West Africa) and T. brucei rhodesiense (East Africa). The vector of the flagellate is the tsetse fly Glossina, which also feeds on cattle, the latter acting as a reservoir for the parasite. African sleeping sickness is not to be confused with encephelitis which is caused by a virus.

***Afterbirth.*** The remains of the placenta and blood that are voided from the uterus of eutherian mammals after the young is born.

***Agammaglobulinaemia.*** Syndrome in humans, most commonly inherited as an X-linked recessive, in which there is an absence of plasma cells and impairment in immunoglobulin synthesis.

***Agamospermy.*** Formation of seeds of the absence of fertilization. Male gametes may not be involved or, if so, purely in a stimulatory capacity.

***Agar.*** 1. Extract of seaweeds, consisting of highly purified polysaccharide and used as an inert solidifying agent in culture media.

2. An extract of certain species of red seaweeds that is used as a gelling agent in microbiological culture media, foodstuffs, medicines, and cosmetic creams and jellies. Nutrient agar consists of a broth made from beef extract or blood that is gelled with agar and used for the cultivation of bacteria, fungi, and some algae.

***Agarose Gel.*** Inert matrix composed of the polysaccharide agarose dissolved in hot water and allowed to gelatinize at room temperature in a suitable mould. Such gels may be prepared using a variety of agarose concentrations (generally in the range 0.2-2 percent wt/vol) and employed as molecular sieves for size fractionation of DNA or RNA by electrophoresis. Gels of high agarose concentration are best suited to the separation of small nucleic acid fragments, and vice versa; speed of fragment migration is inversely proportional to molecular size and is generally retarded by increasing agarose concentration.

***Agar Plate Count.*** Means whereby the number of bacteria in a population is determined by applying serial dilutions of the culture to agar plates (either by spreading the sample over the surface or by incorporating the bacteria into the agar), and counting the number of colonies that develop after a suitable incubation period. The agar plate count, often called the 'viable count', is not necessarily identical to the total number of bacterial cells in the original population (for some cells may be dead) nor to the number of viable cells (cells may be aggregated into clumps or associated into chains; each group forming one colony). The method is also applicable to bacteriophage suspensions, the dilutions being applied to lawns of sensitive bacteria followed by the counting of plaoues.

***Ageing Theories.*** Why organisms age is not well understood; several theories have been proposed to explain ageing and senescence, but none of them is totally satisfactory. Evidence can be cited both for and against all of them, and ageing and senescence are probably caused by a complex, interacting combination of processes.

Random molecular damage and environmental effects, leading to progressively greater deleterious changes at higher organizational levels in the individual form the basis of several theories. Free radical damage may impair molecular or cellular efficiency; somatic mutation of the body cells genome by environmental factors (e.g. ionizing radiation or chemical mutagens) may similarly impair cellular efficiency. Changes in the immune system (perhaps associated with the involution of the thymus gland with age) may render it less able to combat infection; the increased incidence of autoimmune disease in ageing suggests that the immune system's self-censoring mechanism may break down, causing a rise in self-destroying autoimmune phenomena. Cross-linking of DNA molecules and collagen is also associated with ageing. Increased damage to DNA and lowered efficiency of repair mechanisms with age, coupled with errors in the accuracy of DNA transcription and messenger RNA translation, especially concerning those molecules (e.g. RNA polymerases) associated with further transcription and translation, may lead by positive feedback to an error catastrophe.

The theory of programmed ageing and senescence also has its advocates, although evidence tends to be circumstantial. Pleiotropic genes, which had advantageous effects early in life but are deleterious in later life, may persist in a population, and selection against genes that are deleterious in late, post-reproductive life (e.g. huntingdon's chorea) will be weak. There is some evidence that longevity is heritable. The codon restriction theory is based on the degeneracy of the genetic code and on the observation that transfer RNA synthetase spectra change with ageing. The disposable soma theory suggests that investment in reproductive capacity must not be exceeded by investment in repair; when the balance is adversely tilted repair ceases and the organism ages.

The overall effects of these changes in the individual will be increased damage, declining efficiency at progressively higher levels of organization from molecules to the whole organism, imbalances in the internal environment and an inability by homeostatic control mechanisms to rectify them, and an increased vulnerability of the organism to environmental insults leading to decreased vitality, senescence and, ultimately, death.

***Agglutin.*** A type of antibody causing agglutination.

***Agglutination.*** A clumping together of cells, usually as a result of reaction between specific antigens and antibodies in blood and lymph, forming a natural defence against foreign materials, including bacterial cells. Transfusion of blood between persons of different ABO blood groups is also subject to the risk of agglutination.

***Agglutinin.*** Antibody that causes agglutination by binding through its divalent arms to two adjacent cell surfaces, thus attaching the cells to one another.

***Agglutinogen.*** A surface antigen that induces the formation of agglutins in cells (including bacteria) and binds them to produce an agglutination reaction.

***Aggregation.*** A clumping or clustering of individuals of a population in a nonrandom distribution. Such clumping can occur (a) as a response to local habitat differences, e.g. some organisms preferring, say, damp to dry areas; (b) as a response to daily or seasonal weather changes; (c) by reproductive processes, e.g. individuals hatching from the same egg batch in some animals, or poor seed dispersal in plants; (d) as a result of social attraction, e.g. colonial nesting in birds.

***Aggregation Centre.*** Site at which cells, such as the amoebae of Dictyostelium, aggregate following release of a chemostatic signal. Cells adhere to one another within the aggregation centre.

***Aggregation Chimaera.*** Artificial chimaera made by the mixing of cells from two different embryos. Such chimaeras are readily made with mammalian embryos by mixing the inner cell mass and reintroducing the chimaeric embryo to a surrogate mother to permit further development.

***Aggressins.*** Enzymes that are produced by parasitic bacteria. The aggressins dissolve tissues and enable the bacteria to enter the host tissues.

***Aggression.*** A type of behaviour that includes both threats and actual attacks on other animals, though often limited to threat display.

***Agonistic Behaviour.*** A broad grouping of behaviour patterns that not only includes all aspects of aggression, including threat and actual attack, but also the consequent aspects of appeasement and flight.

***Agouti.*** Hair colour in mammals in which, along the length of an individual hair, bands of dark and light brown alternate.

***Agranulocyte.*** A type of leucocyte (white blood cell) with non-granular cytoplasm and a large spherical nucleus. They are produced either in the lymphatic system or the bone marrow. Agranulocytes form about 30% of all leucocytes and are of two types, lymphocytes and monocytes.

***Agrobacterium.*** Genus of bacterium, of which one species Agrobacterium tumefaciens is the causative agent of crown gall, an important disease of many commercial crops, such as raspberries. This disease has come to be recognized in recent years as being caused by a DNA plasmid (Ti plasmid) carried by bacterium and transferred to the plant cells. Once infected by a transient. Agrobacterium attack, the disease will then permit a spread in the plant host by independent replication of a segment of the plasmid integrated in the plant genome, and persistence of the bacterial cells is not required.

Following the discovery of the relationship between crown gall and the Ti plasmid, this plasmid has come to be widely used in plant genetic engineering as a vector, novel plant genetic being spliced into the plasmid sequence by gene manipulation and thus carried into the host plant cells. This offers the possibility of recombination between the novel sequence in the plasmid and the plant genomic DNA. Successful recombination would result in integration of the novel sequence into the plant cell genome and expression of the sequence in the life of the cell. Since many plants can be grown from single somatic cells into complete plants, this system provides the opportunity to develop new and better plant species. Some such success has already been achieved.

*AIDS.* Acronym for Acquired Immune Deficiency Syndrome, a serious human disease caused by a virus that can destroy the body's natural defence system and cause death through the body becoming unable to fight any infection. The level of response to infection varies between different people; not everyone who carries the virus develops AIDS but all infected individuals can pass it on, by two main methods : (a) through sexual intercourse, and (b) by transfer of blood cells, as when drug users share needles. At present there is no known vaccine against the AIDS virus, although several are being developed.

***Albinism.*** An inherited condition found in many organisms, whose chief feature is a lack of melanin pigment in structures that are normally coloured. In humans the syndrome of albinism comprises :

(a) pinkish skin in which the pigment-containing cells (melanophores) are present but contain little or no melanin. The pinkish coloration comes from the underlying blood vessels.

(b) eyes with a deep red pupil and pink iris, both due to a lack of normal pigmentation and heavy vascularization.

(c) Photophobia (fear of light) brought on by excess light entering the eye and reflecting onto the retina. Albinos usually wear dark glasses.

(d) pale yellow hair.

Albinism is an inborn error of metabolism produced by a blockage in tyrosine metabolism due to the absence of a functional tyrosinase enzyme. The condition is controlled by a single recessive gene on an autosome. Approximately 1 in 20,000 of the population are albinos. See Figure A.15.

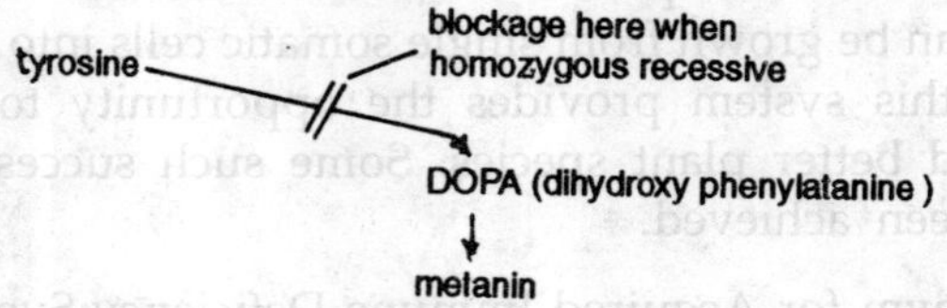


Figure A.15. Albinism. Blockage in tyrosine metabolism.

***Albumen or Egg White.*** A solution of protein in water which is secreted by the oviduct of birds and some reptiles. Albumen surrounds the embryo and yolk which it cushions within the shell of the egg. It is eventually absorbed by the embryo as food.

***Albino.*** Animal or plant lacking obvious pigmentation; more precisely, an animal lacking pigment such as melanin or a plant lacking chlorophyll.

***Albumin Gene.*** Gene coding for serum albumin and present in mammals as a single-copy gene of about 18 kilobases in mouse and rat; Xenopus possesses two copies of the gene. It is a highly complex sequence, found to consist of 15 exons and 14 introns. A related protein, alphafoetoprotein, is closely linked to the albumin gene in the mouse on chromosome 5.

***Albumins.*** Major blood serum proteins in mammals, found at a concentration of 30-50 g/l in humans. Human serum albumin is a simple protein ($M_r$ = 69 000) carrying a negative charge at neutral pH. By maintaining the colloidal osmotic pressure of the blood plasma, it plays an important role in osmoregulation. Ovalbumin, found in the water-soluble part of bird egg white, is a protein that contains a carbohydrate prosthetic group. Albumins are often used as antigens in experimental immunology.

***Alcohol.*** An organic molecule in which a hydrogen atom of a hydrocarbon is replaced by a hydroxyl group (OH). See Figure A.16.

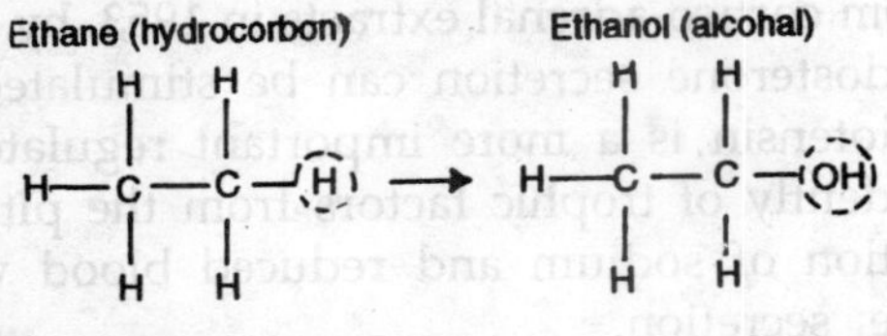


Figure A.16. Alcohol. Molecular structure of an alcohol.

***Alcohol Dehydrogenase.*** Enzyme that catalyses the conversion of ethanol to acetaldehyde. It is important in the metabolism of ethanol and is particularly active in vertebrate liver cells.

***Alcoholic Fermentation.*** A type of cellular respiration found in plants and some unicells which does not require oxygen, resulting in the production of ethanol (an alcohol) from glucose and the release of small amounts of energy. The main details are described under anaerobic respiration but, briefly, fermentation involves glycolysis to produce pyruvic acid and then (in the absence of oxygen) the breakdown of pyruvic acid to ethanol via ethanol with the release of $CO_2$.

***Aldehyde Group.*** Any organic compound containing the group CHO, a carbonyl group fixed to one hydrogen and one oxygen atom.

***Aldose.*** A sugar having an aldehyde group attached to the first carbon atom, e.g. D-glyceraldehyde.

***Aldosterone.*** 1. A hormone of the cortex of the adrenal gland. It is responsible for the relative concentration of sodium and potassium ions in the body. It promotes the reabsorption of sodium ions from the ascending limb of the loop of henle in the kidney, with the elimination of potassium ions, and increases the uptake of sodium ions by the alimentary canal. The concentration of sodium ions in the blood thus rises and potassium ions fall, enabling ionic regulation of body fluids.

2. A potent mineralocorticoid hormone secreted by the adrenal glands of mammals from the cells of the outer cortex (glomerulosa zone) and by the adrenal tissue of many other vertebrates. It was finally isolated and crystallized from cortico-adrenal extracts in 1953, by Simpson and Tait. Aldosterone secretion can be stimulated by ACTH, but angiotensin is a more important regulator, operating independently of trophic factors from the pituitary gland. Deprivation of sodium and reduced blood volumes also stimulate secretion.

***Algae.*** A collective term for several taxonomic groups of plants, namely Charophyta, Chlorophyta, Chrysophyta, Cyanophyta Euglenophyta, Phaeophyta, Pyrrophyta and Rhodophyta. All are relatively simple photosynthetic forms with unicellular reproductive structures. They range from unicellular organisms to non-vascular filamentous or thalloid plants. Algae occur in both marine and fresh water, while others are terrestrial, living in damp situations on walls, trees, etc.

***Algal Bloom.*** An extensive growth of algae in a water body, usually as a result of the phosphate content of fertilizers and detergents.

***Alien.*** An organism, usually a plant, that is not native to the environment in which it occurs, and that is thought to have been introduced by man.

***Alkaline Phosphatase.*** Enzyme commonly extracted from E. coli and used in nucleic acid sequencing and gene manipulation to remove terminal 5'-phosphoryl groups. Alkaline phosphatases are also present in eukaryotes (e.g. in vertebrate intestinal cells).

***Alkaloids.*** A heterogeneous group of basic nitrogen-containing substances that are produced by plants and have potent pharmacological activities. Alkaloids are often of complex structure, typically with heterocyclic rings containing nitrogen; they can be classified according to the type of heterocyclic group present (see table).

Most alkaloids are produced by dicotyledonous plants (ergotamine, obtained from the fungus Claviceps purpurea, is a notable exception) and particular alkaloids are usually restricted to certain families or genera. All members of the family Papaveraceae produce alkaloids; in other families, e.g. Ranunculaceae, Apocynaceae, Solanaceae, alkaloids are produced only by certain genera.

| HETEROCYCLIC GROUP | ALKALOID |
|---|---|
| indole 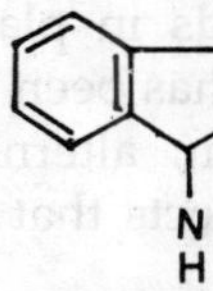 | lysergic acid<br>reserpine<br>strychnine |
| pyridine 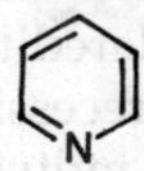 | nincotinic acid<br>nicotine |
| reduced pyridine 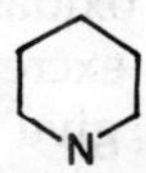 | coniine<br>cocaine |
| quinotine 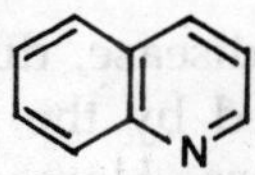 | quinine |
| isoquinoline 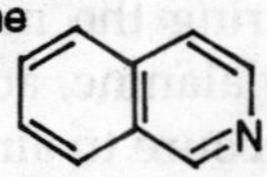 | morphine<br>paparverine |
| pyrimidine 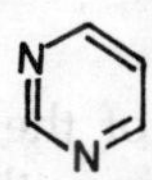 | barbituric acid |
| purine 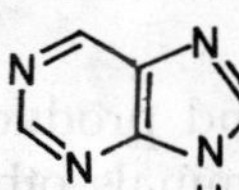 | caffeine |

Figure A.17. Representative alkaloids.

Alkaloids show varied pharmacological activities. They can act as analgesics (e.g. morphine), tranquillizers (e.g. reserpine), respiratory stimulants (e.g. nicotine), vasoconstrictors (e.g. scopolamine), local anaesthetics (e.g. cocaine), muscle relaxants (e.g. strychnine), and psychedelic agents (e.g. psilocybin, LSD). Many alkaloids or their synthetic derivatives are used medicinally, e.g. cinchona (to treat malaria), morphine, and reserpine. Some are poisons, notably coniine (from hemlock) and strychnine.

The function of alkaloids in plants is still a matter of conjecture. For example it has been suggested that they are by-products of metabolism; alternatively they may provide protection against insects that feed on the plants. See Figure A.17.

***Alkaptonuria (Alcaptonuria).*** Hereditary disease of the human caused by an autosomal recessive gene. The disease is relatively benign. Affected individuals are unable to synthesize homogenistic acid oxidase in the liver. The acid remains undegraded and is excreted in the urine. Since the acid is readily oxidized to give a dark product, urine of affected individuals darkens markedly on exposure to air.

***Alkaptonuria.*** A hereditary disease, due to a single recessive gene, that is characterized by the absence of the enzyme homogentisic acid oxidase. Homogentisic acid, normally formed and oxidized during the metabolism of the amino acids tyrosine and phenylalanine, accumulates in the urine, which turns black on exposure to air - the main symptom of the disease. The condition affects about 1 in 1 000 000 individuals.

***Allantoic Chorion.*** The fusion of the allantois with the mesoderm of the chorion which in eutherian mammals develops into the placenta.

***Allantoin.*** The heterocyclic end product of purine catabolism in some reptiles, and mammals other than primates.

***Allantois.*** One of the principal extraembryonic membrane systems fundamental to the evolution of the cleidoic egg. It is a sacular or tubular diverticulum of the hindgut of an amniote embryo; traditionally interpreted as being lined by endodermal epithelium supported by a stroma of splanchnopleural mesoderm. In birds and reptiles, the allantois serves a dual function.

Early in development, it provides a site to sequester potentially toxic wastes arising from embryonic metabolism. Later, it assumes a second and equally vital function. When the outer mesodermal surface of the allantois fuses with the inner mesodermal surface of the chorion to form the richly vascularized chorioallantois, this composite structure is the principal (extraembryonic) respiratory organ of the embryo within the egg. In placental mammals, the allantois is a solid structure, without a cavity, and its excretory and respiratory roles have been superceded by the evolution of the chorioallantoic placenta; nevertheless all the blood vessels and connective tissue of the foetal component of the placenta are derived from allantoic mesoderm.

***Allele (Allelomorph).*** Variant of DNA sequence for a specific gene. In diploid cells a maximum of two alleles will be present, each in the same relative position or locus on homologous chromosomes of the chromosome set. When alleles at any one locus are identical the individual is said to be homozygous for that locus, when they differ the individual is said to be heterozygous for that locus. Since different alleles of any one gene may vary by only a single base, the possible number of alleles for any one gene is very large. When alleles differ, one is often dominant to the other, which is said to be recessive. Dominance is a property of the phenotype and does not imply inactivation of the recessive allele by the dominant. In numerous examples the normally functioning (wild-type) allele is dominant to all mutant alleles of more or less defective function. In such cases the general explanation is that one functional allele out of two is sufficient to produce enough active gene product to support normal development of the organism (i.e. there is normally a two-fold safety margin in quantity of gene product).

The symbols used to designate alleles of a series differ according to the organism. In plants and some animals dominant and recessive alleles of the same gene are distinguished by upper-case and lower-case, respectively (e.g. C for coloured seed and c for white seed in maize). This, in its simplest form, allows for only two alleles per gene, and superscripts have to be used for further alleles. In Drosophila species, and in some fungi, all alleles are given the same lower-case symbol with superscripts as needed and the wild-type allele is distinguished by a + superscript. Thus, in Drosophila, homozygotes for $w^+$, $w^a$ and w have red (wild-type), apricot-coloured and white eyes, respectively. In this system dominance and recessivity are not implicit in the allele symbols except that for some dominant alleles the superscript may be capitalized.

***Allele Frequency or Gene Frequency.*** The proportion of a particular allele of a gene in a population, relative to other alleles of the same gene. For example, if a gene has two alleles. A and a, and the frequency of A is 0.6, then the frequency of a will be 1.0 - 0.6 = 0.4. The allele frequency can be calculated from the genotype frequency.

***Allelic Exclusion.*** Failure of one of the two allelic forms of a gene within one cell to be expressed. It applies to situations in which simple genetic dominance does not explain the lack of expression since the silent allele may be expressed preferentially in other cells. Cases of allelic exclusion in nature are rare. The best known example involves genes coding for antibody, in which any one antibody-producing cell synthesizes only one type of antibody as dictated by one of the two alleles present at that specific locus. Other antibody-producing cells in the same organism will be found to be expressing only the other homologous allele. The mechanism for allelic exclusion is believed to operate at transcription.

***Allelopathic Substance.*** A secretion or excretion of an organism that has an inhibitory effect on others.

***Allelotype.*** Allelic frequency in a population of organisms.

***Allen's Rule.*** A rule stating that in warm-blooded animals (homoiotherms) there tends to be a reduction in size of protruberant parts of the body (such as legs, bill, tail) in cooler climates, for example, bill length within some species of birds, such as the redshank. This size reduction is an extension of Bergmann's Rule and is also a mechanism to reduce heat loss. The rule was devised by J. A. Allen in 1877.

***Allergen.*** Antigen or hapten that induces an allergic reaction, particularly through the production of antibodies of immunoglobulin IgE.

***Allergy.*** Specialized case of immunity, but with a deleterious outcome and described as an immunologically mediated disease. Individuals suffering from allergy display allergic reactions and are hypersensitized to the foreign antigen, which is called an allergen; reactions lead to tissue damage. Allergic diseases are manifested primarily at three sites :

(1) The gastrointestinal tract, when the individual becomes sensitized to certain ingested foods, additives and drugs or their breakdown products (e.g. milk, chocolate, fish, wheat), leading to vomitting and diarrhoea.

(2) The skin, following injection of drugs, stings, infection with bacteria or parasites, or simply contact with a variety of chemical agents. When the reaction is immediate (characterized by a reddening of the skin, termed erythema, and wheal formation) it is referred to as urticaria (e.g. reaction to penicillin injection). Contact dermatitis involves a delayed reaction and often represents a response to simple chemicals present in the environment (e.g. sensitivity to nickel present in thimbles, necklaces and garter clasps) and also to substances present in poison ivy, detergents and cosmetics.

(3) The respiratory tract, where a variety of noxious agents including dust, pollen, moulds and animal dander may be inhaled and lead to inflammatory reactions of the mucous membranes (e.g. hay fever, pigeon breeders' disease — sensitization to proteins present in pigeon

droppings — asthma and farmers' lung — sensitization to fungi present in mouldy hay).

In many types of allergy, the cause is an exaggerated IgE response and the antibodies are then termed reagins. Mast cells and basophils have high-affinity receptors for the Fc region of IgE and the reagins bind to these cells. Minute quantities of allergens that enter the body crosslink the antibody-receptor complex which then leads to degranulation of the mast cell and liberation of histamine, heparin and leukotrienes. The substances in turn cause increase in vascular permeability and contraction of smooth muscles and can act locally at the site of entry of the allergen or more systematically, due to basophil involvement, in which case fatal anaphylactic shock may result. Contact sensitivity reactions involve sensitized lymphocytes, not antibodies as such.

Treatment is with antihistamines, or by immunotherapy, where attempts are made to desensitize the individual by injecting the allergen repeatedly in order to either produce IgE antibodies that compete for binding or to induce specific suppressor T lymphocytes which block synthesis of IgE directed against the allergen.

***Allochronic Species.*** Species which do not occur together in terms of time, i.e. species which occur in different geological times.

***Allocycly.*** Differences in coiling behaviour or condensation shown by different chromosomes or chromosome segments. For example, Y chromosomes and condensed X chromosomes show positive allocycly.

***Allogeneic.*** Describing two cell lines within one organism that are antigenically different. Such as organism is most commonly an experimental mammalian chimaera.

***Allometric Growth.*** 1. Unequal growth rate in different portions of the body of an organism that gives rise to the final shape. 2. Growth of a particular structure at a constantly greater rate than the whole.

***Alloparapatric Speciation.*** Development of new species from populations that are initially allopatric, but later become parapatric.

***Allopatric (of a population).*** Being geographically separate (or nearly so) from another population of the same species.

***Allopatric Speciation.*** The genetic differentiation of populations which are geographically separate to the point where they become separate species.

***Allophene.*** Individual with a transplant of foreign cells.

***Allopheny.*** Expression of genes in animals with transplanted cells, in which there is a genetic interaction between host cells and graft cells.

***Allopolyploid.*** 1. Polyploid organism that has resulted from the combination of two genetically distinct chromosome sets.

2. A type of polyploid in which the number of chromosomes is doubled in a hybrid between two species. The resulting allotetraploid or amphidiploid is fertile since homologous chromosomes of both types can now pair at meiosis to produce viable gametes (see Figure A.18). Such a process has been important in the production of new species, particularly in plants. For example, the successful marshland grass Spartina anglica is a fertile allotetraploid developed from an infertile hybrid (S. townsendii) produced originally by a cross between S. alterniflora and S. maritima.

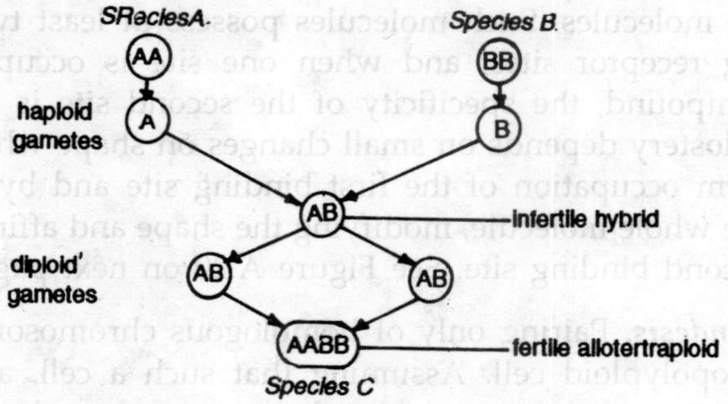


Figure A.18. Allopolyploid. The creation of a fertile allotetraploid.

***Allosteric Enzyme.*** A type of enzyme which has two alternative forms : one active with a functional binding site, the other inactive where the binding site has been altered in shape so as to become non-reactive. Such enzymes have a quaternary protein structure which becomes changed by the addition of a 'modulator' molecule producing the inactive shape, such a process resulting in noncompetitive inhibition. S]ee Figure A.19.

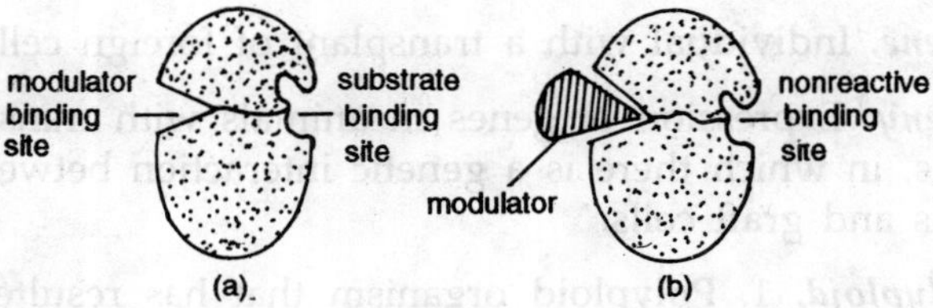


Figure A.19. Allosteric enzyme. Active (a) and inactive (b) forms.

***Allosteric Inhibitors.*** Substances which prevent as enzyme from changing into an active form by combining, not with the active site, but with some other part of the enzyme.

***Allosteric Protein.*** Protein displaying properties of allostery. The protein that regulates the activity of the LAC operon in E. coli repressor is the classical example. When this protein combines with an inducer molecule, its affinity for the operator sequence is abolished. The operon then becomes active because its transcription is no longer blocked by the repressor.

***Allostery.*** Type of behaviour displayed by some large biological molecules. Such molecules possess at least two differing receptor sites, and when one site is occupied by a compound, the specificity of the second site is modified. Allostery depends on small changes on shape which result form occupation of the first binding site and by affecting the whole molecule, modifying the shape and affinity of the second binding site. See Figure A.20 on next page.

***Allosyndesis.*** Pairing only of homologous chromosomes in an allopolyploid cell. Assuming that such a cell, at mitosis, has two sets of a particular chromosome, one derived from each parent or species, then in allosyndesis the homologous chromosomes from one parent always associate with one another and not with the homologous but less closely related chromosomes from the other parent. If pairing between homologous chromosomes from the two parents or species occurs, this is termed autosyndesis, reflecting the similarity of DNA sequences in the two lines of chromosomes.

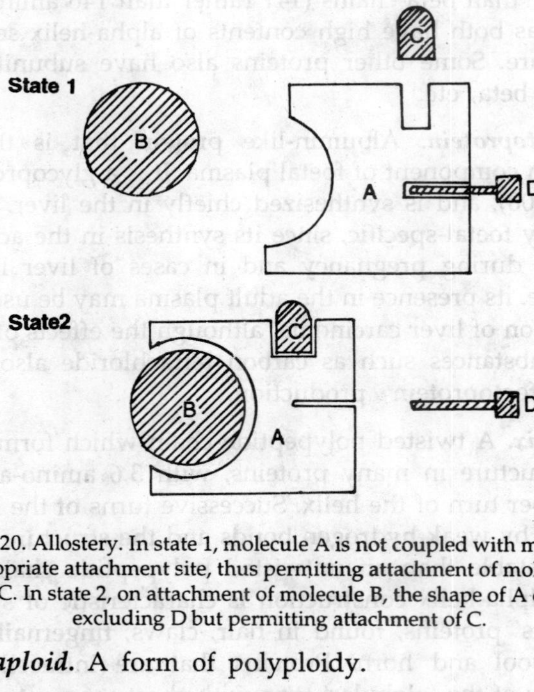


Figure A.20. Allostery. In state 1, molecule A is not coupled with molecule B at the appropriate attachment site, thus permitting attachment of molecule D but excluding C. In state 2, on attachment of molecule B, the shape of A changes, thus excluding D but permitting attachment of C.

***Allotetraploid.*** A form of polyploidy.

***Allotype.*** One of a range of antibodies containing different sequences of amino acids but all having an area with an identical amino acid sequence and thought to be produced by different alleles of the same gene.

***Allozygote.*** Organism that is homozygous at a particular locus, but the two homologous genes are of independent origin.

***Allozyme.*** A form of protein coded by a particular allele at a single gene locus that is detectable by electrophoresis.

***Alluvial Soil.*** A young soil derived from river, estuarine or marine deposits and having a high fertility.

***Alpha-Chain.*** One of the two polypeptide components of vertebrate haemoglobin. Each haemoglobin molecule consists of two alpha- and two beta-chains, put together as two alpha-beta-dimers, and which are in turn the products of distinct alpha- and beta-globin genes. Alpha-chains are shorter than beta-chains (141 rather than 146 amino acids), whereas both have high contents of alpha-helix secondary structure. Some other proteins also have subunits styled alpha, beta, etc.

***Alpha-Foetoprotein.*** Albumin-like protein that is the main protein component of foetal plasma. It is a glycoprotein ($M_r$ = 70 000), and is synthesized chiefly in the liver. It is not entirely foetal-specific, since its synthesis in the adult liver occurs during pregnancy and in cases of liver injury or disease. its presence in the adult plasma may be used in the detection of liver carcinoma. although the effects of poisonous substances such as carbon tetrachloride also include alpha-foetoprotein production.

***Alpha Helix.*** A twisted polypeptide chain which forms a helical structure in many proteins, with 3.6 amino-acid residues per turn of the helix. Successive turns of the helix are linked by weak hydrogen bonds and the structure is much more stable than an untwisted polypeptide chain. Long-chain lpha-helix construction is characteristic of structural 'fibrous' proteins, found in hair, claws, fingernails, feathers, wool and horn. Proteins that are intracellular are usually of the 'globular' type with short segments of alpha helixes.

***Alteration Enzyme.*** Protein associated with the bacteriophage T4 that interacts with bacterial RNA polymerase, preventing recognition of host gene promoters and thus inhibiting transcription of host DNA.

***Alternation of Generations.*** The occurrence within the life cycle of an organism of a sexually reproducing generation followed by an asexual generation. In some coelenterates, such as Obelia, the sexual organs are carried on medusas, and subsequent fertilization gives rise to an asexually producing hydroid stage; here both generations are diploid. See Figure A.21.

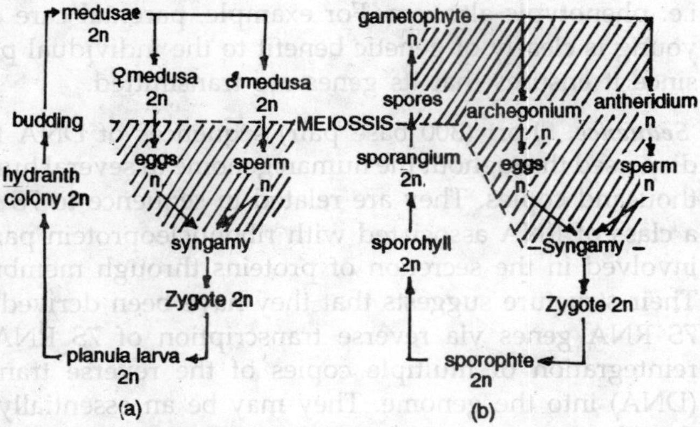


Figure A.21. Alternation of generations. (a) Life cycle of Obelia (Coelenterata). (b) Life cycle of fern (Pteridophyta) n = haploid number of chromosomes.

Amongst the plants, ferns have a diploid sporophyte generation (the plant itself). This undergoes meiosis to form spores that give rise to a haploid gametophyte generation known as a prothallus, which reproduces sexually. Male and female gametes fuse to form a zygote, which then develops into a new fern plant (sporophyte). See Figure. Some definitions of the term require a haploid generation alternating with a diploid generation, so excluding all animal examples.

***Altruism.*** Behaviour by an animal that decreases its chances of survival or reproduction while increasing those of another member of the same species. For example, a lapwing puts itself at risk by luring a predator away from the nest through feigning injury, but by so doing saves its offspring. Altruism in its biological sense does not imply any conscious benevolence on the part of the performer. Altruism can evolve through kin selection, if the recipients of altruistic acts tend on average to be more closely related to the altruist than the population as a whole.

***Altruistic Behaviour.*** Behaviour which involves an unselfish regard for others. In organisms other than man altruism probably only exists where the benefits to the individual performing the behaviour are greater than those to the individual to whom the particular behaviour is directed, i.e. phenotypic altruism. For example, parental care of the young is clearly of genetic benefit to the individual parent, since it ensures that its genes are transmitted.

***Alu Sequence.*** Short (300 base pair) sequences of DNA found dispersed throughout the human genome in several hundred thousand copies. They are related in sequence to 7S RNA, a class of RNA associated with ribonucleoprotein particles involved in the secretion of proteins through membranes. Their structure suggests that they have been derived from 7S RNA genes via reverse transcription of 7S RNA and reintegration of multiple copies of the reverse transcript (DNA) into the genome. They may be an essentially accidental consequence of the presence at some point in time of reverse transcriptase, rather than a result of natural selection of any function beneficial to the cell. At least some of them are transcribed into small RNA molecules.

***Amanitin.*** Drug derived from the highly poisonous fungus Amanita phalloides (death cap). Alpha-amanitin, a cyclic octapeptide, is toxic because of its affinity for RNA polymerase II in eukaryotic cells. Since this enzyme is responsible for mRNA synthesis in the cell, the compound is a potent and selective inhibitor of mRNA synthesis. It is effective at concentrations below I μg/ml, and its specific action has made it a favoured drug in experimental cell biology. It is often used with actinomycin D to block RNA synthesis.

***Amber Codon.*** Nucleotide triplet UAG, which is one of three nonsense codons which cause termination of protein synthesis.

***Amber Suppressor (Am).*** Gene that prevents polypeptide chain termination as a result of an amber mutation. Such genes usually act by coding for transfer RNA which inserts an amino acid at the site of the UAG nonsense codon produced by the amber mutation.

***Ambient.*** Surrounding, prevailing. The term is used most often in connection with temperature levels during experiments.

***Ambulacrum.*** One of the five radial bands on which tube feet occur on the outside surfaces of echinoderms.

***Ames Test.*** A technique devised in the USA by Bruce Ames and an associate that is designed to screen environmental chemicals for mutagenicity. The test uses histidine-requiring mutant strains of Salmonella typhimurium and measures the frequency of back mutations that no longer require histidine supplements in their food supply. The Ames test has been employed widely since 1975 as a check for potential carcinogens, since these chemicals usually act as mutagens.

***Amine.*** An organic base formed by replacing one or more of the hydrogen atoms of ammonia by organic groups.

***Amino Acid.*** A building block of protein, containing a carboxyl group (COOH) and an amino group ($NH_2$), both attached to the same carbon atom. Over 80 amino acids are known to occur naturally, with 20 found commonly in proteins (see Figure Table), each with a different side chain, called an 'R' group (see Figure A.22). Each of these common amino acids is described under its own heading.

Many amino acids can be synthesized in the body from other amino acids by a process called transamination, although most organisms have a number of essential amino acids that must be taken in with the diet. Each amino acid is coded by at least one triplet of DNA bases, and the string of amino acids making up a protein is joined by peptide bonds to form a polypeptide chain. Amino acids are soluble in water but vary considerably in their solubility. When in solution they are ionized and generally are electrically neutral with a pH known as the isoelectric point. They are amphoteric, i.e. acting as acids or bases if the pH is shifted.

| | | | |
|---|---|---|---|
| Ala | = Alanine | Leu | = Leucine |
| Arg | = Arginine | Lys | = Lysine |
| Asn | = Asparagine | Met | = Methionine |

| | | | |
|---|---|---|---|
| Asp | = Aspartic acid | Phe | = Phenylalanine |
| Cys | = Cysteine | Pro | = Proline |
| Gln | = Glutamine | Ser | = Serine |
| Glu | = Glutamic acid | Thr | = Threonine |
| Gly | = Glycine | Trp | = Tryptophan |
| His | = Histidine | Tyr | = Tyrosine |
| Lieu | = Isoleucine | Val | = Valine |

Table. Amino Acid. The 20 amino acids commonly found in protein.

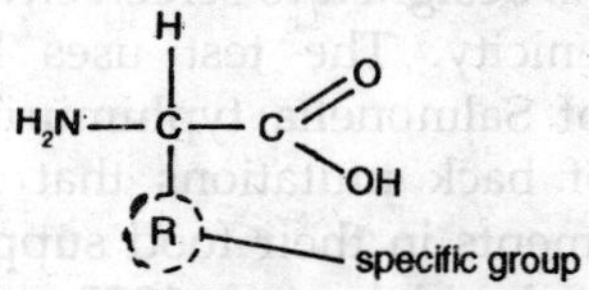


Figure A.22. Amino Acid. Structure of a generalized amino acid.

***Amino-Acid Sequence.*** The order in which amino acids are placed along a protein molecule. Secondary and tertiary protein structure is highly dependent upon amino-acid sequence in the polypeptide chain, which affects the bonding together of the molecule. The 'blueprint' for this sequence is contained in DNA, whose bases contain the amino acid code; three bases provide the code for each amino acid. By the processes of transcription and translation the DNA-base sequence is mirrored in the amino-acid sequence, there being colinearity between DNA and protein.

***Aminoaciduria.*** Spillage of amino acids into the urine as a result of some error in metabolism.

***Aminoacyl-tRNA.*** The molecule produced when an amino acid is activated into its aminoacyl form and attached to its specific transfer RNA molecule, the whole process being catalysed by a specific aminoacyl-tRNA synthetase enzyme.

***Aminoacyl-tRNA Synthetases (activating enzymes).*** Enzymes that catalyse the formation of an aminoacyl-tRNA form an amino acid and its corresponding transfer RNA (tRNA). The reaction consists of an initial activation step in which the aminoacyl-adenylate is formed from the free amino acid and ATP, followed by a transfer step in which the aminoacyl group is transferred to the tRNA. The aminoacyl-adenylate remains firmly bound to the enzyme during the reaction. There is at least one synthetase for each amino acid, and accuracy of translation of the genetic information in the messenger RNA (mRNA) depends on the high degree of specificity of these enzymes.

***Aminopeptidase.*** An enzyme that catalyses the sequential hydrolysis of amino acids in a polypeptide chain from the N-terminal.

***Amino Sugar.*** A monosaccharide in which an amino group has replaced an hydroxyl group on one or more occasions.

***Amitosis.*** Nuclear division in a cell that occurs without the formation of a spindle or the appearance of chromosomes, and from which daughter nuclei with identical chromosome sets are probably not produced. Amitosis occurs for example in the protozoan Paramecium when the macronucleus divides.

***Amniocentesis.*** A technique for the diagnosis of congenital abnormalities before birth. In this procedure a sample of 10-15 $cm^3$ of amniotic fluid surrounding the foetus is extracted through the abdominal wall using a surgical syringe, usually at about the 16th week of pregnancy. The sloughed-off embryonic cells contained in the fluid can be cultured to enable karyotype analysis, which shows the number and condition of the chromosomes. The fluid can also be analysed for the presence of chemicals which indicate biochemical and other defects (e.g. spina bifida). See Figure A.23.

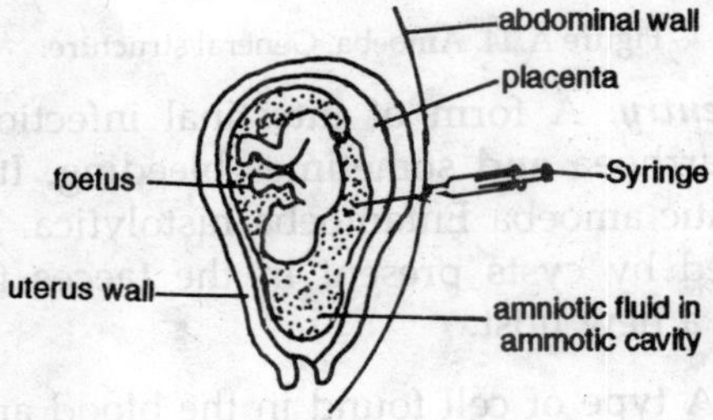


Figure A.23. Amniocentesis. Sampling amniotic fluid by means of a surgical syringe.

***Amniocytes.*** Cells from the membranous lining of the foetal amnion that are recovered during amniocentesis.

***Amnion.*** Extraembryonic or foetal membrane that forms a sac containing the protective amniotic fluid in which the foetus is suspended. The aminon usually fuses with the chorion. Reptiles, birds and mammals have amnions, and these vertebrates classes are grouped together as the amniotes.

***Amniote.*** Terrestrial vertebrate (reptile, bird or mammal) that has embryos with an allantois and amnion.

***Amoeba.*** A genus of unicellular protozoans in the class Rhizopoda. Amoebae are characterized by their changing shape brought about by the projection or pseudopodia which have a locomotory function. Amoeba is often wrongly quoted as an example of a primitive organism, low on the evolutionary scale. However, as in many protista, functions that are carried out by organ systems in so-called 'higher' forms are here carried out within a single cell. Therefore they cannot be considered 'primitive'; they are highly evolved over millions of years, albeit on a different scale from higher organisms. See Figure A.24.

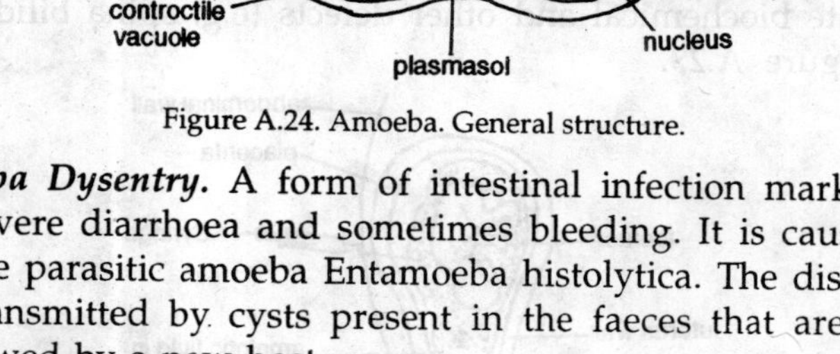


Figure A.24. Amoeba. General structure.

***Amoeba Dysentry.*** A form of intestinal infection marked by severe diarrhoea and sometimes bleeding. It is caused by the parasitic amoeba Entamoeba histolytica. The disease is transmitted by cysts present in the faeces that are swallowed by a new host.

***Amoebocyte.*** A type of cell found in the blood and other body fluids of invertebrates that is capable of amoeboid movement within the fluid, and which often acts as a phagocyte.

***Amoeboid.*** Moving and feeding in the manner of Amoeba, by the action of pseudopodia.

***Amoeboid Movement.*** Movement by means of pseudopodia, being a projection of the surface of a cell caused by alternate formation of sol and gel protoplasm in the region of the temporarily formed 'false foot'.

***Amorph Allele.*** An allele of a gene that appears to code for no detectable product. It can be produced by a deletion mutation.

***AMP (Adenosine Monophosphate).*** A molecule consisting of an adenosine unit onto which is attached a phosphate group with a low-level energy bond. The molecule is important because it functions as the basic structure for ADP and ATP, both of which contain high-energy bonds (34 kJ/mole) that serve as a short-term energy store for the cell.

***Amphimixis.*** True sexual reproduction involving the fusing of a male with a female gamete, fertilization and formation of a zygote.

***Amphipathic.*** Describing compounds that have both a polar group and a hydrophobic portion. Fatty acids and phospholipids are amphipathic compounds.

***Amphiploid.*** A polyploid that is generally fertile, formed by the doubling of chromosomes in a species hybrid, e.g. Primula kewensis (2n = 36) is an amphiploid of P. floribunda (2n = 18).

***Amphoteric (of chemical).*** Capable of acting either as bases or acids. Amino acids and some oxides (such as zinc) are amphoteric.

***Amphotrophic Virus.*** Virus that can replicate both in cells of its normal host and also in cells of other species.

***Ampicillin (Penbritin).*** S. misynthetic antibiotic prepared by acylating 6-aminopenicillanic acid with 2-aminophenylacetic acid. It is acid-stable (and can therefore be administered orally) with a wide-spectrum bactericidal action against gram-positive and gram-negative bacteria. It is one of the most widely used antibacterial agents. See Figure A.25.

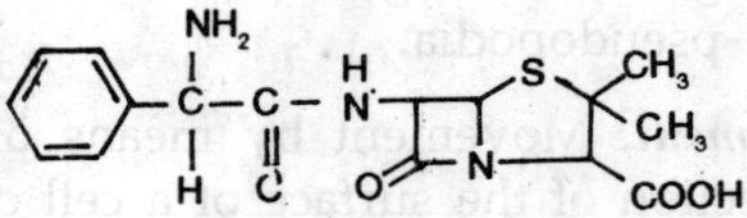

Figure A.25. Ampicillin.

***Amplification.*** Increase in the basic number of a molecule; most commonly applied to the number of a particular gene.

***Amplification, Genetic.*** The synthesis of many copies of DNA from one master region, a mechanism that ensures the rapid production of large quantities of protein when required.

***Amylase.*** A digestive enzyme which enables the splitting of starch into smaller subunits of maltose, usually in alkaline conditions (see Figure A.26).

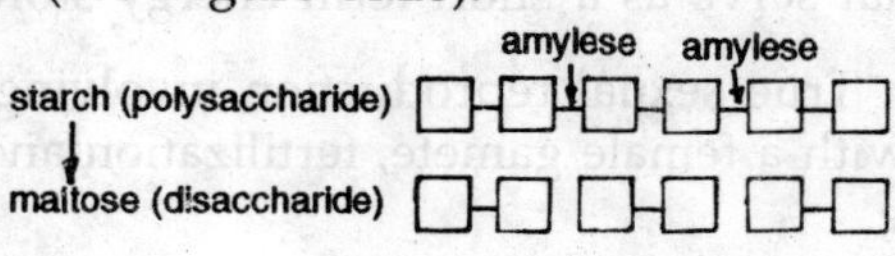


Figure A.26. Amylase. The splitting of starch to form maltose.

Amylases are found in the saliva of most mammals (and were previously called ptyalin), but their functioning is limited to the brief time that food remains in the mouth. Once food is swallowed, the acid stomach conditions prevent further amylase activity. The principal location of starch digestion is in the duodenum, where pancreatic amylase is poured into the gut lumen from the pancreas as part of the pancreatic juice; pancreatic amylase has a greater digestive efficiency than salivary amylase. Amylases are common in plants, particularly in association with the starch stores of seeds and underground perennating organs such as rhizomes, tubers and taproots.

***Amylase Gene.*** Gene for alpha-amylase present in the mammalian genome as at least two copies, designated amy.1 and amy.2. There is evidence that the amy.1 gene produces messenger RNA (mRNA) for two distinct proteins; the amylases of the liver and of the pancreas. The other, amy.2

produces only message for the third protein; the amylase of saliva (ptyalin). The two products of the single amy.1 gene are produced by differential splicing of exon sequences to yield differing mosaic molecules of mRNA which, in the different tissues, are translated into the relevant form of the enzyme.

***Amylopectin.*** A carbohydrate polymer, of high molecular weight, composed of branched chains of glucose units.

***Amyloplast.*** A type of cell inclusion found in many plant tissues, particularly storage organs such as the potato tuber. Amyloplasts contain starch enclosed in a unit membrane, the whole structure being a type of leucoplast. Besides serving as a starch store, amyloplasts are thought by some scientists to function also as a gravity-seeking device, helping the roots to push through the soil in the correct direction.

***Amylose.*** A form of starch composed of unbranched chains of glucose units.

***Anabolism or Synthesis.*** A type metabolism in which complex chemicals are synthesized from simpler building blocks, a process which is endergonic (i.e. requires energy). The classic example of an anabolic process is photosynthesis in which solar energy is incorporated into complex compounds such as glucose and its derivatives. Animals also carry out many anabolic reactions, building up complex molecules such as proteins from simpler subunits (amino acids) obtained from heterotrophic nutrition.

***Anaemia.*** A deficiency in the number of red blood cells, their volume, or the haemoglobin content.

***Anaerobe.*** an organism able to metabolize in the absence of free oxygen, obtaining energy from the breakdown of glucose in anaerobic respiration. Some anaerobes are obligate, i.e. they cannot survive in oxygen, e.g. bacteria causing food poisoning. Others (the majority) can live either in the presence or absence of oxygen and are called facultative. When oxygen is present, respiration in these types is of the aerobic type involving the krebs cycle to release maximum energy; when oxygen is absent they rely solely on energy released in anaerobic respiration.

***Anaerobic Respiration.*** A type of cell respiration that takes place in anaerobes, and in which energy is released from glucose and other foods without the presence of oxygen. The reactions fall into two stages :

Stage 1 : Glycolysis, in which glucose is converted to two molecules of pyruvic acid (pyruvate) in the general cell cytoplasm. The same reactions occur as in aerobic respiration, but in anaerobes the absence of oxygen prevents the two molecules of reduced NAD produced from being oxidized via the electron transport system (ETS) in the mitochondria. Instead, ATP is produced from ADP by substrate-level phosphorylation. Thus the net output of ATP in anaerobic respiration is 2 molecules (4 minus 2 used in the initial phosphorylation).

Stage 2 : Once pyruvate has been produced, two alternative pathways can occurs. In plants and many microorganisms the pyruvate is broken down to ethanol via ethanal (acetaldehyde) in a process called alcoholic fermentation, which requires hydrogen from NADH (see Figure A.27). In animals the pyruvate is changed via a single step into lactic acid, a process called lactic-acid fermentation, which again requires hydrogen from NADH.

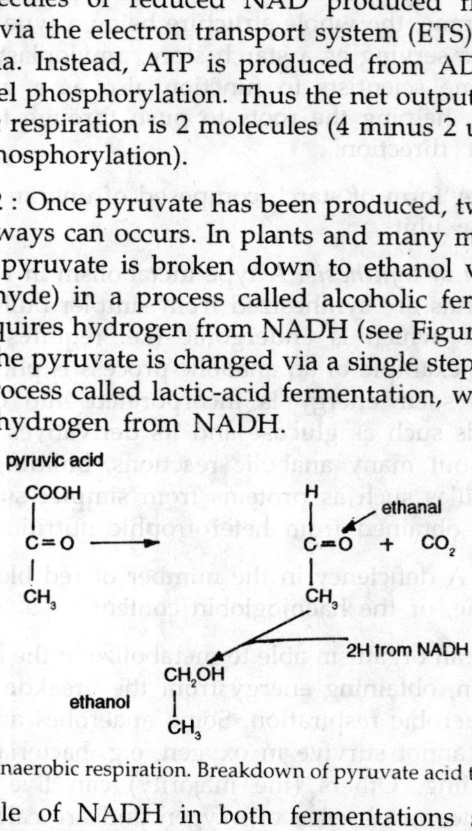


Figure A.27. Anaerobic respiration. Breakdown of pyruvate acid to ethanol.

The role of NADH in both fermentations should be noted. Since the amount of NAD present in the cell is limited, glycolysis would quickly come to a halt if anaerobic respiration stopped at pyruvate. By going on to ethanol or lactic acid, NAD is freed in the fermentations to return to glycolysis and thus allow glucose catabolism to continue. The yield of ATP in anaerobic respiration is poor because, firstly, the ETS cannot be used without oxygen, and, secondly, the end products still contain large amounts of energy. As a result, the free energy released and stored is only a fraction of the amount in the complete oxidation of glucose.

***Anagenesis.*** Progressive evolution.

***Analgesic.*** A substance reducing pain without causing unconsciousness.

***Analogous Organs.*** Organs or parts of the body of different species of animals or plants that have different evolutionary origins but have become adapted to serve the same purpose. For example, the wings of a bat and the wings of an insect are analogous organs.

***Analogous Structure.*** A structure that has the same function as another but different origins, e.g. the eye of man and the eye of the octopus. Analogy between structures does not imply evolutionary relationships but may imply convergence.

***Anaphase.*** 1. A stage of nuclear division in eucaryotic cells, occurring once in mitosis and twice in meiosis. The main process involved is the separation of chromosomal material to give two groups of chromosomes which will eventually become new cell nuclei. This important step is controlled by spindle microtubules (or fibres) which run from the organizing centre at each pole to every chromosome, the point of attachment being the kinetochore of the centromere. Various theories for chromosomal movement have been put forward, including (a) active repulsion of chromosomes, (b) the idea that when sliding past each other the microtubules may act as tiny muscles (the 'sliding filament' theory), and (c) a suggestion that the microtubules are disassembled at the poles, so 'reeling in' the attached chromosomes.

2. Stage in mitosis when the chromosomes, previously aligned more or less centrally by the spindle to form the metaphase plate, begin to move towards the spindle poles. The chromosomes destined to be in each daughter nucleus are therefore recognizable at anaphase.

***Anaphylaxis.*** An abnormal immune response that occurs when an individual previously exposed to a particular antigen is re-exposed to the same antigen. Anaphylaxis may follow an insect bite or the injection of a drug (such as penicillin). It is caused by the release of histamine and similar substances and may produce a localized reaction or a more generalized and severe one, with difficulty in breathing, pallor, or drop in blood pressure, unconsciousness, and possibly heart failure and death.

***Anastral Mitosis.*** Mitosis in dividing cells involving spindle formation without apparent centrioles or asters. Such mitosis occurs normally in cells of higher plants.

***Ancylostomiasis or Ankylostomiasis.*** A human disease in which the lining of the small intestine becomes heavily infested with adults of the hookworm Ancylostoma, causing a lethargic, anaemic state.

***Androdioecious.*** Having male and hermaphrodite flowers on separate plants.

***Androgen.*** One of several types of male hormone that stimulate the development and maintenance of the male's secondary sexual characteristics. Naturally occurring androgens (e.g. testosterone) are steroids which are produced mainly in the testis, but also to a small extent in the ovary and adrenal cortex.

***Androgenesis.*** Development of a fertilized egg into a haploid individual with only paternal chromosomes, due to selective destruction of the maternally derived egg nucleus.

***Androsterone.*** Metabolite of androgens, used as a diagnostic indication of male sex hormone when present in urine.

***Anemophilous.*** Describing plants that are pollinated by the wind. Flowers of these plants (e.g. grasses) have reduced or absent petals and produce no nectar.

***Anemophily.*** Pollination by wind, so that pollen is carried from stamen to stigma by air currents.

***Anencephaly.*** Congenital malformation resulting from defective closure of the neural tube at the head end of the embryo. The vault of the cranium is missing and the hypothalamus defective. Stillbirth or neonatal death is invariable.

***Aneuploidy.*** A condition where more or less than a complete set of chromosomes is found in each cell of an individual. Typically aneuploids have one extra or one missing chromosome. For example, in Down's syndrome affected individuals have three number-21 chromosomes rather than the normal two, a condition known as trisomy.

***Aneusomatic.*** Designating cells or organisms that contain variable numbers of individual chromosomes.

***Angiogenesis.*** Growth of new blood vessels, especially of capillaries in wound healing.

***Angiotensin.*** Either of two polypeptides released from a liver globulin protein in the blood. Angiotensin I is a decapeptide released under the influence of renin, an enzyme secreted by the kidney. Another enzyme removes the two terminal amino acids of angiotensin I to form an octapeptide, angiotensin II. The amino acid sequences were determined, and angiotensin synthesized, in 1956. Angiotensin I is apparently an inactive storage form in the blood, but angiotensin II is a potent vasopressor (i.e. it raises blood

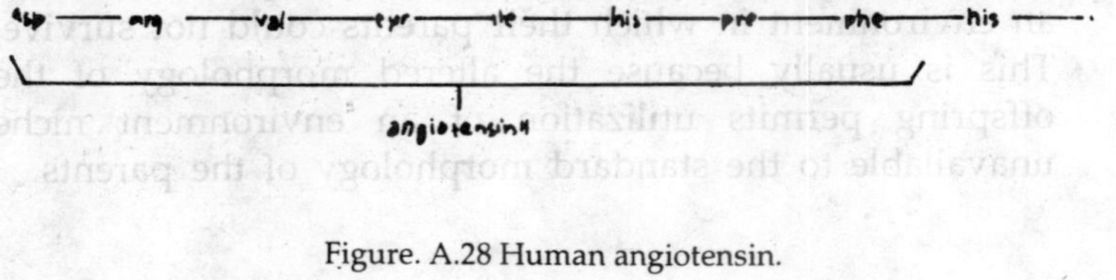


Figure. A.28 Human angiotensin.

pressure), causes contraction of the uterus. and stimulates the secretion of aldosterone from the adrenal cortex. It is found only in the blood of people with high blood pressure. See Figure A.28.

***Angstrom Symbol : A.*** A unit of submicroscopic distance equal to one tenth of a nanometre (one ten thousandth of a micrometre). It is used by biologists for very small distances that can be measured only under the electron microscope; e.g. the width of the double cell membrane is 75 A.

***Anisotropic Band.*** Band of light emitted when material, such as muscle fibre or the metaphase spindle of a cell, is illuminated, due to the birefringence (splitting into two rays) of the light ray as it passes through the highly ordered molecular structures.

***Ankylosing Spondylitis.*** Human disease of the joints for which there is some hereditary predisposition. It is strongly correlated with a particular haplotype of the HLA locus, the major histocompatability locus.

***Ankyrin.*** Protein that helps to bind spectrin molecules to the inner surface of the erythrocyte plasma membrane.

***Anlage.*** Embryonic primordium that gives rise to a specific structure within the animal body following development.

***Annealing.*** Renaturation of nucleic acid molecules following their earlier denaturation or melting. Annealing is a highly specific process involving the formation of precise hydrogen bonds between pairs of bases. This hybridization forms the basis of many techniques in molecular biology and genetic engineering, including the use of probe DNA to identify specific sequence in cells or cot value determination as a means of measuring DNA complexity.

***Annidation.*** Situation in which mutant offspring can survive in an environment in which their parents could not survive. This is usually because the altered morphology of the offspring permits utilization of an environment niche unavailable to the standard morphology of the parents.

***Annulate Lamellae.*** Paired membranes that are organized in stacks within the cell and that posses annulae or pores that show striking similarity to the nuclear pores of the nuclear envelope. Annulate lamellae are commonly found in germ cells and in cells active in protein synthesis.

***Anopheles.*** Genus of mosquitoes that includes many which carry malaria. Anopheline larvae have polytene chromosomes within the cells of their salivary glands.

***Antagonism.*** 1. The inhibiting or nullifying action of one substance or organism on another, e.g. the antibiotic effect of penicillin, or the exhaustion of a food supply by one organism at the expense of another.

2. The normal opposition between certain muscles.

3. The interaction of two substances (e.g. drugs, hormones, or enzymes) having opposing effects in a system in such a way that the action of one partially or completely inhibits the effects of the other. For example, one group of anti-cancer drugs acts by antagonizing the effects of certain enzymes controlling the activities of the cancer cells.

4. An interaction between two muscles in which contraction of one (the antagonist) prevents that of the other (the agonist). The antagonist must relax to enable the agonist to contract and effect movement.

5. An interaction between two organisms (e.g. moulds or bacteria) in which the growth of one is inhibited by the other.

***Anther Culture.*** Technique whereby haploid plants are produced from pollen, following the induction of embryo formation. It is particularly successful in Gramineae and Solanaceae.

***Antheridium.*** Male gametangium, gamete-producing structure, of bryophytes, algae, fungi and pteridophytes. It often consists of a stalked structure with a globular head containing the gametes.

***Antherozoid (Spermatozoid).*** Motile male gamete of fungi and many lower plants, such as algae, bryophytes and a few gymnosperms. They may have one or many flagella.

***Anthocyans.*** Groups of water-soluble flavonoid pigments, comprising the anthocyanidins and their glycosides, and the anthocyanins, found in higher plant vacuoles. They are responsible for the red, violet and blue pigments of flowers, fruits and leaves.

***Anthropomorphism.*** The attribution of human characteristics to animals other than man.

***Antiauxin.*** Any chemical substance that prevents the action of auxins.

***Antibiotic.*** Substance produced by a microorganism that kills or inhibits the growth of other microorganisms. The effective concentration for most antibiotics is in the μg ml range. The term is often extended to include substances obtained by chemical synthesis, especially as some drugs discovered as antibiotics are now prepared or modified (semisynthetic anti-biotics) by this method. Antibiotics are synthesized by both bacteria and fungi. The major groups of bacteria producing antibiotics are Bacillus (gramicidin, polymyxin, bacitracin) and Streptomyces. The latter is the main source from which 60 percent of all antibiotics are obtained, including streptomycin, tetracycline, chloramphenicol and neomycin. The moulds Penicillium and Aspergillus produce antibiotics, including penicillin and griseofulvin (an antifungal agent).

Antibiotics can be classified according to mechanism of action or structure. Penicillins, cephalosporins and bacitracin inhibit the synthesis of the bacterial cell wall; gramicidin and polymyxin disturb the function of the cytoplasmic membrane; mitomycin C and nalidixic acid prevent DNA replication; actinomycin D and rifampicin inhibit the transcription of RNA from DNA; streptomycin, tetracycline, chloramphenicol, neomycin and puromycin are inhibitors or protein biosynthesis. Antibiotics are chemically heterogeneous. For example, penicillins and gramicidin are derived from amino acids (often the D-isomers), the tetracyclines and griseofulvin are biosynthesized from acetyl coenzyme A, the aminoglycoside antibiotics (e.g. streptomycin, neomycin) are sugar derivatives, and puromycin is a nucleoside. Many antibiotics are used as chemotherapeutic agents and have a selectively toxic action against invading pathogenic microorganisms; others are too toxic to the host for general application but are occasionally employed in cancer chemotherapy.

***Antibody.*** Protein molecule found only in vertebrates and synthesized by B cells and with the capacity to bind specifically to an appropriate antigen or hapten. Antibody acts as a cell membrane receptor on virgin B cells (i.e. those that have not previously encountered antigen for which they have specificity). During proliferation and differentiation of B cells to plasma cells consequent on their binding antigenic determinants, antibody molecules with the same specificity as the receptor on the parent cell are secreted as humoral antibody into the lymph and blood and gain entry to other body fluids. Here they act to neutralize toxins and to aid in the removal of bacteria through phagocytosis and lysis.

Antibodies are immunoglobulins. They have a basic structure of two identical light and two identical heavy polypeptide chains joined together by interchain disulphide bonds and forming a Y-shape. See Figure A.29.

Treatment with papain cleaves the molecule into there fragments, two of which are antigen-binding (Fab) and one of which is readily crystallizable (Fc). A flexible hinge region allows movement of the Fab arms. Treatment with pepsin produces a divalent antigen-binding fragment $(Fab')_2$ and destroys much of the rest of the molecule. Each heavy and light chain consists of variable regions and constant regions (relates to amino acid sequences when antibodies of the same class but different specificity are compared with each other). Antibody specificity is governed by differences in amino acid sequences and the antigen-binding site is formed by the variable regions of the light and heavy chains. The constant regions of the heavy chains comprising the Fe fragment control the adjunctive functions of antibody molecules (i.e. properties associated not with specific recognition of antigen, but with the capacity to be transported across the placenta, yolk sac or gut of foetal and newborn animals), to bind complement and to bind to macrophages, mast cells and basophils. Cells able to bind antibody or antibody-antigen complexes do so through the possession of specific Fe receptors; a conformational change in the Fe region provided by binding of the variable region to antigen may be needed before antibody can effect phagocytosis and lysis of bacteria through binding to macrophage and by binding complement. See Figure A.29.

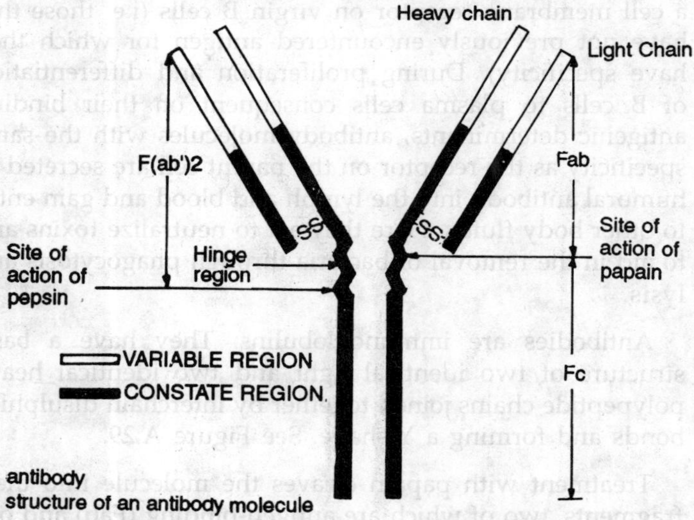


Figure A.29. Structure of an antibody molecule.

***Antibody-Dependent Cellular Cytotoxicity (ADCC).*** Lysis by non-specific K cells of target cells coated by specific IgG antibody. in vitro, ADCC provides a useful assay for very small amounts of antibody (e.g. a system can be set up using $^{51}$Cr-labelled chicken erythrocytes, a rabbit anti-chicken erythrocyte antibody and mouse spleen K cells). In the presence of the antibody, the chicken target cells will be lysed, and radioactivity will be detectable in the culture supernatant; in the absence of antibody no target cell lysis will occur. In vivo, ADCC possibly plays a role in immune surveillance against tumours.

***Anticancer Drug.*** Chemical used in the treatment of cancer, usually because of its ability to block mitosis or reduce cell division. Examples include vincristine and vinblastine.

***Anticlinal.*** (or plant cell division) along a plane at right angles to the outer surface.

***Anticoagulant.*** A substance that hinders agglutination or clotting of blood cells. Blood clotting is a vital reaction to damage in the circulatory system, one of the steps in the process being dependent on the presence of calcium ions. However, the tendency of blood to clot can be overcome by suitable chemicals that remove calcium, such chemicals being used as anticoagulants when storage of blood is required. Many blood-sucking parasites such as mosquitoes secrete anticoagulants into the host's bloodstream, so enabling easy transport of blood into the parasite's digestive system.

***Anticoding Strand (Sense Strand).*** Strand of DNA duplex of a gene that acts as template for the synthesis of message.

***Anticodon.*** In translation, the sequence of three nucleotides in a transfer RNA molecule that pairs with a complementary sequence of three nucleotides (codon) on a molecule of messenger RNA.

***Antigen.*** A substance that stimulates an animal to form a specific antibody. There are three types of antigen : extrinsic (not a constituent of the cell), intrinsic (a constituent of the cell), and occult (a self-antigen that does not reach antibody-forming tissues). The antigenicity of a substance usually depends on the size of the antigen molecule and its chemical configuration; proteins having a molecular weight of less than 10 000 are less effective in producing antibody. Antigen introduced into a animal that is immune to it is rapidly eliminated as a result of complexing with antibody, a process termed immune clearance.

***Antigenic Conversion.*** Change in certain surface proteins on the cells of some protozoan and other parasites, following antibody production by the host organism against the original surface protein.

***Antigenic Determinant.*** Site on an antigenic molecule that is immunogenic (i.e. induces an immune reaction) and to which a specific antibody molecule subsequently binds, Fragmentation of antigens by limited proteolysis reveals that individual antigens may possess several or many such determinant sites or epitopes, depending upon molecular size and complexity of tertiary structure. Those epitopes that are relatively more immunogenic will elicit a stronger immune response and may be described as immunodominant.

***Antigiberellin.*** Any substance that causes the growth of short thick stems, i.e. that has the opposite effect to gibberellins. For example, maleic hydrazide is used to retard grass growth and thus reduce the frequency of cutting.

***Anticistamine.*** Any drug that inhibits the effects of histamine in the body and is therefore used to relieve and prevent the symptoms associated with allergic reactions, such as hay fever. Since one of the side-effects produced by antihistamines is sleepiness, some are used to prevent motion sickness and induce sleep.

***Antilymphocytic Serum.*** A serum produced by injecting lymphocytes into a horse and collecting the antibodies produced. The serum is capable of destroying the original lymphocytes and allowing grafting of tissues to the animal so treated from another.

***Antimessage.*** Messenger RNA molecule made artificially from a complementary DNA strand and so is capable of binding in a complementary way with normal messenger RNA of the appropriate gene sequence.

***Antimetabolite.*** Substance that interferes with the utilization of an essential metabolite by an organism. Antimetabolites are chemical analogues of normal metabolites. The majority compete for enzyme binding sites, thus disturbing metabolism or inhibiting cell division. By substituting for a metabolite the antimetabolite may be incorporated into a cell component. Some of the first antimetabolites to be discovered were the selectively antibacterial sulphonamide drugs. These are analogues of p-aminobenzoate, an essential intermediate in the biosynthesis of folic acid. Other antimetabolities are analogues of purine and pyrimidine bases or of nucleosides. These have a high level of toxicity for humans but, together with the antifolates, are clinically useful in cancer and/or antiviral chemotherapy.

***Antimitotic Drug.*** Agent that blocks mitosis, often by preventing spindle formation. These drugs include colchicine and vincristine.

***Antimycin.*** A poison that blocks the flow of electrons from cytochrome b to cytochrome c in the electron transport system.

***Antiparallel.*** Describing an alignment of two polynucleotide strands when linked together by base pairing, as in the case of native DNA. Polynucleotides have a polarity which arises from the 3'-5' linkage of phosphodiester bonds in their sugar-phosphate backbones each polynucleotide must have one free 3'- and one free 5'-end. Antiparallel alignment occurs when the two linked strands run in opposite directions (i.e. the free 3'-end of one is opposite the free 5'-end of the other). Parallel alignment, with both 5'-ends at the same terminus of double-stranded molecule, is not compatible wit the watson-crick model of DNA and does not occur in nature.

***Antipodal Cells.*** The three haploid cells that remain at the non-micropylar end of the embryo sac subsequent to division of the cells. After the formation of thee egg cell they play little or not further part in seed development.

***Antipodal Nuclei.*** Nuclei formed in the plant embryo sac and situated at the end nearest to the chalaza.

***Antiport.*** Membrane transport protein that functions by pumping a component into cells and simultaneously pumping another out. The sodium/potassium pump in eukaryotic cell membrane functions as an antiport.

***Antiseptic.*** Literally, a substance that counteracts purification; more normally, a substance that prevents infection in a wound. Antisepsis is carried out by disinfection or sterilization using non-toxic, non-injurious substances, and has the effect of killing or inactivating microorganisms which cause infection.

***Antiserum.*** Serum containing antibodies, usually including antibodies directed against a specific antigen. Antiserum may be used to confer passive immunity, but carries the disadvantage that the recipient will raise antibodies against some of the serum proteins.

***Antitermination Factor.*** Protein factor that allows the, RNA polymerase to ignore nonsense codons and so continue transcription beyond the usual terminus of a coding sequence.

***Antitoxin.*** Antibody that, by its specificity for a particular toxin antigen, can neutralize the toxin.

***Anucleate.*** Describing a cell that lacks a nucleus.

***Anucleolate.*** Describing cells that lack a nucleolus. A mutant of Xenopus is known condition, only one nucleolus is present and, in the homozygous condition, the cells are anucleolate. It is designated nu or Onu.

***AP Endonuclease.*** Endonuclease that cuts DNA on the 5'-side of sites devoid of either purines (apurinic) or pyrmidines (apyrimidinic). Such sites are known as AP sites.

***Apert Syndrome.*** Human congenital disorder inherited as an autosomal dominant.

***Aphotic Zone.*** The zone of an ocean or sea into which light does not penetrate and in which, therefore, photosynthesis cannot take place. It is usually below about 100 m.

***Apical Dominance.*** A condition in plants where the stem apex prevents the development of side shoots from lateral buds near the apex. The dominance is controlled by the presence of high concentrations of plant hormones (Auxins) at the apex, producing by the apical bud. Further down the stem the auxin concentration is reduced and strong lateral branches are formed. Removal of the apical bud causes lateral branches to develop (e.g. after pruning rose bushes).

***Apical Growth.*** Growth resulting from an apical meristem.

***Apical Meristem.*** A region of dividing tissue at the growing tips of roots and shoots that is responsible for increase in length of the plant body. Meristem cells are small, with thin walls and cytoplasm containing few vacuoles. They undergo active mitosis when growth is occurring (depending on the season) and the new cells look similar to the parental ones but becomes more vacuolated and elongated. Eventually, further away from the meristem, the cells undergo the process of cell differentiation, taking on the appearance of mature plant cells.

Meristematic tissues are delicate and in need of protection. In shoots the apices are covered by tiny leaves forming apical buds at the tips of the branches and axillary buds at the nodes where the leaves join the stem. Root structures are less complex, each root-tip meristem being protected by a shield of loose cells called a root cap.

***Apical Region.*** A tip of a root or shoot in a plant where growth in length takes place by activity of the apical meristem.

***Aplanospore.*** An asexual, nonmotile spore found in some algae and some fungi.

***Apnoea.*** The absence or suspension of breathing, as occurs in diving mammals.

***Apoenzyme.*** Polypeptide moiety of a conjugated enzyme after removal of its prosthetic group. As the activity of conjugated enzymes depends on their prosthetic groups an apoenzyme is inactive, but its presence can sometimes be demonstrated by binding of specific antibodies raised against the whole enzyme (holoenzyme).

***Apoinducer.*** Specific protein whose presence on the promoter site of a gene permits or enhances binding and consequent transcription by RNA polymerase. It is termed an apo-inducer since it complexes to another molecule — the inducer itself — to effect satisfactory induction.

***Apomict.*** Organism resulting from apomixis.

***Apomixis.*** A type of reproduction in which fusion of male and female gametes does not take place. In angiosperm plants a diploid cell of the ovule (either a cell of the nucellus or a megaspore that has not undergone meiosis) may develop into the embryo and the rest of the ovule develops into the seed. The process therefore mimics sexual reproduction. In some cases a pollen grain is necessary to trigger apomixis, and in these cases it is very difficult to distinguish apomixis from normal sexual reproduction (amphimixis).

***Apomorph.*** A derived character.

***Aporepressor.*** A regulatory protein that inhibits the activity of specific genes when in the presence of a corepressor.

***Aposematic Selection.*** A type of frequency-dependent selection operating on a species that has several morphological forms, at least one of which is a mimic of a different 'model' species that is distasteful.

***Apospory.*** A situation occurring in some plants where meiosis is omitted and an ordinary diploid sporophyte cell gives rise to the spore which produces a diploid gametophyte.

***Apostatic Selection.*** A type of frequency-dependent selection occurring in a species with several morphological forms, and classically used in relation to prey species that are visually polymorphic. The amount of predation of each type is directly related to the relative morph frequencies.

***Apothecium.*** The fruiting body of some ascomycete fungi (cup fungi) and lichens, containing asci. Often lightly coloured, they can reach up to 40 cm in diameter, but are usually only a few millimetres across.

***Appeasement.*** Behaviour that inhibits aggression from another animal of the same species, frequently taking the form of a special posture or display emphasizing the weakness of the performer. Threatening structures (e.g. antlers) and markings are covered or turned away, and vulnerable parts of the body may be exposed. Appeasement is seen in courtship, in greeting ceremonies, and often (from the loser) after a fight.

***Appeasement Display.*** Behaviour designed to pacify or make peace following a display of aggressive behaviour. For example, a defeated dog will turn on its back and present its underbelly to the victor, who then ceases combat.

***Apoplast.*** More or less continuous system of cell walls throughout a plant. Since some 50 percent of cell wall space may be occupied by water, the apoplast may be an important route of water movement in the plant.

***Aporepressor.*** Protein that binds with a specific repressor and, together, they prevent gene transcription by the RNA polymerase.

***Aposematic Coloration.*** Warning coloration, displayed by many species of poisonous snakes and distasteful insects, and resulting from natural selection following the evolution of the toxic or distasteful compound.

***Apposition.*** Addition of multiple layers of cellulose to the inner surface of a plant cell wall.

***Apterous.*** Describing an organism that is wingless.

***Apurinic Acid.*** Polynucleotide devoid of its purines, but still retaining the pyrimidine bases and sugar-phosphate backbone.

***Aquaculture.*** The manipulation of the reproduction, growth rates and mortality of aquatic organisms useful to man to enhance their yield; the aquatic equivalent of agriculture.

***Aquatic Respiration.*** A process in which freshwater and marine organisms carry out gas exchange with the water that surrounds them. Fully saturated water contains only about 0.02% as much oxygen per unit volume as air. However, since the tissues are in direct contact with the gas-carrying medium flowing past, the system is very efficient and often a relatively small respiratory surface is required.

Many aquatic organisms (particularly the less advanced groups) have no special respiratory organs, relying on a large surface area for gas exchange (e.g. protozoa, algae, nematodes). Others have developed specialized structures which are either external (e.g. gills of the ragworm Nereis), or internal (e.g. gills of fish). Gills are richly supplied with blood vessels for transport to and from the body tissues, and many organisms with gills expend large quantities of energy creating a regular flow of water over the respiratory surfaces.

***Aqueous Habitat.*** Any habitat in which water is the medium in which the organisms live.

***Arbovirus.*** One of a large heterogeneous group of RNA-containing viruses that are transmitted from animals to man through the bite of mosquitoes and ticks (i.e. arthropods, hence arthropod-borne viruses). Arboviruses cause various forms of encephalitis (inflammation of the brain) and serious fevers, such as dengue and yellow fever.

***Archaeopteryx.*** The earliest known fossil bird (genus Archaeopteryx) found in the Jurassic period about 140 million years BP. The bird is characterized by the presence of teeth in the jaws, claws on the wing and a tail containing vertebrae.

***Area Effect.*** Patterns of distribution of genetically distinct individuals of a polymorphic species resulting in distributions that cannot be explained in terms of environmental selection and are presumed to result from other underlying genetic effects such as founder effects.

***Arealization.*** Spatial determination. The term has been applied to the differentiation of imaginal discs in Drosophila, in which, by growth of the cells in tissue culture, it can be demonstrated that different groups of cells in different areas of the disc are differentially determined, each area being fated to develop into different substructure of the complete body part produced from the disc.

***Arginine.*** One of 20 amino acids common in proteins. It has an extra basic group, and is alkaline in solution. The isoelectric point of arginine is 10.8

***Arithmetic Mean or Mean.*** A number (symbol : x) that is computed by calculating the sum of a set of numbers (Σx) and dividing the sum by the number of terms (n).

***Arnon, Daniel (1910-) American Biochemist.*** With his co-workers in the 1950s, he first discovered electron passage from one electron-acceptor to another in the electron transport system of photosynthesis, particularly the role of ferredoxin.

***Arsenic.*** A chemical element in the form of a grey metal, more familiar in the extremely poisonous form of arsenious trioxide. It was at one time used in arsenical soap for the preservation of animal and bird skin in museums, so that particular care should be taken in handling old museum skins.

***Artefact.*** Something that appears during preparation or examination of material which is not present in the natural state. Two scientists from the University of Surrey, Harold Hillman and Peter Sartory, have suggested on the evidence provided by solid geometry, that some structures described by electron microscopy, e.g. Golgi apparatus, nuclear pores, endoplasmic reticulum, are artefacts of the preparation of material.

***Artemia Salina.*** Small (1 cm) marine crustacean, the brine shrimp. It is used for genetic experiments, partly because it can be grown in large numbers axenically and partly because its development lends itself to genetic analysis. The so-called 'egg' of a brine shrimp is actually a dormant gastrula which can be kept dry for very long periods, but recommences development when exposed to salt water.

***Artenkreis.*** Group of closely related species within a common geographical area, reproductively isolated from each other by subtle boundaries or behavioural traits. Sometimes such a grouping is called a superspecies.

***Arthrogryposis.*** Congenital condition in humans, characterized by multiple joint contractures, and resulting from various genetic aberrations, including trisomy 18.

***Arthus Reaction.*** Clinically important hypersensitive skin reaction involving swelling and vasodilation, following, for example, the intradermal injection of antigen into a patient already carrying antibody specific to this antigen. Arthus reactions are not necessarily confined to the skin, however.

***Artificial Insemination (AI).*** Artificial introduction of sperm into the female reproductive tract. AID refers to artificial insemination by a donor other than the husband. When sperm is donated by the husband it is then termed AIH (artificial insemination, husband).

***Artificial Parthenogenesis.*** The development of an egg into an embryo stimulated not by fertilization but by artificial means, e.g. cooling, treating with acid, mechanical damage.

***Artificial Selection.*** A selection process in which man chooses particular organisms from which to breed, based upon their phenotype, so aiming to alter the average genotype and phenotype of the resulting progeny (a form of directional selection). This process is carried put by plant and animal breeders whose job is to enhance certain features of the organisms with which they work, e.g. greater resistance to root rot in tomatoes, or higher milk yield in cattle. Such selection depends upon the presence of genetic variability in the chosen population.

***Ascomycete.*** Any fungus of class Asctomycetes (now included in the subdivisions Ascomycotina and Deuteromycotina) characterized by the formation of ascospores during sexual reproduction. The hyphae are septate and the asci are grouped in a visible fruiting body.

***Ascorbic Acid or Vitamin C.*** A water-soluble organic compound, found in citrus fruits, green vegetables and tomatoes. Formula : $C_6H_8O_6$. Its best-known role in the formation of collagen, the chief component of connective tissue. Deficiency in ascorbic acid results in the disease called scurvy which is characterized by changes in collagen leading to many further effects. Ascorbic acid acts as a vitamin in man, but rats and most other mammals can manufacture their own supply from D-glucose.

***Ascospore.*** A haploid spore resulting from meiosis in the ascus within the fruiting body of ascomycete fungi.

***Aseptic Techniques.*** Techniques performed in an environment which is as free of disease-causing microorganisms as possible, e.g. in a hospital operating theatre. To achieve this end the atmosphere is filtered, all instruments and outer clothing are sterilized (usually with high temperatures in an autoclave) and the operators wear face masks and gloves. Such techniques should not be confused with the use of antiseptics.

***Asexual Reproduction.*** A process by which organisms multiply without the formation and fusion of specialized sex cells (gametes). Each feature of asexual reproduction has its advantages and disadvantages.

The genetically identical products of asexual reproduction are called clones. Asexual reproduction is a feature of lower animals and occurs in all groups of plants, including angiosperms, usually in addition to sexual reproduction. Perhaps the fixed location of many plants makes this type of reproduction particularly suitable. There are several types of asexual reproduction. These are dealt with under their own headings but are summarized here :

(a) Fission where the entire organism splits into two (e.g. bacteria).

(b) Budding : new individuals produced as outgrowth of the parent (e.g. yeast, Hydra).

(c) Fragmentation : mechanical separation of the plant body into segments (some algae).

(d) Sporulation : producing asexual spores (e.g. fungi).

(e) Vegetation propagation : parts of higher plants producing new whole organisms (e.g. potato tubers).

***Asexual Spore or Isopore.*** A spore which does not arise through sexual reproduction.

***A Site of Ribosome.*** Site on the larger of the two subunits of a ribosome to which the aminoacyl-tRNA binds.

***Asparagine.*** One of 20 amino acids common in proteins. It has a polar 'R' structure and is water soluble, See Figure A.30. The isoletric point of asparagine is 5.4.

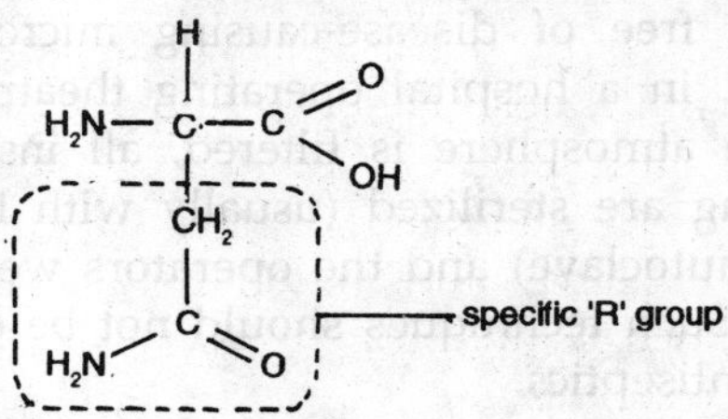


Figure A.30. Asparagine. Molecular structure.

***Aspartic Acid or Aspartate.*** One of 20 amino acids common in proteins. It has as extra carboxyl group and is therefore acidic in solution. The isoelectric point of aspartic acid is 2.8 See Figure A.31.

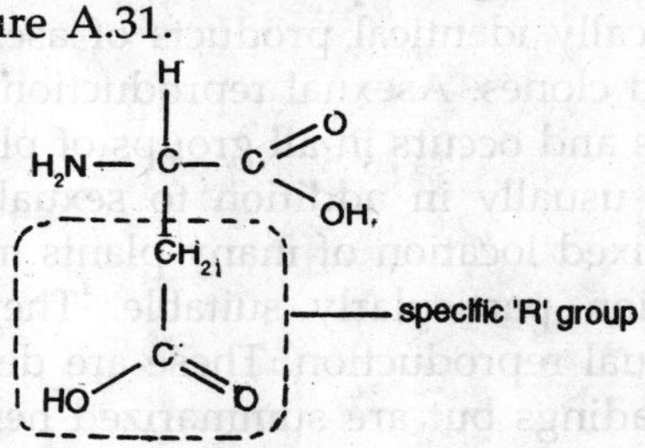


Figure A.31. Aspartic acid. Molecular structure.

***Aspergillus.*** Genus of Ascomycetes; one of the eukaryotic microfungi used in microbial genetics.

***Aspirin.*** Analgesic drug that also reduces fever and tissue inflammation. Effects are believed to result from inhibition of prostaglandin biosynthesis.

***Aspirin or Acetylsalicylic Acid.*** An analgesic that relieves pain without loss of consciousness.

***Assembly Rules (in island biogeography).*** Rules (devised by Diamond) that explain why only certain combinations of species exist on a given island. In some cases this may be due to competition and exploitation of resources, which minimize the amount of unused resources available to potential new invaders.

***Assimilation.*** The intake by organisms of new materials from the outside and their incorporation into the internal structure of the organism.

***Association.*** 1. An ecological unit in which two or more species occur in closer proximity to one another than would be expected on the basis of chance. Early plant ecologists recognized associations of fixed composition on the basis of the dominant species present (e.g. a coniferous forest association). Associations now tend to be detected by using more objective statistical sampling methods.

2. Joint appearance in some individuals in a population of two genetically determined characters at a frequency higher than would be predicted on the basis of their independent frequencies.

***Assortative Mating.*** A type of cross in which the choice of partner is affected by the genotype, i.e. mating is nonrandom. For example, human matings are often assortative with respect to racial features since persons of one racial group may tend to have children by partners of the same group. This choice of mates means that genotypic frequencies predicted by the Hardy-Weinberg law may not be found.

***Assortment.*** In the biological sense, random distribution among gametes of the two homologous copies of each chromosome. One of each pair of homologous chromosomes if paternally derived, but each gamete receives randomly some maternal and some paternal genes. Thus the important principle of genetics that genes assort independently (except when they are linked, that is, carried on the same chromosomes).

***Aster.*** A group of blind-ending spindle microtubules radiating out from the centrioles of dividing cells in lower plants and all animals. The aster function is uncertain, but does not seem to concerned with spindle formation. See Figure A.32.

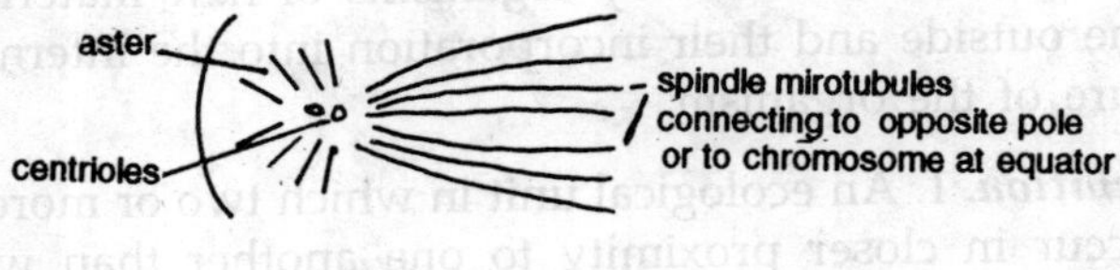


Figure A.32. Aster. Generalized form.

***Asteroidea.*** A class of star-shaped echinoderms which have a basic pentaradiate shape (a five-sided radial symmetry), e.g. starfish.

***Asynapsis.*** Failure of homologous chromosomes to pair during meiosis.

***Atavic Mutation.*** Mutation that restores a primitive condition in a tissue or organism. Homeotic mutations have been designated atavic since the disturbance in segmental organization is normally in the direction of losing a recent or advanced arrangement and replacing it with a more primitive one (e.g. replacement of a haltre by a wing in Drosophila, restoring the primitive four-winged state from the presumably advanced two-winged state of the Diptera).

***Atavism.*** Situation in which a genetic trait, evident in a parent organism, is not expressed in the progeny nor in the immediate future, but is expressed only in a distant generation. The phenomenon is understandable as a pattern of inheritance of a recessive gene. The term is now rarely used.

***Ataxia Telanglectasia.*** Rare inherited disease in humans in which affected individuals develop tumours following exposure to X-rays. It is believed to be due to a congenital defect in a DNA polymerase responsible for DNA repair.

***Atelotype.*** Tissue that is incapable of responding to hormone or lacking in some other function which is normally expressed in the fully differentiated state of an organism or tissue.

***Athlete's Foot or Tinea or Ringworm.*** A fungal disease caused by Epidermophyton floccosum. The fungus can cause irritation of other parts of the body apart from the feet and is parasitic or pathogenic on nails and skin in general. Athlete's foot is most common in adolescent males and infection is caused usually by walking barefoot on infected floors.

***Atmosphere.*** The gaseous envelope surrounding a particular structure, or the gaseous content of a given structure or container.

***ATP (Adenosine Triphosphate).*** A molecule consisting of adenine and ribose sugar onto which are attached three phosphate groups, two being joined by high-energy bonds (See Figure A.33). Hydrolysis of these special bonds results in the release of energy. ATP molecules are formed in two main processes, both involving the addition of inorganic phosphate to ADP via a high energy bond :

$$ADP + P + 34\ kJ\ energy = ATP + H_2O$$

ATP can be formed during cellular respiration, either in the general cytoplasm during glycolysis or in the mitochondria via the krebs cycle and the electron transport system if oxygen is present. ATP is also formed during photosynthesis in the chloroplasts of green plants, again using an

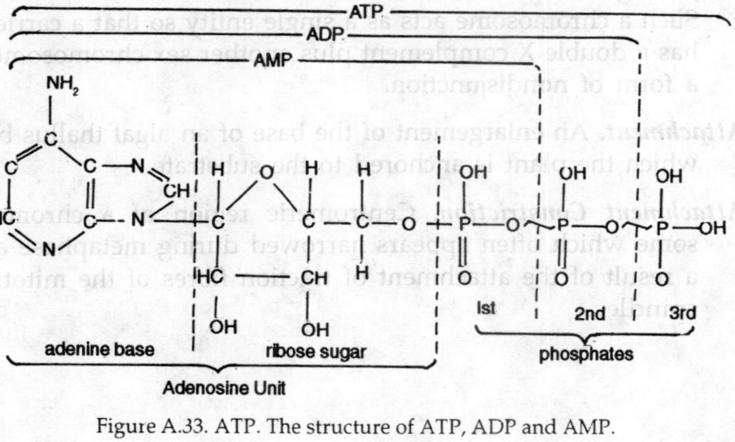


Figure A.33. ATP. The structure of ATP, ADP and AMP.

electron transport system. ATP molecules act therefore as short-term 'biological batteries', retaining energy until required for such processes as active transport, synthesis of new materials, nerve transmission, and muscle contraction. An active cell requires more than two million molecules of ATP per second to drive its biochemical machinery.

***ATPase.*** Enzyme that hydrolyses ATP. ATPases are involved in the ionic pumping of the plasma membranes of eukaryotic cells.

***ATP Synthetase.*** Enzyme found in plasma membranes of aerobic bacteria and in the inner membranes of mitochondria and chloroplasts, that catalyses the synthesis of ATP from ADP and phosphate.

***Atrichia.*** Hairlessness; a congenital condition in many mammals, such as the nude mouse mutation. In the dog it is inherited as an autosomal dominant gene or trait, and homozygous individuals are stillborn.

***Atropine.*** A poisonous chemical obtained from the deadly nightshade that prevents depolarization of the postsynaptic membrane and therefore prevents synaptic transmission, in a similar way to curare. It is used medicinally in preanaesthetic medication and to treat peptic ulcers, renal and biliary colic, etc.

***Attached-X Chromosome.*** A single chromosome formed by the joining of two X-chromosomes at a common centromere. Such a chromosome acts as a single entity so that a carrier has a double X complement plus another sex chromosome, a form of nondisjunction.

***Attachment.*** An enlargement of the base of an algal thallus by which the plant is anchored to the substrate.

***Attachment Constriction.*** Centromeric region of a chromosome which often appears narrowed during metaphase as a result of the attachment of traction fibres of the mitotic spindle.

***Attachment Plaque.*** Specialized area of the inner surface of the nuclear envelope of eukaryotic cells to which chromosome ends are attached, especially in the early stages of meiotic division.

***Attenuation.*** The loss of virulence of a microbial pathogen so that although still alive, it is no longer pathogenic. In this state it is able to stimulate beneficial antibody production when used as a vaccine. Various procedures are used to attenuate the virulence of a pathogen, e.g. the ageing of cultures, or passing the pathogen through an unnatural host.

***Attenuator.*** A regulatory nucleotide sequence occurring in the leader region of an operon and containing a transcription stop signal. The attenuator acts as a fine control mechanism for the activity of structural genes, sometimes being operative, sometimes not, depending on conditions in the cell.

***Att Site.*** Site within the bacterial genome and any infecting bacteriophage genome at which integration of excision of the phage may occur, through a process of recombination.

***Aureomycin.*** 7-Chlortetracycline.

***Australian Antigen.*** Diagnostic antigen present in the serum of patients suffering from the viral disease hepatitis B (infectious hepatitis). Originally discovered in an Australian aboriginal and now more commonly referred to as hepatitis B antigen (HB-Ag), it is thought to represent a subunit of the surface protein of the virion.

***Autocatalysis.*** Phenomenon whereby the product of a reaction catalyses the reaction and so effects positive feedback.

***Autocatalytic (of a substance).*** Catalysing its own production. The more substance is made, the more catalyst is available for further production.

***Autochthonous (of peat).*** Derived from plants that lived on the site of its formation.

***Autoclave.*** 1. An apparatus in which objects or materials are sterilized using air-free saturated steam under pressure at temperatures in excess of 100°C. 2. A sealed vessel in which chemical reactions can occur at high pressure.

***Autocoid.*** An alternative name for hormone.

***Autogamy.*** Self-fertilization; frequently applied in botany, but has also been used to describe the self-fertilization that occurs in some strain of Paramecium aurelia, in which the micronucleus divides to form a zygote nucleus. This diploid nucleus then proceeds to divide to provide both micronuclei and macronuclei in the daughter cells following cell division.

***Autogenous Control.*** Pattern of gene regulation in which proteins control their own synthesis.

***Autograft (Autologous Graft).*** Tissue that is grafted back onto the donor and is normally not rejected.

***Autoimmune Disease.*** Result of an immune reaction to self components that are not normally recognized as foreign. Autoimmune diseases can arise : (1) Due to autoantibody production; for example, against acetylcholine receptors leading to impairment of neuromuscular transmission (myasthenia gravis), and to antigens on erythrocytes leading to their destruction through agglutination and lysis (autoimmune haemolytic anaemia); (2) As a result of cell-mediated immunity in which autoreactive T lymphocytes become directed against self antigens in organs such as the thyroid (Hashimoto's thyroiditis) and adrenal gland (Addition's disease) and against myelin sheaths on central and peripheral nerves (multiple sclerosis), leading to inflammatory reactions and cell destruction.

***Autoimmunity.*** A situation where the immunological defences of the body become sensitized to parts of the same body, resulting in self-destruction in that area. In other words, 'self' antigens become mistaken for 'foreign' antigens, so setting up an immune response. Such an occurrence is clearly dangerous and may be associated with ageing. An example is rheumatoid arthritis in man.

***Autolysis.*** The breakdown of tissues, usually after death, by their own enzymes.

***Automimicry.*** Mimicry within a single species, such that all look alike to a predator, but some, due to their chosen food plant, are toxic or distasteful, whereas others, reared on distinct food plants, are palatable. The polymorphism therefore affects only the character of palatability, and the palatable members of the population gain protection by their resemblance to unpalatable members. The North American monarch butterfly displays such a pattern of mimicry.

***Autonomously Replicating Sequence (ARS).*** Extra chromosomal DNA molecule that replicates independently of host chromosomal DNA synthesis.

***Autophagic Vacuole.*** Lysosome that contains mitochondria or other cellular organelles and is thus involved in digesting parts of the cell in which it resides or of neighbouring cells.

***Autophagy.*** Special type of controlled autolysis in which cellular constituents are selectively degraded by inclusion within a specialized lysosome or autophagic vacuole. Autophagy is most active during embryonic development or senescence.

***Autopolyploid.*** A type of polyploid in which there has been duplication of the number of each chromosome, all chromosomes coming from the same original species. For example, in Figure A.34. A represents one complete set of chromosomes. Like an allopolyploid, an autopolyploid is a mechanism for creating new species, particularly in plants.

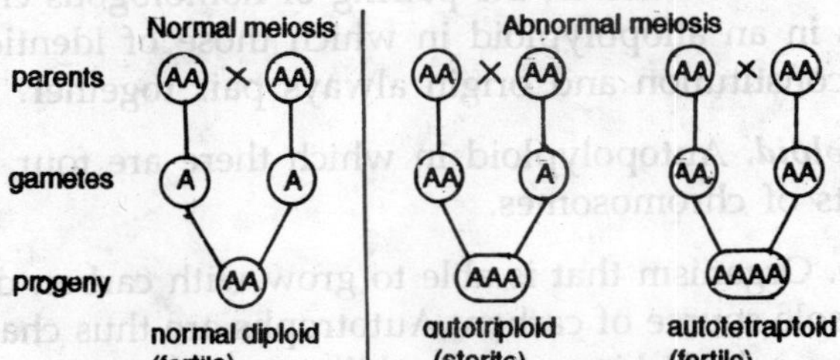


Figure A.34. Autopolyploid. Types of autopolyploid compared with normal diploid.

Allopolyploids are more successful, perhaps because autopolyploid chromosomes have pairing difficulties at meiosis.

***Autoradiograph.*** A photographic representation of radioactive areas in a tissue. Tissues labelled with an isotope (e.g. $^{14}C$) are placed on a photographic plate which is irradiated in the same way as photographic film is exposed to light. Radioactive areas can be seen in the photographs.

***Autosexing.*** A technique by which the sex of an offspring can be determined without examination of the genitalia. For example, the sex of young poultry chicks is difficult to determine anatomically. However, a 'Barring' gene allows the colour of females (one X-chromosome) to be distinguished from that of males (two Xs).

***Autosomal Gene.*** A gene found on an autosome.

***Autosomal Inheritance.*** A pattern of transmission of alleles that are located on autosomes, i.e. not on sex chromosomes, so that the sex of the parent does not affect the result of a mating, reciprocal crosses giving identical results.

***Autosome.*** A type chromosome found in all cells not concerned with sex determination. Chromosomes are of two types : autosomes and sex chromosomes. Autosomes carry the major part of genetic information in cells, including information on sexual characteristics.

***Autosyndesis.*** Situation in the pairing of homologous chromosomes in an allopolyploid in which those of identical genetic constitution and origin always pair together.

***Autotetraploid.*** Autopolyploid in which there are four identical sets of chromosomes.

***Autotroph.*** Organism that is able to grow with carbon dioxide as its sole source of carbon. Autotrophs are thus characterized by a high biosynthetic ability; green plants are the most obvious examples. In the majority of autotrophs, the carbon dioxide is assimilated (or 'fixed') into cell material by the ribulose bisphosphate pathway (ribulose diphosphate pathway), but in a few photosynthetic bacteria a reversed citric acid cycle operates. In the methanogens, carbon dioxide is assimilated by a novel partially known route involving acetyl coenzyme A. Autotrophs grow in the absence of reduced carbon compounds; energy for growth is therefore obtained from light (photoautotrophs) or by oxidation of inorganic compounds such as hydrogen, ammonia, nitrite, sulphide, sulphur, thiosulphate or ferrous ions (chemolithotrophs). Most autotrophs are obligate, but some are facultative and able to grow as heterotrophs.

***Auxin.*** A type of plant hormone involved in the growth of cells and several other functions. The most important auxin is indolacetic acid, but many other substances have been classified as auxins, using a bio-assay method developed by Fritz Went.

The effects of auxins depend on their concentration in the plant. They are most concentrated at the shoot tip and least concentrated in the root, except for small amounts at the root tip. The major effects of auxin are summarized below :

(a) Encourages cell growth by elongation, producing a softening of the middle lamellae of cell walls.

(b) Stimulates cell division in the phloem of the vascular bundles, so encouraging new growth.

(c) Promotes positive phototropism in shoots by growth of tissues towards the light source.

(d) Promotes geotropism in all parts of the plant (positive in roots, negative in shoots, due to unequal distributions of the hormone).

(e) Induces apical dominance by suppressing lateral buds.

(f) Induces lateral root formation.

(g) Stimulates fruit development, enabling seedless fruits to be produced artificially.

(h) Suppresses abscission in leaves and fruit.

(i) Encourages the formation of wound tissues in injured or diseased plants.

***Auxocyte.*** Cell whose nucleus is about to enter meiosis and therefore including cells such as primary oocytes and spermatocytes, microsporocytes and megasporocytes.

***Auxotroph.*** A mutant strain of microorganism that requires growth factors in addition to those required by the wild type, i.e. will not grow on minimal medium.

***Avena Test.*** Test used to assay for auxin, and involving measured curvature of the Avena (oat) coleoptile following its exposure to a block of tissue impregnated with the test solution.

***Avery, Oswald T (1877-1955).*** American physician, who with Colin Macleod and Maclyn McCarty in 1944, demonstrated that the 'transforming principle' suggested by Griffith to explain bacterial transformation was DNA. Thus DNA alone could cause a heritable change in bacteria, strongly suggesting that DNA (rather than protein) is the basic genetic material of cells.

***Avian Leukosis.*** Virally induced leukaemia of the chicken.

***Avian Myeloblastosis Virus.*** RNA virus that causes leukaemia in chickens.

***Avidin.*** Substance present in uncooked white of the fowl's egg, which may include deficiency of the coenzyme biotin, since it specifically binds to and inactivates this compound.

***Avidity.*** Total affinity of an antibody for its specific antigen as a summation of all possible binding sites.

***Avogadro's Number.*** Number of atoms in one gram atomic weight of an element ($6.025 \times 10^{23}$). It also signifies the number of molecules in the gram molecular weight of a compound.

***Axenic Culture.*** Pure culture containing only one type of micro-organism.

***Axolotl.*** Mexican axolotl Ambystoma mexicanum; an amphibian of the order Urodela. It is a facultative neotene (i.e. it exhibits neoteny or the persistance of larval features, such as external gills) into sexually mature adulthood. Under drought conditions or after stimulation of the pituitary-thyroid axis by thyrotrophin, metamorphosis to a salamander is induced. The axolotl may also be said to show paedogenesis. Formerly known as Siredon mexicanum, axolotls have been used in experimental embryology and in limb-regeneration studies.

***Axon.*** Long extension of a neurone, normally conducting impulses away from the nerve cell body. Axons vary greatly in length from less than 1 mm to more than 1 m. As well as being responsible for the conduction of a nerve impulse in the form of an action potential, axons also have an important transporting role involving the so-called axon flow. This is a steady movement of molecules from the neurone cell body along the axon towards the terminal branches and. to a lesser extent, a somewhat slower returning passage of molecules. Axon transport is greatly facilitated by the cytoskeleton of neurofilaments and microtubules. See Figure A.35.

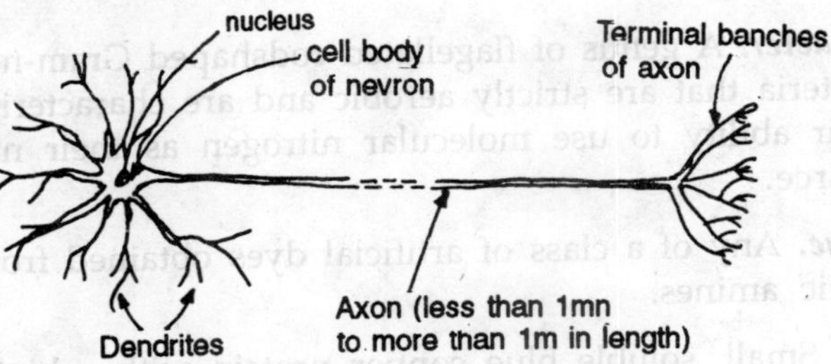


Figure A.35. Axon

***Axonal Membrane.*** In a general sense, the plasma membrane covering the axon, but more specifically, the presynaptic membrane at the synapse, where it has a central role in adhesion and in the release of neurotransmitter substances into the synaptic cleft, thus affording communication with either a second neurone or a muscle cell.

***Axonal Transport (Axon Flow).*** Transport of molecular aggregates and vesicles along axons, both away from the cell body (anterograde transport) and back towards the cell body (retrograde transport). The former moves at a speed of about 400 mm day and the latter at 200-300 mm day.

***Axoneme.*** Central strand of the eukaryotic cilium or flagellum, comprising a characteristic arrangement of nine pairs of microtubules surrounding an inner core of two microtubules.

***Axoplasm.*** Cytoplasm contained in axons.

***5'-Azacytidine.*** Chemical analogue of the naturally occurring nucleotide cytidine in which -CH = at position 5 in the base ring is replaced by -N =. Cells incorporate 5'-azacytidine into RNA in place of normal cytidine, but protein synthesis is impaired as a result. The 2'-deoxy derivative is also incorporated into DNA, but again the cells may be ultimately killed in consequence.

***8'-Azaguanine.*** Purine Analogue.

***Azolla.*** Genus of aquatic fern widely used in work on plant cell physiology.

***Azotobacter.*** A genus of flagellated rodshaped Gram-negative bacteria that are strictly aerobic and are characterized by their ability to use molecular nitrogen as their nitrogen source.

***Azo Dye.*** Any of a class of artificial dyes obtained from aromatic amines.

***Azurin.*** Small, soluble blue copper protein with a high mid-point redox potential that is involved in nitrite reduction in bacteria.

# B

***B₁, B₂, B₃, etc.*** First and subsequent generations resulting from a backcross. A first backcross is made by mating an individual with its parents, or with another individual with identical genotype to that of a parent. Offspring from such a cross are designated the $B_1$ generation. Crossing of individuals of the $B_1$ generation with the parents, or others of identical genotype to parents, is designated a second backcross $B_2$ and produces the $B_3$ generation.

***Bacillus.*** Genus of rod-shaped bacteria; includes the aerobic, gram-positive, sporeforming bacilli.

***Backbone.*** Linear, supporting back of a polymer molecule from which the sidechains project. The backbone of DNA consists of two antiparallel strands of alternating sugar and phosphate groups to which the bases attach and from which they gain support. In the case of DNA, the formation of hydrogen bonds between the bases within the helix gives further strength to the structure.

***Backcross.*** A genetical term describing a mating between a hybrid organism and one of the original parental types. The results of a backcross depend upon the parental type. A backcross to the recessive parental is diagnostic (since it reveals the genotype of the hybrid) and is called a testcross.

***Background Radiation.*** Radiation from natural sources, such as cosmic radiation and granitic rocks, as compared to radiation from radioisotopes involved in experimental situations. Fall out from atomic explosion may contribute considerably to background radiation, as will accidental leaks from atomic power stations.

***Back Mutation.*** An inherited change (mutation) in a mutant gene that causes it to regain its wild type function.

***Bacteria.*** (Sing bacterium) unicellular or (more rarely) multicellular procaryote organisms. Some are autotrophic, contain bacteriochlorophylls and bacterioviridin, carrying out photosynthesis anaerobically. Bacteria have various shapes, occurring as cocci (spherical), bacilli (rod-shaped) and spirilla (helical) which range in size from 1 μm to about 500 μm, but usually 1-10 μm in diameter. They are present in soil, water, air and as free-living symbionts, parasites and pathogens. While some bacteria are useful in nitrogen and sulphur cycles, many cause diseases of plants, animals and man, e.g. anthrax, tetanus. Reproduction occurs asexually but genetic transfer can take place by conjugation; other genetic changes may be brought about by mutation or the acquisition of a plasmid (See Figure B.1). Identification usually involves biochemical tests rather than visual study and classification often involves the use of numerical taxonomy.

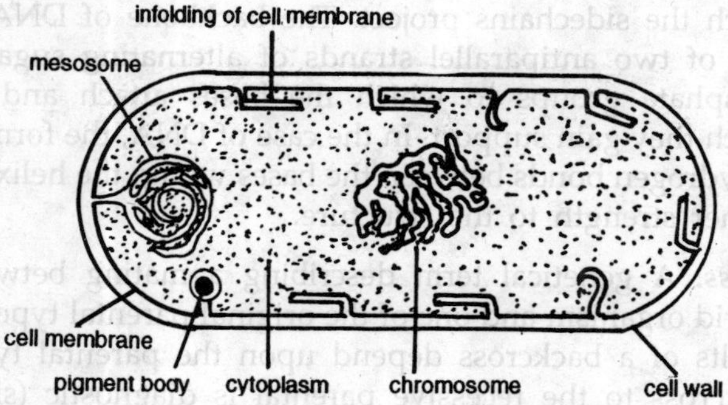


Figure B.1. Bacteria. A generalized bacterium.

***Bacterial Conjugation (Bacterial Mating).*** Directional transfer of genetic material (DNA) by cell contact between donor (male) and recipient (female) bacteria. Conjugation is one mechanism by which plasmids are spread through bacterial populations and is also the basis of the classical approach to genetic analysis of bacteria. First discovered for E. coli in 1946, conjugation has since been observed for other gram-negative bacteria including species from Azotobacter, Klebsiella, Pseudomonas, Salmonella, Shigella and Vibrio, and between species from different genera (e.g. E. coli × Salmonella, Salmonella × Shigella).

Donor character is conferred by an intracellular plasmid sex factor. The plasmid is of the conjugative (self-transmissible) type (e.g. the F factor, resistance factor or certain larger colicin factors). In $F^+$ donor cells, the F factor is present as one or two extrachromosomal copies. Recipient ($F^-$) cells lack the F factor. Donor-recipient mating pairs are formed following random collisions shortly after mixing cultures of $F^+$ and $F^-$ bacteria. The cells are then connected by the F pilus, a proteinaceous appendage of the donor. The tip of the pilus interacts with a specific recognition site on the surface of the $F^-$ cell (a major outer membrane protein, the product of the ompA gene, may be involved in this recognition process). The role of the pilus may be to bring the cells together by pilus retraction through depolymerization.

During conjugation, $F^-$ bacteria gain the F factor and are thus converted to $F^+$. Transfer of the F factor is dependent on DNA synthesis. One strand of the circular, double-stranded F factor is cut at a specific site oriT (origin of transfer) by a plasmid-coded endonuclease (product of the traY and traZ genes). Unidirectional DNA synthesis, using a membrane-bound DNA polymerase, is initiated at this site, the unbroken circular strand acting as a template. The newly synthesized strand displaces the cut strand, which then enters the recipient (5'-end first). The transferred donor strand is replicated in the recipient cell to form a double-stranded F factor. All the $F^-$ cells in a culture may be converted to $F^+$ donors in this fashion, whereas the original donor cells retain their donor character.

In about one in 100 000 $F^+$ cells the F factor is stably integrated into the chromosome, thereby losing its autonomy and behaving as a single replicon with the chromosome. These Hfr bacteria rarely confer the donor state on $F^-$ recipients, but Hfr x $F^-$ crosses give a high frequency of recombination of donor markers. In a given Hfr strain integration of the F factor has occurred, with particular orientation, at one of several specific sites scattered around the chromosomes. These sites show some sequence homology with F-DNA. The integration process is reversible leading to reconstruction of the circular autonomous F factor. Mobilization of the chromosome is similar to F transfer. During conjugation, a cut is made is one DNA strand at oriT within the integrated F factor, whereupon the 5'-end unwinds and enters the recipient. This results in the immediate entry of part of the F factor followed by oriented transfer of chromosomal genes, proximal to the leading end, at a uniform rate of about 1 percent of the chromosome length per minute. The donor remains viable because DNA synthesis replaces the trans ferred strand DNA synthesis in the recipient also converts the transferred single strand into double-stranded DNA. The order in which the donor genes are transferred is determined by the position and orientation of F within the chromosome. Only when the entire length of the chromosome is transferred (about 100 minutes) is the complete F factor transmitted and Hfr character conferred on the recipient. Complete chromosome transfer occurs very rarely (from about one in 10 000 donor cells); strand breakage normally terminates transfer prematurely.

The presence of donor DNA within the recipient creates a merozygote, which is diploid for the genes carried on the fragment. The fragment is not an independent replicon and is lost at cell division unless it becomes integrated into the recipient chromosome by crossing-over at two or more sites to create a stable recombinant.

Intermediate donors carry F′ factors. F′ factors are excised from the chromosomes of a Hfr strain and consist of the F factor together with adjacent regions of the donor chromosome (up to one-third of the chromosome may be attached). F′ formation occurs in primary F′ donors, which thereby undergo chromosome deletion. During F′ X F″ conjugation (F duction). F′ is transferred in a manner analogous to F transfer; the recipient becomes a secondary F′ donor and is diploid for the chromosomal genes carried by the F′ factor. F′ can be reversibly integrated into the chromosome within the diploid region so that cultures of intermediate donor strains are about 90 percent F′ and 10 percent Hfr bacteria. F′ factor are used conveniently to map gene loci on the bacterial genome and for complementation analysis of genes.

***Bacterial Lawn.*** Continuous, uniform layer of bacteria growing on the surface of a solid medium such as an agar plate. Lawns are prepared by flooding the agar plate with a suspension of bacteria, followed by an incubation period to allow bacterial growth. Inhibition of growth within a lawn is an indication of sensitivity of the organism to agents applied to the lawn (e.g. antibiotics, bacteriophages).

***Bacterial Slant (Bacterial Slope).*** Slants are used for storing stock cultures of bacteria, yeasts and other microorganisms in the laboratory. Microorganisms are grown on the surface of a suitable nutrient medium solidified at 45° from horizontal in a small, airtight vial. The method is most suitable for aerobes, but slants of anaerobes can be covered with sterile liquid paraffin.

***Bacterial Stab.*** Stabs are used for storing stock cultures of bacteria and other microorganisms in the laboratory. The microorganisms are inoculated into a soft medium (e.g. 0.6 percent wt/vol nutrient agar) contained within a small, airtight vial using a straight wire. The method is suitable for anaerobes and facultative anaerobes.

***Bacterial Transposon.*** Any one of a number of different DNA sequences found in some strains and species of bacterial cells that are characterized by their mobility in the genome, since they can move from one site to another within the circular chromosome. They own their mobility to the existence of short insertion elements at each end of the transposon, and they may carry bacterial coding sequences within the transposon itself. Transposons betray their presence in bacteria by the movement of a coding sequence within a transposon (as revealed by mapping the gene sequence through an interrupted mating experiment) or by the altered expression or mutation rate of other bacterial genes adjacent to the site of insertion of a transferable sequence.

***Bactericide.*** A substance causing death to bacteria, for example an antibiotic.

***Bacteriochlorophyll.*** A form of chlorophyll possessed by photosynthetic bacteria (green and purple types). In addition to small amounts of bacteriochlorophyll, green bacteria mostly possess another type of chlorophyll called bacterioviridin.

***Bacteriology.*** The study of bacteria.

***Bacteriocidal.*** Designating toxic chemicals that destroy bacteria. Bacteriocides, which include phenol and its derivatives, hypochlorite ($OCL^-$), mercuric chloride, and organic mercury compounds, are often called disinfectants.

***Bacteriocin.*** Any of a group of antibacterial proteins produced by bacteria. Different bacteriocins are produced by different groups of bacteria and are often designated by the name of the producing organism, e.g. colicins are derived from E. coli and staphylococcins from some Staphylococcus species. These proteins are coded by genes carried on distinct plasmids (rather than in the main bacterial genome). Certain bacteriocins tend to aggregate into large complexes, some of which show a striking similarity in the electron microscope to the tails of bacteriophages.

***Bacteriocin.*** Protein secreted by certain bacteria and lethal (i.e. bactericidal) for other closely related bacteria. Bacteriocins are mostly named after the producing strain (e.g. colicins are produced by E. coli and other enteric bacteria). They bind initially to cell surface receptors on the bacterial outer membrane. They have potent killing action; often one molecule is sufficient to render a susceptible bacterium non-viable.

Many bacteriocins are enzymes acting, for example, on the cell wall mucopeptide (e.g. pesticin from Yersinia pestis, colicin M) or on cellular nucleic acids (e.g. colicin E2 is a DNase, colicin E3 is RNase) or on membrane components (e.g. megasin from Bacillus megaterium is a phospholipase). Other bacteriocins destroy the integrity of cell membranes. Colicins A, E1, Ia, Ib and F form ion-permeable channels leading to collapse of the membrane proton motive force. Pyocin R1 (produced by Pseudomonas aeruginosa), which resembles a contractile bacteriophage tail and contains over 20 protein subunits, also damages the energy-transducing membrane. Most bacteriocins are encoded by plasmids, some of these being conjugative. Bacteriocin production is mostly repressed; they are formed because a cell occasionally escapes from repression (this causes the cell to lyse). The remaining bacteriocinogenic bacteria in the culture are immune to their own bacteriocin, some may have an immunity protein that irreveribly binds to and inactivates the bacteriocin. Bacteriocins may confer a selective advantage on the producing strain in its natural environment by inhibiting the growth of closely related species with similar nutritional requirements.

***Bacteriolysis.*** Rupture of bacterial cells. Bacteriolysis can be caused by the action of enzymes (e.g. lysozyme), by complement, bacteriophage multiplication or chemical agents (e.g. penicillins, some disinfectants) or mechanical means (e.g. ultrasonically).

***Bacteriophage (Phage).*** A virus whose host is a bacterium. Bacteriophages range in size and complexity from Qβ, a tiny icosahedral particle with a molecular weight of $4 \times 10^6$ daltons, to the T-even phages (T2, T4, T6), with a complex head and tail structure and 50 times the molecular weight of Qβ. Qβ contains a single-stranded RNA chromosome that carries only three genes, whose products are involved in replication of the phage RNA and capsid production. T4 contains a double-stranded DNA chromosome coding for about 60 genes whose products are either structural components of the phage particle or are needed for synthesis of phage nucleic acid. T4 has a complex structure. The DNA is wound inside the head, and after the phage becomes attached to the bacterial surface, the tail core is forced through the cell wall by contraction of the sheath, so that the infecting DNA can pass through it into the bacterium. After injection of the DNA a lytic cycle follows : the host cell switches its metabolism entirely to the production of new bacteriophages, leading ultimately to lysis of the host cell and the release of new viral particles. Some phages do not induce an immediate lytic cycle. Instead their DNA becomes inserted into the host chromosome and remains dormant, only occasionally leaving the host DNA and initiating a lytic cycle.

Unlike viruses that infect eukaryotes, almost no bacteriophage enters its host cell as a whole particle. Most insert only their RNA or DNA into the host cell. Like other viruses, bacteriophages are parasitic in the RNA, DNA, and protein-synthesizing machinery of their hosts. See Figure B.2.

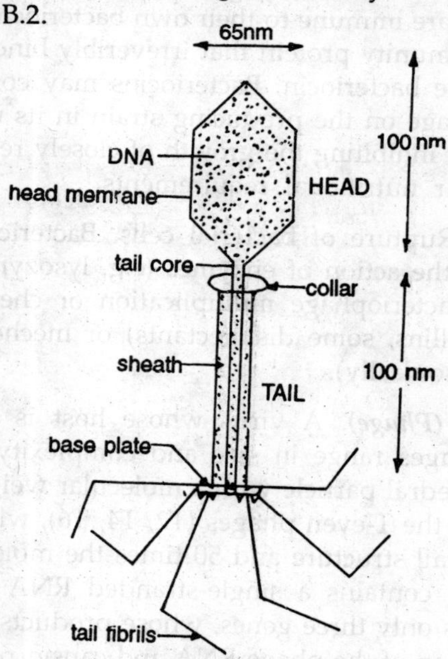


Figure B.2. Structure of a bacteriophage.

***Bacteriophage Packaging.*** Assembly of novel genes into phage genomic DNA, usually of lambda phage, together with the inclusion of these recombinant molecules into phage heads, followed by the growth of such phage in host E. coli bacterial cells and the consequent formation of phagê plaques.

***Bacteriorhodopsin.*** Bacterial protein ($M_r$ = 25 000) that is located in a specialized region of the cell membrane of halobacteria, known as the purple membrane. The protein converts light into a transmembrane protein gradient that is used to synthesize ATP.

***Bacteriostatic.*** Describing any chemical or physical agent that reversibly inhibits the growth of at least some types of bacteria.

***Bacteroid.*** Bacterium-like cells such as those of Rhizobium found in root nodules.

***Bal 31 Exonuclease.*** Exonulease from the bacterium Brevibacterium albidum, which is able to digest DNA at both the 5'- and 3' -ends and can be used to introduce deletions into cloned molecules of DNA.

***Balance.*** The maintenance of stability and specific orientation by an organism in relation to the immediate environment. Organs of balance occur at the end of each semicircular canal in the inner car where there is a swelling, an ampulla; this is a reçeptor which has a group of sensory cells, hairs from which are embedded in a gelatinous cap - the cupula. Since the semicircular canals are at right angles to each other the ampullae are sensitive to movement in any plane, as the canal fluid moves the cupula in a direction opposite to that of the movement of the head. Head position is given by receptors containing calcareous otoliths in the utricle and saccule, and these react to gravity in relation to the position of the head. Nerve fibres lead to the brain from ampullae, saccule and utricle.

***Balanced Chromosome.*** Chromosome having several overlapping inverions which impede recombinations with a homologous chromosome.

***Balanced Lethal System.*** Strain of organisms that are heterozygous for at least two non-linked, recessive genes that are lethal in the homozygous condition. When two such individuals are interbred there is a dihybrid cross, with a normal 9:3:3:1 ratio of genotypes. All nine of the first category survive because they are heterozygous for both lethal genes, but all remaining progeny the since they are homozygous for at least one of the two lethals. Because the lethals die they are often undetected, and the strain appears to breed true, thus the term balanced lethal.

***Balanced Polymorphism or Stable Polymorphism.*** A genetic polymorphism in which the various morphs are maintained in a stable frequency over several generations due, possibly, to constant natural selection pressures.

***Balanced Stock.*** Heterozygous genetic stock or population that can be maintained for many generations without artificial selection. Such stocks often contain balanced lethal genes or some other genetic balancing mechanism, such as sterility of homozygous females.

***Balbiani Chromosome.*** Polytene chromosome found in the salivary glands of Drosophila and some other Diptera flies; so-called because they were discovered in Chironomus By E. G. Balbiani in 1881.

***Balbiani Ring.*** Certain giant puffs of the polytene chromosomes of Chironomus; so-called because of their discovery by E. G. Balbiani in 1881. They represent highly active genes and are sites of intense RNA synthesis, the genes concerned coding for proteins secreted in the salivary secretion.

***Bam HI Restriction Enzyme.*** Type II restriction enzyme isolated from Bacillus amyloliquifaciens that recognizes the hexanucleotide target sequence.

5' ... G—C—A—T—C—C ...3'

3' ... C—C—T—A—G—G ...5'

***Band III Protein.*** Protein that is found in the plasma membrane of erythrocytes. It is a transmembrane protein and is believed to be responsible for the gaseous exchange of oxygen and carbon dioxide across the membrane. The protein is named as a result of its electrophoretic position relative to other membrane proteins.

*Banding.* Distinctive patterns appearing on chromosomes. The term is applied to two quite different phenomena. (1) Pattern of staining that can be induced in spreads of metaphase chromosomes when giesma staining is preceded by treatment of the preparation with elevated temperature, trypsin digestion or extraction with strong alkali. Such bands are termed giemsa or G bands. Other distinct banding patterns can be revealed on mitotic chromosomes by exposure to quinacrine (Q bands) or to treatments that strain the heterochromatin at the centromeres (C bands). Chromosome banding techniques, especially G banding, have revolutionized cytogenetics because they permit unequivocal identification of the separate chromosomes, as well as accurate assignment of genes to particular chromosomes. (2) Pattern that is a distinctive feature of the giant polytene chromosomes found in some tissues of the larvae of dipteran flies (e.g. Drosophila and Chironomus). The banded pattern is visible within nuclei of living cells, and may also be visualized by phase contrast microscopy or orcein staining. The bands, also known as chromosomes, are stretches of relatively condensed chromatin, whereas the lighter interband regions are stretches of uncondensed chromatin. Interbands are believed to be stretches of DNA containing house-keeping genes, which are transcribed and expressed constantly, whereas the bands, which contain at least 70 percent of the chromosomal DNA, contain non-coding sequences and luxury gene sequences. When a band is transcribed and expressed, as when a luxury gene is active, the band is dramatically decondensed and is then termed a puff.

***Banks, Barbara.*** Biochemist who, in the early 1970s, argued that ATP when hydrolysed required rather than gave up energy to break covalent bonds. Most biologists consider that energy is provided when ATP is hydrolysed but it is not thought to be stored simply in the terminal phosphate bond.

***Banting, Sir Frederick Grant (1891-1941).*** Canadian physician and Nobel prizewinner. He is best-known for his discovery, with C. H. Best, of the hormone insulin, in 1921, during his work on the internal secretion of the pancreas.

***Barbiturate.*** Any ureide such as phenobarbital, amytal, seconal, etc. Barbiturates have a depressant effect on the CNS, usually producing sleep.

***Barr Body.*** Sex chromatin particles found in the interphase nucleus of buccal epithelial cells in some female mammals and probably derived from an X-chromosome. First described by Murray Barr in 1949, Barr bodies can be used as a sex marker, always occurring in numbers one less than the total number of X-chromosomes. Thus normal human males and turner's syndrome females have no Barr bodies, whilst Klinelfeter's syndrome males have two. See Figure B.3.

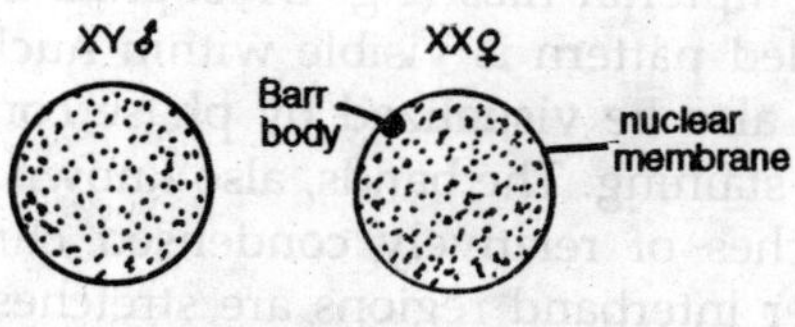


Figure B.3. Barr body. Sex chromatin in nuclei from human male and female buccal epithelial human cells.

***Basal Body.*** A structure similar to (and homologous with) a centriole connected to the axial filament of the flagellum and cilium, e.g. in sperms.

***Basal Metabolic Rate (BMR) or Basal Metabolic Level (BML).*** The minimal rate of metabolism in a resting organism in an environment with a temperature the same as its own body heat, whilst not digesting or absorbing food. The rate is commonly expressed in terms of energy per unit surface area per unit time, usually as kJ $m^{-2}$ $h^{-1}$.

***Base.*** A chemical substance which has a tendency to accept protons ($H^+$), the base dissolves water with the production of hydroxyl ions and reacts with acids to form salts.

***Base Analogue.*** Any chemical that has a similar structure (i.e. analagous) to one of the purine or pyrimidine bases in DNA or RNA. Such analogues can become incorporated into the nucleic acid and may act as a mutagen. For example, 5-bromouracil (5Bu) is an analogue of thymine and can be incorporated into DNA in place of thymine. In its normal state 5Bu acts like thymine and pairs with adenine but the analogue sometimes undergoes a chemical change called a tautomeric shift and now pairs with guanine. At the next DNA replication an incorrect base will be incorporated into the DNA, causing a transition substitution mutation (adenine-guanine). See Figure B.4.

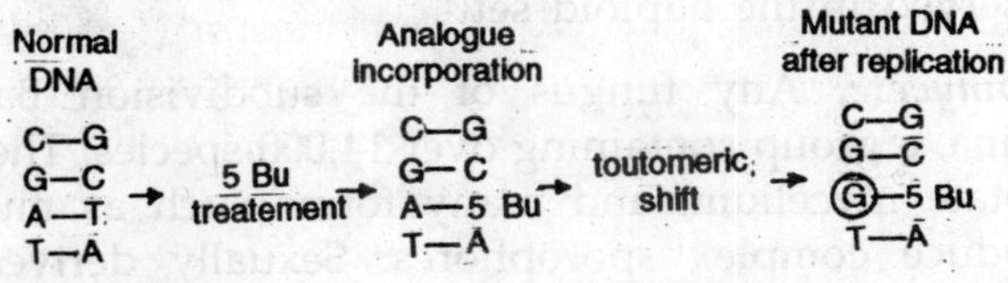


Figure B.4. Base analogue. The action of 5-bromouracil on DNA.

***Base Deletion.*** Removal of a nucleotide base, a purine or a pyrimidine from the DNA structure, producing a deletion mutation that can have serious consequences for the related protein.

***Base Pairing.*** The chemical linking of two complementary nitrogenous bases in DNA and in certain types of RNA molecules. Of the four such bases in DNA, adenine pairs with thymine and cytosine with guanine. In RNA, thymine is replaced by uracil. Base pairing is responsible for holding together the two strands of a DNA molecule to form a double helix and for faithful reproduction and reading of the genetic code. The links between bases take the form of hydrogen bonds.

***Base Ratio.*** The ratio of the number of adenine and thymine bases (A + T) to the number of guanine and cytosine bases (G + C) in the DNA of a particular species. For any one species the amount of adenine is equal to the amount of thymine, similarly the amount of guanine is equal to the amount of cytosine; furthermore the ratio of A + T to G + C is constant. The base ratio varies widely between different species; for example among bacteria it ranges from 0.35 to 2.7.

***Base Substitution.*** The replacement of a nucleotide base in a DNA molecule with another base, possibly producing a substitution mutation.

***Basic Dyes.*** Dyes with a basic organic grouping which strain when coloured with an acid; they are used mainly for nuclear staining where they combine with nucleic acids, e.g. fuchsin as used in the Feulgen stain for DNA.

***Basic Number.*** Basic haploid number of chromosomes. In species where there is variability of chromosome number in the karyotype, the basic number is the lowest number observed in the haploid set.

***Basidiomycete.*** Any fungus of the subdivision Basidiomycotina, a group containing over 14,000 species. They have a septate mycelium, and many forms such as mushrooms produce complex sporophores. Sexually derived spores (basidiospores) are produced externally on basidia, usually in groups of four, and this is characteristic of the group Basidiomycotina. Members are important as food (mushrooms), in plant diseases (rusts and smuts) and in dry rot of timber.

***Basidium.*** The (microscopic) structure on which the sexually produced basidiospores of basidiomycete fungi are formed during sexual reproduction. See Figure B.5.

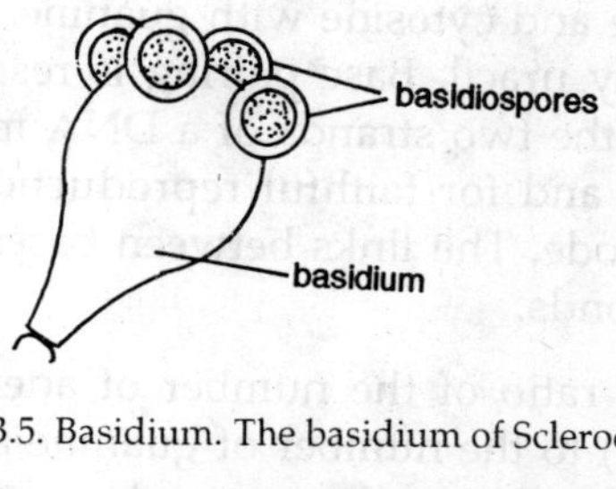


Figure B.5. Basidium. The basidium of Scleroderma.

***Basifixed (of anthers).*** Joined by the base and not capable of independent movement.

***Basophil.*** Type of polymorph with cytoplasmic granules which stain with basic dyes such as methylene blue. They comprise about 0.5 percent of the leucocyte population of human blood and are responsible for release of histamine and serotonin in certain immune reactions. Together with neutrophils and eosinophils, they are classed as granulocytes.

***Basophilic.*** Describing a cellular or tissue component that binds to a basic (cationic) dye (e.g. methylene blue, toluidine blue, carmine, basic fuchsin, haematoxylin).

***Basophil Leucocyte.*** A type of white blood cell (of the granulocyte group) which takes up the stain of a basic dye. Basophils form a tiny proportion of the adult human leucocytes (about 1%), being produced in the bone marrow and have a function which is probably associated with the immune response, e.g. in chickenpox infection.

***Bateson's Rule.*** When an appendage is abnormally duplicated, the supernumerary copy will usually be double, and one of these two will have a reversed orientation. Two versions of the appendage will thus be found behind the normal organ, one a mirror image of the other. It is named after the geneticist William Bateson who published the rule in 1894.

***Bateson, William (1861-1926).*** British pioneer of genetics. He 'rediscovered' Mendelian inheritance in 1900, using, for example, poultry and sweet peas.

***Bayes' Theorem.*** Theorem in human genetics used to predict risk of inheriting an X-linked recessive trait or being at risk for a late onset autosomal dominant trait, using pedigree data and information from normal progeny.

***B Chromosomes (Accessory Chromosomes).*** Supernumerary chromosomes found in maize, rye, grasshoppers, and many other animal and plant species. B chromosomes appear to be dispensable genetically and they are normally composed of highly condensed chromatin.

***B DNA.*** Normal form of the double-helical molecule of DNA. It differs from the other right-handed helical form of DNA

— the A form — and from the left-handed helical form of DNA — Z form — in terms of base stacking and helical pitch.

***Beadle, George Wells (1903-).*** American geneticist. With Edward Tatum, he began the modern study of biochemical genetics using the red bread mould Neurospora crassa. They investigated nutritional mutants in the fungus (auxotrophs), and coined the one gene/one enzyme hypothesis.

***Behaviour.*** 1. The total activities of a living organisms (usually an animal) ranging from simple movement to complex patterns involved with courtship, threat, camouflage, etc. 2. The observable response of an organism to stimuli from the environment.

***Behavioural Genetics.*** 1. The branch of genetics concerned with determining the relative importance of the genetic constitution of animals as compared to environment factors in influencing animal behaviour.

2. Aspect of genetics that involves the inheritance of behaviour patterns.

***Belt Desmosome.*** Type of adhering junction in animal cells, forming a continuous band around each interacting cell in an epithelial sheet and located near to the apical end of the cell. Contractile bundles of actin filaments run along the belts just under the plasma membrane.

***Bence-Jones Protein.*** Immunoglobulin light chain present in the urine of patients suffering from multiple myelomatosis; originally discovered by H. Bence-Jones in 1847 as proteins that coagulated on heating the urine to 60°C. They arise as a result of an excess synthesis of light chains by the mutant B lymphocytes and their subsequent passage from the blood across the kidney into the urine because of their relatively low molecular weight ($M_r$ = 23 000). These proteins were of paramount importance in elucidating the variable region and constant region structure, since they are unique in having a high degree of homogeneity, enabling amino acid sequences of one Bence-Jones protein to be compared with another.

***Benedict's Test.*** A procedure used to detect the presence of reducing sugars in a solution. Benedict's Reagent consists of a single solution of copper sulphate, sodium citrate and sodium carbonate in water. The reagent is added to the test solution and heated. A red precipitate of Cu(I) oxide indicates the presence of a reducing sugar.

***Benign.*** Describing non-invasive tumours or those not spreading by metastasis; commonly, though not exclusively, applied to neoplasms.

***Benlate.*** Commonly used systemic fungicide, readily absorbed by growing plants.

***Benzidine.*** Potent carcinogen, used as a stain for haemoglobin. It is not absolutely specific for haemoglobin, since it also reacts with other haem-containing molecules.

***Benzpyrene.*** Potent carcinogen; most important carcinogenic factor in polycyclic hydrocarbons.

***Bergmann's Rule.*** A rule stating that the individuals from populations of warm-blooded species of animals (homoiotherms) which occur in cooler climates tend to be larger on average than individuals of the same species in warmer climates. This is because the surface area/volume ratio in large animals is smaller, so that heat loss is consequently reduced. The rule is named after the German biologist W. Bergmann, and was formulated in 1847.

***Beri-Beri.*** A human disease caused by vitamin $B_1$ (thiamine) deficiency in which affected individuals suffer from wasting of muscles, paralysis, mental confusion and sometimes heart failure.

***Bernard, Claude (1813-78).*** French physiologist. He was the father of modern experimental physiology, and the first person to appreciate the importance of the internal environment in the functioning of organisms.

***Beta-Chain.*** One of the polypeptides found in the adult haemoglobin of many vertebrates, including man. Two molecules of beta-globin, with tow molecules of alpha-globin, together with their attached haem groups, go to form the tetramer of the haemoglobin molecule.

***Beta-Decay.*** Gradual loss of radioactivity from a radioisotope with emission of beta-particles. The rates of decay are characteristic for different radioisotopes and are conventionally considered in terms of their half-lives. Half-lives of beta-emitters commonly used in biological studies range from 14 days for phosphorus ($^{32}P$) to 5100 years for carbon ($^{14}C$).

***Beta-Particles.*** Electrons emitted by one category of radioisotope. The radioisotopes of carbon ($^{14}C$), phosphorous ($^{32}P$) and hydrogen ($^{3}H$ tritium) are beta-emitters. The electrons emitted by different radioisotopes have a characteristic distribution of kinetic energies; measurement of the energy of the electrons allows the radioisotopes to be distinguished. This permits double-labelling experiments in which different precursors labelled with different radioisotopes may be used simultaneously.

***Beta-Pleated Sheet.*** A regular folding of polypeptide chains that constitutes the secondary and tertiary structure of some proteins. The polypeptide chains are linked to each other by hydrogen bonds between the carbonyl (—C = O) and imino (—NH) groups. See Figure B.6.

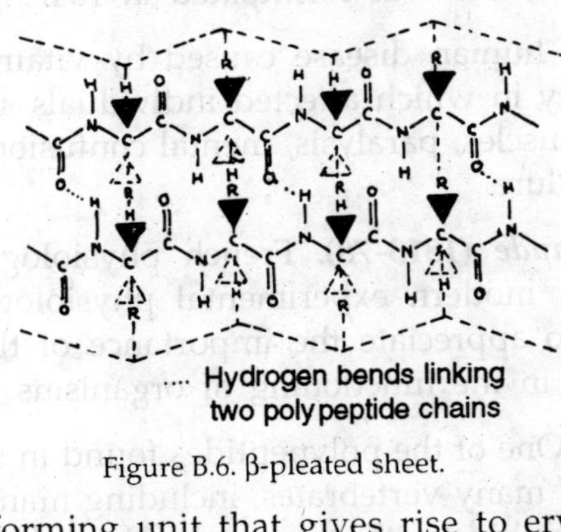


Figure B.6. β-pleated sheet.

***BFU-E.*** Burst-forming unit that gives rise to erythrocytes.

***BHK Cells.*** Established cell line derived from the kidneys of newborn hamsters.

***Bidirectional Replication.*** Mechanism of DNA replication commonly found in both prokaryotes and eukaryotes, in which two DNA replication forms move out in either direction from a single site of initiation, the replication origin.

***Bifid.*** Divided into two distinct arms or projections.

***Bilateral Cleavage or Radial Cleavage.*** The type of cleavage which gives rise to bilateral symmetry. It occurs in echinoderms and chordates.

***Bilharzia or Schistosomiasis.*** A human disease common in Egypt and other warm parts of the developing world, in which affected individuals suffer from body pains followed by severe dysentery and anaemia, leaving them weak and highly susceptible to other diseases. The disease is caused by the miracidium larva of the blood fluke Schistosoma, which lives as an adult in the abdominal veins and has a water snail as a secondary host, transmission being effected via urine.

***Bimodal Distribution.*** A statistical pattern in which the frequencies of values in a sample have two distinct peaks, even though parts of the distribution may overlap. For example, the sexual differences between men and women for such characters as height and weight produce a bimodal distribution. See Figure B.7.

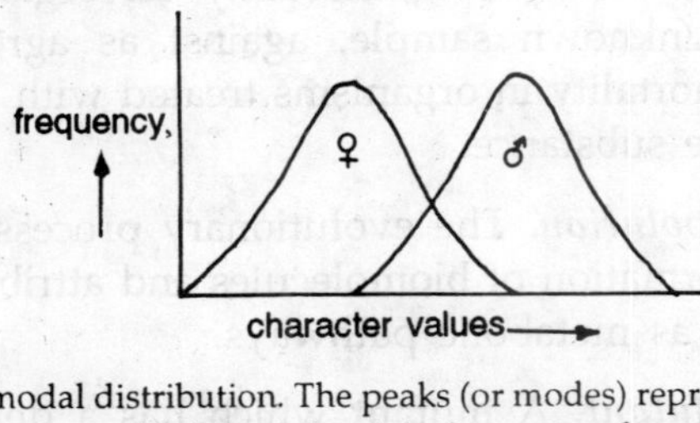


Figure B.7. Bimodal distribution. The peaks (or modes) represent the character values of height and weight for men and women.

***Binary Fission.*** An asexual method of cell reproduction carried out by procaryotes and some primitive eucaryotes, in which the chromosomal material is replicated and then the cytoplasm splits by cytokinesis. Such processes differ from mitosis and meiosis in that the chromosomal separation does not involve cellular microtubules forming a spindle.

***Biochemistry.*** The study of the chemistry of living organisms, especially the structure and function of their chemical components (principally proteins, carbohydrates, lipids, and nucleic acids). Biochemistry has advanced rapidly with the development, from the mid-20th century, of such techniques as chromatography, X-ray diffraction, radioisotopic labelling, and electron microscopy. Using these techniques to separate and analyse biologically important molecules, the steps of the metabolic pathways in which they are involved (e.g. glycolysis and the krebs cycle) have been determined. This has provided some knowledge of how organisms obtain and store energy, how they manufacture and degrade their biomolecules, how they sense and respond to their environment, and how all this information is carried and expressed by their genetic material. Biochemistry forms an important part of many other disciplines, especially physiology, nutrition, and genetics, and its discoveries have made a profound impact in medicine, agriculture, industry, and many other areas of human activity.

***Bio-Assay.*** A technique in which the presence of a chemical is quantified by using living organisms, rather than by carrying out chemical analysis. For example, the amount of a toxic substance (such as an insecticide) in a sample could be estimated by comparing mortality on organisms treated with the unknown sample, against as agreed standard figure of mortality in organisms treated with known quantities of the substance.

***Biochemical Evolution.*** The evolutionary processes concerned with the formation of biomolecules and attributes of living cells, such as metabolic pathways.

***Biochemical Mutant.*** A mutant which has a defect in a biochemical pathway, such as an auxotroph.

***Bioengineering.*** 1. The use of artificial tissues, organs, and organ components to replace parts of body that are damaged, lost, or malfunctioning, e.g. artificial limbs, heart valves, and heart pacemakers. 2. The application of engineering knowledge to medicine and zoology.

***Biogenesis.*** The principle that life is propagated only by existing life, rather than by spontaneous generation. The principle's original formulation was that organisms are able to generate only other forms similar to themselves, but where alternation of generations occurs the statement is not entirely true; biogenesis has thus come to mean that a species gives rise only to similar forms and these forms can only be derived from parents which are similar.

***Biogeographical Region.*** The regions of the earth's surface which contain distinctive groups of animals and plants that are normally prevented from moving out of those regions by various natural barriers.

***Biokinetic Zone.*** The temperature range over which organisms can survive (5° -60°C).

***Biological Clock or Internal Clock.*** An internal mechanism (as yet poorly understood) by which many plants and animals keep a sense of time, making possible a rhythmic pattern of behaviour. Many organisms have such 'clocks' producing activity cycles of approximately 24 hours (circadian rhythms) which, however, can be affected by external influences that 'set' the clock (entrainment). An individual's clock can be re-entrained if placed in a new time zone, as happens with rapid, long-distance travel.

Biological clocks affect not only whole organisms activities (e.g. sleeping) but also cellular patterns of activity (e.g. varying metabolic rates).

***Biological Control.*** A method of pest control using natural predators (harmless to other organisms) to regulate the size of pest populations. The technique has been mainly used against arthropod pests causing economic or medical problems. For example, red spider mites (Tetranychus urticae), which are pests of glasshouse crops such as cucumbers, are routinely controlled by application of commercially available samples of predatory mites (Phytoseilus persimilis) that feed on the red spider mites, thus reducing their numbers below an economically harmful level.

***Biological Indicator.*** Any organism which can be used to characterize particular environmental properties, e.g. pollution, oxygenation. For example, Sagitta elegans characterizes oceanic waters, S. setosa characterizes the continental shelf.

***Biological Magnification.*** The increasing concentration of a substance such as a pesticide in organisms from their predecessors in the food chain.

***Bioluminescence.*** Production of light by living organisms. It is a widespread phenomenon in nature, occurring in some bacteria, some fungi, many deep-sea crust-aceans and coelenterates, and insects, such as glow-worms and fireflies. Bioluminescence is produced by the action of luciferase on luciferin. Activated luciferin emits light as it returns to the ground state following combination with ATP.

***Biomass.*** Total amount of living material in a region or locality of study.

***Biometrical Genetics.*** Genetical analysis applied in animal and plant breeding, in which variable phenotypic characters are carefully quantified and their underlying patterns of inheritance determined.

***Biometry or Biometrics.*** The analysis of biological data by means of statistical or mathematical techniques.

***Biopsy.*** The surgical removal of small amounts of tissue for examination to aid a diagnosis.

***Biosphere.*** That part of the earth's surface and its immediate atmosphere which is occupied by living organisms.

***Biosynthesis.*** The process by which more complex molecules are formed simpler ones by living organisms, e.g. photosynthesis.

***Biota.*** The living organisms present in a specific region or area, ranging in size from a small puddle to a biome or larger.

***Biotechnology.*** The use of organisms, their parts or processes, for the manufacture or production of useful or commercial substances. The term denotes a wide range of processes, from using earthworms as a source of protein, to the genetic manipulation of bacteria to produce human gene products such as growth hormone.

***Biotic Community.*** All the organisms living on and contributing to a specific region (a biota).

***Biotic Factor.*** The influences which occur within an environment (on both the physical environment and the organisms living there) as a result of the activities of living organisms.

***Biotic Potential.*** The theoretical maximum rate of increase of a species of organism in the absence of any adverse environmental factors such as predators or disease.

***Biotrophic (of microorganisms).*** Feeding on living organisms, parasitic.

***Biotype.*** (1) Particular physiological form of an organism or an individual produced by a specific physiological adaptation. A plant species that is salt-tolerant might be found to vary in its vegetative form depending on whether it was collected in freshwater marshland or in brackish marshland. The two variant forms could be referred to as biotypes. (2) Group of organisms forming a genetically identical population or clone.

***Bipolar Cell.*** Neurone of the vertebrate retina that is specialized to stretch perpendicularly so that it provides connections between two layers of the retina.

***Bipolar Molecule.*** Molecule with two separate polar or hydrophilic groups, most often at opposite extremities.

***Birefringence.*** Property of anisotropic materials such that a ray of plane-polarized light is split into two separate rays by the internal architecture of the material.

***Birth.*** The act of bringing forth young from the female animal, usually from the uterus of a female mammal, but also denoting the birth of any animal where eggs develop inside the adult and young are produced as independent organisms, e.g. seahorses.

***Birth control.*** Any method used to limit the size of the human population, which usually involves the prevention of fertilization of the ovum by the sperm but can also include abortion of the foetus. Behavioural methods include (a) abstention from copulation, (b) the so-called 'rhythm method' which takes advantage of less-fertile phases of the menstrual cycle, (c) coitus interruptus. Other methods involve the use of contraceptive devices, hormonal treatment and sterilization.

Many countries have government-sponsored birth control programmes, initiated in an attempt to control the rapidly increasing human population. For example, China not only encourages one child per family but is also attempting to produce a longer period between generations (over 25 years) by favouring marriages at a late date.

***Birth rate.*** The average number of offspring produced by a female in a given time. This is calculated as the total number of new individuals added to the population during the time in question, divided by the number of mature breeding females in the population at that time.

***Bisexual.*** Of or referring to (a) hermaphrodite individuals, (b) a population that contains both males and females.

***Bithorax complex.*** DNA sequence that is a complex locus of at least nine genes in Drosophila, each gene being defined by the mutations that affect it. All nine genes, when in mutant form, lead to partial or complete loss of a function necessary for normal segmentation. The first genes in the complex to the investigated were found to induce, in mutant form, the development of characteristics of the second thoracic segment (i.e. a wing) in the position of the third thoracic segment, the normal third thoracic segment appendage being a haltere.

***Bittiner's mouse milk factor.*** Virus carried in the milk of certain strains of mice that induces mammary tumours in a high percentage of the suckled progeny.

***Biuret reaction.*** A chemical change used as a quantitative method for protein determination. The reaction takes place when dilute copper sulphate solution is added to a protein solution which is then made alkaline by the addition of sodium hydroxide. A copper hydroxide precipitate forms and a purple/ violet colour is produced, the strength of which indicates the quantity of protein present. The reaction only works if at least two peptide bonds are present in the protein. Thus single amino acids and dipeptides with only one peptide bond will not give a positive Biuret reaction.

***Bivalent.*** (of a pair of homologous chromosomes) being paired during prophase I of meiosis.

***Blastema.*** Aggregation of apparently undifferentiated mesenchyme cells, covered by epidermis, that forms at the end of the stump of an amputated limb in amphibians (e.g. axolotls and newts). The blastema grows and differentiates in a precise way to develop into the parts of the limb that lie distal to the stump. Thus, if the forelimb is amputated at the wrist, blastema cells will grow and differentiate to form a hand. Treatment of the blastema with retinoic acid disturbs this organization: for example, a whole arm may regenerate from the retinoic acid-treated blastema on an amputated wrist.

***Blastocoel.*** Central, fluid-filled cavity of the blastula, which arises as a space between blastomeres towards the end of the cleavage stage of many animal embryos. (In mammalian embryos it is analogous with the blastocelic cavity.)

***Blastocyst.*** The blastula of mammals, differing from that of lower

***Blastoderm.*** The layer of cells formed by cleavage of the fertilized egg in the presence of large amounts of yolk, e.g. in birds, so that the blastoderm forms on one side of the yolk mass, initially as a small blastodisc.

***Blastodisc.*** Blastula stage of development in a meroblastic system, prior to morphogenetic movements and epilbolic overgrowth of the yolk (e.g. in teleost). In avian development the related term, blastoderm, is used after epiboly has commenced.

***Blastokinesis.*** The movement of an embryo within an egg during the course of development.

***Blastomere.*** One of the cells produced by the early cleavage of an egg. When great size differences occur between different blastomere cells, they may be styled macromeres and micromeres.

***Blastoporal lip.*** Dorsal lip of the blastopore, which functions as an embryonic organizer region, inducing the formation of neural tube in later development.

***Blastopore.*** Point on the surface of a gastrulating embryo, vertebrate or invertebrate, at which superficial cells are being internalized from the surface into the interior of the embryo. As a result, the blastocoel will be occluded, totally, or in part, and the internationalized cells reorganize to form new tissue layers within the embryo. The blastopore is thus a dynamic structure, being comprised of different cells at different stages of gastrulation. In many forms the blastopore persists, in modified form as the proctodaeum or embryonic anus.

***Blastula or Blastophere.*** A stage in the development of an embryo, where the embryo consists of a hollow ball of cells with a central cavity (a morula) formed by a process of cleavage. Invagination (in-pushing of the ball at one side) of cells into the blastula gives rise to the gastrula. See Figure B.8.

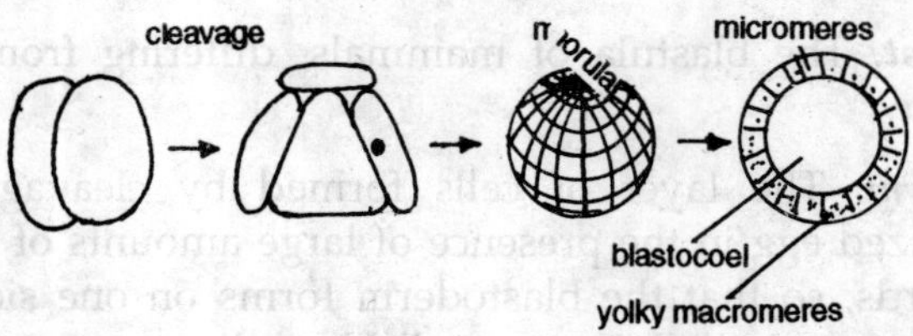


Figure B.8. Blastula. Formation of the blastula by cell cleavage.

***Bleb.*** Extrusion of the cellular plasma membrane or nuclear membrane, often but not always as a result of insult or injury.

***Blending inheritance.*** A pre-20th century theory that the male and female gametes each contained essences from the various parts of the parental body, which were mixed at fertilization to produce offspring showing some features of both parents. The theory was backed up by results from crosses involving quantitative characters in which there was an apparent mixing of phenotypes due to segregation of polygenes. However, the idea of blending was overtaken by the discoveries of mendel and his laws of particulate inheritance.

***Blight.*** Any of various plant diseases caused by microorganisms, where the entire plant is infected and soon dies.

***Blood.*** A connective tissue with a liquid matrix called blood plasma. Suspended in the plasma are three types of cell which form about 45% of total blood volume : (a) red blood cells or erythrocytes, (b) white blood cells or leucocytes and (c) cell fragments or platelets. See Figure B.9.

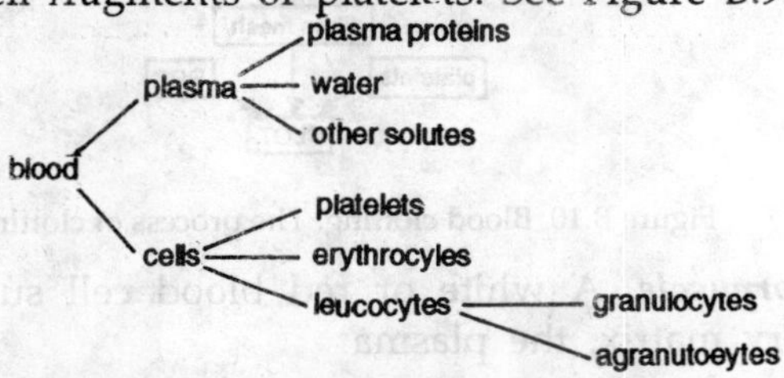


Figure B.9. Blood. The constituents of blood.

***Blood Clotting.*** A condition where elements in the blood plasma change consistency from a liquid to a gel-like structure, causing a 'clot' to form at the site of damage. The process of clotting is complex, but can be summarized as follows:

(a) damage to the blood circulatory system causes both blood platelets and the blood vessels to secrete thromboplastin.

(b) thromboplastin, in the presence of calcium ions, causes prothrombin (a globulin type of plasma protein produced in the liver when vitamin K is present) to change to thrombin.

(c) thrombin acts as an enzyme, causing fibrinogen (another type of plasma protein) to be changed to fibrin which, when it contracts, forms a mesh of fibres in which blood cells become trapped. The final result of clotting is a hard lump which can plug the damaged area (if not too large) thus preventing further loss of blood and entry of microorganisms from outside. See Figure B.10.

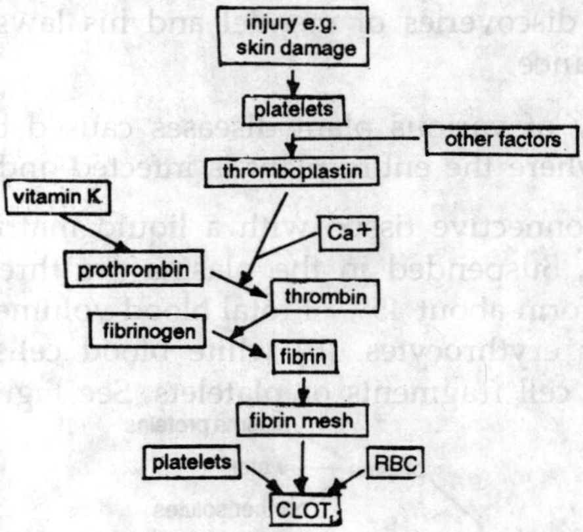


Figure B.10. Blood clotting. The process of clotting.

***Blood corpuscle.*** A white or red blood cell suspended in a watery matrix, the plasma.

***Blood Film.*** A smear of blood made on a microscope slide that is subsequently fixed and stained for examination.

***Blood grouping.*** A method in which blood is characterized by the presence or absence of particular antigens on the surface of red blood cells. The antigens can be recognised by their reaction to specific antibodies which causes agglutination to occur. Two well-known blood groupings are the abo blood group and rhesus blood group systems.

***Blood Pigments.*** The complex protein molecules found in blood and other tissues, which contain metal atoms in their structure. Such pigments have a high affinity for oxygen, functioning in oxygen transport, e.g. hemoglobin in vertebrates (containing iron) and haemocyanin in molluscs and arthropods (with copper), and in oxygen storage within tissues, e.g. myoglobin (iron) found in muscle cells.

***Blood plasma.*** The watery matrix of blood in which the blood cells are suspended. Plasma consists of about 90% water, acting as a solvent, and the following solutes :

(a) plasma proteins. The largest component (about 7% by weight), which is divided into three groups; albumin (55%), globulin (44.8%) and fibrinogen (0.2%). Plasma proteins are important in the maintenance of correct blood osmotic potential, the regulation of blood pH and (fibrinogen only) in blood clotting.

(b) nitrogenous waste substances that are carried from their site of production to the kidneys. These excretions consist mostly of urea, but also have small amounts of ammonia and uric acid.

(c) inorganic salts of sodium, calcium, magnesium and potassium, the most common being sodium chloride. These salts form about 0.9% by weight and are responsible for maintenance of correct osmotic pressure and pH in the blood as well as maintenance of the proper physiological balance between the tissues and blood.

(d) organic nutrients. Among the most important are : (i) blood sugar, mainly glucose, derived from the breakdown of foods, either directly from the gut or from glycogen stored in the liver (glycogenolysis). The precise level of blood sugar is critical for the maintenance of homeostatis and is controlled by a negative feedback mechanism in which insulin plays a major part. (ii) blood lipids such as fats and cholesterol, derived from dietary intake or activity of the liver.

(e) hormones manufactured in the endocrine glands.

(f) dissolved gases such as nitrogen (physiologically inert), small quantities of oxygen (mostly carried by hemoglobin in the erythrocytes) and carbon dioxide carried as bicarbonate ($HCO_3^-$) in the plasma.

***Blood Platelets or platelets or thrombocytes.*** disc-like components of mammalian blood, consisting of non-nucleated cytoplasmic fragments of large bone-marrow cells 3 m in diameter called megakaryocytes that have entered the blood circulatory system. Platelets play an important part in blood clotting.

***Blood serum or serum.*** A fraction of the blood consisting of blood plasma from which fibrinogen (a clotting factor) has been removed.

***Bloom.*** An overabundant growth of algae, often resulting from nutrient enrichment.

***Bloom syndrome.*** Human disease, inherited as an autosomal recessive, an characterized by fragility of the chromosomes.

***Blotting.*** General procedure (either by electrophoresis or capillary action) for transferring DNA, RNA or proteins to solid supporting matrices.

***Blue baby.*** A rare condition in human infants where there is incomplete separation of oxygenated and deoxygenated blood in the heart. Some deoxygenated blood enters the aorta rather than the pulmonary artery, resulting in an inadequate oxygen supply to the body tissues and a 'bluish' appearance to the skin. The problem arises because of incomplete closure of two routes which cause bypassing of the lungs during foetal life: (a) ductus arteriosus, a blood vessel connecting the pulmonary artery and the aorta and (b) foramen ovale, a hole in the septum which divides left and right atria. The condition is a serious one which can, however, be rectified by surgery.

***Blue copper proteins.*** Small, soluble proteins having a single copper atom. They act as electron transfer proteins in bacteria and plants.

***Blue-green algae.*** A division of algae-like organisms (Myxophyta or Cyanophyta) whose members are procaryotes and live in marine or freshwater. They are usually blue-green in colour and propagate mainly by asexual reproduction. Some blue-green algae are filamentous, with no well-defined nucleus or chromatophores, and reproduce by fission, or fragmentation if filamentous. Some blue-greens live in very inhospitable environments, for example hot springs, where the temperature is in excess of 85°C. The pigments produced are chlorophyll (green) phycocyanin (blue) and phycoerythrin (red).

***Blunt-end ligation.*** Joining of non-cohesive ends of DNA by means of DNA ligase.

***Blunt ends.*** (flush ends, non-cohesive ends). Ends of pieces of DNA, usually fragments from digestion of DNA with restriction enzymes, which are cut evenly so that neither strand of the duplex has a free, single-stranded portion.

***B lymphocyte.*** (B cell). Vertebrate white blood cell involved in the production of antibody. Mature virgin B lymphocytes (i.e. those that have not encountered antigen) are characterized by the presence of the following surface markers: monomeric IgM receptors for antigen; Fc receptors for IgG; receptors for the activated form of the C3b component of complement. Stem cell precursors of B lymphocytes undergo an antigen-independent phase of differentiation, which takes place in haemopoietic areas of the liver and spleen in the case of foetal mammals and in bone marrow in adults. In birds, where this process was first discovered, the main site of antigen independent differentiation is the bursa of fabricius, hence the designation B. Stimulation of virgin B lymphocytes by antigen leads to their differentiation into plasma cells and memory B lymphocytes (B cells with the same surface receptors for antigen as the parent cell). This antigen-dependent phase of B cell differentiation takes place in peripheral lymphoid organs where B lymphocytes predominate in the follicles (referred to as B lymphocyte dependent areas).

***Bobbed.*** Describing a Drosophila mutant allele that, in the homozygous condition, leads to the formation of dwarf bristles, together with a reduction in the number of copies of the genes for ribosomal RNA. The locus of the bobbed gene is near to the centromere of the X chromosome and is also the nucleolus organizer. Bobbed mutants, of which there is a range, are believed to represent partial deletions of the rRNA cistrons following unequal crossing-over.

***Bohr effect or Bohr shift.*** A phenomenon named after its discoverer, the Danish physiologist Christian Bohr (1855-1911), who showed that the oxygen-carrying capacity of blood haemoglobin varies with ph. At high pH values haemoglobin has a high affinity for oxygen, but more acid conditions cause haemoglobin to release its oxygen, as in tissues with a high concentration of dissolved carbon dioxide.

***Bolting.*** An unusual lengthening of plant steams, due to elongation of cells, which can be induced by plant hormones called gibberellins producing a stem with long internodes. Bolting can occur naturally, as when biennials such as cabbage and sugar beet produce elongated flower stalks in their first year rather than flowering in the second year. The problem arises when such plants are subjected to winter conditions in their first year (usually having been planted too early in the spring) which induces growth typical of the second year.

***Bombay blood type*** A rare blood type in which individuals appear to be Group O and yet can produce offspring of a type normally impossible for a Group O parent. It appears that Bombay types are homozygous for a pair of recessive h alleles that inactivates the production of the ABO blood group antigen, even though they have the genes to manufacture these antigens, a form of epistasis. See Figure B.11.

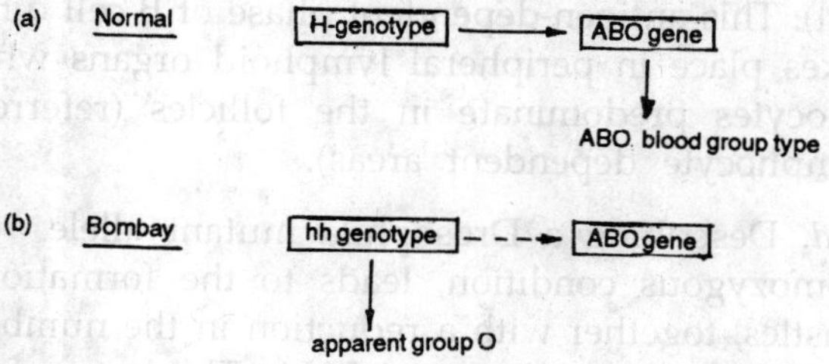


Figure B.11. Bombay blood type. (a) Normal and (b) Bombay blood group types.

***Bombay phenotype.*** Phenotype displayed by individuals homozygous for a recessive mutation associated with absence of alpha-L-fucose from the carbohydrate precursor of the ABO antigens of erythrocytes. Such individuals, whatever their genotype, have total absence of ABO characteristics on their erythrocytes.

***Bombyx mori.*** Commercial silk moth; widely used in genetic research and also for studies on the synthesis of fibroin.

***Bordered pit.*** Pit in the secondary wall of some plant cells, in which an extension of the wall surrounds and arches over the pit cavity. Bordered pits occur in vessel elements, tracheids and fibres of the xylem, but may also be found in some sclerenchyma cells outside of the xylem.

***Bottleneck.*** A period in the history of a population during which the number of individuals is reduced to a low number, perhaps by disease or extreme environmental conditions. As a result random genetic drift may occur in the population.

***Botulism.*** A dangerous type of food poisoning, caused by toxins from the bacterium Clostridium botulinum, an obligate anaerobe that grows well in airtight containers (e.g. tins) which have not been properly sterilized before being filled. The toxin acts against the nervous system, particularly the cranial nerves, producing weakness and sometimes paralysis. The disease is named after the Latin botulus for sausage, a common source of the bacterium.

***BP.*** Before Present, a term used in geological time scales to denote any time before the present.

***Bradykinin.*** A hormone formed from a kininogen in the blood plasma that has the effect of rapid vasodilation in the skin.

***Bradymetabolism.*** The pattern of thermal physiology in which an animal possesses a relatively low basal metabolic rate when measured at a body temperature of 37°C. In such animals a fall in core temperature simply results in a reduction of BMR. Although usually poikilothermic and ectothermic, many bradymetabolic forms are able to attain varying degrees of homoiothermy. All living lower vertebrates and invertebrates are bradymetabolic.

*Branch migration.* Ability of a partially paired DNA strand to displace the resident strand and so increase the length of base pairing with its complement.

*Breakage and reunion.* Process presumed to occur in crossing-over in which the DNA of neighbouring homologous chromatids breaks and a crossways reunion of the strands within the chromosome tetrad follows.

*Bread mould.* The fungus Mucor or a related form (e.g. Rhizopus) which grows on bread. The term can also denote Neurospora crassa, a member of the class Pyrenomycetes which is associated with decomposing or burned vegetation. This organism was used by beadle and Tatum in their work on which the one gene/one enzyme hypothesis is based.

*Breast-feeding.* (in humans) the direct feeding of an unweaned child on breast milk from the mammary gland, as opposoed to bottle-feeding.

*Breed.* A domesticated variety of an animal or rarely, a cultivated variety of plant. Cultivated plants are more often simply called varieties or, more correctly, cultivars. Examples of animal breeds are Friesian cattle and Shetland sheepdogs.

*Breeding range.* The geographical area within which a species breeds.

*Breeding true.* An organism that is not genetically variable for a particular character. Thus, crossing two parents (or self-pollinating one parent) of this type would produce offspring that were all identical with the parents. Such types are also knows as 'pure-breeding' and were, for example, used by mendel in his experiments with the garden pea. In more precise terms, parents breed true when they are homozygous for a pair of alleles of a particular gene.

*Breeding value.* The (economic) worth of an individual's genotype, as judged by the average performance of its offspring.

From the size of the breeding value it is possible to choose suitable parents for future crosses.

***Bristle mutant.*** One of a range of mutants that affect bristle morphology or pattern in Drosophila. Large chaetae (macrochaetae) are present on the body surface and legs. There are also finer chaetae referred to as microchaetae or hairs.

***Britten-Davidson model.*** Model of eukaryotic gene regulation proposed by Roy Britten and Eric Davidson in 1969. It is to an extent an extrapolation of the operon model of prokaryotic gene regulation, and proposed that four distinct types of DNA sequence would be involved in eukaryotic gene regulation. Firstly, sensor genes would be sensitive to effector substances bringing signals to the genome from the cytoplasm or from outside the cell. On such stimulation, as integrator gene adjacent to the sensor gene would be activated, releasing RNA products which would move to other sequences in the genome, the receptor genes, which would all be sensitive to the integrator RNA. Receptor genes are deemed to be adjacent to producer genes, of variable sequence, each of which would be activated by the receptor gene response to integrator RNA. Producer gene product would be messenger RNA responsible for protein synthesis. Although many gene sequences in eukaryotes are not characterized by this proposed coordinate expression, cellular responses to hormone do have many of the qualities inherent in the Britten and Davidson proposal.

***Broad-sense heritability.*** The widest estimate of the role of genes in influencing total phenotypic variability, measured by the ratio of total genotypic variance to total phenotypic variance.

***Brown earth soil.*** Any mull soil typically found on loams or clays under deciduous forest. Most British agricultural soils fall into this group.

***Brownian movements.*** A random movement of microscopic particles suspended in liquids or gases which results from the impact of molecules in the fluid around the particles.

Such movements can be seen in colloids in a solid state or in a suspension of microorganisms. Named after Robert Brows (1773-1858).

***Brown rot.*** Any fungal or bacterial disease of plants where browning and tissue decay occur.

***Brucellosis.*** A feverish disease caused by the bacterium Brucella that occurs commonly in cattle, sheep and goats. Infection of B. abortus in cattle can cause spontaneous abortion of calves and an attenuated live vaccine has been developed in decrease the prevalence of the pathogen.

***Bryophyte.*** Any plant of the division Bryophta, a division containing the liverworts and mosses (Musci). These plants do not possess a vascular system and there is always an alternation of generation with distinct sporophyte and gametophyte generations.

***Bubble.*** Structure that can be visualized by electron microscopic examination of spread films of replicating DNA. It represents the separate replicated duplexes which lie between the sites of DNA replication during the bidirectional replication of DNA.

***Bubble respiration.*** Respiration by means of a bubble attached to the rear end of an insect, e.g. a water beetle, which enables the insect to stay below water until the oxygen is used up, when the insect surfaces and takes on a new bubble.

***Budding.*** A method of asexual reproduction common in some lower animal groups (e.g. coelenterates) in which part of the body wall bulges outwards and eventually forms a new individual which becomes detached from the parent. Budding can also take place in single-celled organisms such as yeasts, but here the process is more akin to mitosis with daughter cells of unequal size being produced. The production of 'plantlets' from the leaf margins of Bryophyllum is also called budding by some biologists.

***Budding yeast.*** Type of yeast that can reproduce by budding as well as by sexual means. The common budding yeast used for banking and brewing in Saccharomyces cerevisiae.

***Buffer.*** A solution that resists change in pH when an acid or alkali is added or when the solution is diluted. Acidic buffers consist of a weak acid with a salt of the acid. The salt provides the negative ion $A^-$, which is the conjugate base of the acid HA. An example is carbonic acid and sodium hydrogencarbonate. Basic buffers have a weak base and a salt of the base (to provide the conjugate acid). An example is ammonia solution with ammonium chloride. In the hydrogen-carbonate buffer, for example molecules $H_2CO_3$ and ions $HCO_3^-$ are present. When acid is added most of the extra protons are removed by the base:

$$HCO_3^- + H^+ \dashrightarrow H_2CO_3$$

When base is added, most of the extra hydroxide ions are removed by reaction with undissociated acid :

$$OH^- + H_2CO_3 \dashrightarrow HCO_3^- + H_2O$$

Thus, the addition of acid or base changes the pH very little.

Natural buffers occur in living organisms, where the biochemical reactions are very sensitive to change in pH. The main natural buffers are $H_2CO_3/HCO_3^-$ and $H_2PO_4^-/HOP_4^{2-}$. Buffer solutions are also used in the laboratory (e.g. to keep microscopical preparations at their original pHs in order to prevent the formation of artefacts), in medicine (e.g. in intravenous injections), in agriculture, and in many industrial process (e.g. dyeing fermentation processes, and the food industry).

***Burkitt's lymphoma.*** Fairly common tumour of the lymph glands in the neck, almost entirely confined to people living in Central Africa. It is caused, at least partially, by the Epstein-Barr virus and is also associated frequently with a specific translocation between chromosomes 8 and 14. Since the pattern of distribution of the disease coincides with the malaria belt, it is postulated that malaria may be a predisposing factor to the onset of the disease. Although EB virus is prevalent throughout the world as the causative agent of mononucleosis, only in Africa does it lead to development of Burkitt's lymphoma.

***Bursa of Fabricius.*** Lymploid organ of birds, associated with the lower gut. Removal of the bursa at hatching impairs later production of antibody but not cellmediated immunity. It has given its name to the B lymphocyte, meaning the bursa-derived lymphocyte, although so called B lymphocytes occur in animals without a bursa.

***Burst-forming unit.*** (BFU). Cells in the erythropoietic pathway that give rise, through a series of cell divisions to the end cells of the pathway (e.g. erythrocytes or granulocytes). They are categorized according to the cell type which they produce (e.g. BFU-E cells give rise to erythrocytes). They appear to be intermediate in the erythropoietic pathway between the pluripotent stem cell and the colony-forming unit cells which in turn produce the final differentiated cell type.

***Busulfan.*** Mutagen; an alkylating agent. It is used as a cytotoxic drug in some cancers and polycythaemia.

# C

**$C_3$ and $C_4$ plants.** A grouping of higher plants, related to the carbon content of the compound produced when carbon dioxide is fixed during photosynthesis. In $C_3$ plants (the most common type), carbon dioxide combines with 5-carbon ribulose diphosphate to produce two molecules of 3-carbon phosphoglyceric acid (pga). In $C_4$ plants (e.g. maize), there is a special kranz anatomy in which mesophyll cells are adjacent to bundle sheath cells containing large chloroplasts. Carbon dioxide combines with 3-carbon phosphenol pyruvate (PEP) in the mesophyll cells to form 4-carbon oxaloacetic acid and malic acid which are then

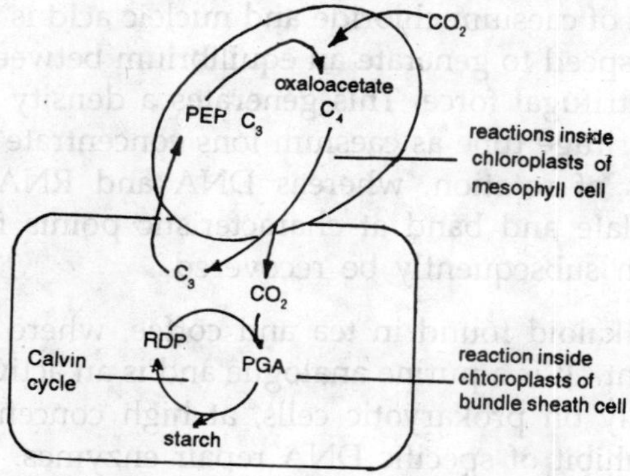


Figure C.1. $C_3$ and $C_4$ plants. Starch formation in $C_4$ plants.

transported to the bundle sheath cells where carbon dioxide is released to go into the calvin cycle. The advantage of using PEP is that $C_4$ plants can fix carbon dioxide even when in low concentration in the atmosphere (e.g. in dense tropical vegetation). The system is also used in some xerophytes as a $CO_2$ source during the day when the stomá is closed. See Figure C.1.

***C57 mouse cells.*** Cells from mice of the inbred, genetically defined C57 strains. C57BL mice originated from a mating in 1921, which also gave rise to C57BR and C57L strains. C57BL mice are the most widely used of all inbred mice, the C57BL/6 subline accounting for 14 percent of occasions when an inbred strain is used. A number of standard cell lines, derived from C57 mouse neoplasms, are available for in vitro study.

***Cacodylate buffer.*** Buffer commonly used to prepare fixatives for electron microscopy containing an organic arsenical salt.

***Cadaverine.*** Polyamine containing two amino groups.

***Caenogenetic (of larval features).*** Evolved because of use in the larval stage, being absent in the adult form.

***Caesium chloride gradient centrifugation.*** Technique for separating macromolecules, especially nucleic acids, on the basis of their buoyant densities. An initially homogeneous solution of caesium chloride and nucleic acid is centrifuged at high speed to generate an equilibrium between diffusion and centrifugal force. This generates a density gradient in the centrifuge tube as caesium ions concentrate distal from the axis of rotation, whereas DNA and RNA molecules accumulate and band at characteristic points from which they can subsequently be recovered.

***Caffeine.*** Alkaloid found in tea and coffee, where it acts as a stimulant. It is a purine analogue and is an active mutagen, especially on prokaryotic cells, at high concentration due to its inhibit of specific DNA repair enzymes.

***Calamites.*** An extinct group of reed-like plants found in the upper Devonian, Carboniferous and Triassic periods. They are usually classified with equisetales.

***Calcareous.*** Of, containing, or resembling calcium carbonate; chalky.

***Calcicole.*** A plant usually found on or limited to soils containing free calcium carbonate, such as Fragaria vesca, the wild strawberry.

***Calcifuge.*** Lime-hating; describing plants that grow best on acid soil.

***Calcitonin.*** (thyrocalcitonin). One of the hormones that controls the level of calcium in the blood, the others being parathyroid hormone (parathormone, PTH) and a vitamin D derivative 1,25-dihydroxycholecalciferol (1,25-DHCC). Calcitonin, which is released from the C cells of the thyroid, induces hypocalcaemia by inhibiting the release of calcium from bone.

***Calcium ion pump.*** Chemical pump, which in some cases is operated by atpases, that is responsible for : (a) keeping the calcium concentration of the cytosol lower than the extracellular concentration by a ratio of approximately $10^{-7}$ M inside to $10^{-3}$ M outside; (b) pumping calcium ions from the cytosol through the sarcoplasmic reticulum of muscle cells to balance the loss of calcium due to nerve impulse depolarization of the muscle cells membranes.

***Callose.*** Polysaccharide; a β-1, 3-linked polymer of glucose and found in plants, particularly enveloping the connecting strands in sieve areas and sieve plates of sieve elements and around tetrads of microspores during pollen development in angiosperms.

***Calorie.*** The quantity of heat required to raise the temperature of 1 gram of water by 1°C (1K). The calorie, a c.g.s. unit, is now largely replaced by the joule, an SI unit. I calorie = 4.1868 joules.

***Calorie (kilogram calorie; kilocalorie).*** 1000 calories. This unit is still in limited use in estimated the energy value of foods, but is obsolescent.

***Callus.*** A mass of immature plant cells which can differentiate into mature tissues, depending upon the relative concentrations of plant growth hormones present. Callus can develop from explants in laboratory tissue culture experiments but also occurs naturally at the end of cut or wounded surfaces of shoots and roots.

***Calmodulin.*** Calcium-binding protein found in all animal and plant cells and responsible for regulation of such enzymes as ADENYL CYCLASE because of their dependence on calcium. A typical animal cell may contain $10^7$ molecules of this protein (1 percent of total cell protein). It is a single polypeptide of 148 amino acids and binds allosterically, to calcium ions.

***Calorie.*** The heat required to raise 1 g (1 $cm^3$) of water through 1°C (i.e. from 14.5°C to 15.5°C). A Calorie (with a capital C) is used sometimes to denote a kilocalorie. Used as a unit of energy content or output, but now largely superseded by the S.I. unit joule (4.19 J = 1 cal).

***Calorimeter.*** An instrument for measuring quantities of heat, e.g. a bomb calorimeter measures the heat output on burning a sample of material. Calorific values used in energetics are now measured in joules rather than calories.

***Calvin, Melvin*** (b. 1911) American biochemist best known for this work on $CO_2$ fixation in photosynthesis. In his experiment he labelled $CO_2$ with $^{14}C$ and, using the 'Lollipop apparatus' (for exposing algal cells to light), and chromatography of cell extracts after varying time intervals, was able to isolate the various steps from $CO_2$ to starch, a sequence later called the calvin cycle. He was awarded a Noble Prize for this work in 1961.

***Calvin cycle.*** A series of chemical reactions, first described by Melvin calvin, which take place in the watery matrix of chloroplasts, where carbon dioxide is incorporated into more complex molecules and eventually carbohydrate. Energy for the reactions is supplied by ATP with NADPH acting as a reducing agent, both having been produced in the light reactions of photosynthesis. Since light is not required for the Calvin cycle to continue (provided $CO_2$, ATP and NADPH are present) the steps are called the 'dark' reactions. See Figure C.2. Every turn of the cycle fixes one molecule of carbon dioxide by producing two molecules of PGA and then two molecules of PGAL; three turns are necessary to release one molecule of PGAL ($C_3$) for the glucose pathway with the remaining five PGAL molecules remaining within the cycle. Thus six turns produce sufficient quantities of PGAL for the production of one molecule of glucose ($C_3 + C_3 = C_6$).

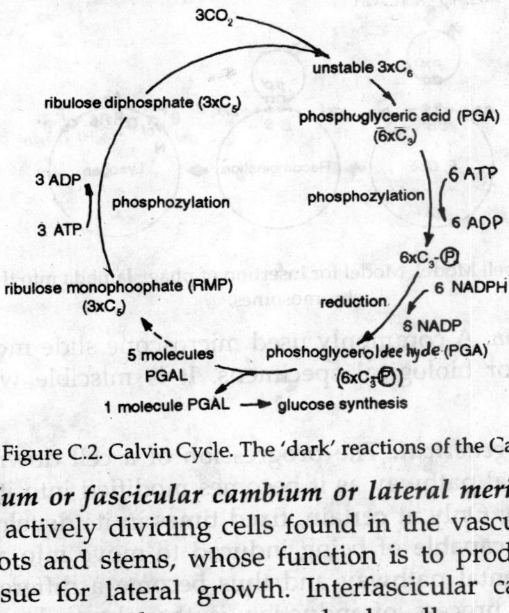


Figure C.2. Calvin Cycle. The 'dark' reactions of the Calvin cycle.

***Cambium or fascicular cambium or lateral meristem.*** A group of actively dividing cells found in the vascular bundles of roots and stems, whose function is to produce new plant tissue for lateral growth. Interfascicular cambium sometimes occurs between vascular bundles.

***Cambrian period.*** A geological period which began about 515 million years ago and ended 445 million years ago. At this time the British Isles lay in the southern hemisphere and the Sahara was at the South Pole and subject to extensive glaciation. Trilobites and Brachiopods flourished and most invertebrate phyla had evolved. The first graptolites appeared in the mid-Cambrian, but few traces of plants have been found and these are largely limited to simple algae.

***Campbell model.*** Mechanism proposed by A. Campbell to account for integration of lambda phase into the E. coli genome without a reciprocal loss of bacterial DNA (as would be expected in conventional recombination). The mechanism, which has proved to be that operative in nature, assumes the initial circularization of the linear lambda phage DNA, followed by precise breakage and reunion of the phage and bacterial DNA at specific sites. See Figure C.3.

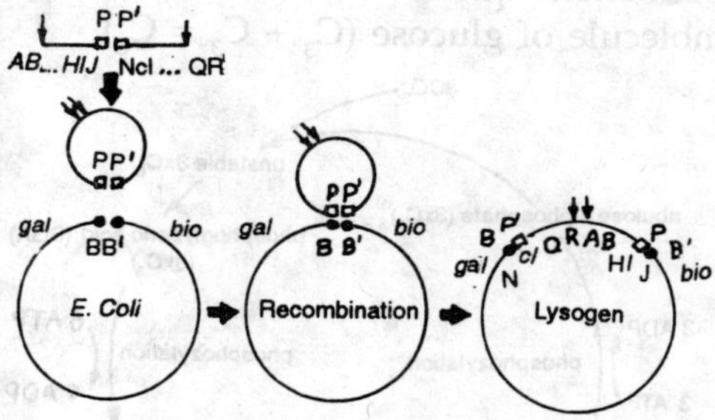


Figure C.3. Cambell Model. Model for insertion of phage lambda into the E. coli chromosomes.

***Canada balsam.*** A commonly used microscope slide mounting material for biological specimens. It is miscible with xylene.

***Canalization, genetical.*** The progression of a cell down a developmental pathway as it becomes modified into its final, adult form. Only at certain, fixed times in its development is the cell capable of being induced to move into another developmental pathway and thus become a different end type. The process of induction is thought to be due to chemicals secreted by tissues surrounding the developing cell.

***Canalizing selection.*** Gene selection that stablizes developmental pathways so that the phenotype is less affected by genetic and environmental disturbances.

***Cancer.*** A disease affecting the growth rate of affected tissues, in which the control mechanisms of cells become altered and the cells divide to form neoplastic growths or tumours.

'Benign' tumours consist of well-differentiated cells similar to those in the surrounding tissues and are usually harmless unless located in regions where no operation is possible. 'Malignant' tumours are dangerous and usually contain embryonic cells, which are capable of floating away and forming a new malignant growths in other sites.

Little is known of the cause of cancer, though exposure to carcinogens such as nicotine and mustard gas or the presence of certain microorganisms are possible causes. Radiation, surgery and chemotherapy are all used in the treatment of different cancers.

***Canker.*** A plant disease giving a limited necrosis of affected tissue and caused by bacteria or fungi.

***CAP (catabolite activator protein).*** A molecule that, together with cyclic AMP, binds to the CAP site of the lac operon in E. coli. The presence of CAP protein plus cyclic AMP facilitates the binding of RNA polymerase to the promoter sequence and thus greatly increases the efficiency of transcription of the lac operon.

***Capacitation.*** Process that mammalian spermatozoa must undergo before they can attain fertilizing capacity and that is normally effected by secretions within the female reproductive tract. The exact mechanism is not understood, but is believed to involve removal of seminal plasma proteins that coat the sperm surface. This enables the acrosome reaction to take place and therefore fusion with the egg membranes. Capacitation can also be effected in vitro by incubation in various chemically defined hypertonic media.

***Capping.*** 1. The modification of most eukaryotic messenger RNA molecules after transcription by the addition of a methylated guanosine residue to the 5' ends.

2. An energy-dependent concentration of a specific protein at a localized region of the cell surface. When measured by the use of fluorescent antibodies, the antibody often binds initially to all parts of the surface, but is eventually swept to one end of the cell along with the specific antigen.

***Capsid.*** The protein coat of a virus. The chemical nature of the capsid is important in stimulating the body's immune response against the invading virus.

***Carbaminohaemoglobin.*** The compound formed by the reaction of haemoglobin with carbon dioxide, which forms one of the methods of transportation of $CO_2$ in blood.

***Carbohydrase.*** An enzyme that catalyses the hydrolysis of carbohydrates.

***Carbohydrate.*** A family of organic molecules with the general formula $(CH_2O)_x$, ranging from simple sugars such as glucose and fructose to complex molecules such as starch and cellulose. All complex carbohydrates are built up from simple units called monosaccharides which cannot be hydrolysed to a simpler structure.

***Carbol-fuchsin.*** Stain, soluble in alcohol, that is used diagnostically to stain bacterial cells.

***Carbon.*** The element which is the basis of organic structure. Carbon has a valency of four, each atom forming four covalent bonds in its compounds. Long chains may be formed which give rise to the complexity of many organic compounds.

***Carbon cycle.*** The circulation of carbon by the metabolic processes of living organisms in an ecosystem so that it always returns to an arbitrary starting point. See Figure C.4.

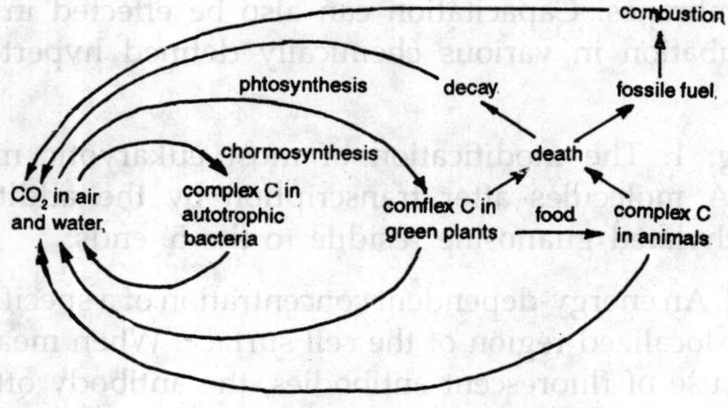


Figure C.4. Carbon Cycle. The main steps.

***Carbon dating.*** The dating of organic remains by measuring the radioactive carbon content. Atmospheric carbon dioxide contains carbon atoms of two types, ordinary carbon $^{12}C$ and radioactive carbon $^{14}C$. Like other radioactive isotopes, $^{14}C$ decays with age, so that the proportion of radioactive carbon present in, say, peat gives an indication of its age, assuming no more $^{14}C$ has been incorporated in it since it was a live plant, and also that the amount of $^{14}C$ in the atmosphere has remained constant. $^{14}C$ has a HALF-LIFE of 5,570 years and one carbon atom in every million million in the atmosphere is radioactive. Dating organic remains by the use of $^{14}C$ is a well-used and valuable technique, but not entirely accurate due to variations in atmospheric $^{14}C$ over long periods of time. Comparisons with tree ring dates have shown errors in the order of 900 years in 5,000.

***Carbon dioxide.*** A colourless, odourless gas, heavier than air, produced in respiration of organisms, and utilized to form sugars in photosynthesis. Formula: $CO_2$.

***Carbon dioxide sensitivity.*** Condition affecting some genetic strains of Drosophila which are unusually sensitive to carbon dioxide and will die when exposed to moderate concentrations of the gas. It is known to be correlated with the presence of sigma virus in the tissues of affected flies.

***3'-Carbon end.*** End of a polynucleotide molecule (DNA or RNA) where the C-3 of the pentose (i.e. deoxyribose or ribose) is not involved in phosophodiester bond formation.

***Carbon fixation.*** Incorporation of atmospheric carbon (from carbon dioxide) into carbohydrate in photosynthesis.

***Carbonic anhydrase.*** An enzyme that accelerates the reaction between carbon dioxide and water to form carbonic acid in the red blood cells.

***Carboniferous period.*** A geological period that began about 370 million years ago and ended 280 million years ago. It is often divided at about 325 million BP into Lower and Upper Carboniferous; the coal measures from which the period derives its name occurred mainly in the latter period. Club mosses, horsetails and ferns were the dominant plants during the period, and amphibians the commonest vertebrates, though this was also the time of the emergence of the reptiles. Britain crossed the equator.

***Carboxyhaemoglobin.*** A stable compound produced when carbon monoxide combines irreversibly with haemoglobin in the red blood cells, giving the blood a bright red colour. A consequence of the reaction is that haemoglobin is less able to combine freely with oxygen. This can lead to poisoning by lack of oxygen in the blood and eventually death if there is sufficient carbon monoxide in the atmosphere.

***Carboxylase.*** An enzyme that assists in the carboxylation or decarboxylation of a substrate (3).

***Carboxylation.*** The addition of carboxyl (COOH) or carbon dioxide into a molecule as, for example, when carbon dioxide is added to ribulose diphosphate ($C_5$) in the calvin cycle to give an unstable $C_6$ product.

***Carboxyl group.*** The monovalent group -COOH, found in aldehydes and ketones.

***Carboxypeptidase.*** An exopeptidase that catalyses the hydrolysis of amino acids in polypeptide chains from the C-terminal.

***Carcinogen.*** Any agent that causes cancer. Chemical carcinogens include benzpyrene, aflatoxin $B_1$ (produced by certain moulds growing on foodstuffs), and mustard gas (sulphur mustard) used in World War I to gas troops. Ultraviolet light and other ionizing radiation (such as X-rays) are also carcinogens. The former can cause skin cancer while high doses of X-rays can cause leukaemia and other cancers. Most, possibly all, carcinogens are also mutagens (i.e. they cause genetic mutations).

***Carcinoma.*** Any malignant tumour that arises in epithelial tissue.

***Carcinoma.*** Malignant tumour or neoplasm, derived from an epithelial or endothelial tissue. Over 90 percent of human cancers are carcinomas, and of those 56 percent occur in 'external', surface-covering epithelia (i.e. skin, gut and respiratory tract) and 36 percent in 'internal', glandular epithelia (i.e. breast, pancreas, thyroid, etc.).

***Carotene.*** An orange plant pigment of the carotenoid group which is usually present in the chloroplasts, and sometimes occurs in pigment containing structures called chromoplasts which are found in yellow/ orange leaves, vegetables and fruits. Carotene is necessary for the production of vitamin A in man and has an absorption spectrum of about 450 nm.

***Carotenoids.*** A group of yellow/ orange pigments found in plants which are subdivided into carotenes (orange) and xanthophylls (yellow).

***Carpogonium.*** The female sex organ of red algae which contains the egg in the swollen base. The male gamete enters the narrower mouth or trichogyne.

***Carrier.*** 1. An individual plant or animal that is infected with pathogenic organisms internally or externally without showing signs of disease, and which is capable of transferring them to others, thus causing disease. 2. An individual with a genotype containing a deleterious recessive gene that does not show in the phenotype. For example, a carrier of phenylketonuria.

***Carrier-free radioisotope.*** Radioisotope preparation to which no CARRIER has been added; often used generally to describe radioactive material that is of high specific activity.

***Carrier molecule.*** A molecule that is lipid-soluble and carries other molecules with a lower mobility within biological membranes.

***Carrion feeder or necrophagus feeder.*** Any organism that feeds on dead animals.

***Carrying capacity.*** The capacity of a particular habitat with reference to the maximum number of organisms which that habitat can normally support, e.g. the maximum number of wading birds an estuary can support.

***Casparian strip.*** (casparian band). Specialized sealing barriers in the apoplast between adjacent endodermal cells of the plant root. The function of these strips is analogous to the tight junctions between animal epithelial cells, since they prevent leakage of solutions back from the central vascular tissue of the root to the outer parenchyma.

***Cassette mechanism.*** Genetic mechanism proposed to explain the switching of mating type in the budding yeast Saccharomyces. Two distinct mating types exist - a and α - but cells of one strain have the capacity to switch spontaneously to the other mating type, a switch that appears to require transposition of DNA sequences within the yeast genome.

***Caste.*** Group of individuals within a species of social insect (e.g. ants or bees) which are structurally and functionally specialized for a particular role (e.g. soldiers or workers). The term derives from the strictly separate classes of society into which India was once devided.

***Catabolism.*** Production of simpler molecules from more complex molecules. Catabolism is exergonic and usually oxidative, giving rise to NADH whose oxidation is coupled by oxidative phosphorylation to the generation of ATP.

***Catabolite.*** Product of catabolism.

***Catabolite activating protein.*** (CAP). Dimeric protein composed of two identical subunits ($M_r = 2 \times 22\ 500$), the product of the crp gene of E. coli CAP is active only when cyclic AMP is bound to it, when it facilitates the trascription of certain genes regulated by catabolite repression.

***Catabolite repression (glucose effect).*** A phenomenon in mierobial metabolism in which glucose (or metabolites produced from glucose) inhibits pathways of enzyme synthesis. The role of this control system is to permit preferential catabolism of glucose whenever it becomes available, glucose being the preferred carbon source for growth. There is some evidence to suggest that at least in bacteria, catabolite repression depends on reduction by glucose of cellular levels of cyclic AMP, and thus on the effective operation of CAP protein.

***Casual.*** An introduced plant that has not become established in an area but which may occur away from cultivation.

***Catabolism or katabolism.*** A type of metabolism in which biochemical processes taking place in a cell result in the breaking down of complex compounds into simpler ones to release energy. Catabolism usually involves a series of step-by-step reactions, each catalysed by its own enzyme, for example aerobic respiration.

***Catadromous.*** (of fishes such as the eel) migrating down river to the sea to spawn.

***Catalase.*** An iron-containing enzyme found in tissues such as liver and potato tubers whose function is to catalyse the breakdown of toxic hydrogen peroxide into water and oxygen:

$$H_2O_2 \dashrightarrow H_2O + 1/2O_2$$

Catalase has a very high turnover rate and works by reducing the activation energy required from about 80 kj to less than 10 kj.

***Catalyst.*** A compound which is able to increase the speed of a reaction by lowering the activation energy needed for the reaction to start. Protein catalysts are called enzymes and are found in all living cells.

***CAT box.*** Consensus sequence of conserved DNA, most commonly consisting of the sequence CAAT, and occurring some 75 base pairs upstream from the initiation site of eukaryotic genes. As with the tata box, it is believed to act as a recognition site for RNA polymerase II enzymes.

***Cat cry syndrome.*** Cri-du-chat syndrome.

***Catecholamine.*** Any catechol-derived compound such as adrenalin or dopamine, which exert an action similar to that of the sympathetic nervous system.

***Catenated.*** Joined together like the links of a chain. Some minicircles of mitochondrial DNA are joined in this way to form a concatamer.

***Catharrhini.*** The primate group containing the Old World apes and monkeys and man. Members of this group have an internasal septum and a bony external ear passage.

***Cathepsin or kathepsin.*** The intracellular, proteolytic enzymes that bring about autolysis.

***Cattanach's translocation.*** Translocation in the mouse, discovered by B.M. Cattanach, involving the insertion of a segment of chromosome 7 into an x chromosome. During inactivation of the appropriate copy of the X chromosome it has been found that inactivation of the autosomal genes also occurs, but usually partially and depending on distance from the sex chromatin.

***C-banding.*** A technique of chromosomal staining in which chromosomes are exposed to alkaline and then acid conditions, in order to reveal bands of constitutive heterochromatin that are identified with Giemsa stain.

***C cell.*** Type of cell found in the thyroid and parathyroid glands of vertebrates that secretes calcitonin. In embryonic development, the C cells are derived from the last pair of gill pouches.

***cDNA clone.*** Cloning vector carrying a Complementary DNA sequence.

***Cell.*** The structural unit of most orgnisms, consisting of a microscopic mass of protoplasm bounded by a membrane and containing one or more nuclei (in Eucaryotes) or pieces of chromosome material (in pocaryotes). Cell size is roughly constant in all tissues and organisms, being limited by the physical restraints of unfavourable surface area/volume ratios as size increases.

***Cell adhesion.*** Process by which adjacent cells adhere to one another and by which isolated cells or sheets of cells attach to particular surfaces. Cell adhesion involves a variety of different mechanisms; tissue cells, which are more or less permanently associated, are bound together by cell junctions of various kinds. One important component of the extracellular matrix is fibronectin, which seems to play a role in the adhesion of many tissue cells. Such phenomena as contact inhibition in the movement of cells in culture are a function of cell adhesion, and the lack of contact inhibition, which characterizes many neoplastic or transformed cells, is largely a function of the lack of adhesion between the cells.

***Cell ageing.*** As a culture of cells ages, the times between successive mitoses become longer, the G1 phase of the cell cycle being more and more extended. Eventually division ceases and the cells become disorganized and die. The reasons why cells age, in vivo or in vitro, are not known. It has been suggested that mutations and damage may occur in the cells' DNA and the effectiveness of repair mechanisms may decline, that the efficiency of cellular processes may be inhibited by the build-up of errors in the machinery responsible for DNA replication, transcription of messenger RNA from DNA and translation of messenger RNA at the ribosomes, and that waste products (e.g., lipofuscin) may build up to critical levels. There is also circumstantial evidence to suggest that differentiated cells may be, in some way, programmed to undertake a finite number of cell divisions, after which they can no longer divide.

***Cell aggregation.*** (1) Formation of clumps of cells in a cell suspension or following deposition of cells on a surface, resulting from selective adhesion. If cells of different kinds are mixed together they may display a sorting out phenomenon, where the aggregates are made up specifically of one cell type or another. (2) In the life cycle of some organisms (e.g., Dictyostelium), there is a stage at which the free-living single amoebae aggregate together, followed by fruiting body formation. Such aggregation is mediated by specific attractant molecules; in the case of Dictyostelium this is cyclic amp.

***Cell body.*** The enlarged region of a neuron containing the nucleus.

***Cell commitment.*** More or less synonymous with cell determination. It signifies the fact that, at a certain time in the development of a cell, especially evident in embryonic life, the cell is committed to a particular fate (i.e. it will at the end of its differentiation become, say, a liver hepatocyte or a ciliated epithelial cell). Although commitment is remarkably stable, it can in certain circumstances by changed. One of the distinctive features of commitment is that it is often not morphologically detectable and may precede the overt differentiation to the particular cell fate by long periods of time. The precise mechanisms involved in cell commitment are not well understood, but are often assumed to involve a genetic switching mechanism in which a regulatroy gene within the cell becomes specifically activated.

***Cell compartmentalization.*** Subdivision of the cell interior into distinct compartments, for the most part membrane-bound. They include nuclei, endoplasmic reticula, lysosomes, mitochondria, vacuoles and, in plant cells and chloroplasts.

***Cell culture.*** General term used to indicate the growing of cells in vitro, either in tissue culture or as single cells. Cells in culture are not normally organized into tissues. Cells may be established in culture by making an explant of cells from a living organism under sterile conditions and placing the explant in a suitable sterile tissue culture medium. Many cells will grow only for a few generations and then die out, and there is evidence to suggest that many or most vertebrate cells that become established in culture are virally transformed cells. Established cells in culture are referred to as a cell line. Cells may be cultured either in a stirred suspension, on a glass or plastic surface of a roller tube or petri dist, or, in a recently developed technique, on the surfaces of inert minispheres which are themselves maintained in suspension.

***Cell culture medium.*** (tissue culture medium). Any one of a range of media used for the in vitro maintenance of animal or plant cells in culture. Such media commonly consist of a suitably buffered balanced salt solution, together with amino acids, nucleotides and vitamins. Many cells are particularly fastidious and will only grow well in media fortified with additional components such as foetal calf serum.

***Cell cycle.*** The series of stages through which a cell progresses when it is actively dividing, consisting of three subdivisions of interphase (G1, S and G2) plus mitosis. See Figure C.5.

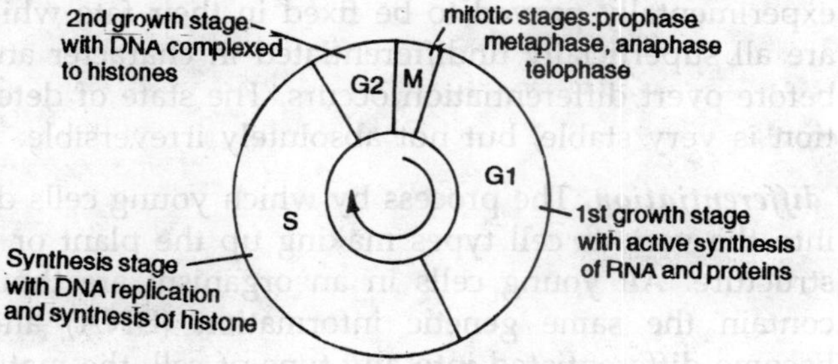


Figure C.5. Cell Cycle. The Interphase stages.

***Cell death.*** Normal cells die after a limited number of divisions (e.g., cultured mammalian lung fibroblasts die after 20-50 divisions), depending upon the age of the source animal. Ageing cultures of cells take longer and longer to go through their cell cycles until division eventually ceases, the cellular contents become disorganized and obstructed with waste materials, and the cells die. The reason why such cell strains die is not known. It has been suggested that as cells differentiate they may become programmed to die after a specified, finite number of divisions. This number of divisions is sometimes called the Hayflic limit, after its discoverer, and the phenomenon has been called programmed cell death. Cancerous cell lines (e.g., HeLa cells) will go on dividing indefinitely, as will some apparently normal, non-cancerous cell strains which are described as immortalized. In vivo, cell death after a fixed number of divisions may ensure that 'rogue' cells that have escaped normal cell division control processes do not grow in an unbridled way.

***Cell determination.*** Process through which the ultimate differentiated fate of a cell becomes fixed. It is often used synonymously with cell commitment, but in the latter phrase the distinction from cell differentiation is less clear. Determined cells are committed, but have not as yet gained the complete morphology or biochemistry characteristic of the cell type to which they are destined to belong. They clearest distinction between determination and differentiation is found in the imaginal discs of insects, the disc cells being experimentally proved to be fixed in their fate while they are all superficially undifferentiated in character and long before overt differentiation occurs. The state of determination is very stable, but not absolutely irreversible.

***Cell differentiation.*** The process by which young cells develop into the various cell types making up the plant or animal structure. All young cells in an organism are thought to contain the same genetic information (DNA) and may become differentiated into any type of cell, the mature cell being produced by gene switching rather than loss of DNA.

***Cell division.*** The division of a cell into two new cells during growth or reproduction. The new cells are called daughter cells. In procaryotes, two identical cells are produced by binary fission. In eucaryotes, cell division is more complicated because the genetic material is located on chromosomes inside the nucleus, being composed of two distinct processes that usually occur together; (a) nuclear division (Mitosis producing two identical nuclei, or meiosis producing four nuclei with a halving of the genetic complement) and (b) cytoplasmic division (cytokinesis).

***Cell fusion.*** Formation of one cell by the coalescence of two or more cells. Cell fusion occurs naturally in the fusion of gametes to form a zygote. The natural fusion of somatic cells is less frequent, although it does occur as in the fusion of myoblasts to form a myotube. Cell fusion can also be induced to occur artificially by treating cells with a fusogen. Such experiments have usually been carried out on cultured animal cells; when it is required to fuse plant cells it is first necessary to remove the cell wall to produce an isolated protoplast. For cell fusion to occur it is necessary to bring about an interaction or destablization at the plasma membrane with the formation of cytoplasmic bridges between adjacent cells. These cytoplasmic bridges will then expand allowing the mixing of the cytoplasms of the two cells. Treatment with inactivated sendai virus will induce the fusion of mammalian cells; polyethylene glycol will also induce fusion in both animal cells and plant protoplasts. It will also fuse bacterial spheroplasts and fungal protoplasts and is regarded as a universal fusogen. Cells can also be fused by passing a brief pulse of electric current through them. When two cells of the same genotype fuse a homokaryon results and when the cells have different genotypes a heterokaryon is formed. A hybrid cell forms when the two genomes of a heterokaryon are integrated into one nucleus. This somatic hybridization is a technique that provides information on the interaction of genomes and has led to the development of somatic cell genetics.

***Cell junction.*** Connection between cells. Plant cells often have substantial cytoplasmic connections - plasmodesmata - and many embryonic cells are connected by cytoplasmic bridges. Other cell junctions function as communicating connections (e.g., gap junctions, synapses), as impermeable junctions controlling chemical communication and providing tissue integrity (e.g. Tight juncions, septate junctions) and adhering junctions to provide tissue strength and elastic adhesion (e.g. belt desmosomes, spot desmosomes, hemidesmosomes).

***Cell line.*** Population of cells established in tissue culture from a single explant and most frequently showing characteristics of unlimited growth because of transformation. Cell lines retain their differentiated character through many rounds of division, although after many years of culture chromosome anomalies and aberrant growth characteristics may become noticeable in the cells.

***Cell-mediated immunity.*** One of two systems of adaptive immunity in which the effector agents of the response are T lymphocytes (not secreted antibodies). Cellmediated immunity is generated in particular against intracellular viral infections, cancer cells, fungi, parasites and foreign tissue. It involves recognition of self-histocompatablity antigens, as well as foreign antigens, in order to effect lysis of infected cells.

***Cell membrane or plasma membrane.*** The outer boundary of cells, the structure of which is visible only under the electron microscope and which is still not clearly understood. Two major models have been pproposed for membrane structure: the unit membrane model and the fluid-mosaic model structures. The cell membrane gives shape and sȯme protection to the cell, and also acts as a regulatory filter for transport of materials in and out of the cell. Higher plants, fungi and bacteria have a cell wall outside the cell membrane.

***Cell memory.*** Phenomenon by which cells retain a commitment to a particular path of specialization (determinatin) even in the absence of overt differentation. The memory is presumed to reside in complex feedback loops between nucleus and cytoplasm which, once established, are very stable, even through many rounds of cell division. Established lines of cells in tissue culture will retain their differentiated character through many successive rounds of cell division, whereas the imaginal disc cells of insects, although embryonic in character, can be experimentally proved to be highly determined.

***Cell plate.*** A membrane of differentially staining material in plant cells that appears at the equator of the spindle in telophase of mitosis, and is concerned with the formation of the middle lamella between the two new cells.

***Cell polarity.*** Referring to the fact that many cells such as fibroblasts have, at least in the short term, an anterior and posterior end, and that both movement across the substratum and movement of molecules in the plasma membrane may reveal such polarization.

***Cell sap.*** A watery liquid contained in the vacuoles of plant cells which is usually hypertonic to the external medium.

This causes the vacuoles to take in water by osmosis, maintaining turgor in the cell.

***Cell sorting out.*** Phenomenon in which a mixture of two or more distinct cell types separate from one another and ultimately form discrete aggregates of the separate cell types. The sorting out may result simply in the formation of separate rough aggregates or, with appropriate mixtures, one cell type may be internalized to form a central core or sphere, the outer layer of the sphere being made up entirely of the other cell type. Cell sorting out can be dramatically demonstrated using a mixture of disaggregrated sponge cells from species of different colours. The mechanism that results in sorting out is believed to be the differential adhesion existing between cells of the same type as compared to that between cells of differing types. Some cell movements during early development may be analogous to sorting out.

***Cell surface.*** Outer side of the plasma membrane of animal cells. Specific receptor molecules are present on the surfaces of some cells, and most animal cells have some accumulation of polysaccharide material—the glycocalyx—on their outer surface.

***Cell surface antigen.*** Antigen, often a protein or a polysaccharide, inserted into the plasma membrane (or attached to a plasma membrane insert), and protruding from it in such a way as to elicit an immune reaction by non-self immunocompetent cells. Cell surface antigens include histocompatibility antigens, allotypically and idiotypically non-self surface immunoglobulins, and blood group antigens such as those derived from H substance on erythrocytes.

***Cell synchronizaiton.*** Derivation of a population of cells which are synchronized so that all of the cells are precisely in the same stage of the cell cycle. Natural cell synchrony occurs in some embryonic tissues in the growing root tip and in the syncitium of Physarum. Artificially synchronized cells are widely used for studies on the cell cycle and are obtained either by the administration of heat shock, or mitotic-blocking agents (e.g., colchicine) or by cell selection techniques. These techniques consist of washing off cells in the process of mitosis from a randomly growing adherent population: the fact that mitotic cells round up and adhere less strongly to a substratum permits their selective removal.

***Cell theory.*** The idea that all living things are composed of cells, first proposed by the German biologists Mattias Schleiden and Theodor Schwann in 1838/39. The cell theory is also used to suggest that all living cells come from pre-existing living cells and do not arise by spontaneous generation.

***Cellular respiration or cell respiration.*** A catabolic process occurring in cells where complex organic molecules are broken down to release energy for other cellular processes. Cell respiration usually occurs in the presence of oxygen but some organisms can respire without oxygen.

***Cellulase.*** An enzyme capable of splitting cellulose into glucose, used particularly in the softening or digestion of plant cell walls. Most animals are not capable of producing cellulase and therefore of digesting plant material themselves, relying instead on a variety of gut micro-organisms to produce the enzyme and then absorbing the glucose product. Cellulase is also produced in large quantities in the abscission layer formed in leaf stalks of higher plants, causing a weakening of cell walls prior to leaf fall.

***Cellulose.*** A type of unbranched polysaccharide carbohydrate composed of linked glucose units which can be hydrolysed by the enzyme cellulase. Cellulose is the main constituent of plant cell walls and is the most common organic compound on earth.

***Cell wall.*** A thick, rigid coat formed outside the cell membrane of plants, fungi and bacteria, that is composed mainly of cellulose secreted by the protoplasm of the cell. Older cells may also produce a secondary wall inside the primary wall which is thicker and contains lignin for extra strength. Such cells often die after producing the secondary wall, e.g. xylem vessel cells.

***Cenozoic or Cainozoic period.*** A geological era that includes the quaternary period and tertiary period, beginning some 65 million years ago and extending up to the present time.

***Centimorgan.*** Chromosome map distance equal to 0.01 of a morgan unit. A recombination fraction of 0.1 indicates a map distance of 10 centimorgans.

***Central dogma.*** The hypothesis (based on weismannism) that genetical information flows only in one direction, from DNA to RNA to protein, and not in the opposite direction. Thus, in general, changes to protein structures produced by external forces are not inherited.

***Centric fission.*** The splitting of a chromosome at or near the centromere to produce two chromosomes.

***Centric fusion.*** The joining together of two acentric chromosomes to produce one metacentric chromosome.

***Centrifugation.*** A process in which particles in suspension are subjected to centrifugal forces by being spun in a centrifuge, so forming a sediment. Subsequent removal of the supernatant fluid from the sediment and subjecting it to higher speeds of centrifugation can enable particles of different sizes to be separated out and collected. Eventually the supernatant fluid will contain only soluble materials.

***Centriole.*** One of a pair of small organelles lying at right angles to each other just outside the nucleus of lower plants and all animals. Centrioles are self-replicating, dividing into two during the 'S' phase of the interphase of the cell cycle and then separating into two pairs, one pair migrating to each pole of the future mitotic spindle, from which an aster

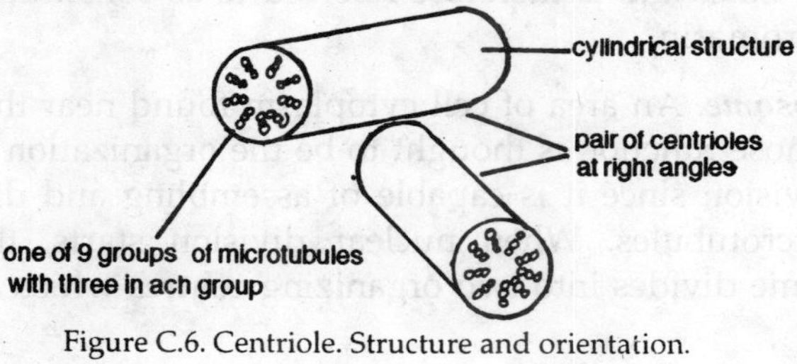


Figure C.6. Centriole. Structure and orientation.

forms. The role of centrioles in nuclear division is unclear, since they are absent from most plant cells and laser-beam irradiation of centrioles has no effect on division. See Figure C.6.

***Centromere.*** A structure occurring along the length of a chromosome, often visible under the light microscope as a bump or a constriction whose location can help to identify the chromosome. The centromere contains a complex system of fibres called kinetochore which becomes duplicated when the chromosomes divide into chromatids. The kinetochore attaches to spindle microtubules during nuclear division. Damaged chromosomes without centromeres (acentric chromosomes) fail to move normally during nuclear division. Chromosomes often have centromeres that are more or less centrally placed (metacentric chromosomes), but some have the centromere located of centre (acrocentric chromosomes) or even terminally (telocentric chromosomes). Centromeres are composed of heterochromatin and the DNA found in and around the centromere consists of short highly repetitious sequences, the so-called centromeric DNA.

***Centromere interference.*** Inhibitory effect exerted by the centromere on crossing over in the chromosome region immediately adjacent to be centromere.

***Centromeric DNA*** (simple sequence DNA). DNA located in the centromeric regions of chromosomes. It consists of highly repeated short sequences of DNA without a gene-coding function, and due to its anomalous structure it may be recovered as a centromeric satellite fraction on DNA centrifugation. Centromeric DNA is also highly condensed at all times and is therefore referred to as constitutive heterochromatin.

***Centrosome.*** An area of cell cytoplasm found near the nucleus, whose function is thought to be the organization of nuclear division since it is capable of assembling and dissembling microtubules. When nuclear division starts, the centrosome divides into two organizing centres which migrate to each pole (along with the centrioles, if present) and the spindle develops between them.

***Cephalic index.*** An anthropological measurement obtained by dividing the maximum head width by the maximum length (back to front) and expressing it as a percentage.

| | | |
|---|---|---|
| dolichocephalic | <75% | (long head) |
| mesocephalic | 75-80% | |
| brachycephalic | >80% | (short head) |

The ratios of one index to another vary between populations and have been used in studies of race.

***Cephalization.*** The development of the head of an organism during evolution. The development is largely associated with a concentration of sense organs at the front of an animal. The complexity of the head region depends on the habits of the animal; highly active, free-living animals have the best-developed cephalization requiring maximum detection of the environment at the front, whereas sedentary forms normally have less well-developed heads.

***Cercaria.*** The last larval stage of the liver fluke. It lives in the fresh water snail Limnaea, produces a cyst round itself and develops into the adult fluke after ingestion by a sheep or another primary host.

***C gene.*** Gene coding for the constant region of immunoglobulin chains.

***Chagas's disease.*** Human disease produced by Trypanosoma cruzi and transmitted by blood-sucking bugs. It is common in South America, and Darwin is thought to have contracted the disease there during his travels with HMS beagle.

***Chalaza.*** (1) In plants, region of the ovule in which nucellus, funcile and integuments merge. (2) In animals, an albuminous structure of twin cords which attach the yolk to the egg membrane in eggs of birds.

***Chalcone.*** Yellow flavonoid pigment found in plant cell VACUOLES and providing colour in many flowers.

***Chalones.*** Substances that act as growth regulators but, unlike hormones, they are effective against the tissue that produces them. They therefore constitute a mechanism of inhibition of growth by positive feedback. They are postulated to be glycorproteins, although some doubt continues to surround claims for their activity. Many different tissues such as epithelial tissue, liver parenchyma and erythrocytes are said to have effective chalones, which prevent the growth of these tissues beyond certain limits. They are assumed to be released ihnto ciruclation and to act as mitotic inhibitors on the target tissue. Thus, if an animal is subjected to partial hepatectomy (removal of part of the liver) and then the liver growth is monitored post-operatively, it is found that there is a burst of mitosis in the liver tissue so that the organ rapidly recovers its original tissue mass. It is postulated that, on hepatectomy, the level of ciruculating liver chalone drops (since there are fewer liver cells releasing it into circulation and it is presumed to have a very short half-life). This drop in circulatory level allows cell division in the liver cell population to increase dramatically until such time as the normal mass size of that tissue is restored when, as a result of higher chalone concentration, growth would be reduced to the more normal low level.

***Channel-forming ionophore.*** Small hydrophobic molecule, dissolved in the lipid bilayer of the plasma membrane, that increases ion permeability by providing a shielded channel through the membrane so that the charge of the transported ion does not interact with the hydrophobic interior of the lipid bilayer.

***Channel protein.*** Transport protein located in the plasma membrane that permits solutes of appropriate size and charge to cross the lipid bilayer by simple diffusion.

***Chaotrope.*** Substance that causes chaos, in this instance within the plasma membrane, for example, 3M KCI acts as chaotropic agent.

***Character.*** A genetic feature of an individual that can be assessed in some way. Such features often appear in various alternative 'forms', each controlled by different alleles. For example, the height of a pea plant is a `character', with tall plants (2m high) and dwarf plants (0.3 m high) as alternative forms. Characters sometimes display a continuous range of forms, as in human height, which may be influenced strongly by environmental conditions.

***Character displacement.*** The divergence of characteristics in sympatric species, as a result of the selective effects of competition.

***Character index.*** A value made up of the sum of the ratings of several cenetic characters which is used in numerical taxonomy to indicate degrees of difference between related taxa.

***Chagaff's rule.*** Rule originally set out by E. Chargaff, which states that in a DNA sample of duplex molecules, the ademine residues will numerically equal the thymines, and the guanines will equal the cytosines. Correspondingly the total pyridines (T+C) will equal the total purines (A+G).

***Charged tRNA.*** Transfer RNA already conjugated with its specific amino acid molecule.

***Charon vectors.*** Cloning vectors based on lambda phage.

***Charophyta.*** A group of the ALGAE, including the stoneworts, which inhabits ponds.

***Chasmogamic.*** (of a flower) opening before pollination.

***Checklist.*** A list of the organisms contained within a group which can be used for quick reference in the arrangement of collections, for example, a list of the organisms' presence in various habitats.

***Chemical dating.*** An absolute dating technique that depends on measuring the chemical composition of a specimen. Chemical dating can be used when the specimen is known to undergo slow chemical change at a known rate. For instance, phosphate in buried bones is slowly replaced by fluoride ions from the gorund water. Measurement of the proportion of fluoride present gives a rough estimate of the time that the bones have been in the ground. Another, more accurate, method depends on the fact that amino acids in living organisms are L-optical isomers. After death, these racemize and the age of bones can be estimated by measuring the relative amounts of D- and L- amino acids present.

***Chemical fossils.*** Organic molecules of biological origin, sometimes recovered from fossils themselves. Most frequently the chemicals involved are breakdown products of the original molecules and include alkanes, which are saturated hyrocatons and porphyrins. Such molecules can also be recovered from old non-fossiliferous rocks of pre-Cambrian strata and are believed to represent evidence for the existence of simple cellular organisms at the time of depositions of thse strate.

***Chemical sequencing.*** One of the two main methods currently in use for determining primary sequences of DNA molecules. Single-stranded DNA is labelled with $^{32}P$ at one end using polynucleotide KINASE and is then cleaved by four separate types of chemical treatment in reactions run in parallel. The chemistry is designed to cleave preferentially adjacent to one of the four types of nucleotide and gives rise to populations of fragments ending at all the possible places and all radiolabelled at one end. These fragments are then separaed by electrophoresis, autouadiography and the sequence deduced from the patterns of bands observed.

***Chemiosmotic hypothesis.*** Mechanism first proposed by P. Mitchell to explain the coupling of electron transport to the synthesis of ATP and inoganic phosphate, and to the transport of solute across membranes. The components of the electron transport chain are arranged so that electron carriers (e.g. iron-sulphur proteins) and hydrogen carriers (e.g. ubiquinone) alternate so that when electrons flow from one type to the other, protons are taken up or released. The electron transport components are arranged asymmetrically in the mitochondrial, chloroplast or bacterial membrane so that protons are always removed from one side of the membrane and released on the opposite side. The reaction of oxygen with protons to form water (catalysed by terminal oxidases) also contributes to the asymmetry of reactions involving protons. These vectorial reactions lead to a proton gradient across the membrane and to a transmembranous electrical potential. These two components together constitute an electrochemical potential known as the proton motive force. It should be noted that the occurrence of a proton motive force is well established, but the mechanism of proton translocation or proton pumping remains a matter of debate. The membrane-bound ATP synthetase (or ATPase) is arranged so that protons cross the membrane through this enzyme down the electrochemical gradient (an exergonic process) concomitant with the phosphorylation of ADP to ATP (an endergonic process). The proton motive force may also be used to drive the uptake of solutes. Cations can be taken up in response to the electrical component of the proton motive force; anionic or neutral components are taken up in response to both of its components. The proton motive force can also be used to drive bacterial flagellar rotation and 'reverse electron transport' (e.g., the reduction of $NAD^+$ to NADH).

***Chemoattractant.*** Compound that induces chemotaxis by cells due to interaciton with surface-located chemoreceptors. Thus cyclic AMP is a chemoattractant for the migrating cells of Dictyostelium.

***Chemoautotrophic or chemotrouphic.*** (of an organism) capable of manufacturing organic molecules from carbon dioxide and water by a process of chemosynthesis. For example, Thiobacillus oxidizes hydrogen sulphide to sulphur in order to produce the energy for chemosynthesis. Chemoautotrophic organisms are one form of autotroph, the other form displaying phototropism.

***Chemoreceptor.*** A receptor that is stimulated by contact with molecules and is capable of reacting to and differentiating between different chemical stimuli, for example in taste and smell.

***Chiasma.*** Junction points between non-sister chromatids visible during the first diplotene of meiosis. Although chiasmata are visible as distinct crosslinks between the chromatid of one chromosome and the chromatid of its homologue in the tetrads which can be seen at this stage of meiosis, they are not representative of the true positions of crossing-over. Chiasma frequence varies greatly between nothing and four or five for different chromosomes, and they are absent in some situations (e.g., in males of Drosophila melanogaster). Crossing-over is a mechanism that increases genetic variation and diversity, but a chiasma also exerts a physical effect in holding homologous chromosomes together during meiosis. Chiasma frequency varies greatly from species to species and even in different populations of the same species.

***Chiasma interference.*** Greater than expected frequency of chiasma occurring in a chromosome bivalent, most often used when more than one chiasma occurs in a situation where only one is normal.

***Chiasmata.*** Plural of chiasma.

***Chiasmatype theory.*** Theory that chiasma formation is a result of crossing-over between non-sister chromatids. Originally advanced by Janssens and Darlington, the theory not only emphasizes that the events of DNA recombination and chiasma formation are linked, but that the former precedes and cuases the latter.

***Chickenpox.*** An acute, contagious disease distinguished by slight fever and skin vesicles, and caused by the herpes varicella-zoster virus. The same virus can cause shingles in adults, a painful inflammation along the path of a major nerve, frequently across the back or sides.

***Chimaera.*** An organism composed of tissues that are genetically different. Chimaeras can develop if a mutation occurs in a cell of a developing embryo. All the cells arising from it have the mutation and therefore produce tissue that is genetically diffeerent from adjacent tissue, e.g. brown patches in otherwise blue eyes in humans. Graft Hybrids are examples of plant chimaeras.

***Chimaeric plasmid.*** plasmid that, by dint of having a novel gene sequence spliced into it by genetic engineering, now contains two covalently linked DNA sequences, one of which is the original plasmid molecule.

***Chimaeric vector.*** Bacteriophage or plasmid cloning vector carrying a novel DNA sequence integrated into it DNA.

***Chironomus.*** Genus of gnat-like dipteran flies, the larvae of which, like Drosophila, contain giant polytene chromosomes in some tissues.

***Chi-sites.*** Cross-over hot-spot instigators; short DNA sequences that stimulate DNA crossing-over.

***Chi-squared test.*** A statistical routine which is a test of significance, comparing the observed results of an experiment or sample against the numbers expected from a theory or prediction. The test produces a value called chi-squared ($\chi^2$) which is :

$$\chi^2 = \text{sum of } \frac{(\text{observed no. in class} - \text{expected no. in class})}{\text{expected no. in class}} \text{ for each class}$$

The $\chi^2$ number is then converted to a proability value (P) using an $\chi^2$ table. If the P value is larger than 5% we can conclude that there is 'no significant difference' between the observed results and those expected, any deviation being due to chance. If, however, the probability is less than 5%, it must be concluded that there is a 'signficant difference' between the observed results and those expected from theory. Note that the $\chi^2$ test can only be used with data that fall into discrete categories, e.g. heads or tails, long or short, yellow or orange.

***Chlamydomonas.*** A flagellate, unicellular gree alga now normally placed in the division chlorophyta but in many (older) texts regarded as a protozoan and placed in the class mastigophora. It is characterized by the presence of two flagella and, because of the presence of chromatophores (1), is referred to as a phytoflagellate (often given subclass status: Phytoflagellata). Reproduction is by repeated fission or varies between species from an asexual method to a sexual method of conjugation where ISOGAMETES rather than differentiated male and female gametes are produced. See Figure C.7.

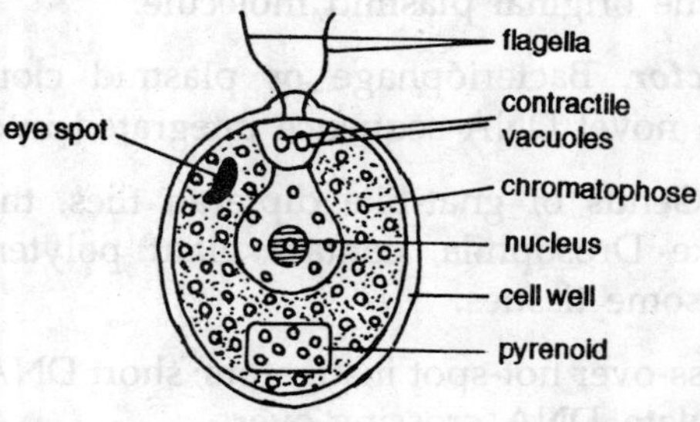


Figure C.7. Chlamydomonas. Generalized structure.

***Chlamydospore.*** An asexually produced, thick-walled fungal spore which is capable of surviving adverse conditions that are unfavourable to the main body of the fungus.

***Chloramphenicol.*** (Chloromycetin). Antibiotic produced by certain species of Streptomyces, but now prepared commercially by complete chemical synthesis. It was the first broad-specturm antibiotic (active against both gram-positive and gram-negative bacteria) to be used clinically, mostly to treat typhoid fever and dysentery. However, serious side-effects (damage to bone marrow) have limited its use as a general antibacterial agent. The bacteriostatic action of chloramphenicol is due to inhibition of protein biosynthesis on the 70S ribosome; it is inactive against the 80S ribosome of eukaryotic cells. Present evidence suggests that chloramphenicol inhibits peptidyl transferase activity by binding to the 50S ribosomal subunit. See Figure C.8.

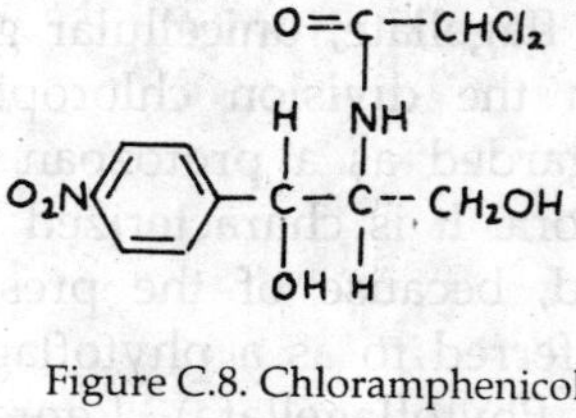

Figure C.8. Chloramphenicol.

***Chlorella.*** Genus of green algae used extensively in studies on the physiology and genetics of photosynthesis.

***Chlorophyll.*** Major photosynthetic pigment found in all photosynthetic organisms. The chlorophyll molecule has a roughly square planar porphyrin head with magnesium at its centre and a long phytol chain tail. Chlorophyll is anchored to membrances by this phytol chain. There are a number of forms of chlorophyll, differing in the structure of the side chains. Chlorophyll a is found in all eukaryote photosynthetic organisms and in the blue-green algae. In addition, chlorophyll b is found in higher plants and green algae, chlorophyll c in brown algae, diatoms and dinoflagellates, and chlorophyll d in some red algae. Purple and green bacteria possess bacteriochlorophyll. Chlorophyll absorbs mainly red and blue-violet light and reflects green, hence giving organisms that possess it a green colour. The light energy absored by chlorophyll is used for photosynthesis. See Figure C.9.

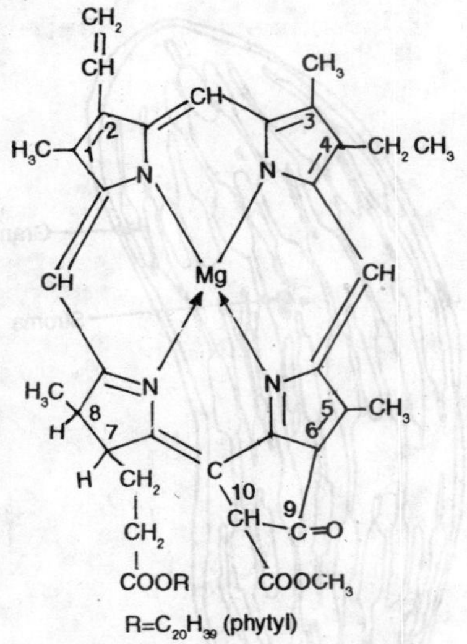

Figure C.9. Chlorophyll.

***Chloroplast.*** Plastid that contains photosynthetic pigments and in which photosynthesis takes place. All eukaryote organisms that undertake photosynthesis possess chloroplasts, but in photosynthetic prokaryotes the photosynthetic pigments are not contained within a plastid. In land plants there may be over a hundred chloroplasts in a single cell. These chloroplasts are typically lens-shaped and generally have a diameter of 3-10 p.m. They are thought to develop from proplastids present in meristematic cells. In the algae, the chloroplasts are more variable in shape and are often larger than those of land plants, with many algal cells containing only one chloroplast. Frequently, algal chloroplasts are associated with a pyrenoid. Chloroplasts are bounded by a double membrane, with the interior consisting of a complex hyrophilic proteinaceous sol, the stroma and a series of membranes forming the lamellar system. Within the stroma are found particles of various kihnds, some of which, such as starch grains, plastoglobbulin and crystals, develop as a result of photosynthesis, whereas others are ribosomes and polysomes. Chloroplast ribosomes are smaller than those in the cytoplasma

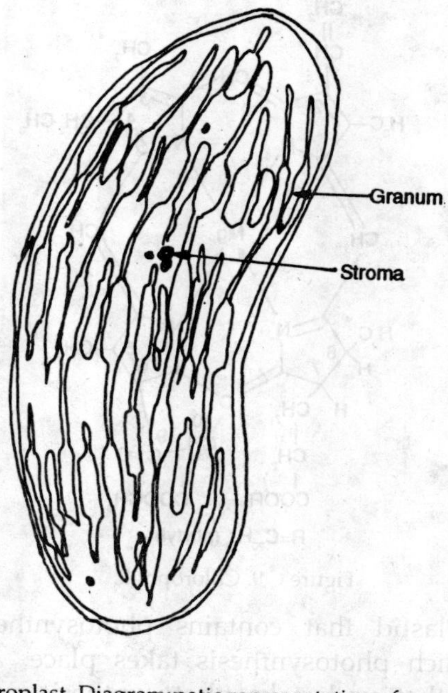


Figure C.10. Chloroplast. Diagramınatic representation of cross-section through a chloroplast.

and both in their size and reaciton to various antibiotics they resemble prokaryote ribosomes. Within the stroma are also found fibrils of DNA and the enzyme complex ribulose bisphosphate carboxylase and other enzymes concerned with the dark reactions of photosyntheis. The lamellar system consists of a series of flattened circular sacs known as thylakoids. At intervals, a number of thylakoids are stacked together to form grana, which are linked by intergrana lamellae. The photosynthetic pigments are located in the lamellar system, and this is the site of the light reactions of photosynthesis. See Figure C.10.

***Chloroplast DNA.*** (cpDNA). Single circular molecule, like the mitochondrial DNA, containing numerous coding sequences. It is found in all green plants and is responsible for photosynthetic function. cpDNA is normally ciruclar. It is some 10 times larger than circular DNA of animal mitochondria.

***Chlorocruorin.*** Red/green respiratory pigment resembling haemoglobin found in some species of polychaete worms.

***Chlorosis.*** Conditiion in green plants in which levels of chlorophyll are reduced, leading to a pale green or yellow colour in the leaves. Chlorosis may be caused by a number of factors, including a deficiency of iron, magnesium or copper, poor light conditions or infection with virus or other pathogens.

***Choanocyte.*** Cell having a single flagellum with a delicate protoplasmic rim or collar at its base. These cells line the body mass of sponges. The beating of their flagella cause water circulation and food particles in the water to adhere to the basal collar and to be ingested.

***Choanoflagellate or collar flagellate.*** Any stalked protozoan that occurs either singly or in branching colonies, possessing a flagellum surrounded by a cup-like structure into which food particles are wafted by flagellar movement. They are very similar to choanocyte cells.

***Cholecystokinin-pancreozymin (CCK-PZ).*** A single hormone secreted by the wall of the duodenum in mammals when food enters the small intestine. CCK-PZ causes contraction of the gallbladder muscle, resulting in the bile being pumped into the duodenum via the bile duct, and stimulates the pancreas to secrete pancreatic juice containing large quantitites of digestive enzymes, which enter the duodenum via the lower part of the bile duct. At one time it was considered that cholecystokinin and pancreozymin were separate, different hormones. CCK-PZ causes vasodilation of the intestinal blood vessels.

***Cholera.*** A serious human disease caused by gut infection of the bacterium Vibrio cholerae that results in severe diarrhoea, vomitting and abdominal cramps. Up to 15 litres per day of fluid may be lost from the gut, resulting in extreme dehydration and even death. Treatment is effected by replacement of the lost body fluids and salts. Cholera is endemic in certain. Third World countries, occurring more often where natural resistance of the host is impaired, particularly by malnutrition.

***Cholera toxin.*** (choleragen). Protein complex ($M_r$ - 87 000) that increases adenylcyclase activity in the gut mucosa, resulting in loss of water and ions by the gut epithelial cells into the gut. It is produced by the causative organism of cholera Vibrio cholerae.

***Cholesterol.*** A steroid that occurs in the cell membrances of animal cells, but not in plants. Cholesterol is produced in the liver and when in excess is excreted in the bile but is partly reabsorbed by the ileum. It may precipitate gallstones in the gallbladder or bile duct. Alternatively, if there is excess cholesterol in the blood, it may be deposited on the walls of the blood vessels, obstructing them and often leading to an intravascular clot which if it occurs in the region of the heart gives rise to a 'heart attack' or coronary thrombosis. Cholesterol is the precursor of animal steroid hormones and bile acids.

***Choline.*** Important constituent of some phospholipids, such as lecithin (phosphatidylcholine) and the neurotransmitter acetylcholine. It is a basic compound with the formula $HOC_2H_4N(CH_3)_3OH$. Although it can be synthesized by the human, it is an essential nutrient for some animals and microoganisms.

***Cholinergic.*** (of nerve fibres) secreting acetylcholine as a transmitter substance; in vertebrates these include motor fibres to striated muscle, parasympathetic fibres to involuntary muscle and fibres to sympathetic ganglia from the central nervous system.

***Cholinesterase.*** An enzyme that hydrolyses and destroys excess acetylcholine after it has been liberated and has produced its effect on specific sites on the postsympatic membrane.

***Chondriome.*** Collective term for all of the mitochondria within a cell. The number of mitochondria per cell varies from less than 10 (in some yeast cells and erythrocytes, for example) to a few thousand.

***Chondrocyte.*** Cell type occurring within the extracellular matrix material (i.e. cartilage). Chondrocytes are derived from chondroblasts.

***Chondroitin sulphate.*** Major glycosaminoglycan of the extracellular matrix, it consists of repeating disaccharide subunits of D-glucuronic acid and N-acetyl-D-galactosamine ($M_r$ = 5000 - 5000, depending upon the number of subunits). Like all other glycosaminoglycans, except hyaluronic acid, it is typically found covalently bound to a core protein to form a proteoglycan . Such chondroitin sulphate rich proteoglycans are found in abundance in cartilage, cornea, skin, bone and arterial walls. Two principal sulphated forms are known - chondroitin 4-sulphate and chondroitin 6-sulphate, with 0.2-1.0 and 0.2-2.3 sulphate groups per disaccharide subunit, respectively.

***Chorea.*** Disorder of the nervous system, characterized by so-called choreic movements (i.e. irregular and involuntary contractions of the facial and limb muscles). An example in huntingdon's chorea.

***Chorioallantoic grafting.*** An experimental process of culturing tissues in eggs, whereby the tissue is introduced to the surface of the chorion (2) of a live chick embryo, the blood vessels of which enter the tissue and maintain it after sealing the egg shell.

***Choriocarcinoma.*** Carcinoma of the trophoblast epithelium in the foetus, commonly found in hydatidiform moel.

***Chorion.*** 1. The superficial outer coat of the insect egg which is non-cellular and secreted by the ovary around the ovum. 2. An embryonic membrane of amniotes formed from an outer ectodermal layer and an inner mesodermal layer. In birds and mammals it forms the outer membrane covering the amniotic cavity, and in mammals the mesodermal component of the chorion fuses with the allantois to form the chorioallantoic placenta. Here the chorion develops finger-like outgrowths, the chorionic villi, which project into blood spaces in the uterus of the mother.

***Chorion gene.*** Family of genes that code for the proteins of the egg coat or chorion in insects and some other animal species. The genes have been studied in some detail in Drosophila, where they are found to be active for a few hours only in the cells of the ovarian follicle. An unusual feature of these genes is that they are preferentially amplified within the follicle cells. Some of the genes in the family have been studied in detail (four out of approximately 20) and have been found to be short sequences of between 700 and 850 bases, each with a short intron of between 50 and 150 bases.

***Chorionic biopsy.*** A technique that enables the prenatal assessment of a foetus between the 7th and 11th week of pregancy, involving the sampling of cells from the chorionic villus. These villi are small, finger-like outgrowths of the chorion (2) that, at the time of the sampling, are full of rapidly dividing foetal cells. A biopsy of the villus is taken with a small tube inserted through the vagina and cervix. No anaesthetic is needed and no amniotic fluid is collected. The large number of dividing foetal cells in the sample means that chromosomal and biochemical studies can be quickly completed, so that termination (if required) is usually before the 10th week, a significantly less traumatic period of gestation than termination after amniocentesis.

***Chorionic gonadotrophin.*** Glycoprotein hormone that maintains the early corpus luteum in mammals. The hormone is secreted by the chorionic villi of the placenta in higher mammals and can be detected in the urine of pregnant women. The immunological detection of the hormone in urine has been widely used as a test for pregnancy. Animals such as Xenopus can be induced to mate and lay eggs by injection of the hormone.

***Christmas disease.*** (haemophilia B). Form of haemophilia, caused by a deficiency in Factor IX (gamma-thromoboplastin component). The disease is sex-linked and determined by a distinct gene from the sequence involved in the commoner haemophilia A, in which deficiency of Factor VIII occurs.

***Christmas tree.*** Form in which transcriptionally active genes are visualized when spreads of chromatin are viewed using an electron microscope. The most dramatic christmas trees are seen on the tendemly repeated copies of the large ribosomal. RNA (rRNA) genes, the branches of varying length being rRNA molecules at differing stages of completion. Rather looser christmas trees of heterogenous nuclear RNA can also be visualized on transcriptionally active structural genes.

***Chromaffin tissue.*** Tissue, thought to be derived from modified postganglionic neurones, found in the medulla of the adrenal glands. There are two populations of cells within the chromaffin tissue, one producing andrenaline and the other producing noradrenaline. These catecholamines are associated with a carrier protein - chromagranin - and are located in membrane-bound granules within the chromaffin tissue cells.

***Chromatid.*** One of a pair of duplicated chromosomes produced during the 'S' phase of the cell cycle, which are joined together at the centromere. During nuclear division the centromere splits (in anaphase of mitosis, anaphase 2 of meiosis) to produce two separate chromosomes. See Figure C.11.

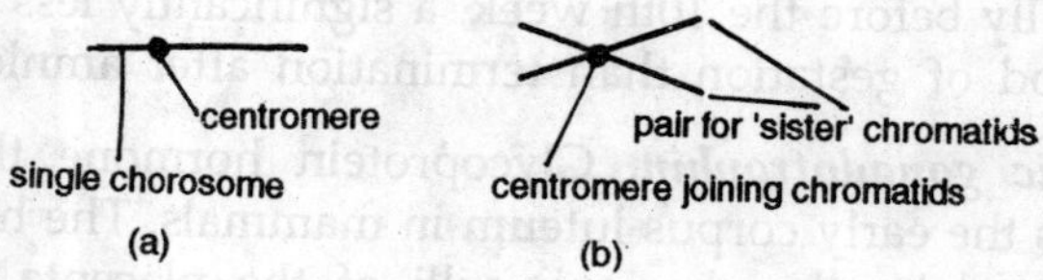


Figure C.11. Chromatid. (a) Before duplication. (b) After duplication.

***Chromatin.*** Material of which chromosomes are composed. The main constituents of chromatin are DNA and protein, in approximately equal amounts, most of the protein being histone. DNA and histone are organized in chromatin as strings of small subunits termed nucleosomes, each nucleosome consisting of eight molecules of histone around which two coils of DNA are looped. Adjacent nucleosomes are linked together by DNA, the DNA forming a continuous long molecule looping around the outside of the histone octamers and then running on to the next nucleosome. Within chromatin the nucleosomes are further compacted so that a solenoid of closely packed nucleosomes, the so called 30-nm fibre, is formed. Depending on the degree of compaction of chromatin, the genes on the DNA are rendered more or less accessible to the RNA polymerase molecules which transcribe the genes. Very highly condensed chromatin is genetically inert and is styled heterochromatin, the less condensed chromatin being termed euchromatin. See Figure C.12.

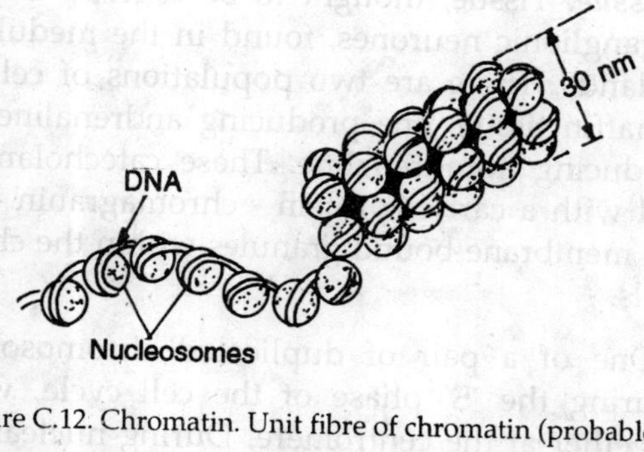


Figure C.12. Chromatin. Unit fibre of chromatin (probable structure).

***Chromatin-negative.*** Descriptive of an individual whose cell nuclei lack the highly compacted X chromosome called the barr body. Normal males in the human are chromatin-negative.

***Chromatin-positive.*** Descriptive of an individual whose cell nuclei exhibits the highly compacted X chromosome called the barr body. Normal females in the human are chromatin-positive.

***Chromatogram.*** A record obtained by chromatography. The term is applied to the developed records of paper chromatography and thin-layer chromatography and also to the graphical record produced in gas chromatography.

***Chromatography.*** A technique for analysing or separating mixtures of gases, liquids, or dissolved substances, such as mixtures of amino acids or chlorophyll pigments. The original technique (invented by the Russian botanist Mikhail Tsvet in 1906) is a good example of column chromatography. A vertical glass tube is packed with an adsorbing material, such as alumina. The sample is poured into the column and continuously washed through with a solvent (a process known as elution). Different components of the sample are adsorbed to different extents and move down the column at different rates. In Tsvet's original application, plant pigements were used and these seprated into coloured bands in passing down the column (hence the name chromatography). The usual method is to collect the liquid (the eluate) as it passes out from the column in fractions.

In general, all types of chromatography involve two distinct phase - the stationary phase (the adsorbent material in the column in the example above) and the moving phase (the solution in the example). The separation depends on competition for molecules of sample between the moving phase and the stationary phase. The form of column chromatography above is an example of adsorption chromatography, in which the sample molecules are adsorbed on the alumina. In partition chromatography, a liquid (e.g. water) is first absored by the stationary phase and the moving phase is an immiscible liquid. The separation is then by partition betwen the two liquids. In ion-exchange chromatography the process involves competition between different ions for ionic sites on the stationary phase Gel filtration is another chromatographic technique in which the size of the sample molecules is important.

***Chromosomal aberration.*** Abnormal chromosome complement that follows from the duplication, loss or rearrangement of the genetic material within the chromosome set. Single chromosome duplications or deficienccies may occur, leading to the states of monosomy, trisomy, etc. Changes within individual chromosomes, such as inversions or deletions, may change the arrangement or presence of individual gene loci, whereas translocations involve the movement of a section of a chromosome so that its position in the chromosome set alters, usually by its union with another chromosome. Chromosomal aberrations constitute one class of mutations, being gross or chromosomal mutations in distinction to the intragenic mutations involving single base changes within a DNA sequence. Gross chromosomal aberrations may often be defectable by light microscopy of mitotic chromosomes (karyotype analysis) and inversions or deletions in polythene chromosomes are accompanied by the appearance of an inversion or deletion loop, being the looped out homologous chromosome which can no longer lie in proper register with the invested or defected version.

***Chromomere.*** One of many small beadlike granules that occur along the length of a chromosome, staining most deeply at prophase of mitosis and meiosis. When chromosomes pair during zygotene of meiosis, chromomeres of homologous chromosomes are specifically aligned, chromomere to chromomere. Chromomeres probably represent regions of tightest coiling of euchromatin during mitosis and meiosis. They can be readily visualized at meiotic prophase and are also apparent at the bases of the loops of lampbrush chromosomes; they are also probably homologous to the condensed bands of the giant polytene chromosomes found in some insect tissues.

***Chromonema.*** Any of the coiled threadlike strands that make up a chromosome. Each chromonema consists of a DNA double helix conjugated with his tone.

***Chromosomal mutation.*** Any genetic change in the structure of a chromosome, usually of a fairly type and often causing severely adverse effects. Such mutations are classified into various types: (a) inversion, the rearrangement of a chromosomal segment so that it has the reverse sequence e.g. ABCDE ---> ABCBE; (b) deletions, the removal of a segment; (c) duplication, the repeating of a segment either next door to the original or elsewhere along the chromosome; (d) translocation, the exchange of segments between nonhomologous chromosomes. Sometimes the loss or gain of whole chromosomes occurs, which is an extreme example of chromosomal mutation.

***Chromosomal sterility.*** Situation in which sterility results from lack of homology or incompatibility between the separate chromosomal lines in a hybrid.

***Chromosome.*** A coiled strucutre found in the nucleus of eucaryote cells which contains DNA (the genetic material making up the genes), basic proteins called histones, and nonhistone acidic proteins which may regulate the activity of DNA. Each species of organism has a typical number of chromosomes (e.g. 46 in man, 20 in maize) which come in identical homologous pairs in diploid (1) types, although lower types such as some fungi have only one chromosome of each type. Chromosomes are not visible during the interphase parts of the cell cycle, but during mitosis and meiosis they shorten and thicken and, after suitable preparation, may be observed under the microscope. Individual chromosomes can be recognized by their overall length and the position of the centromeres.

In procaryotes, the chromosome consists of an intact DAN molecule lacking a centromere and is often circular. In viruses, the chromosomal material can be DNA or RNA. The number of chromosomes in the nucleus is always constant for any one species, although chromosomes may be present in the haploid, diploid, or polyploid state, depending on the type of cell or organism. Chromosomes differ from each other in length, shape, and position of the centromere; pairs of homologous chromosomes in diploid cells are identical in these respects. The chromosomes determining sex are known as sex chromosomes; the others are called autosomes.

***Chromosome condensation.*** Condensation of chromatin during early mitosis or meiosis, so that the chromosomes become shorter, fatter and more readily visibly by microscopy.

***Chromosome loss.*** Process in which, following formation of artificial cell hybrids chromosomes are spontaneously lost. Such loss may also occur spontaneously at a very low incidence in normal cell division.

***Chromosome map (linkage map).*** A plan showing the relative positions of genes along the length of the chromosomes of an organism. It is constructed by making crosses and observing whether certain characteristics tend to be inherited together. The closer together two allele pairs are situated on homologous chromosomes, the less often will they be separated and rearranged as the reproductive cells are formed. The proportion of offspring that show recombination of alleles concerned thus reflects their spacing and is used as a unit of length in mapping chromosomes.

***Chromosome puffs or puffs.*** Cloudy areas visible on specific chromomeres of salivery gland chromosomes at certain times, which contain DAN and RNA and are thought to represent gene transcription. This idea is reinforced by teh fact that such puffs occur at regular intervals, suggesting that gene swithcing is in operation.

***Chromosome rearrangement.*** Chromosomal aberration that involves novel association of sequences due to inversion or translocation.

***Chromosome scaffold.*** Basic architecutral form that persits after histones have been removed from chromosomes. In this form, revealed by electron microscopy of spread films of such chromatin, long loops of DNA appear to be subtended by a persisting framework of non-histone proteins. These are loosely referred to as the scaffold proteins, but the identity of these proteins has not been established. During interphase, when chromosomes cannot normally be optically resolved, the basic scaffold structure is presumed to persist; the individual chromosomes are also believed to be retained in roughtly the same relationship to one another by their separate attachments to the nuclear cage.

***Chromosome set.*** Complement of chromosomes that together contribute the entire haploid genome of a species.

***Chronic granulocytic leukaemia.*** Human disease in which the granulocytic blast cells of the blood proliferate in an uncontrolled way.

***Chrysophyta.*** A division of the algae. The colouring is caused by the presence of carotenoid pigments that are present with the chlorophyll. This very diverse group of freshwater and marine forms includes the golden-brown algae (Chrysophyceae), yellow-green algae (Xanthophyceae) and the diatoms (Bacillariophyceae).

***Chymotrypsin.*** An enzyme found in the pancreatic juice of mammals that functions as an endopeptidase, catalysing the hydrolysis of peptide bonds. It attacks the carboxyl groups of specific amino acids (phenylalanine, tyrosine, leucine, tryptopha, and methionine) and so produces large peptides. The enzyme works in the alkaline medium of the small intestine and is secreted by the pancreas in an inactive form.

***Chymotrypsiongen.*** The inactive precursor of chymotrypsin.

***Cillary movement.*** Cilla normally occur in sheets, often made up of parallel rows. Fields of cilia bend together in coordinated waves, each cilium moving with a whip-like motion in which a forward driving stroke leads to full extension, followed by a recovery stroke in which the cilium bends to reduced viscous drag on returning to its original position. Adjacent cillia have cyles that are almost, but not quite, in synchrony, so producing the metachronal rhythm of coordinated ciliary movement.

The movement of an individual cilium is ATP-dependent in which the microtubules that make up the ciliary structure slide past one another. The sliding motion involves the small projections called dynein arms which extend from each microtubule doublet in the outer ring of the cilium.

***Circular linkage map.*** Gene map displayed as a continuous circle. The map corresponds to the physical structure of the underlying genetic material which is a covalently closed circle of DNA double or single-stranded. The first circular linkage map was suggested for E. coli to explain the permuted linear maps generated by different Hfr donor bacteria. The physical basis for the circular map was revealed by autoradiographs of DNA from E. coli which showed DNA molecules as continuous loops. Circular linkage maps have been prepared for other bacteria (e.g. Salmonella Pseudomonas, Bacillus, Streptomyces), for plasmids (including the F factor and varies R factors), and for DNA of the mitochondrion and chloroplast. A circular linkage map of a different type (e.g. the linkage map of bacteriophage T4) is generated when linear concatemers of simiilar DNA molecules are cut into pieces (corresponding to genomes) slightly longer than the repeat period of the concatemer. The segments of DNA thus produced are a collection of linear molecules with terminally permuted reptitious markets. The linear molecules can be accommodated within a single circular map.

***Circular overlap.*** A naturally occurring arrangement of contiguous and intergrading populations which interbreed, curving round geographically until the beginning and end overlap and behave as good species. A species that behaves in this way is called a ring species.

***Cirrhosis.*** Disease of the liver in which fibrous connective tissue proliferates at the expense of the hepatocytes, often as a consequence of insult to the liver cells by alcohol or other poisons.

***Cis-acting locus.*** Gene or DNA sequence that affects other sequences on the same DNA molecule. Such effects are usually due to DNA folding or to position effect as compared to trans-acting effects which are modulated through RNA or protein products.

***Cis configuration.*** Location of two mutations or two DNA sequences on the same chromosome as defined by the CIS, transtest. Two mutations in cis are either distinct mutations of the same gene sequence or of other sequences upstreat or downstream from one another on the same chromosome. Thus cis-acting factors are deemed to be factors, normally other DNA sequences, that are present on the same chromosome and so exert influecnce by impeding the movement of RNA polymerase molecules or other similar effects. Mutations or sequences on the other homologous chromosome are said to be in the trans configuration.

***Cis-dominant.*** Ability of a locus to affect other genes on the same DNA molecule in a dominant way.

***Cisterna.*** Vesicle of the endoplasmic reticulum and gogli apparatus, often in the form of a long finger of somewhat flatened form, and involved in storage and transport within the cell.

***Cis-trans isomerization.*** The conversion of the configuration of a 'cis' isomer with similar atoms or groups on the same side of the molecule to a `trans' form, with the similar atoms or groups on opposide sides.

***Cis-trans test.*** A genetic complementation test to determine if two mutations have occurred within the same cistron or in adjacent cistons. The test depends upon the two mutations beging introduced into a cell at the same time. If they 'complement' each other by producing a wild type phenotype the mutations are in different cistrons (i.e. nonallelic). If a mutant phenotype is produced this shows the two mutations to be noncomplementary and therefore to be located in the same cistron (i.e. allelic). Two arrangements are possible in the cis-trans test which can be carried out in a double heterozygote individual (a heterokaryon in a haploid type). The more important is the transconfiguratin, which is diagnostic, since two normal cistrons are present if the mutations are nonallelic (giving wild type) whereas the same cistron is mutuant on both chromosomes if the mutations are allelic (giving a mutant phenotype). See Figure C.13.

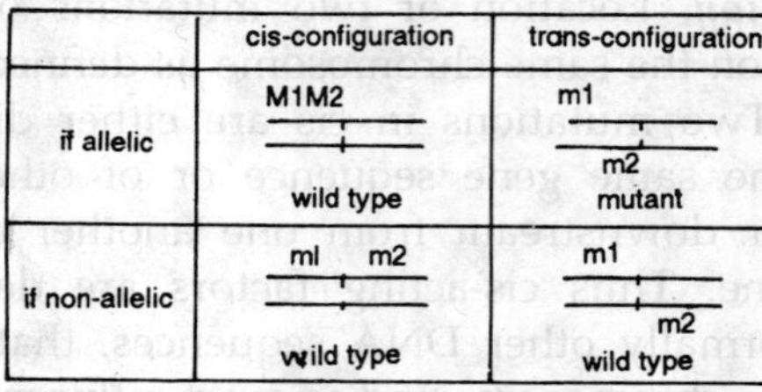


Figure C.13. Cis-trans test. The cis-trans test configurations. m1 and m2 are mutations. The two lines represents two homologous chromosomes.

***Cladistics.*** The study of evolutinary groupings and relationship that have arisen from cladogenesis, including the method of classification based on this type of evolution. In a cladistic classification, organisms are placed into taxonomic groups called clades when they share characteristics that are thought to indicate common ancestry. It assumes that two new species are formed suddenly, by splitting from a common ancestor and not by gradual evolutionary change. A diagram indicating these relationships therefore consists of a system of dichotomous branches, each point of branching representing divergence from a common ancestor. The opponents of neo-Darwinism argue that the major branching patterns of cladograms correspond to large-scale evolutionary events that cannot be explained by orthodox neo-Darwinism, which postulates a series of small changes occurring over a long period of time.

***Cladogenesis.*** The separation of a particular evolutionary sequence into two or more separate lineages. Study of such evolutionary groupings and divisions is termed cladistics.

***Cladoselachii.*** An order of the Elasmobranchii containing extinct sharklike fishes, e.g. Cladoselache, that flourished in the Devonian and became extinct in the Carboniferous. They typically had broad-based paired fins, a heterocercal tail, and amphistylic jaw suspension.

*Clearing.* A process used in the preparation of materials for microscopic examination when, after dehydration using alcohols, clearing in benzene or xylene is carried out as these are miscible with the mountant and alcohols whilst the alcohols are immiscible with the mountant.

*Cleavage.* The division of the cytoplasm during nuclear division following fertilization of the egg to form the zygote. Holoblastic cleavage occurs in animals where there is little yolk, and here the entire zygote fials to divide, only part of the zygote undergoing cleavage. Bilateral cleavage gives rise to a bilaterially symmetrical arrangement of blastomeres, as opposed to spiral cleavage which gives rise to a spiral arrangement of blastomeres. Bilateral cleavage occurs in chordates, echinoderms and a few smaller groups, indicating their common origins whereas most other invertebrate phyla have spiral cleavage. See Figure C.14.

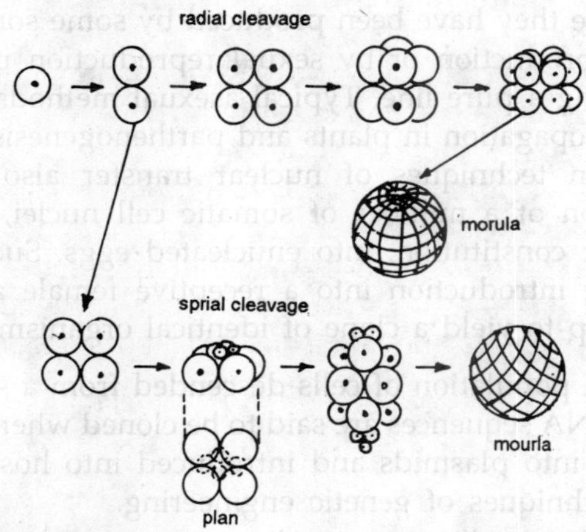


Figure C.14. Cleavage. Radial and spiral cleavage.

*Climax.* (in ecology). The final steady state of a community that has developed in a formerly uninhabited area. Colonization results in successions of plants and animals, which eventually end in a stable climax community. Because of the widespread effects of man on the natural environemnt, true climax communities, such as the Caledonian forest in Scotland, are confined to very small areass of relatively unspoiled habitat. A climax community is only relatively permanent, since in the long term it is subject to further changes as result of such factors as climate changes, wchich bring about organic evolution.

***Cline.*** A smooth gradation of characteristics from one end of the range of a species to the other, usually brought about by gradients of climate, soil, or other environmental variables. It is difficult to place members of a cline in suitable taxa. Although the individuals at each end of the cline differ from each other sufficiently to be given subspecies status, the variation within the cline is too gradual to establish discontinuities by means of which each subspecies could be separated from the next.

***Clisere.*** A succession of climax communities in a particular region, each formed as a result of changes in climate in that region.

***Clone.*** 1. A group of organisms that are genetically identical because they have been produced by some sort of nonsexual reproduction or by sexual reproduction involving inbreeding a pure line. Typical asexual methods are vegetative propagation in plants and parthenogenesis in animals. Modern techniques of nuclear transfer also permit the injection of a number of somatic cell nuclei, of identical genetic constitution, into enucleated eggs. Such eggs, following introduction into a receptive female animal, then develop to yield a clone of identical organisms at birth.

2. A population of cells descended from a single parent cell. DNA sequences are said to be cloned when they are inserted into plasmids and introduced into host bacteria in the techniques of genetic engineering.

***Closed community.*** A plant community that is so dense on the ground that new species cannot colonize.

***Closed population.*** A population into which there is no gene input from outside, i.e. the only possible genetic change is through mutation.

***Clustering methods.*** The means by which groups of related or similar species are arranged in species groups or into higher taxonomic groupings.

***Coacervate theory.*** A theory expressed by the Russian biochemist A.I. Oparin in 1936 suggesting that the origin of life was preceded by the formation of mixed colloidal units called 'coacervates'. These are particles composed of two or more colloids which might be protein, lipid or nucleic acid. Oparin proposed that whilst these molecules were not living, they behaved like biological systems in the ancient seas. They were subject to natural selection in terms of constant size. They were subject to natural selection in terms of constant size and chemical properties, there was a selective accumulation of material and they reproduced by fragmentation. Subsequent work by the American biochemists Stanley Miller and Harold Urey shows that such organic materials can be formed from inorganic substances under the conditions prevailing on the prebiological earth. They synthesized amino acids by passing a spark through a mixture of simple gases in a closed system.

***Cobalamin or cyanocobalamin or vitamin $B_{12}$.*** One of the B-complex of water-soluble vitamins, containing cobalt and required for red blood cell formation. A deficiency of $B_{12}$ can lead to pernicious anaemia especially amongst old people. The vitamin is synthesized by bacteria in the gut rather than being obtained from the diet.

***Co-dominance.*** The condition that arises when both alleles in a heterozygous organism are dominant and are fully expressed. For example, the human blood group AB is the result of two alleles, A and B, both being expressed. A is not dominant to B, nor vice versa.

***Codon.*** The basic coding unit of mesenger RNA, consisting of a triplet of nucleotides that determines the incorporation of a particular amino acid into a polypeptide chain. The complementary triplet of nucleotides on transfer RNA is called the anticodon. Codon-anticodon pairing provides the specificity for translating genetic information - transcribed from DNA into messenger RNA - into protein.

***Coefficient of inbreeding.*** The probability that any two gametes fusing to form a zygote will carry the same allele of a gene from a common ancestor. Symbol: F.

***Coefficient of variability.*** The standard deviation as a percentage of the mean.

***Coenocyte.*** A multinucleate mass of protoplasm formed when nuclei divide without the division of the cytoplasm of the original cell, as in many fungi.

***Coenospecies.*** A group of species which may be capable of forming hybrids with each other.

***Coenzyme.*** An organic cofactor molecule smaller than protein that bonds with a specific enzyme while the reaction is being catalysed. Like enzymes, coenzymes are not altered or used up in the reaction and can be used many times, but a minimal quantity is required for normal level of enzyme function and thus normal health. This explains why vitamins, which often act as coenzymes, are so essential.

***Coenzyme A (CoA).*** A complex organic compound that acts in conjunction with enzymes involved in various biochemical reactions, notably the oxidation of pyruvate via the Krebs cycle and fatty-acid oxidation and synthesis. It comprises principally the B vitamin pantothenic acid, the nucleotide adenine, and a ribose-phosphate group. See Figure C.15.

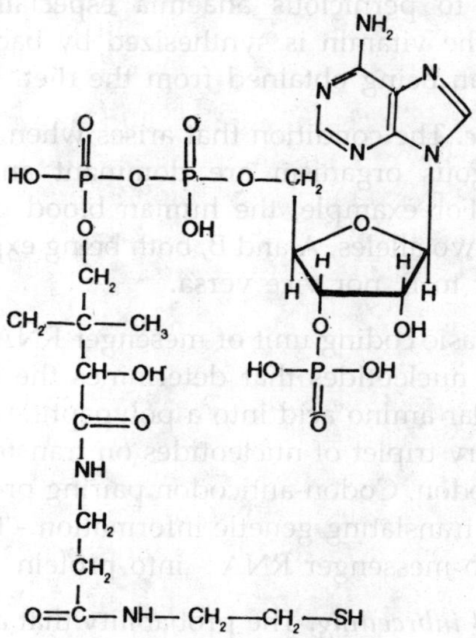

Figure C.15. Coenzyme A.

***Coenzyme Q (ubiquinone).*** Any of a group of related quinone-derived compounds that serve as electron carriers in the electron transport chain reactions of cellular respiration. Coenzyme Q molecules have side chains of different lengths in different type of organisms but function in similar ways. See Figure C.16.

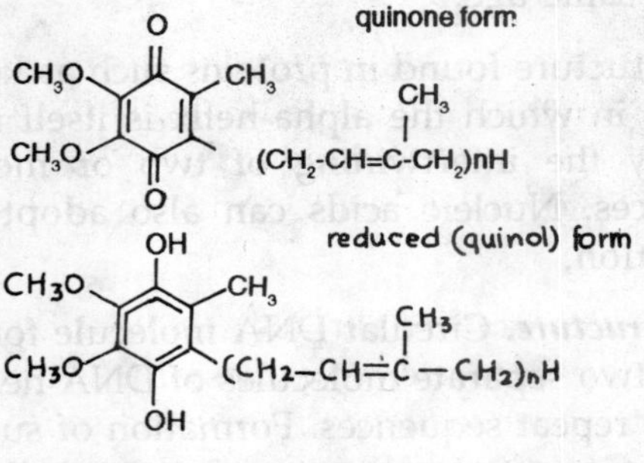


Figure C.16. Coenzyme Q.

***Coevolution.*** The evolution of unrelated organisms that has taken place together because of the special link between them, e.g. insects and the flowers they pollinate, parasites and their host, members of a symbiotic relationship. The arumlily is a notable example.

***Cofactor.*** A substance that is essential for the catalytic activity of some enzymes, binding to the enzyme only during the reaction. Cofactors can be metallic ions, or nonprotein organic molecules (coenzymes) such as vitamins in the B-complex.

***Coincidence, coefficient of.*** The proportion of double recombinant types observed in a progeny as compared to the number expected. A value less than 1.0 indicates that chromatid interference has taken place.

***Coitus.*** The act of copulation between male and female animals during which sperm is transferred from male to female.

***Colchicine.*** A poisonous alkaloid extracted from the corms of Colchicum autumnale that acts as a spindle inhibitor during nuclear division and can thus be used to produce cells with double sets of chromosomes, due to nondisjunction.

***Cognate tRNA.*** Transfer RNA recognized by a particular aminoacyl-tRNA synthetase.

***Cohesive ends.*** Single-stranded termine on DNA molecules that have complementary nucleotide sequences.

***Cohort.*** Group of individuals within a population all of which are of the same age.

***Coiled coil.*** Structure found in proteins such as keratin, myosin and fibrin in which the alpha-helix is itself further coiled, usually by the intertwining of two or more individual alpha-helices. Nucleic acids can also adopt a coiled coil configuration.

***Cointegrate structure.*** Circular DNA molecule formed by association of two separate molecules of DNA held together by two direct repeat sequences. Formation of such cointegrate structures seems to be a necessary intermediate step in the functioning of transposable elements.

***Colcemid.*** Trade name for demecolcine (N-deacetyl-N-methylcolchicine). Like colchicine it binds to tubulin and prevents polymerization of tubulin to form microtubules.

***Colchicine.*** Alkaloid derived from the autumn crocus Colchicum, a member of the Liliaceae. Colchicine is a mitotic poision, inhibiting aggregation of microtubules to form the mitotic spindle. It is widely used to yield a large number of cells in mitosis by mitotic arrest (since the cells can not progress beyond metaphase) and has also been used to produce polyploid varieties in horticulture. See Figure C.17.

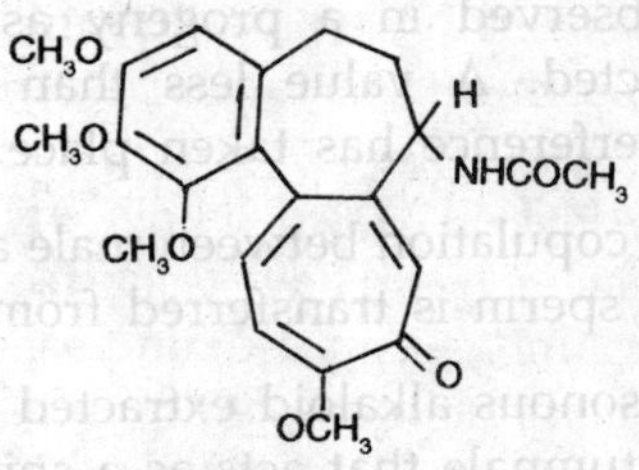


Figure C.17. Colchicine.

***Col factors.*** Plasmids that carry genes for colicins, in contrast to, for example, sex factors which carry sex-determining genes.

***Colicins.*** Group of protein antibiotics ($M_r$ = 40 000-80 000) produced by certain enteric bacteria (e.g., Escherichia, Salmonella, Shigella) which are bactericidal for other closely related bacteria. Each colicin is encoded by a plasmid colicin (Col) factor. In a population of colicinogenic bacteria only a small proportion of the cells produce colicin (usually a lethal event); the remaining cells are immune. Col E2 is a DNase (endonuclease), and Col E3 a RNase that cleaves 16S ribosomal RNA 49 nucleotides from the 3'-end. These two colicins are complexed with specific inhibitor subunits which confer immunity. The inhibitor subunit dissociates in the growth medium, and the nuclease component can penetrade the surface layers of susceptible bacteria. Colicins A, E1, Ia, Ib and K are not complexed to any other protein. These colicins act by forming ion-permeable aqueous channels spanning the bacteerial cytoplasmic membrane, leading to collapse of the proton motive force and leakage of potassium and magnesium ions. Col M acts on an enzyme involved in peptidoglycan formation at the bacterial cell wall.

***Coliform bacteria.*** Facultative gramnegative rod-shaped bacteria that inhabit the intestinal tract of man and other animals, usually without causing disease. They include species from the following genera: Escherichia, Klebsiella and Enterobacter. They ferment lactose forming acid and gas. Sometimes the term is extended to include certain lactose non-fermenters (e.g., Serratia).

***Colinearity.*** The order of amino acids in polypeptide chain corresponds to the order of nucleotides in the gene sequence that specifies its structure. Although originally an hypothesis, it is now so strongly supported by observation (such as the correspondnece between the position of an altered base in a DNA sequence and the position of a new amino acid in the protein sequence, e.g., in sickle cell globin) that it is regarded as rule. Because of the existence of intron sequences within eukaryotic genes, however, the genetic code should be understood as an interrupted colinear code rather than a simple colinear one.

***Coliphage.*** Bactereophage that has a hostrange that is restricted to the bacterial species E. Coli.

***Collagen.*** One of the most abundant animal proteins, and an important structural compeonent of fibrous tisssues (e.g., skin, tendoncartilage). Collagen is synthesized, promarily by fibroblasts, as tropocollagen ($M_r$ = 360 000; lenght = 280 nm). About one-third of the molecule is glycine and about one-third is proline or hydroxyproline. The secondary structure of collagen is a triple helix. The macromolecule polymerizes to form native collagen fibres which have a repeating period of 70 nm due to the overlapping arrangement of the collagen macromolecules.

***Collagenases.*** Group of enzymes that deave peptide bonds located in the helical regions of collagen. Some are endogenous in vertebrate tissue and are important in wound healing and development (e.g., resorption of the tail of a tadpole).

***Collenchyma.*** Plant tissue that is composed of closely compacted cells with thickened cell walls. Although it is retained as a supporting tissue by herbaceous plants, it is frequently replaced by sclerenchyma in trees and shrubs.

***Collloid.*** A mixture of two substances which are immiscible, but where the particles of one are too small to settle out, and so remain suspended indefinitely. Glue is a colloid of animal gelatin in water; the water is defined as the matrix and the gelatin as the inclusion. Colloid particles measure $1 \times 10^{-4}$ to $1 \times 10^{-6}$ mm in diamter, forming either a SOL or GEL structure which does not diffuse through cell membrances. Colloids are common in cells, where their alrge surfaces are important for chemical changes constantly in progress there.

***Colony.*** 1. (in zoology) A group of animals of the same species living together and dependent upon each other. Some, such as the corals and sponges, are physically connected and function as a single unit. Others, such as insect colonies, are not physically joined but show a high level of social organization with members specialized for different functions. 2. (in microbiology) A group of microorganisms, usually bacteria or yeasts, that are considered to have developed from a single parent cell. Colonies that grow on "agar plates differ in shape, colour, surface texture, and translucency and can therefore be used as a means of identification.

***Colony-forming unit (CFU).*** Cell type found in the erythropoietic (blood-forming) pathway that is committed, but still largely undifferentiated. It gives rise to differentiated blood cells by division, but only to cells of one specific type. Thus if it produces erythrocytes it is termed a CFU-E, colony forming unit - erythrocyte. The CFU is itself a product of the burst-forming unit, and both have been identified by the help of the spleen colony-forming cell technique.

***Colony hybridization.*** Method used in screening gene libraries held in bacterial host cells. A replica plate from a'pteri dish of discrete colonies is blotted on to a filter and, following fixation, in situ hybridizaiton with a radioactive DNA probe is carried out. Autoradiography is then used to identify the colony containing the specific gene and its location on the filter is used to identify it on the original plate.

***Colour blindness.*** A condition in which certain colours cannot be distinguished, due to a lack of one or more colour-absorbing pigements in the retina. In humans the most common example is red/ green colourblindness which can be considered as being controlled by a single locus on the x-chromosome (although at least two, closely linked loci are known to influence the character). The 'normal vision' allele is dominant to the 'colour blindness' allele; colour-blind females must therefore be homozygous for the colour-blindess allele, while males will be affected if they carry only one colour-blindness allele. Consequently, colour blindness is more common in males than females.

***Colour change.*** A process in which certain animals (e.g. squid, sole) can alter their colours or shade by changing the concentration of pigement in their pigement cells under nervous or hormonal control.

***Colour vision.*** The ability of some animal groups to detect colour in an object, due in vertebrates to activity of cone cells˙ in the retina of the eye. Examples of animals with colour vision include primates, many fishes, most birds and the insects. Animals without colour vision probably see objects in shades of grey (monochrome vision).

***Comma-less code.*** Referring to the fact that the genetic code is typified by a series of continuous codons, so that there is no information inherent in the code to indicate where one codon stops and another begins. As a result, deletion of a single base can lead to a reading frame shift and, on translation, production of a protein with a profoundly different amino acid sequence.

***Commensualism.*** Association between two or more organisms of distinct species in which one, the commensal, derives benefit from the other, the host; the host organism neither suffers nor benefits.

***Common ancestor.*** A relative occurring in the family trees of both parents in a cross. For example, cousin matings have grandparents as common ancestors.

***Communication.*** The transmission of information from one individual to another of the same or different animal species, which receives and understands it. Any of the five senses can be used in communication. Many higher organisms use sound, but posturing in specific displays, e.g. courtship in birds and primates, dancing in bees, touch and smell are other important means of conveying information.

***Community.*** A naturally occurring group of different species of organisms that lives together and interacts as a selfcontained unit, relatively independent of inputs and outputs from adjacent communities. Ideally, it is selfcontained in terms of food relationships, and usually the only energy required from outside is that of the sun.

***Compartment.*** (1) Developmental concept arising from studies attempting to produce a map of determination in Drosophila embryos. X-Irradiation of embryos will induce genetic recombination in somatic cells. From each cell so affected, a mutant CLONE will arise and the size attained by each clone in the adult will depend largely upon the developmental stage at which the mutation was originally induced. By using clones that express a detectable phenotypic aberration (e.g., changed bristle number per cell or changed bristle form) and which are therefore in effect 'marked', clonal composition of the organism can be mapped. Analysis of the shape of such clones induced in embryonic stages or in isolated imaginal discs prior to transplantation reveals that, irrespective of clone size or growth rate, clones always occur within certain domins and never cross certain invisible interfaces. These domains have been called compartments and the otherwise undertectable interfaces compartment boundaries'. By mapping the shape of successive mutant clones onto the form of the adult fly, a latent image of compartment boundaries can be built up. They exist not only between major anatomical features, such as segments, which are certainly specified very early in development, but also are found regularly within anatomical entities, dividing them into anterior/posterior, dorsal/ventral compartments for instance. The boundaries are usually sharply defined and often quite straight, and, importantly, don't necessarily follow any obvious anatomical feature (e.g., in the Drosophila wing, there are two compartments - anterior and posterior - with a straight boundary between them, the line of which is highly precise, and doesn't follow the central vein which it in fact intersects a number of times). In fact cells isolated from different embryonic compartments do not aggregate even though they will aggregate with like cells from their own compartment, suggesting that adhesivity differences may be responsible for boundary maintenance.

The existence of such compartments is seen as a kind of determination map, but it is important to note that this is not necessarily a determination to a particular cell type but a determination to form a particular part of the larva/adult. Within a compatment, the fate of individual cells is not necessarily precisely defined at all; in fact, evidence suggests that each compartment is polyclonal and the determination state is finally fixed not in a single founder cell but in a small group of such cells. Thus the fly is viewed as an assemblage of compartments each having a unique determination state different from all other compartments.

(2) Where cell lineage is known, it has been suggested that the cells in different commitment states along a particular lineage exist within compartments. (n.b. This is not a topographical entity, unlike the previous definition.) For cells in erythropoietic lineages in the multiple sites of marrow formation, within a compartment proliferative mitoses may occur. However, to move along the lineage a cell has to undergo a 'quantal' mitosis, as a result of which, its daughters have a new pattern of transcriptional genes, a new commitment state and have therefore entered the next compartment.

***Compatibility group.*** Assortment of plasmids, some of which cannot exist together with others in the same bacterial cell.

***Compensator gene.*** Gene present on the x chromosome OF Drosophila, which in the female reduces the activity of other sexlinked genes that the possesses in double dose. No X chromosome interaciton occurs in Drosophila. Since the male only possesses one X chromosome, no activity on the part of the compensator gene is necessary.

***Competence.*** 1. A period when a differentiating cell or tissue is capable of switching to an alternative developmental pathway. 2. A state in bacteria when they are able to receive DNA from other bacteria in a process called transformation.

***Competition.*** The interaction between organisms striving for the same end. Such interaction may adversely affect their growth and survival. This includes competition for resources (food, living space), mates etc.

***Competitive exclusion.*** The principel that two species cannot coexist if they have identical ecological requirements.

***Competitive inhibition.*** A form of enzyme control in which an inhibitor molecule very similar in structure to the normal substrate of an enzyme becomes reversibly bound to the active site, thus reducing the quantity of enzyme available. However, if excess substrate is present the inhibitor can be forced out by the substrate molecule which takes its place and the reaction proceeds.

***Complement.*** A group of proteins present in blood plasma and tissue fluid that aids the body's defences following an immune response. Following an antibody-antigen reaction, complement is activated chemically and becomes bound to the antibody-antigen complex (complement fixation); it becomes involved in destroying foreign cells and attacting scavenging white blood cells (phagocytes) to the area of conflict in the body.

***Complement males.*** The small males of certain animals that live in or on the females and are usually more or less degenerate apart from the reproductive organs. They occur in certain crustaceans (e.g. some brancles), in which the normal individuals are hermaphrodite but the complemental males have suppressed ovaries, lose their alimentary canal, and lead to semiparasitic existence in the mantle cavity of the larger partner. This may ensure that cross fertlization occurs.

***Complementary base sequence.*** Sequence of bases in a single-stranded molecule of DNA or RNA that is precisely complementary to that on another single strand and therefore capable of specific hybridization to it with consequent hydrogen bonding.

***Complementary bases.*** Bases that normally pair up when DNA or RNA adopts a double-stranded configuration. Guanine pairs with cytosine, and adenine with either thymine or uracil (depending on whether DNA or RNA is involved), the former pair having three hydrogen bonds between the bases, and the latter two pairs having only two hydrogen bonds between the bases.

***Complementary DNA.*** (cDNA). DNA synthesized in vitro using RNA as a template and RNA-dependent DNA polymerase. The reaciton requires a primer, usually a synthetic oligonucleotide capable of base pairing to the RNA, and generates a DNA molecule complementary in sequence to the RNA template. Complementary DNA can be made highly radioactive for use as a probe in nucleic acid hybridization studies, or rendered double-stranded by a further round of polymerization and then cloned into a bacteriophage or plasmid vector.

***Complementary genes.*** Non-allelic genes that complement one another in their expression in the phenotype. This may occur in either the dominant or recessive condition. When dominant complementarity is involved, the dominant alleles of two or more genes are essentially involved in the expression of some trait (e.g., the ability of an organism to synthesize a complex molecule). In the case of recessive complementarity, the trait is only apparent in the homozygous double recessive since the dominant expression of either gene will prevent expression.

***Complementation.*** Phenomenon in which two separate homologous chromosomes, when brought together by genetic manipulation in a diploid cell, complement one another. The complementation is defined by the production of a wild-type phenotype, despite the fact that each chromosome carries a mutant allele. Complementation results from the mutants being in different gene loci and is the basis for the definition of a coding sequence as a complementation group, that is, a length of DNA within which different alleles in the trans position will not show complementaiton.

***Complementaiton map.*** Representation of the complementation pattern of a series of mutations occurring in a short chromosomal segment of DNA. Definition of the limits of a coding sequence plus any sequences upstream or downstream from the coding sequence that are genetically essential for its correct expression can be derived from such a map. It therefore helps not only to delineate one coding sequence from another, but also to define adjacent non-coding regulatory sequences.

***Complementation test.*** A genetical test to determine the precise location of mutations in one area of DNA.

***Complementary base pairing.*** The arrangement of nucleotide bases so that purines bond with pyrimidines, as occurs in the two polynucleotide chains of DNA (ademine with thymine, guanine with cytosine) and between DNA and messenger RNA nucleotides during transcription.

***Complementary bases.*** Bases that normally pair in opposite strands of double-stranded DNA or RNA, i.e. guanine-cytosine, adenine—thymine, and admine—uracil. Complementary DNA or RNA strands are those with compelemtary base sequences.

***Complementary DNA (cDNA).*** DNA synthesized in vitro from a messenger RNA template and used in cloning.

***Complementation.*** The phenomenon in which two homologous mutant chromosomes brought together in a diploid cell or fungal heterokaryon produce a wild-type phenotype. The mutations are assumed to be in different cistrons, the deficiency of one being supplied by its wild-type allele in the homologous chromosome.

***Complement fixation.*** The ability of certain antigen-antibody complexes to bind (fix) the components of complement. This property is utilized in the complement fixation test, which enables antibodies to be detected in the presence of known antigens, and vice versa. The test is used in the diagnosis of symphilis and certain viral infections.

***Complexity of DNA.*** Summations of the length of different types of sequence in a given sample of DNA.

***Complex loci.*** DNA sequences that may be interpreted as including more than one structural gene with a common regulatory element They have been found in a wide range of eukaryotic organisms and are normally discovered as a series of mutants which behave as alleles by the CIS, transtest, that is they do not complement one another in trans, but they are readily separated by crossing-over, implying a substantial length of DNA. For these latter reasons, these sequences have also been termed psecudoalleles. An example of such a complex locus is the white (w) locus in Drosophila, within which mutations cause loss of pigment from eyes and other body tissues.

***Composite transposon.*** DNA sequence flanked by insertion sequences which facilitate its transposition.

***Concanavalin A (Con A).*** Protein found in the jackbean (Conavalia ensiformis) that has properties, when purified, of specific adhesion to transformed cells, resulting in their agglutination. The surface residues to which Con A binds are known to be glucose and mannose. It is therefore classified as a lectin.

***Concatemer.*** Number of DNA molecules or sequences covalently linked in series. In animal cells, for example, genes coding for ribosomal RNA are often present as mutltiple, tendemly linked copies and thus form natural concatemers. Components need not however be identical, and during cloning into bacteriophage lambda concatemers of the two phage arms and a DNA insert between them are constructed in vitro.

***Concatenates.*** Multiple circular DNA molecules linked in a chain-like arrangement. Concatenates can arise as a result of the normal processes of DNA replication with circular genomes and cannot be separated without strand breakage. Plasmids in bacteria and kinetoplast DNA in trypanosomes frequently form concatenates. See Figure C.18.

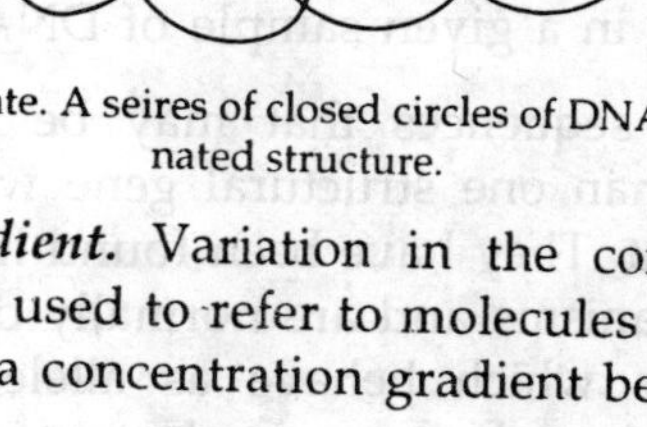

Figure C.18. Concatenate. A seires of closed circles of DNA forming a concatenated structure.

***Concentration gradient.*** Variation in the concentration of a molecule; often used to refer to molecules in solution, such as ions, where a concentration gradient between two sides of a membrane may exist. Molecules will tend to move randomly and thus on average to move from higher to lower concentration points, but ion pumps may act to reverse or modify such a trend.

***Concerted evolution.*** Situation in which two or more related genes evolve together as if occupying the same locus.

***Concordance.*** Exhibiting the same or similar properties. Identical twins are described as being concordant for a particular trait if both exhibit it.

***Conditioned lethal mutation.*** Situation in which a particular mutation will only prove lethal if certain environmental conditions occur. Many conditioned lethal mutants are temperature-sensitive, for example, and affected individuals will die if certain temperatures are encountered during development. Mutations in genes coding for heat shock genes behave in this way.

***Cone cell.*** Type of photosensitive cell found in the vertebrate retina, involved idn bright light vision and colour reception. Cones are also responsible for precise visual acitivty, each being connected to the brain by a single fibre of the optic nerve. Different populations of cones occur in the retina with maximum absoroption in the red, green and blue regions of the visible spectrum.

***Confluent cell culture.*** Culture of cells grown as a monolayer on a flat surface, such as a petri dish, in which, by dint of growth and cell replication, the cells form a continuous layer and are all in intimate cell-to-cell contact with one anoher. Most cells undergo a marked reduction in growth rate when they become confluent, due to contact inhibition, but some transformed cell lines continue to grow rapidly and to move over one another following the development of confluence.

***Conformation.*** Three-dimensional configuration of a molecule or multimolecule strucutre.

***Congenic strain.*** Genetic strain of an organism that differs only in a restricted area of its genome.

***Congenital.*** Present at birth. Congenital disorders of the body may be due to genetic factors, e.g. "Down's syndrome, or caused by injury or environmental factors, e.g. drugs (such as thalidomide) and chemicals (such as dioxin).

***Conjugation.*** 1. The fusion of two reproductive cells, particularly when these are both the same size. 2. A form of sexual reproduction seen in some algae (e.g. Spirogyra), some bacteria (e.g. Exchericha coli), and ciliate protozoans. Two individuals are united by a tube formed by outgrowths from one or both of the cells. Genetic material from one cell (designated the male) them passes through the tube to unite with that in the other (female) cell. See Figure C.19.

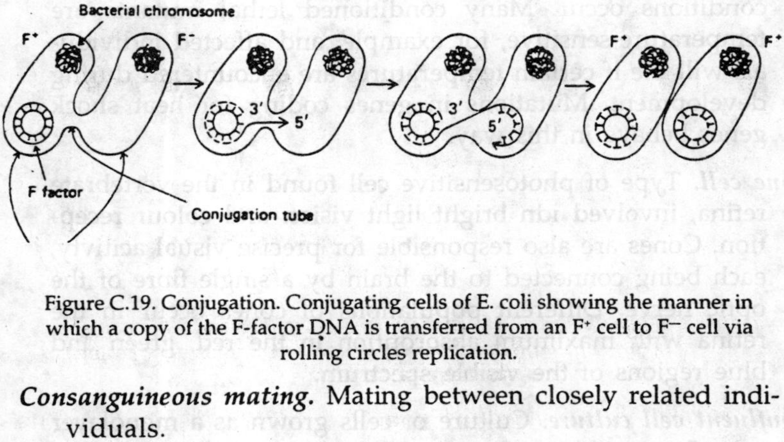


Figure C.19. Conjugation. Conjugating cells of E. coli showing the manner in which a copy of the F-factor DNA is transferred from an $F^+$ cell to $F^-$ cell via rolling circles replication.

***Consanguineous mating.*** Mating between closely related individuals.

***Consanguinity.*** Literally means 'common blood': used to denote genetic relationship. Consanguineous individuals share at least one relative in preceding generations.

***Consensus sequence.*** Nucleic acid sequence that is shared between a number of gene sequences. Consensus sequences need not be identical. For example, the promoter regions of eukaryotic structural genes share certain consensus sequences, such as the TATA BOX, generally assumed to be recognition sites for RNA polymerase molecules, but differing slightly by one or two base pairs in different gene promoters. Consensus sequences are now readily detected by computer analysis of known sequences.

***Conservation.*** The preservation, protection and management of an environment which takes into account recreational and aesthetic needs, in addition to preserving as much as possible of the natural fauna and flora and allowing for the harvesting of natural resources and agriculture. This necessitates the sensible planning of what is taken from the environment in terms of the yield of plants, animals and materials, whilst at the same time maintaining as much natural habitat as possible, and thus the largest possible gene pool.

***Conservative recombination.*** Breakage and rejoining of existing strands of DNA without any net synthesis of new DNA.

***Conservative replication model.*** A model of DNA synthesis, now disproved, in which both chains of the original molecule act as a template for a new daughter molecule. The semiconservative replication model is now accepted as the correct method of DNA replication.

***Consociation.*** A climax vegetation in which one species is dominant, e.g. oakwood, as opposed to association where there are several dominant species.

***Conspecific.*** (of animals or plants) belonging to the same species.

***Constant (C) region.*** An area of an immunoglobulin molecule that shows little variation between molecules with different specificities.

***Constitutive enzyme.*** (housekeeping enzyme). Enzyme that is present as part of the normal metabolic make-up of a cell and does not require any special stimulus to evoke its synthesis. Such enzymes (e.g., those involved in glycolysis are constitutive in many cell types). Enzymes that are normally inducible may become constitutive in mutants or other cells where the normal control mechanism regulating enzyme production is defective or absent.

***Constitutive heterochromatin.*** Heterochromatin, which is invariably in this conformational state, as is, for example, the chromatin of the centromere regions of chromosomes.

***Constriction.*** Visibly narrow region of a metaphase chromosome. Centromeres appear as constricted areas on many chromosomes.

***Contact guidance.*** Cell response to small scale, topographical irregularities in the substratum, by changing shape or polarity, and (usually) displaying oriented movement. Thus, cells cultured on a substratum of parallel groves, or in a matrix of aligned fibrils, will align with a long axis parallel to the grooves or fibirls and tend to move along rather than across them. However, although contact guidance will orient cells (e.g., north/ south), it will not provide a directional stimulus for subsequent movement (i.e. north or south); for that a vectorial cue is necessary, such as chemical attractant or contact inhibition of movement. In its purest form, contact guidance is simply a response to the physical character of the substratum. However, in practice, it has been notoriously difficult to separate this from any possible adhesive differences eliciting a haptotacitic response.

***Contact inhibition.*** (1) Mutually exclusive relationship in vitro between cell contact and cell division. Thus cells cultured at low densities will continue to proliferate until a confluent mondolayer is formed, at which point cell division decreases or is arrested. Çhange in cell density, caused by subculturing or by 'wounding' of the monolayer, will result in a resumption of division until confluence is again achieved. Transformed or neoplastic cells tend not to respond to cell density in this way and may continue to proliferate at high densities. (2) Contact between moving cells, or between a moving cell and a stationary one, will cause a localized paralysis of the contractile apparatus in that part of the cytoplasm, resulting in temporary arrest of motility and a subsequent resumption of movement in a direction away from the point of contact (initiated by a site of cytoplasmic motility elsewhere on the cell). Contact inhibition of movement is typically displayed by dispersed populations of non-epithelial cells grown at low densitites on a planar substratum. Following contact, epithelial cells first show paralysis but then form stable adhesions and, as a result of accumulated encounters, reconstruct epithelial sheets in vitro. Contact inhibition of movement may be expressed either on a small scale, where only localized cytoplasmic paralysis occurs and the non-contacted part of the cell continues to display motility, or on a larger scale where the entire cell contracts onto the point of contact and remains paralysed for varying periods before movement is resumed. As a result of contact inhibition of movement, normal cells grown on planar substrata tend to move away from arteas of high cell density and, at unavoidable high densities, form a confluent monolayer as they are inhibited from moving over one another (they will also stop dividing - see definition (1). Transformed or neoplastic cells show varying degrees of deviation from this behaviour, displaying an apparent lack of contact inhibition due to their reduced adherence to the substratum and consequent tendency to underlap. This abnormal behaviour in culture often correlates with the degree of invasiveness shown by a particular transformed/ neoplastic cell type in vitro.

***Contact site.*** Localized contact between two cells (typically in culture) and related particularly to the concept of contact inhibition. A cultured, non-epithelial cell with only a single contact site might proceed to migrate away from that point and might subsequntly divide, whereas a cell with numerous contact sites around its periphery might consequently be inhibited from both moving and dividing.

***Containment.*** Safety procedure in the handling of microorganisms, viruses and parasites in which the dangerous material is cultured within defined areas of complete isolation such that no particles or oranisms can escape to the outside. Various categories of containment are recognized as essential for different classes of material and microorganisms.

***Contingency table.*** A method of presenting results so as to show relationships between two characters which can then be tested statistically by a modified chi-squared test (the heterogeneity chi-square test). For example, eye colour and hair colour might be measured in a sample population and the results presented in a contingency table. See Figure C.20.

| | | Eye Colour | | | |
|---|---|---|---|---|---|
| | | Blue | Grey | Brown | total |
| Hair Colour | Blonde | 96 | 42 | 37 | 175 |
| | Brown | 58 | 61 | 107 | 226 |
| | Black | 17 | 32 | 93 | 142 |
| | total; | 171 | 135 | 237 | 543, |

Figure C.20. Contingency table. A contingency table for eye and hair colours in a sample population

***Continuity.*** The principle in taxonomy that continued usage of a particular scientific name should have priority over date of publciation. Normally in scientific classification the date of publication has priority.

***Continuous variation.*** A feature of certain characters, e.g. height, in which there is a complete spread of forms across a range, often producing a bell-shaped, normal distribution curve when sampling in a population.

***Convergence or convergent evolution or parallelism.*** A form of evolution which results in unrelated organisms independeltly producing similarities of form, usually because they become adapted to living in similar types of environment. For example, fish and cetaceans have evolved similar streamlined body shapes and fins.

***Coomassie brilliant blue.*** Blue dye widely used for staining proteins after electrophoresis through agar or polyacrylamide gels. Staining is followed by destaining in buffered solution until the appropriate staining density is achieved.

***Coordinated enzyme.*** Enzyme of a metabolic pathway that retains a constant concentration ratio with another enzyme whatever the degree of induction or repression of the pathway. Coordinated enzyme synthesis is associated with those bacterial enzymes produced from a common messenger RNA molecule transcribed from a cluster of genes in an operon.

***Coordinate regulation.*** Regulation of a group of genes in a coordinate fashion, so that all become active or inactive simultaneously.

***Copia.*** Small, mobile genetic element of Drosophilla. It has general structural features very similar to those of the integrated forms of retrovirus proviruses, including an internal DNA segment several kilobases long flanked by two direct terminal repeats.

***Copolymer.*** Polymeric molecule made up from more than one subunit (i.e. monomers).

***Copy nuymber.*** Number of copoies of a specific gene sequence in a GENOME.

***Cordycepin.*** (3' -deoxyadenosine). Compound that inhibits the attachment of polyadenosine residues to the 3'-terminus of RNA.

***Core enzyme.*** RNA polymerase of E. coli without the sigma subunit. Together they would be termed the holoenzyme.

***Core particle.*** Central particle of the nucleosome, composed of eight moleucles of the basic protein - histone - the octamer containing two molecules of each of the core histones H2A, H2B, H3 and H4. The core particle, together with the double coil of DNA that loops around it, form the basic subunit of all eukaryotic chromatin.

***Corepressor.*** Molecule involved in the functioning of one class of operon in bacterial gene regulation. Such molecules function by binding with the product of a regulatory gene, the aporepressor, and together the two molecules form an effective repressor to prevent transcription of the appropriate operon. Corepressors are often themselves end-products of the metabolic pathway that they help to regulate, and so their repressing function is an example of end-product inhibition.

***Correlated response.*** A change in the phenotype resulting from selection for a completely different character, e.g. selection for more bristles, which in some insects can also cause sterility.

***Correlation.*** A statistical association between two variables, calculated as the correlation coefficient r. The coefficient can range from r = 1.0 (a perfect positive correlation) to r= -1.0 (a perfect negative correlation), with an r value of 0 indicating no relationship between the two variables. Height and weight in humans are positively correlated (as values for height increase so do values for weight), whereas other variables give a negative correlation, e.g. as human age increases so mental agility tends to decrease.

***Cortisol (hyrocortisone).*** A hormone produced by the, adrenal glands, that promotes the synthesis and storage of glucose and is therefore important in the normal response to stress, supresses or prevents inflammation, and regulates deposition of fat in the body. It is used as treatment for various allergies and for rheumatic fever, certain skin conditions, and adrenal failure (Addison's disease).

***Cortisone.*** A glucocorticoid hormone secreted by the adrenal cortex, whose function is to combat stress. It causes shrinkage of lymph nodes and lowers the white blood cell count, reduces inflammation, promotes healing and stimulates gluconeogenesis. Cortisone controls its own production which is triggered by the adrenocorticotropic hormone in a negative feedback mechanism.

***Cosmic rays.*** A stream of atomic particles entering the earth's atmosphere from outer space at nearly the speed of light. Cosmic rays are thought to be a cause of spontaneous mutations.

***Cosmid.*** Type of plasmid cloning vector into which cos sites from lambda phage have been inserted. The presence of the cos sites allows their packaging within phage coats in vitro, and they are specially useful for the cloning of large DNA molecules.

***Cos site.*** Cohesive ends of the linear genome of bacteriophage lambda are able to hybridize, forming a circular molecule. These cohesive ends constitute the COS site, and are used together with other foreign DNA sequences to form cosmids, which can be packaged in phage heads and cloned into bacterial cells.

***Cosynthèsis.*** Synthesis of two compounds together, as of enzymes that are coordinately regulated as in the products of the lacoperon of E. coli.

***Cot.*** Concentration of a DNA sample multiplied by time of incubation in a reaction in which strand reassociation is permitted.

***Cot 1/2.*** Cot required for one-half of the total reassociation to occur in a sample. It is proportional to the length of unique sequences in the DNA.

***Cot plot.*** (Cot curve). Graph showing the extend of reannealing of previously denatured DNA molecules as a function of cot value. Cot plots indicate the relative amounts of unique sequence, moderately repetitive and highly repetitive DNA in a genome, as well as giving some idea of the total sequence complexity. See Figure C.21 on next page.

***Cotransduction.*** Simultaneous transduction of two or more bacterial genes by a single bacteriophage particle. The cotransduction frequency is inversely related to the distance between the genes on the chromosome.

$$\text{Contransduction frequence} = (1 - d/L)^3$$

where d = distance between markers and L = length of the transduced gene (exogenote).

***Cot value.*** A measure of DNA complexity based on hybridization (annealing) of single-stranded DNA. 'Co' refers to DNA concentration; 't' to the time of hybridization in seconds. Cot values are derived from Cot curves, which are obtained by heating a sample of purified DNA until the double helices have come apart and the molecules are single-stranded. When the sample is placed in renaturing conditions, the rate of annealing for any particular sequence present is dependent on its complexity or its frequency in the DNA sample. Short, simple, and highly repeated sequences will renature very quickly, while long, complex and scarce sequences (the so-called unique sequences) will renature very slowly, if at all. Thus DNA fractions with low Cot values are likely to contain abundant and simple short sequences, whereas those with high Cot values are likely to be scarce and relatively complex. A Cot curve of mammalian DNA will reveal four or more separate fractions, each a distinct type of DNA sequence. They are, going from low to high Cot value, (1) foldback DNA, usually indicating palindromic sequences; (2) highly repetitious DNA; (3) moderately repetitious DNA; and (4) unique-sequence DNA.

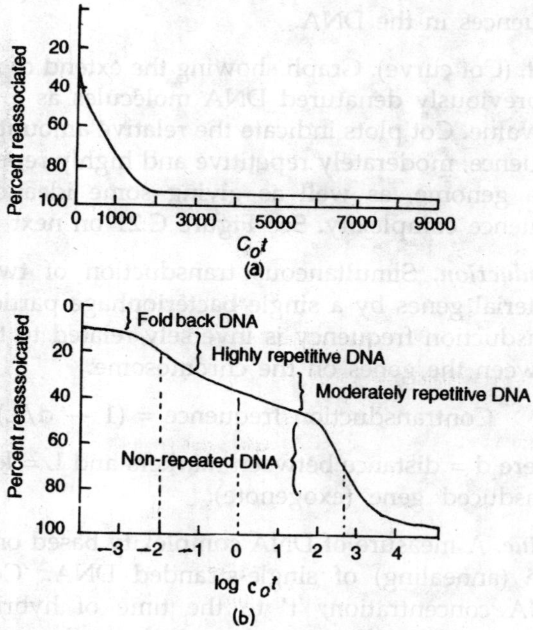


Figure C.21. Cot plot. Reassociation profile of highly sheared human DNA. Four kinetic classes is the minimum number consistent with the data, but other repetition frequencies may be present. (a) $c_0t$ on a linear scale (approximate values). (b) $c_0t$ on a log scale.

***Countercurrent exchange.*** A bilogical mechanism designed to enable maximum exchange between two fluids. The mechanism's effect is dependent on the two fluids flowing in opposite directions, and having a concentration gradient between them.

fluid ONE high concentration ---> low concentration

fluid TWO high concentration <--- low concentration

Such mechanisms occur, for example, in oxygen exchange between water and the blood vessels in fish gills, and in the ascending and descending tubules of the loop of henle in the mammalian kidney.

***Countercurrent multiplier.*** The amount of corss-transport in a countercurrent-exchange system per unit distance, being a function (-multiplication) of the total distance over which the exchange takes place.

***Coupling.*** An arrangement in a double heterozygote where wild type alleles of two genes are located on one chromosome with mutant alleles of these two genes on the other homologous chromosome. Such an arrangement of linked genes is usually referred to as in coupling. Such arrangements are important when considering the implications of genetic linkage. See Figure C.22.

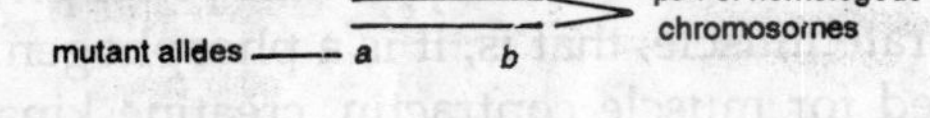


Figure C.22. Coupling. The arrangement of genes in coupling.

***Courtship.*** Behaviour in animals that plays a part in the initial attraction of a mate or as a prelude to copulation. Courtship often takes the form of displays that have evolved through ritualizaiton; some are derived from other contexts (e.g. food begging to some birds). Chemical stimuli are also important in many mammals and insects.

As well as ensuring that the prospective mate is of the same species, the male's courtship performance allows females to choose between different males. The later stages of courtship may involve both partners in an alternating series of displays that inhibit aggression and fear responses and ensure synchrony of sexual arousal.

***Covalently closed circle.*** Circle of DNA which is without intervening linker regions and is therefore a continuously covalent DNA sequence.

***Covalent modification.*** Activation of an enzyme by covalent insertion of a small molecule group (e.g., activation of enzymes by serine phosphorylation).

***Covariance.*** Statistical tactic used to compute the correlation coefficient between two variables.

***Cracking.*** In genetics, determination of which codons are specific coding triplets for each amino acid.

***Cretaceous period.*** The geological period which began about 135 million years BP and ended 65 million years BP. It is usually divided into Lower (135-95 million years) and Upper (94-65 million years) periods. The dominance of flowering plants began during this period and large reptiles (e.g. dinosaurs) and ammonities were extinct by its end. By the end of the period, London was at 40ºN and Britain was still moving northwards.

***Creatine phosphate.*** (phosphocreatine). Compound that acts as a reservoir of high-transfer potential phosophyoryl groups in vertebrate muscle; that is, it is a phosphogen. When ATP is required for muscle contractin, creatine kinase catalyses the transfer of phosophoryl groups from creatine phosphate to ADP. The same enzyme regenerates creatine phosphate from ATP and creatine when ATP is plentiful.

***Creatline.*** Produced as a result of a ring closure reaction of creatine. The creatinine cannot be converted back to creatine and is therefore excreted. Small quantities of creatinine are ususally excreted in mammalian urine. The excretion of this compound increases markedly in conditions characterized by the breakdown of muscle tissue.

***Cretinism.*** Disease due to genetically determined metabolic disorders resulting in failure of the thyroid gland to form the hormones thyroxine and throdothyreonine. The disease is characterized by severe mental and physical retardation.

***Cri-du-chat syndrome.*** (cat cry syndrome). Genetically determined disorder due to a deletion of part of the short arm of chromosome 5. A number of congenital malformations are manifested in the condition, one of the most noticeable in early life being a peculiar cry which resembles the mewing of a cat.

***Crinophagy.*** Breakdown of secretory granules by fusion with lysosomes in secretory cells. Such breakdown is used as a means of preventing overproduction of the secretory product in these cells.

***Crippled strain.*** Genetically enfeebled strain of a bacterium that will grow only in highly complex media. Such strains are used for any potentially hazardous experiments in gene manipulation to ensure that the bacteria would not survive in the wild; in the case of E. coli, crippled strains are unable to survive in the human intestinal tract.

***Cristae.*** Folds of the inner membrane of mitochondria. This membrane has a typical trilaminar structure, but bears in addition the elementary of $F_1$ particles. The inner membrane carries the enzymes of the respiratory or electron transport chain. The elementary particles contain, in a precise arrangement, the components of the oxidative phosphorylation system. The morphology of the mitochondrial cristae changes with and is characertistic of the functional state of the mitochondrion, and thus can be used as in indicator of the physiological or pathological state of the cell.

***Crohn's disease.*** Non-infectious inflammatory bowel disease in the human with numerous environmental trigger factors in addition to an inherited factor.

***Crick, Francis.*** (1916- ) English biochemist best known for his work with James Watson and Maurice wilkins on the structure of the DNA molecule, for which they shared a Noble Prize in 1962. They were able to suggest a modle for DNA structure and how it replicates which is widely accepted today. Crick also proposed the wobble hypothesis which refers to the fact that the third base of each DNA codon often can be varied without changing the amino acid coded for by that codon.

***CRM (cross-reacting material).*** A protein, usually without an enzymic function, that can be recognized in serological tests.

***Cro protein.*** A protein found in bacterial cells infected with bacteriophage and responsible for determining the choice of the lytic cycle of viral replication instead of lysogeny. The cro protein has the effect of blocking synthesis of a repressor molecule that would normally prevent commitment to the lytic cycle (the name is an acronym for control of repressor and other things).

***Cross.*** 1. A mating between a male and a female of a plant or animal species, from which one or more offspring are produced. 2. A hybrid produced by mating two unlike parents.

***Cross-fertilization or allogamy.*** The production of an offspring by the female gamete being fused with a male gamete from a different plant.

***Cross-linking.*** Formation of covalent bonds by bases in two complementary and opposite DNA strands by mitotic poisons such as the nitrite ion or the antibiotic mitomycin C.

***Cross-over fixation.*** Spread through a series of tandem sequences of a mutation in one member as a result of unequal crossing-over.

***Crossing over.*** A process occurring in the diplotene stage of Prophase 1 of meiosis in which there is exchange of nonsister chromatids, producing genetic recombination. See Figure C.23 on next page.

***Cross-over region.*** Section of a chromosome situated between two distinct marker genes in which crossing-over of the DNA length between the two marker loci has been detected.

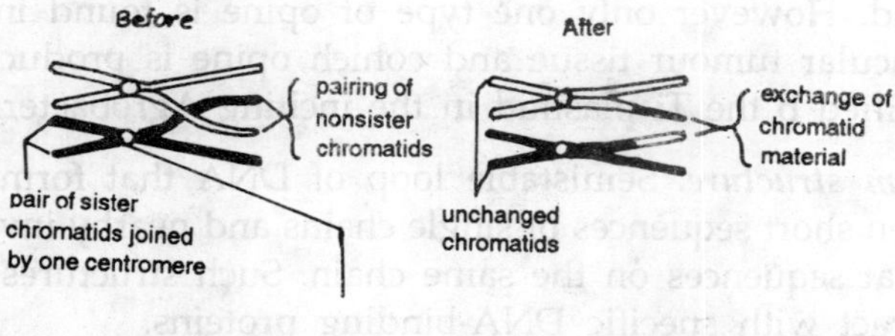


Figure C.23. Crossing over. The exchange of chromatid material.

***Cross-reaction.*** Antibody binding to antigen other than that used to stimulate its production.

***Crown gall.*** Plant tumour formed as a result of infection of wounded tissue by a soil-borne bacterium Agrobacterium tumefaciens. The condition derives its name from the fact that these tumours usually appear near the plant crown (i.e. the region where the stem and root merge). The disease occurs in a wide variety of dicotyledonous plants, but not in monocotyledons. Virulent strains of A. tumefaciens possess a large plasmid of about 150-230 kilobases, the Ti plasmid, which is essential for the initiation of the tumour. Part of this plasmid, known as the T-DNA, is transferred to the plant cells where it is incorporated into the nuclear DNA. This T-DNA specifies or induces a change in the phenotype of the cells. Infected cells in the region of the wound proliferate in an unorganized manner leading to the formation of the gall. Gall tissue will continue to grow in the absence of the initiating bacterium, and therse tumours have the ability to form an overgrowth when grafted on uninfected tissue. In addition, when cultured in vitro the tumour cells, unlike those of the non-tumour host tissue, will grow without the inclusion of growth substances in the nutrient medium. The tumour cells have, therefore, undergone an oncogenic transformation. Usually these transformed cells are also characterized by the capacity to synthesize opines. These are amino acids not found in non-transformed plant cells and which can not be metabolized by plant tissues. Opines can, however, be metabolized by Agrobacterium, and they can serve as their sole carbon and/or nitrogen source. There are several different opines of which octopine and nopaline are the most commonly found. However only one type of opine is found in any particular tumour tissue and cohich opine is produced is specified b the Ti plasmid in the inciting Agrobacterium.

***Cruciform structure.*** Semistable loop of DNA that forms between short sequences of single chains and nearby inverted repeat sequences on the same chain. Such structures may interact with specific DNA-binding proteins.

***Cross-over value.*** The percentage of recombinants (the products of recombination) in the total number of offspring from a given corss. This figure indicates the amount of crossing over between two genes and thus the degree of linkage between them. Cross-over values are used in making genetic (or linkage) maps, which show the relative positions of the genes on the chromosomes, as the values are roughtly proportional to the distnace between the genes. If two genes are far apart on a chromosome crossing over is very likely to occur between them, and a high corss-over value is obtained. There is much less chance of crossing over occurring between two genes that are close together on a chromosome, and a lower cross-over value is obtained. Cross-over values are not precisely proportional to the distance apart of genes because of interference (the fact that corssing over does not occur in certain regions of the chromosome) and because the formation of chiasmata is affected by environmental conditions.

***Cryobilology.*** The study of the effects of very low temperatures on living organisms. Applications of this study include cryopreservation, in which cells and tissues can be frozen and stored for long periods. In this way sperm can be stored for artificial insemination and blood for transfusion. Cryosurgery is the use of extreme cold to destroy unwanted tissues.

***Cryptic coloration.*** The type of colouring in an animal that causes it to be camouflaged in its environment. The coloration may resemble that of the surroundings, causing the animal to merge with its background, or it may contain disruptive patches of colour, which obscure the outline of the animal.

*C value paradox.* The paradox presented by comparisons of C value among eukaryotic organisms. C value is the amount of DNA present in the haploid genome of an organism, usually expressed in picograms per cell (1 picogram = $10^{-12}$ g). Generally, the C value increases with the complexity of the organism, but in some cases the C value is very variable in closely related organisms and certain genera, such as Protopterus (lungfish) and Lilium, have very much larger genomes than man. A further aspect of the paradox is that the higher eukaryotes appear to have much higher C values than they can utilize for strictly genetic purposes; the human genome, for example, theoretically has enough DNA in the haploid state for about 3 million genes but it is unlikely that more than 50 000 different genes are actually utilized. The following is a selection of C values (in picograms) for different species:

| | |
|---|---|
| E. coli | 0.0044 |
| Neurospora | 0.017 |
| Drosophila | 0.18 |
| Chicken | 1.25 |
| Xenopus | 3.15 |
| maize | 3.9 |
| Protopterus | 142.0 |
| Lilium | 32.8 |
| man | 3.4 |

*Cybernetics.* The study of the comparison of control in the workings of the living body with man-made mechanical systems such as are used in robots.

*Cyclic AMP.* A derivative of ATP that is widespred in animal cells as an intermediate messenger in many biochemical reacions included by hormones. Upon reaching their target cells, the hormones activate the enzyme that catalyses cylic AMP production. Cyclic AMP ultimately activates the enzymes of the reaction induced by the hormone concerned. Cyclic AMP is also involved in controlling gene expression and cell division, in immune responses, and in nervous transmission.

***Cysterine.*** One of 20 amino acids common in proteins that has a polar 'R' structure and is water-soluble. See Figure C.24. The isoelectric point of cysteine is 5.1.

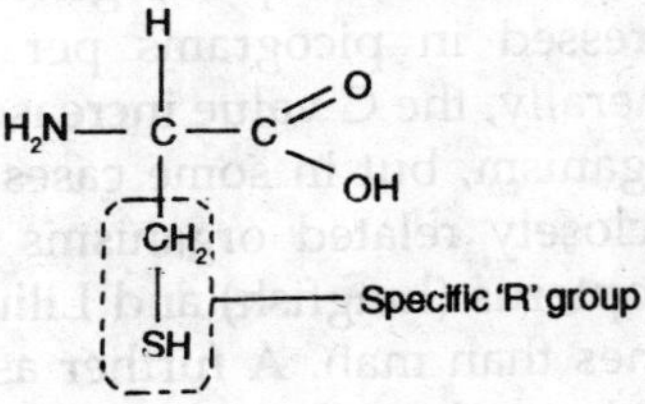


Figure C.24. Cysteine. Molecular structure.

***Cystic fibrosis.*** A rate disease of humans (affecting one child per 2,000 live births) in which various mucus-secreting glands, particularly in the pancreas and in the lungs, become fibrous, producing an abnormally thick mucus. Symptoms of the disease include intestinal blockage and pneumonia which, despite modern medicines, can still be fatal. The condition is inhertied as an autosomal recessive gene on the long arm of chromosome 7, so that affected children are homozygous receissive, a mutant allele having been passed on by both parents. At present there is no cure for the disease, but in 1986 a gene probe prenatal test was announced involving chorionic biopsy of the foetus at 9-11 weeks. If the result of the test is positive, the parents have a choice of whether to terminate the pregnancy or not.

***Cystine.*** A molecule resulting from the oxidation reaction between the sulphydryl (-SH) groups of two cysterine molecules. This often occurs between adjacent cysteine residues in polypeptides. The resultant disulphide bonds (-S-S-) are important in stablizing the structure of protein molecules.

***Cytidine.*** A nucleoside comprising one cytosine molecule linked to a D-ribose sugar molecule. The derived nucleotides, cytidine mono-, di-, and triphosphate (CMP, CDP, and CTP respectively) participate in various biochemical reactions, notably in phospholipid synthesis.

***Cytochrome.*** A protein pigement containing iron that is capable of being alternately oxidized and reduced, acting as an electron carrier in the electron transport system of a mitochondrion.

***Cytogenetics.*** The study of the inheritance of cells and their chromosomes. Cytogenetic analysis of foetal cells is used to assess potential risks tö the baby.

***Cytokinin (kinin).*** Any of a group of plant growth substances chemically related to the purine adenine. Cytokinins stimulate cell division in the presence of auxin and have also been found to delay senescence, overcome apical dominance, and promote cell expansion. Zeatin is a naturally occurring cytokinin.

***Cytology.*** The study of cells, especially by means of light or electron microscopy.

***Cytolysis.*** The disruption of a cell, usually by destruction of the plasmalemma.

***Cytomegalovirus.*** A virus belonging to the herpes group. In man it normally causes symptoms that are milder than the common cold, but it can produce more serious symptoms in those whose immune response is disturbed (e.g. cnacer patients). Infection in pregnant women may cause congenital handicap in their children.

***Cytoplasm.*** The jelly-like material surrounding the nucleus of a cell. It can be differentiated into dense outer ectoplasm, which is concerned primarily with cell movement, and less dense endoplasm, which contains most of the cell's structures.

***Cytoplasmic inheritance or extranuclear inheritance.*** The control of certain characters by genetic factors located in the cytoplasm of eucaryotes. These cytoplasmic mechanisms can show themselves as general 'maternal' influences (since the female gamete contains more cytoplasm than the male) as in the control of shell coiling in the snail Limnaea. DNA has also been located in several cytoplasmic organelles, such as a mitochondrion or a chloroplast, which can replicate and function independently of the nucleus.

***Cytoplasmic streaming or cyclosis.*** The movement of cytoplasm from one region of a cell to another, often in definite currents, thought to be controlled by microfilaments composed of protein similar to actin. Such streaming has several possible functions: (a) transport of substances from one part of the cell to another (e.g, during translocation in sieve tubes); (b) cellular movement (e.g. in pseudopodia of white blood cells); (c) maintenance of optimal temperature; (d) provision of optimal light conditions for chloroplasts (e.g. in mesophyll cells of leaf).

***Cytosine.*** One of four types of nitrogenous bases found in DNA, having the single-ring structure of a class known as pyrimidines. Cytosine forms part of a DNA unit called a nucleotide and always forms complementary pairs with a DNA purine base called a guanine. Cytosine also occurs in RNA molecules.

***Cytosol.*** Soluble phase of cytoplasm, in which small particles, such as ribosomes, and many molecules are suspended or dissolved. It excludes the structured parts of the cytoplasm such as mitochondria, chloroplasts, lysosomes and endoplasmic reticulum, and may be separated from them by ultracentrifugation.

***Cytostatic agent.*** Agent that stops, or supresses, cell growth. The drugs that inhibit bacterial growth are referred to as cytostatic or bacteriostatic antibiotics in contrast to bacteriocidal drugs, which kill bacteria,. Drugs that actually kill eukaryotic cells are termed cytotoxic agents.

***Cytotoxic drug.*** Drug that kills cells. Many antitumour drugs widely used clinically are cytotoxic drugs, and owe their selective antitumourigenic properties to the fact that they are most effective against rapidly dividing cells.

***Cytotoxic T cell.*** T lymphocyte that has the capacity to recognize and kill foreign tissue cells, as in a graft, or cells infected with virus, and therefore carrying novel antigen on its surface.

# D

***2,4-D.*** 2,4-dichlorophenoxyacetic acid: a synthetic auxin frequently used as a weedkiller of broad-leaved weeds. See Figure D.1.

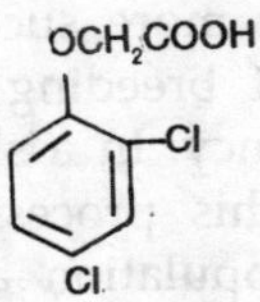


Figure D.1. 2,-4D.

***Dalton.*** A unit of mass used to express molecular weight, based on 1/12 of the mass of the isotope carbon 12 and equal to 1.660 33 x $10^{-27}$ kg. It is also known as the atomic mass unit (amu).

***Dark repair.*** DNA repair carried out by a special type of DNA polymerase in the absence of visible light. The repair involves the enzymatic removal of dimers from the DNA molecule (thymidine dimer formation is a common result of exposure of DNA to radiatin) and synthesis of normal segments to replace those excised.

***Dart sac.*** A sac branching from the vagina of snails which contains a dart that is shot out prior to copulation between two snails, so that the darts from each penetrate the tissues of the other.

***Darwinian selection.*** Selection of organisms within a population on the basis of their increased fitness as compared with the rest of the population. Thus natural selection is deemed to accomplish the 'survival of the fittest'.

***Darwin, Charles Robert.*** (1809-92) English naturalist. His works include: Voyage of the Beagle (1839), On the Origin of Species by means of Natural Selection (1859), and The Descent of Man (1871). He was with wallace, the originator of modern evolutionary theory.

***Darwinism.*** The theory of evolution proposed by Charles Darwin in 1859, in The Origin of Species. His argument runs as follows. All organisms produce more offspring than actually survive; these offspring differ from each other, i.e. they show variations, some of which are heritable. Certain variations enable the individual to survive when the population is acted upon by the forces of natural selection Individuals showing these variations are able to combat the environment more successfully and therefore have a better chance of breeding and passing on their variations to their progency. In a slowly but continuously changing environment this process results in a gradual change in the whole population and, ultimately, in the evolution of new species. Darwin also suggested the importance of sexual selection in evolution.

He based his theory on findings acquired during his voyage around the world in the Beagle (1831-36), compiling evidence from comparative anatomy, palaeontology, geographical distribution, and embryology. A.R. Wallace (1823-1913), working independently of Darwin, arrived at the same theory using evidence from the distribution of related groups of organisms and their natural classification.

Darwin knew nothing of the patterns of Mendelian heredity and the source of the variation on which his theory is based. The modern version of Darwinism, neo-Darwinism, incorporates subsequent discoveries in genetics and cytogenetics. It elucidates the source of variation and stresses the nature and importance of isolating mechanisms and genetic drift in the formation of new species.

The essential points of Darwin's theory are :

(a) in organsims that reproduce sexually there is a wide range of variability, both within and between species.

(b) all living forms have the potential for a rapid rise in numbers, increasing at a geometric rate.

(c) the fact that populations usually remain within a limited size must indicate a 'struggle for existence' in which those individuals unsuited to the particular conditions operating at that time are eliminated or fail to breed as successfully as others.

(d) the struggle for existence results in natural seleciton that favours the survival of the best-adapted individuals, a process described by Herbert Spencer (1920-93) as the 'survival of the fittest' in his Principles of Biology (1865).

***Darwin's finches (Galapagos finches).*** The 14 species of finch, unique to the Gàlapagos Islands, that Charles Darwin studied during his journey on HMS Beagle. Each is adapted to exploit a different food source. They are not found on the mainland because competition there for these food sources from other birds is fiercer. Darwin believed all the Galapagos finches to be descendants of a few that strayed from the mainland, and this provided improtant evidence for his theory of evolution.

***Dauermodification.*** Phenotypic change in a cell that has been environmentally induced (and is therefore not genetic), but persists at least for a time in the daughter cells produced vegetatively. The change will finally disapper by dilution. Damage to mitochondria or chloroplasts by irradiation may persist as a dauermodification.

***Daughter cell.*** Cell resulting from the mitotic division of a parent cell; two daughter cells are formed.

***Davson and Danielli model.*** Model proposed for the strucuture of plasma membranes, which suggested that a unit membrane consisted of a lipid bilayer, with the lipid polar groups facing outwards and each polar surface associated with an outermost layer of protein. The model, although useful in its day, was later superceded by the fluid mosaic model of Singer and Nicholson, in 1972.

***DDT.*** A chlorinated hydrocarbon (dichlorodiphenyltrichloroethane) which acts as a powerful insecticide with long-lasting effects. DDT was the first major insecticide in use. Although DDT is cheap to manufacture, it has produced adverse ecological consequences. Its lack of biodegradability and the fact that it tends to accumulate in fatty tissues has resulted in its transfer from one consumer to another up the food chain, becoming concentrated at each step. One effect of this has been to endanger the top carnivorous birds whose eggshells have become paper-thin because DDT has prevented the mobilization of calcium in the oviduct, so reducing the reproductive potential of many rare species. While these processes have been occurring the target insects have been subjected to strong selection pressure from the DDT, with the result that highly resistant populations now exist, making the insecticide useless in many parts of the world.

***Deamination.*** The removal of the amino group ($NH_2$) from a molecule, as in the release of ammonia ($NH_3$) from amino acids, the residue of which can then enter the krebs cycle, usually via acetyleoenzyme A. The amino group then enters the ornithine cycle.

***Dedifferentiation.*** Reversal of differentiation, in which cells that have been committed and modified to fulfil a particular specialized function lose their specialized character and return to a relatively unspecialized structure and function. Well authenticated examples of dedifferentiation are rare, but the production of poorly differentiated cells of the amphibian limb is widely reported during the formation of a blastema following partial limb amputation. Dedifferentiation, followed by redifferentiation, is commoner in plants than in animls and is evident in callus formation and in many cases of plant vegetative propagation.

***Defective virus.*** Virus that is unable to complete its replicative cycle in the host cell unaided. This may be as a result of a genetic mutation which blocks some part of the replicative process, but some viruses are sytled defective in the wild-type state since they only successfully replicate when another helper virus is also present in the host cell. Such dependence on a second virus involves utilization of some biochemical catalyst such as a polymerase molecule produced only by the second virus.

***Deficiency disease.*** Any condition exhibiting abnormalities produced by lack of a particular component in the diet. Examples include beri-beri (vitamin $B_1$), scurvy (Vitamin C), kwashiorkor (protein deficiency), rickets (vitamin D). Plants can also exhibit conditions brought about by deficiency of minerals. For example, magnesium is required in the synthesis of chlorophyll a lack of the mineral producing chlorosis of the leaves.

***Definitive host.*** Host in which a parasite finally gains sexual maturity. It contrasts with other non-definitive host organisms, in which development can only proceed to a contain stage, at whicht it is blocked by a biochemical or morphological impediment.

***Degeneracy.*** A situation in the genetic code when most amino acids are coded by more than one triplet of DNA nucleotide bases. For example, arginine is coded by CGU, CGC, CGA and CGG codons.

***Degenerate code.*** Genetic code in DNA and RNA in which many words (i.e. amino acids) are each coded for by more than one ODON: for example, both UAC and UAU code for tyrosine. Degeneracy of the code is permitted because there are 64 possible permutations of triplets made from the four different bases, but only 20 amino acids and the 'stop' signa to be coded. In most cases, an observation which has led to the wobble hypothesis, which, in essence, suggests that the molecular recognition site on appropriate transfer RNA moleucle, when associating transiently with the appropriate triplet of bases on the messenger RNA, has some inherent imprecision which can compensate for changes in the third base of the triplet.

***Degrees of freedom (d.f.).*** The number of unrestrcited variables in a frequency distribution, a factor that is of great importance in statistical testing. For example, in a simple chi-squared test the number of degrees of freedom is one less than the number of classes (types) of individuals, one d.f. having been lost due to the assumption that a certain proportion of each class is expected. Thus in testing a 9:3:3:1 ratio there are three degrees of freedom.

***Dehydrogenase.*** An enzyme, such as any of the respiratory enzymes, that catalyses a reaction in which hydrogen is remvoed from a molecule (often to be taken up by the electron transport system). For example, in the krebs cycle the conversion of suiccinice acid to fumaric acid is catalysed by succinate dehydrogenase, the hydrogen released being passed on to FAD.

***Dehydrogenation.*** The removal of hydrogen atoms from a donor molecule, which is oxidized, to a receptor molecule which is reduced, a reaction involving dehydrogenases.

***De Lange Syndrome.*** Congenital malformation in the human characterized by severe mental retardation, limb malformations and early death.

***Deleterious gene.*** An allele of a gene whose effects on the phenotype are likely to result in a reduced fitness. Such genes are often recessive, so that they can be transmitted through families without being detected unless two occur together in the same individual.

***Deletion.*** Loss of a part of a DNA molecule or of a protion of chromatin from a larger molecule or a chromosome. Deletions may range from individual nucleotides to large chromosomal segments, including many gene loci. Loss of part of a chromosome is termed intercalary if it is within the chromosome, or terminal if at the end of a chromosome. Most deletion mutations are lethal if homozygous, but many are viable in the heterozygous condition. Drosophila salivary gland cells in the larva have both homologous chromosomes lying together in register and dletions in the heteroszygous condition can be detected by deletion loops, where the non-deleted part of the homologue is visible as an unpaired loop of chromosome opposite to the deleted segment.

***Deletion mapping.*** The use of overlapping deletions to locate the position of a gene on a chromosome map.

***Deletion method.*** Procedure for isolating messenger RNA (mRNA) specific to a particular gene, involving hybridization of total cellular mRNA to the DNA from a particular cell line, under conditions favouring such hybridization. When the DNA is derived from a cell line with a deletion at a particular locus, the population of mRNA that fails to hybridize is likely to be specific for the gene or genes involved in the deletion.

***Deletion mutation.*** A type of gene mutatin in which genetic material is removed from chromosomes. The deletion can be as small as a single DNA base (which can cause a misreading of the base sequence during protein sunthesis,) to a large peice of chromosome containing many genes. For example, if a chromosome contains the genes ABCDEFGH, the deletion of seciton CD results in the gene sequence ABEFGH. Some deletions can be recognized when chromosomes pair at prophase of meiosis. A loop is formed to allow normal pairing on either side of deleted portion. See Figure D.2.

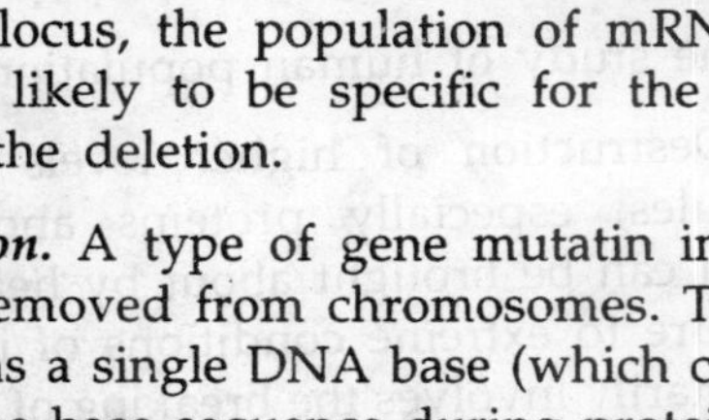


Figure D.2. Deletion observed during pairing of homologous chrmosomes.

***Delta-haemoglobin.*** ($HbA_2$) Comprises between 1.5 and 3.2 percent of the haemoglobin in healthy adult humans. $HbA_2$ has two alpha-globin protein chains and two delta-globin chains, giving an $\alpha_2\delta_2$ formula. The delta-globin gene is found close to the beta-globin gene on chromosome 11.

***Deme or local population.*** A group of individuals within a species that is largely isolated genetically from other individuals of the species, with clealry definable genetical, cytological and other characteristics.

***Demographic transition.*** A theory of demography which states that, as a nation industrializes, it goes through a series of populational changes, starting with a decline in infant and adult mortality and followed later by a reduction in birth rate. The time lag between the decline in deaths and births produces a rapid population growth in 'developing' nations. In 'developed' nations births and deaths become approximately equal, giving a stable population structure.

***Demography.*** The study of human populations.

***Denaturation.*** Destruction of higher levels of structure in macromolecules, especially proteins and nucleic acids. Denaturation can be brought about by heating in solution or by exposure to extreme conditions of ionic strength or pH, and primarily involves the breaking of hydrogen bonds and disruption of hyrophobic interactions. Covalent bonds holding the polymers together are not normally affected. Proteins vary in susceptibility to denaturation depending on their amino acid sequence; nucleic acids are less variable and generally need more extreme conditions than proteins before they denature. Denaturation of nucleic acids amounts to strand separation and is readily reversible, whereas denaturation of proteins is usually irreversible.

***Denatured protein.*** Protein in which secondary, tertiary and quaternary structures have been disupted. A denatured protein consists of polypepitide chains randomly dispersed and not folded into the precise conformations necessary for biological activity. Denatured proteins only very occasionally renature spontaneously when returned to physiological conditions. The best example of protein renaturation after prologned boiling is ribonuclease.

***Denitrification.*** A chemical process in which nitrates in the soil are reduced to molecular nitrogen, which is released into the atomosphere. This process is effected by the bacterium Pseudomonas denitrificans, which uses nitrates as a source of energy for other chemical reactions in a manner similar to respiration in other organisms.

***De novo.*** (1) From a new or unknown source, (2) Indicating synthesis of a complex molecule from simple precursors, as in protein synthesis from AMINO ACIDS, rather than formation of the complex moleucle by small modifications to pre-existing, large molecules.

***Dense bodies.*** Membrane-bound vesicles in cytoplasm of animal cells. They are thought to result from fusion of phagocytotic vacuoles and other pinocytotic vacuoles.

***Density-dependent factor.*** Any factor that regulates the size of a population under natural circumstances by acting more severely on a population when it is large than when it is small. Such factors can affect either the birth rate or the mortality, but the latter is more usual. At high densities of populations some organisms have fewer young, or the mortality rate (brought about by predation, disease or food shortage) might be higher than at low densities. The factors tend to cause population numbers to be maintained at a relatively constant level over long periods of time.

***Density-dependent inhibition of growth.*** Reduction in cell division in vitro and in vivo that results from dense packing of cells due to contact inhibition of movement and ultimately of cell division. In some situations, negative feedback by specific growth inhibitors called chalones may occur.

***Deoxyribonucleoside.*** Compound consisting of a purine or phrimidine base attahced to 2-deoxyribose. When the deoxyribose is phosphorylated the compound is known as a deoxyribonucleotide.

***Deoxyribonucleotide.*** Compound consiting of a purine or pyrimidine base attahced to 2-deoxyribose which is in turn bonded to a phosphate group at either the 3'- or 5'- position. The ability of one phosphate group to form a phosphodiester link between two deoxyribose molecules is the basis for stringing nucleotides together in the polymer DNA. The ends of the polymer are thus charactterized by whether the 3'- or the 5'-position is free. The four commonly occurring bases in deoxyribonucleotides are the purines adenine and guanine and the pyrimidines cytosine and thymine.

***Deoxyribose.*** Sugar which, complexd to a phosphate group and to either a purine or pyrimidine base, goes to form the deoxynucleotides of the DNA molecule.

***Dependent differentiation.*** The differentiation of embryonic tissue initiated from other tissue by organizers. For example, the eye lens on a frog develops under the influence of organizers from the optic cup.

***Depolarization.*** The process of reversing the charge across a cell membrane (usually a neuron), so causing an action potential. In depolarization, the inside of the mebrane, which is noramlly negatively charged, becomes positive and the outside negative. This is brought about by positive sodium ions rapidly passing into the axon. The resisting potential is restored by the sodium pump mechanism. See Figure D.3.

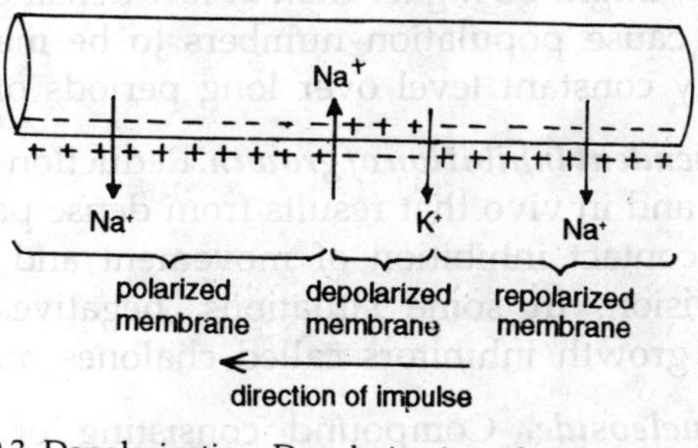


Figure D.3. Depolarization. Depolarization of a nerve fibre.

***Depression.*** Initiation of or increase in transcriptional activity of a gene sequence resulting from the removal of a repressor molecule from the sequence or a neighbouring control sequence. In the case of induced enzyeme synthesis in bacteria, derepression occurs by induction, an inducer molecule binding to the repressor molecule, and so reducing or eliminating its affinity for the controlling operator region of the operon. Depression is an excample of negative control of gene activity, in contrast to positive control in which the inducer or other regulatory molecule interacts with the regulatory or operator sequence and positively induces or enhances the activity of the gene or genes.

***Derived character.*** A characteristic that is considerably altered from the ancestral condition.

***Desensitization.*** In broad terms, loss of sensitivity to a molecule that previously elicited a cellular response; most often applied to situations in which cells lose responsiveness to chemical signal molecules (e.g., hormones or growth factors) to which they previously reacted. Such desensitization (called adaptation in some situations) is believed to result from loss of surface receptor proteins or of other molecules involved in transducing the signal from the cell surface.

***Desmin.*** Accessory protein of muscle myofibrils that probably functions as a bond between adjacent sarcomeres, keeping myofibrils in register in the region of the Z disc of the striated muscle fibre.

***Desmosome.*** (macula adherans). Junctional complex that exists between cells, especially those in tissues such as epithelia which require considerable elastic strength. Two opposed button-like dense plaques exist in each of the two cell membranes, separated by a space of about 25 nm. Bundles of cytoplasmic keratin filaments converge on each of the plaques, and are linked via the junction to the cytoskeletal filaments in adjoining cells. Desmosomes are of three specialized types; belt desmosomes, spot desmosomes and hemidesmosomes.

***Detached x.*** In Drosophila a free X chromosome formed by detachment of the X chromosome arms of a previously attached X chromosome.

***Detergent.*** Amphipathic molecule (i.e. molecule having both lipophilic and hydrophilic parts) that is used in biology to disrupt lipid membrane and solubilize the component lipids and hyrophobic proteins into aqueous media. Non-ionic detergents (e.g. Triton X-100 and octyglucosides) form mixed micelles of detergent-lipid and detergent-lipid-protein, often preserving the native conformaiton of the proteins. Ionic detergents (e.g., deoxycholate, cetyltrimethylammonium bromide and sodium dodecylsulphate (SDS) have a greater tendency to denature enzyems and carrier prteins with consequent loss of activity. However, SDS is deliberately used to denature proteins prior to determination of their molecular weights or subunit composition by SDS-polyacrylamide gel electrophoresis (SDS-page).

***Determinant.*** Part of an antigen molecule that has been responsible for instigating the production of a specific antibody, and which is therefore recognized in binding of such specific antibody.

***Determined.*** Describing cells that are committed to a particular pathway of differentiation; often applied to cells in which there is experimental evidence of commitemnt, but little or no sign of overt differentiation. A striking case of cell determination is found in imaginal disc cells of insect larvae, in which transplanation experiments indicate that commitment to a particular fate can proceed actual differentiation by long periods of time. Determinatin is often assumed to have a molecular basis in gene reguation, but this remains uncertain.

***Deterministic theory.*** (1) In developmental biology, states that after embryonic cells have passed beyond the stage of competence, their fate and differentiation are irreversibly determined and cannot be influenced by external, environmental factors. (2) In general bilogy, states that all expression of the bilogy of an individual, including behaviour and interactions by higher animals, is encoded in the genome.

***Detoxication.*** (detoxification). Chemical modification of toxins in the body by breakdown or by conjugation with other molecules prior to excretion. The liver and kidney are the major orgns of detoxication; within these tissues the peroxisomes are important. The term can be misleading as some compounds are rendered more toxic by metabolic processes (e.g., the 'lethal synthesis' of fluorocitrate from fluoroacetate).

***Deuteranopia.*** Green colour blindness.

***Deuterium oxide.*** ($D_2O$, $^2H_2O$). Heavy water; composed of the hydrogen isotope - deuterium - combined with oxygen. It has been widely used in cytological experimentation, especially in the determination of the structure and function of microtubules and the mitotic spindle.

***Development.*** Broad range of complex changes undergone by an organism during its life-time from its inception, at fertilizaiton, to death. It is not simjply a synonym for embryogenesis, but it includes gametogenesis, fertilization, embryogenesis, growth, regeneration, cell ageing and even some aspects of tumour bilogy. Moreover, the term is now interpreted as being equally applicable to plants and animals. There are several reasons underlying this move towards a collective and integrated approach, but the principlal one has been the general trend away from 19th century descriptive, phenomenological study to experimental investigation seeking to identify causal mechanisms. Conseuqnetly, as developmental phenomena are analysed at the cellular/molecular level, it becomes increasingly apparent that some of the underlying mechanisms and principals are common to all, or most, of the pheonomena.

***Developmental genetics.*** Any or all aspects of genetics within a developmental context. Given the diveristy of meaning of the word genetics and the fact that all the major issues of development ultimately have a genetic basis, the term lacks any precise meaning.

***Devoret test.*** More sensitive version of the ames test, used for detection of potential carcinogens of relatively weak toxicity. The test assay uses lambda phage lysis of previously lysogenic E. coli.

***Dexamethasone.*** Glucocorticoid hormonelike drug often used clinically for suppression of inflammation and inhibition of acth secretion in adrenal hyperplasia.

***DiGeorge syndrome.*** Condition associated .in some patients with a small deletion of chromosome 22. The thymus is absent and some structural abnormality of the aortic arch is common.

***Devonian period.*** A geological period lasting from about 415 to 370 million years ago. Many freshwater fish existed during this period and plants became established on land. True seed plants evolved and lycopods reached the size of trees. Amphibians evolved, the first known insects, spiders and mites occurred and most graptolites became extinct. Britain still lay south of the equator with London at 10°S.

***De Vriesianism.*** The hypothesis that evolution has taken place as a result of drastic mutations, particulary at the species level. The hypothesis was suggested c. 1900 by the Dutch botanist, H. de Vries (1848-1935), who was also responsible for the rediscovery of mendelian genetics.

***Dextran.*** Mucilaginous polysaccharide in the capsule of certain bacteria. Dextrans are polymers ($M_r$ = 30 000 - 250 000) of D-glucose largely a-1.6-linked with a-1.4-links at about every five units and have considerable resistance to enzymic hydrolysis. Dextrans have a variety of uses commercially, therapeutically and in biochemical analysis.

***Dextrin.*** A polysaccharide carbohydrate that may form an intermediate step in the hydrolysis of insoluble starch to soluble glucose, ready for cell respiration, translocation or further synthesis.

***Dextrorotatory.*** (of a crystal, liquid or solution) having the property of rotating a plane of polarized light to the right (e.g. glucose).

***Diabetes (diabets mellitus).*** A disorder of sugar metabolism caused by a lack of the pancreatic hormone insulin. Unutilized glucose accumulates in large quantitites in the blood (hyperglycaemia) and is excreted in the urine (glycosuria) The use of alternative energy sources leads to loss of weight and disturbances in the acid-base balance. There appears to be a hereditary tendency to the disorder, which may be triggered by various factors.

***Diakinesis.*** The final stage in Prophase I of meosis, where the chromosomes reach maximum contraction with the homologous chromosomes tending to separate from each other. The nucleolus disappears, the nuclear membrane degenerates and a spindle is formed of microtubules produced by the centrosomes.

***Dialysis.*** A process by which small molecules can be separated from larger ones using a fine membrane, e.g. collodion, to contain the larger, but which allows the smaller molecules to pass through into the excess water on the other side. The kidney functions by means of this principle, which is also the basis for kidney machines used in cases of kidney disease or failure.

***Diapause.*** A period of suspended development or growth occurring in some insects during which metabolism is greatly decreased. It is often triggered by seasonal changes and regulated by an inborn rhythm and enables the insect to survive unfavourable environmental conditions so that its offspring may be produced in more favourable ones.

***Diastase.*** An enzyme mixture common in seeds such as barley, that is responsible for starch hydrolysis. The mixture contains amylases for conversion of starch to maltose (sometimes via dextrin) and maltase for conversion of maltose to glucose.

***Dichogamy.*** The condition is which the male and female reproductive organs of a flower mature at different times, thereby ensuring that self-fertilization does not occur.

***Dicentric.*** Chromosome or chromatid that possesses two centromeres.

***Dictyosome.*** Complex of cisternae and associated vesicles which together form the golgi apparatus; most often used in relatin to plant cells.

***Dictyostelium discoideum.*** Widely studied organism sometimes referred to as a cellular slime mould and belinging to the Acrasiales. It is probably only distantly related, if at all, to the acellular slime moulds of Myxomycetes (e.g., Physarum). Dictyostelium exists for much of its life history as single-celled amoebae living freely in forest soils, but in the event of desiccation, the amoebae aggregate into a multicellular motile grex or slug, which eventually produces a stalked fruiting body with spores. The differentiation of Dictyostelium cells to make the stalk or the spores of the fruiting body is often cited as one of the simplest models of cell differentiation.

***Dictyotene.*** Prolonged diplotene stage of meiosis which occurs in oocytes during yolk production and accumulation. Chromosomes exhibiting chiasmata may remain in this configuraiton for many months in some species when present in such oocytes.

***Dideoxy sequencing.*** Method for determining the primary sequence of DNA. Single-stranded DNA is copied by DNA polymerase I using the four deoxynucleoside triphosphates, including one radiolabelled with $^{32}P$ and another in the presnence of trace amounts of its 2'-3'-dideoxy equivalent. Four reactions are run in parallel with the four different precursors. Phosphodiester bonds cannot form in the absence of the 3'- hydroxyl group so the reaciton yields oligomers terminating at all the possible sites where the corresponding normal nucleotide should have been incorporated. The reaction products are then separated by electrophoresis into gels, which resolve single nucleotide size differences, and by autoradiography, and the DNA sequence of the original template deduced from the four 'step ladders' of bands thus revealed. Primary sequences several hundred nucleotides long can be determined by a single experiment.

***Dieldrin.*** A chlorinated hydrocarbon that is a powerful insecticide, with long-lasting effects. However, it has become ecologically damaging and is banned from many countries.

***Difference equation.*** (in ecology). An equation that models changes in an organism's population in a stepwise way, often showing generation-by-generation changes. A basic form is : $N_{t+1} = F(N_{tt})$, where $N_t$ is the number of individuals in the population at time t and $N_{t+1}$ is the number at the next stage. F is a function such as a fecundity or mortality parameter. Difference equations are used in population models for orgaisms with distinct generations, such as some insects. For this reason, they are not appropriate for populations of mammals, birds, fish, etc., in which individuals, from several generations exist at the same time.

***Differentiation.*** 1. A phase of growth during which unspecialized cells become specialized for particular functions. The young unspecialized cells of organisms, particularly embryonic or regenerating cells of animals and meristematic cells of plants, adopt specialized functions and structures during growth depending partly on their position in relation to other cells. In this way the tissues and organs of the mature organism are built up. The mechanisms of differentiation are poorly understood; factors such as physical constraints and chemical gradients are probably involved. The fact that a mature differentiated cell can, under suitable conditions, revert to an embryonic undifferentiated state when isolated from its neighbours indicates that differentiation invlves no actual loss of information (in the form of DNA), but rather a masking of irrelevant information.

2. A process used in the preparation of microscope slides of organisms or tissues. It consists of the removal of excessive stain after the staining process and is done by placing the overstained section in acid alcohol.

***DiGeorge syndrome.*** Condition associated in some patients with a small deletion of chromosome 22. The thymus is absent and somje structural abnormality of the aortic arch is common.

***Dihybird.*** 1. An organism that carries two different ALLELES of one gene and two different allels of another gene. For example, character A (controlled by alleles A1 and A2) and character B (alleles B1 and B2). The dihybrid would have the genotype A1A2, B1B2 ie. a double heterozygote. 2. (of a cross) having two parents that have been mated to produce dihybrids that are then also mated. A single dihybrid plant is self-fertilized. Mendel, formulated his law of independent assortment from the results of a dihybrid cross involving pairs of contrasting characters in the pea plant.

***Dihydrofolate reductase.*** (dihydrofolarte dehydrogenase DHFR). Enzyme that catalyses the NADPH-dependent reduction of folate to tetrahydrofolate, an essential cofactor in the synthesis of glycine, purines and thymidine. It is the target of the anticancer drug mèthotrexate. Cells resistant to this drug tend to have the gene coding for DHFR amplified to high copy number.

***Dihydroxyphenylalanine (DOPA).*** Precursor of melanin, and, through the intermediate dopamine, of noradrenaline and adrenaline.

***Dikaryon.*** A fungal hypha with two types of nuclei in an unfused state in the same cells, so that cytologically they are n+n. When the nuclei are from different genetic strains the individual or cell is called a heterokaryon. 2. a single animal celi with two nuclei, each from a different species, e.g. mouse and man.

***Dimethylsulphoxide.*** (DMSO). Compound that destabilizes and partially denatures the double helix of DNA, DMSO has been used to 'induce' activity of specific genes, previously unexpressed, in tissue culture cells.

***Diminution.*** Reduction in the chromosome number of particular cells or tissues. In certain nematodes of the genus Ascaris, some small flies of the family Cecidomyiidae, and in the crustacean Cyclops, the complete chromosome set is retained in the germ line cells but is drastically reduced by chromosome elimination in somatic cells.

***Dimorphism.*** The occurrence of an organism in two forms, e.g. the male and female. Dimorphism can occur in body form or in colour phases, e.g. the two-spotted ladybird which has brown form with four red spots, and a red form with two dark spots dinosaur. An extinct terrestrial reptile belonging to a group that constituted the dominant land animals of the Jurassic and Cretaceous periods, 190-65 million years ago. There were two orders. The Ornithischia were typically quadrupedal herbivores, many with heavily armoured bodies, and included Stregosaurus, Triceratops, and Iguanodon. They were all characterised by bridlike pevic girdles. The Saurischia included many bipedal canivorous forms, such as Tyrannosaurus (the largest known carnivore), and some quadrupedal herbivores forms, such as Apatosaurus (Brontosaurus) and Diplodocus. They all had lizard-like pelvic gridles. Many of the herbivorous dinosaurs were amphibious or semiaquatic.

***Dinosaur.*** Any extinctreptile of the orders Saurischia and Ornithischia. Dinosaurs (the name means 'fearful lizard') were the dominant form of land vertebrates during the jurassic and cretaceous periods.

***Dinucleotide.*** A compound formed of two nucleotides.

***Dioecious.*** (of plants) the occurrence of male flowers in one individual and female flowers in another individual, for example, willow. The term literaly means 'two homes'.

***Dipeptide.*** The product of joining together two amino acids by a condensation reaction forming a peptide bond. See Figure D.4.

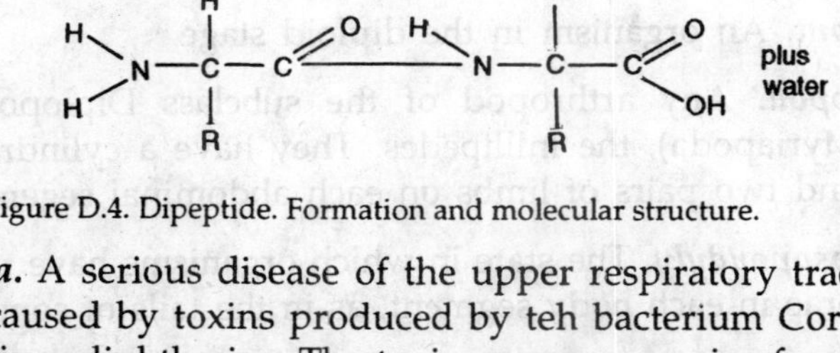


Figure D.4. Dipeptide. Formation and molecular structure.

***Diphtheria.*** A serious disease of the upper respiratory tract in man caused by toxins produced by teh bacterium Corynebacterium diphtheriae. The toxins cause necrosis of epithelial cells in the throat, resulting in the production of a greyish exudate that gradually forms a membrane on the tonsils and can spread upwards into the nasal passages, or downwards into the larynx causing suffocation if not treated.

***Diplochromosome.*** Aberrant chromosome consisting of four chromatids resulting from failure of the centromere to divide and consequent failure of the daughter chromosomes to separate.

***Diploid.*** Describing cells, tissues and organisms in which each chromosome is present as two copies (except for the sex chromosomes). Diploidy results from fusion of the haploid egg and sperm cells and is maintained as the normal state in most eukaryotic cells other than some groups of fungi and algae. Some cells become polyploid in certain specialized tissues of some organisms.

***Diploid.*** (of a cell nucleus) containing two of each type of chromosome in homolgous paris and formed as a result of sexual reproudction. 2. An organism in which the main life stage has cell nuclei with two of each type of chromosome, written as 2n. Diploid stages occur in all eucaryotes, apart from certain fungi, and allow a greater degree of genetic variability in individuals than the haploid (2) state (n).

***Diploid condition.*** State of being diploid; frequently applied to certain stages of the life cycle of some primitive plants such as mosses and ferns in which there is a conspicuous alternation of generation between a diploid phase and a haploid phase.

***Diplonema.*** Chromosome structure during the diplotene stage of meiosis.

***Diplont.*** An organism in the diploid stage.

***Diplopod.*** Any arthropod of the subclass Diplopoda (class Myriapoda), the millipedes. They have a cylindrical body and two pairs of limbs on each abdominal segement.

***Diplosopondyly.*** The state in which organisms have two vertebrae in each body segment, as in the tails of some fish.

***Diplotene.*** A stage of meiosis near the end of Prophase 1, in which the chromatids become separated (except at the chiasmata), and the chromosomal material is contracting. The chiasmata indicate that crossing over is taking place.

***Directed mutation.*** Selective mutation of a particular gene sequence or class of sequences. Such mutations may be achieved by the use of drugs which have a particular affinity for the sequence in question (e.g., active as compared to inactive gene sequences) or which tend to alter permanently the stage of differentiation of cells in culture. Site-directd mutation refers to the.manipulation of cloned DNA sequences by enzymic means so that specific base changes are intorudced into a defined sequence.

***Direct repeat sequence.*** Identical or near athentical sequence of DNA present as two or more copies in the same orientation in the same molecule. Such sequences need not be adjacent.

***Directional selection.*** The selection of a character in one direction, e.g. towards larger size, that may occur as a result in a change in environment. For example, if another ice age was imminent then temperature would fall and the overall size of warm-blooded vertebrates living in a particular region would probably increase.

***Disaccharide.*** A 'double' sugar, such as maltose or lactose, with the general formula $C_{12}H_{22}O_{11}$, synthesized by a condensation reaction joining together two monosaccharide sugars. See Figure D.5.

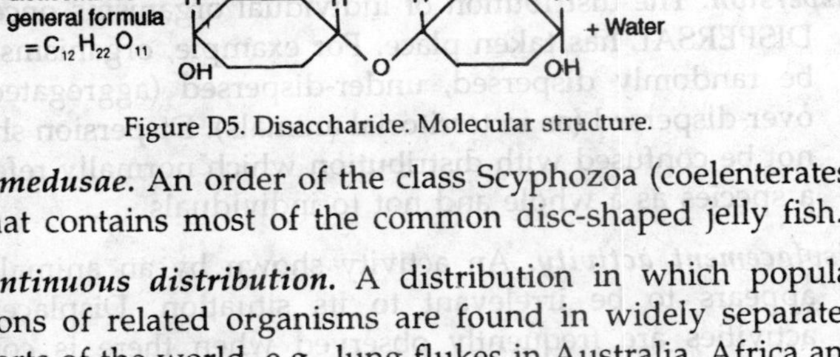


Figure D5. Disaccharide. Molecular structure.

***Discomedusae.*** An order of the class Scyphozoa (coelenterates) that contains most of the common disc-shaped jelly fish.

***Discontinuous distribution.*** A distribution in which populations of related organisms are found in widely separated parts of the world, e.g., lung flukes in Australia, Africa and

South America. Such a distribution is thought to indicate the great age of the group, with intermediate populations having become extinct.

***Discontinuous variation.*** A variation in which different forms of a character fall clearly into a particular grouping without overlapping each other, and are often controlled by a small number of major genes. For example, white and red eye colours in fruiflies.

***Discordance.*** Any difference in a character between individuals due to genetic differences, as may occur in dizyogotic twins, but not usually in monozygotic twins.

***Disease.*** An abnormality of an animal or plant caused by a pathogenic organism that affects performance of the vital functions and usually gives diagnostic symptoms.

***Disease resistance.*** The ability of some organisms to withstand the attach of pathogens and remain virtually unaffected. The resistance can occur naturally but may be enhanced in a population by artificial selection, as in plant and animal breeding. For example, the breeding of varieties of tomatoes resistant to the fungal disease that produces brownroot rot.

***Disjunction.*** The separation of homologous chromosomes to opposite poles during anaphase of nuclear division, particularly meiosis. Abnormalities in disjunction can lead to a chromosomal mutation in which daughter cells possess too many or too few chromosomes. In humans extra autosomes can result in severely abnormal individuals.

***Dispersion.*** The distribution of individual organisms once any DISPERSAL has taken place. For example, organisms may be randomly dispersed, under-dispersed (aggregated) or over-dispersed (as in territorial animals). Dispersion should not be confused with distribution which normally refers to a species as a whole and not to individuals.

***Displacement activity.*** An activity shown by an animal that appears to be irrelevant to its situation. Displacement activities are frequently observed when there is conflict between opposing tendencies. For example, birds in aggressive situations, in which there are simultaneous tendencies to attach and to flee, may preen their feathers as a displacement activity.

***Display behaviour.*** Stereotyped movement or posture that serves to influence the behaviour of another animal. Many displays in courtship and aggression are conspicuous and characteristic of the species; special markings or parts of the body may be prominently exhibited (for example, the male peacock spreads its tail in courtship). Other displays are cryptic and make it harder for a predator to recognize the displaying animal as potential prey. For example, geometer moth caterpillars, which look like twigs, hold themselves on plant stems with one end sticking into the air.

***Disruptive selection.*** The selection in favour of phenotypic extremes in a population. Disruptive selection produces divergence between subpopulations.

***Disassortative mating.*** Mating system within a variable population in which an individual of one phenotype preferentially chooses to mate with individuals of differing phenotype.

***Discoidal cleavage.*** Cell cleavage in early embryos where the cells rest as a flat disc on top of a very large mass of yolk.

***Discontinuous replication.*** Synthesis of short okazaki fragements of DNA on the lagging strand during DNA replication.

***Disjunction.*** Separation of chromosomes at the anaphase stage of mitosis or meiosis.

***Disposable soma.*** A geting theory, proposed by Kirkwood and Holliday, which states that an organism's investment in reproductive capacity must not be exceeded by its investment in repair processes. Natural selection tends to favour cessation of repair processes (resulting in senescence) when investment in repair exceeds investment in reproduction.

***Dissociation constant.*** (pK). The relationship between protondonor and protonacceptor molecules in solution. The pK equation allows determination of the ratio of ionized to non-ionized groups in solution.

***Dissociation element.*** ($D_5$). Transposable genetic element identified in maize; socalled because in addition to producing variegation of colour pattern of maize kernel, it also causes chromosome breakage.

***Diversifying selection.*** (Disruptive selection). Mating system in which matings between dissimilar phenotypes are favoured, leading to increased heterozygosity in the population and persistence or spread of phenotypic variation.

***Diversity.*** An attribute of ecological communities. Diversity can be measured credely by the number of species present but this takes no account of their relative rarity or abundance. One type of diversity measure records the number of individuals and the number of species (e.g. the a-index of Williams). Others quantify the apportioning of individuals between species (e.g. the Shannon-Wiener index).

***Diversity (D) region.*** A sequence of amino acids that is unique to particular immunoglobulins, enabling the molecule to act as an antibody against specific antigens.

***Diversity index.*** A single integrated measure that expresses the diversity of a particular community of organisms, e.g. freshwater invertebrates. The index can be related to the level of pollution in an ecosystem, and the greater the diversity, the less the pollution.

***Division.*** 1. A major grouping in plant classification. 2. The process of the formation of daughter cells from a parent cell.

***Dizygotic twins or fraternal twins.*** A pair of children born at the same time to the same mother but each developing from a different egg. Such twins are therefore nonidentical, being equivalent to normal siblings, and can be of the same or different sexes.

***D-loop (displacement loop).*** A structure occurring in DNA at the beginning of replicaiton in which a short length of DNA is displaced from its complementary strand by a length of newly synthesized DNA. The structure is visible in the electron microscope as a 'bubble', single-stranded on one side and double-stranded on the other. See Figure D.6.

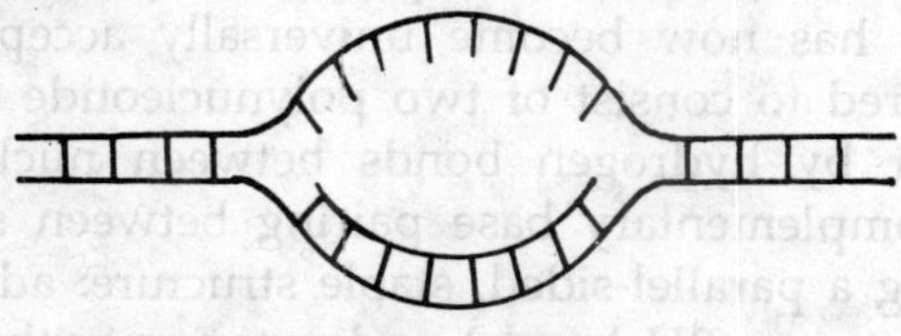

Figure D.6. D-loop.

I ***loop.*** (displacement loop). Structure produced in replicating DNA when 'bubble' or 'eye' of DNA is formed and cna be visualized in the electron microscope. The production of the loop results from the DNA being double-stranded on one side of the bubble and single-stranded on the other, and it is exploited as a technique to demonstrate hybridization of an exogenous sequence to one of the complementary strands, leaving the other displaced strand looping out from the helix. See Figure D.7.

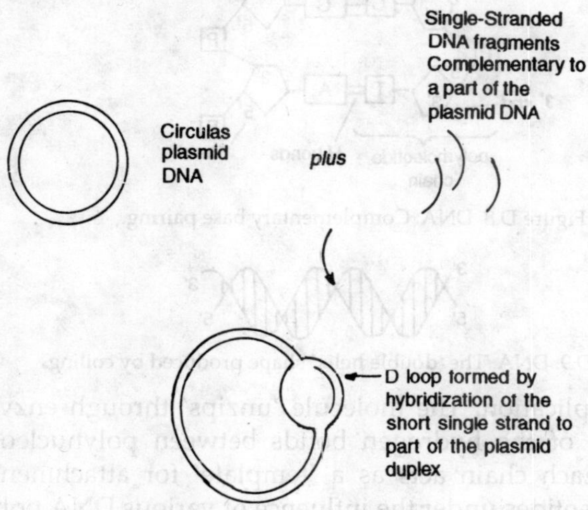


Figure D.7. D loop.

I ***A (deoxyribonucleic acid).*** A complex nucleic acid molecule found in the chromosomes of almost all organisms, which acts as the primary genetical material, controlling the structure of proteins and hence influencing all enzyme-driven reactions.

(a) Structure. The model proposed by Watson and Crick in 1953 has now become universally accepted. DNA is considered to consist of two polynucleotide chains joined together by hydrogen bonds between nucleotide bases, with complementary base pairing between specific bases ensuring a parallel-sided, stable structure: adenine pairing with thymine (2H bonds) and cytosine with guanine (3H bonds). See Figure D.8. The two polynucleotide chains each have an opposite polarity due to the way the phosphates are attached to the sugar, and the whole, molecules is twisted into a double helix shape, with a complete turn every 10th base. See Figure D.9.

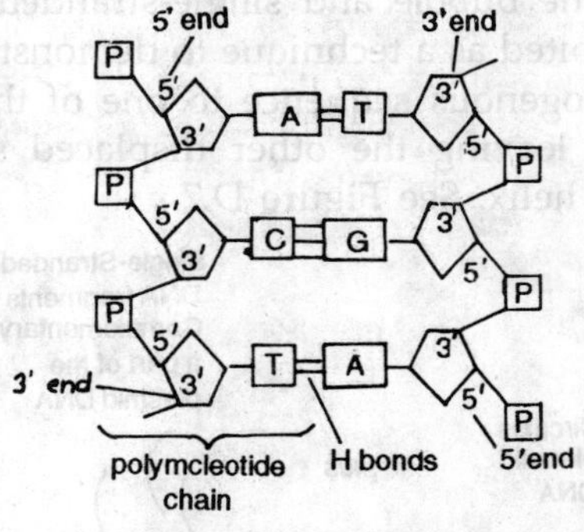


Figure D.8. DNA. Complementary base pairing.

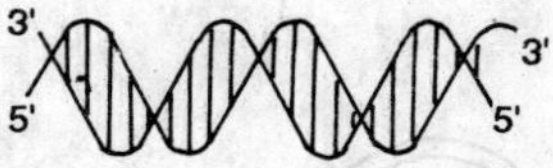


Figure D.9. DNA. The 'double helix' shape produced by coiling.

(b) Replication. The molecule 'unzips' through enzymic breakage of the hydrogen bonds between polynucleotide chains. Each chain acts as a 'template' for attachment of free nucleotides under the influence of various DNA polymerases working in the 5' to 3' direction only. See Figure D.10.

(c) Location. DNA is found in all chromosomes except those of certain viruses (e.g. tobacco mosaic virus, TMV), where the heritable material is RNA. In procaryotes, DNA is in the form of a single coiled molecule in a continuous loop and may also occur as extra-chromosomal material in the cytoplasm. In eucaryotes, the DNA is also highly coiled but is complexed with basic and acidic proteins. There is probably only one very long DNA molecule per chromosome. DNA is also found in chloroplasts and mitochondria of eucaryote cytoplasm.

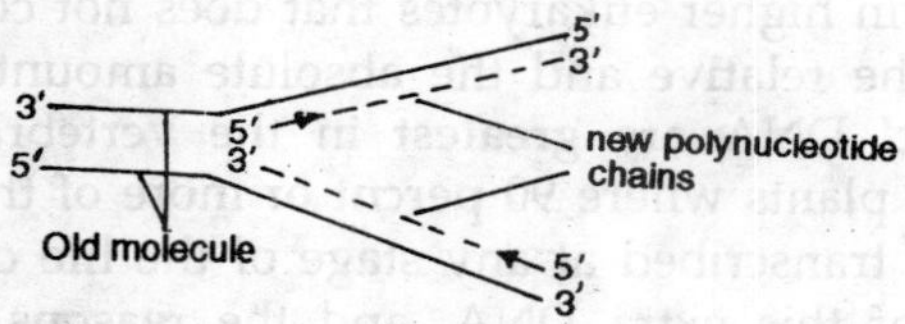


Figure D.10. DNA. Replication.

(d) DNA as a genetic material. there are several pieces of evidence to suggest the role of DNA in inheritance; (i) transformation experiments with Pneumococcus in 1928, by F. Griffith; (ii) the identification of 'transforming principle' as DNA by Avery, MacLeod and McCarty in 1944; (iii) the fact that the wavelength of ultraviolet light which causes most mutations in various procaryotes and eucaryotes matches the absorption spectrum of nucleic acids (260nm); (iv) Hershey and Chase's experiment with labelled bacteriophage. DNA has several features which make it an ideal genetic material: great stability; accurate replication so that all cells contain an identical copy of information; four nucleotide bases providing storage of coded information; it is capable of mutation by altering the base sequence; it may be broken and rejoined to form new genetic combinations; stored information can be accurately 'read' by other cell molecules.

*DNA, genomic.* DNA of the genome, which, in bacteria, is a single, circular loop, and in eukaryotic cells is the entire haploid nuclear complement of DNA. Non-genomic DNA includes, in bacteria, the DNA of plasmids, and in eukaryotes the DNA of viruses or other contaminants. Note that in eukaryotes the mitochondrial genome and chloroplast genome are often considered separately from the nuclear genome.

***DNA, native.*** Double-stranded, non-denatured DNA in a preparation that has been extracted from a particular known biological source - viral, bacterial, or eukaryotic tissue - as distinct from any additional material added as a probe or marker.

***DNA, selfish.*** Speculative term for some or all of the DNA found in higher eukaryotes that does not constitute genes. Both the relative and the absolute amounts of this 'non-genetic' DNA are greatest in the vertebrates and some higher plants where 90 percnt or more of the genome may not be transcribed at any stage of the life cycle. The functions of this extra DNA, and the reasons underlying its persistence and evolutionary expansion in hgiher organisms, have become matters for debate and speculation. Replication of so much nucleic acid represents a considerable burden to the cell in terms of supplying nucleotide substrates and the provision of energy for polymerizaiton and packaging into chromatin with histones and other chromosomal proteins. Such a burden would probably only be borne if this DNA has a function as yet unrecognized, or if the cell has no mechanism for preventing the proliferation of inherently useless sequences. It is in the latter context that Crick and others have coined the term selfish DNA. The idea is that such sequences may have evolved by selection for an intrinsic propensity to be replicated by the host cell's polymerization machinery and not because they yield any benefit to the cell or organism in which they exist. They would thus be parasitic, surviving and spreaidng up to a limit beyond which their replication would adversely affect the host's survival prospects.

***DNA cloning.*** Technique whereby DNA from one source is inserted into a cloning vector and then introduced into a host bacterium. The DNA for cloning may be prepared by partial or total digestion with restriciton endonucleases and inserted into a cloning vector that has been cleaved by the same restriction endonuclease, or an enzyme that yields complementary single-stranded termini. Alternatively DNA may be prepared for insertion by mechanical shearing, deoxyribonuclease digestion or tailing. Losse ends are religated using DNA ligase to produce a coherent recombinant DNA molecule. Recombinant DNA molecules are introduced into a host bacterium (usually E. coli) by transformation if a plasmid vector is used, or if the cloning vector is bacteriophage-based by transfection or infection (following in vitro pack.)

***DNA-driven reaction.*** Reaction in which nucleic acid hybridization is utilized in an experimental situation, and complementary DNA is greatly in excess of a radioactive tracer RNA. The RNA is thus forced to compete with a much greater proportion of hybridizing DNA, and thus will bind cheifly to highly repetitious DNA sequences.

***DNA duplex.*** Double helix of DNA. Single-stranded DNA can be produced by the controlled denaturation of double-stranded DNA.

***DNA fingerprinting.*** Technique in which the banding pattern of DNA fragments is compared and can be used in many species including the human, to indicate relatedness. DNA is digested with restriction enzymes, run on an electrophoretic gel, and blots made from the gel. Such blots are then hybridized with radiolabelled probe DNA consisting of cloned sequences of the short interspersed repeat sequences (such as the alu sequences in the human) which are common in vertebrate genomes. Autoradiography then provides a distinct banding pattern of DNA fragments containing such DNA sequences.

***DNA gyrase.*** (swivelease). Enzyme that increases or introduces positive supercoiling in covalently closed circular DNA molecules generated by DNA replication. This is achieved by breakage of at least one DNA strand followed by untwisting and subsequent resealing of the duplex. DNA gyrase is an alternative term for a type II topoisomerase.

***DNA polymerase.*** A group of three types of enzymes that are responsible for the attachment of free nucleotides onto the unzipped DNA molecule during DNA replication. The first DNA polymerase was discovered by A. Kornberg in

1957 (for which work he received the Noble Prize), although it now appears that this enzyme is not the main one in the group, but rather helps to repair DNA after damage.

***DNA hybridization.*** A method of determining the similarity of DNA from different sources. Single strands of DNA from two sources, e.g. different bacteiral species, are put together and the extend to which double hybrid strands are formed is estimated. The greater the tendency to form these hybrid molecules, the greater the extent of complementary base sequences, i.e. gene similarity. The method is one way of determining the genetic relationships of species.

***DNA library.*** (DNA bank). Collection of cloned DNA fragments that represents part or all of the genome of an organism. Most libraries are partial simply as a result of the method of formation and the comparative rarity of some gene sequences. Genomic and cDNA libraries differ in that the former comprises pieces of genomic DNA and therefore include introns and non-coding sequences, whereas the latter, being complementary to mRNA, contain only coding sequences.

***DNA ligase.*** An enzyme responsibel for bonding the newly inserted nucleotides together during cellular DNA synthesis, so yielding a long polymer of nucelotides. The enzyme is now widely used in genetic engineering to join together reassociated DNA with overlapping ends.

***DNA ligation.*** Joining of adjacent nucleotides in a strand of DNA by the formaiton of a phosphodiester bond. The prcess is catalysed by DNA ligases and occurs during DNA replication and DNA repair, and in recombinant DNA technology.

***DNA melting.*** Denaturation of double-stranded DNA to yield single-stranded DNA. Melting, which can be induced by increased temperatures when DNA is dissolved in a suitable salt solution, results in a reduction of viscosity and an increase in ultraviolet absorption. This increase in light absorption is the hyperchromic effect. Melting can be followed by annealing or renaturation, which involves specific hybridization between sister strands and is used in the derivation of cot plots.

***DNA methylation.*** Attachment of a methyl group to cytosine residues of eukaryotic DNA to form 5-methylcytosine. Usually the cytosine residues that become methylated are in a C-G pair in the DNA. In prokaryotes and lower eukaryotes, some adenine residues are also methylated. DNA methylation is a post-replicational modificaiton to the DNA, and in bacterial cells the methylation of the genomic DNA serves to preserve it from the attack by native restriction endonucleases which rapidly degrade invading viral DNA. Thus the restriction/modificaiton system of bacteira uses DNA modification system of bacteria uses DNA methylation as a protective measure to ensure preservation of the genome and destruction of foreign DNA.

In cells of some eukaryotes (e.g. Drosophila) no methylation has been detected, but in higher eukaryotes much of the DNA contains a proportion of methylcytosine residues. There is a strong, but not absolute, correlation between high levels of methylation and transcriptional inactivity. The pattern of methylation in a sequence is normally passed on faithfully at DNA replication (through preference of DNA methylase for half-methylated sites), but can be inhibited by the addition of the base analogue 5'-azacytidine.

There is also evidence that methylation of cytosine residues in DNA may fundamentally change the conformation of the double helix, leading to a preferential transition from B form to Z form (left-handed DNA).

***DNA modification.*** Alteration of DNA in which particular bases have additional side groups added to them by the action of specific enzymes. The best-known modificaiton to DNA is methylation, which is used to protect genomic DNA from attack by restriction endonuclease enzymes in bacteria. In eukaryotes, methylation of certain bases is involved in the synthesis of transfer RNA and there is also evidence that rarely transcribed sequences are frequently rich in methylated bases.

***DNA-protein interaction.*** Molecular interaction that is a crucial aspect of living systems, both to form stable complexes such as nucleosomes, and transient ones involving RNA polymerases and DNA polymerases and gene regulatory proteins.

***DNA repair.*** A process carried out by specific enzymes (including DNA polymerases and ligases) that reducés the damage to a DNA base sequence inflicted by radiation and other mutagenic agents. The fact of DNA repair implies that the genetically effective mutation rate is much lower than the initial rate of mutation. DNA repair is a rather complex process involving different mechanisms, some being enhanced by light and others occurring in the absence of light.

***DNA replication.*** Process of DNA synthesis whereby a parent DNA molecule is faithfully copied, giving rise to two identical daughter molecules. DNA replication is semiconservative.

Polymerization of the nucleotides forming the new strand is catalysed by DNA polymerase, and a number of steps are involved. Firstly, the double helix is destablized and opened up to permit each strand to serve as a template for the polymerase enzyme. Secondly, a short primer sequence of RNA is synthesized first, followed by the DNA sequence. The RNA primer is later cleaved out and replaced with DNA,. Lastly the DNA is replicated only in one direction since the DNA strands are polarized, synthesis proceeding from a 5'-to a 3'-direction, that is the parent strand is read in the 3'- to 5'-direction. The last observation introduces a complication, since only one of the two parent strands can continuously read in the required direction. In order to overcome this the new DNA on the so-called lagging strand is synthesized discontinuously in short okazaki fragments, later to be joined up by DNA ligases. Synthesis on the leading strand appears to be continuous. This pattern of DNA replication is followed in both prokaryotes and eukaryotes but, in prokaryotes, where the bacteirla genome is circular, synthesis poceeds from a single initiation point in both directions round the circle. DNA synthesis is also continuous throughout the prokaryotic cell cycle. In contrast, eukaryotic DNA synthesis is discontinuous, and proceeds only during the S phase of the cell cycle. The DNA is replicated from many separate initiation points along the length of a chromosome, again in both directions, and eventually the separate replicons join up to yield the two complete daughter strands. See Figure D.11.

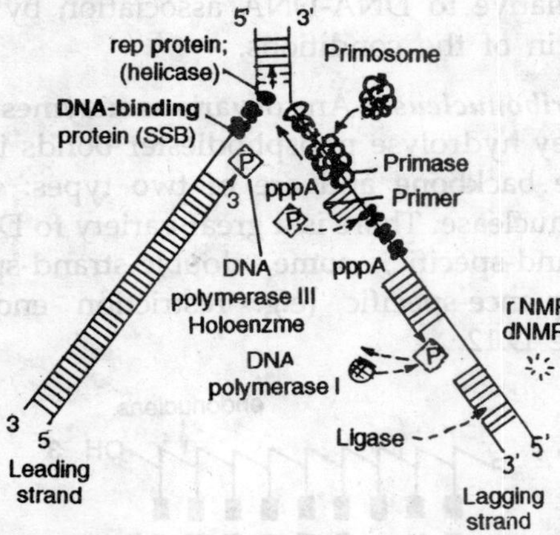


Figure D.11. DNA replication. Scheme for enzymes operating at one of the forks in the bidirectional replication of an E. coli chromosome.

***DNA restriction endonuclease.*** Most important class of restriction 'endonucleases, class II, which cut double-stranded DNA molecules only at sites characterized by a specific nucleotide sequence. Restriction enzymes are isolated from bacterial cells, and are tools for molecular biologists. Several hundred restriction enzymes are now known, each with a specific sequence requirement dictating where it will cut DNA. Most recognize sequences between four and six base pairs long, which in turn are likely to occur by chance once every few hundred to once every few thousand nucleotides along a DNA molecule. Some, such as Hin dIII, make staggered cuts leaving 'sticky ends' three nucleotides long protruding on one strand from each severed terminus; others make clean cuts in both strands at the same place and thus generate 'blunt ends'. Digesting DNA with a restriction enzyme therefore creates a characteristic set of fragments, which can be isolated by electrophoresis and subsequently analysed.

***DNA-RAN hybridization.*** Pairing of DNA with RNA molecules by specific hydrogen bonding between complementary bases. DNA-RNA association by annealing can be favoured relative to DNA-DNA association by appropriate manipulatin of the conditions.

***DNase (deoxyribonuclease).*** Any of various enzymes that degrade DNA. They hydrolyse phosphodiester bonds in the sugar-phosphate backbone and are of two types: exonucleases and endonuclease. There is a great variety fo DNases, some single-strand-specific, some double-strand-specific, and some sequence-specific (e.g. restriction endonucleases). See Figure D.12.

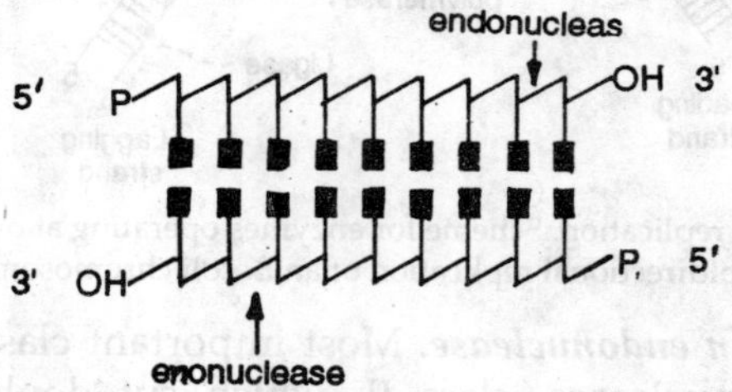


Figure D.12. Sites of action of DNases.

***DNA sequencing.*** The determination of the sequence of bases along a length of DNA. The first complete nucleotide sequence of a naturally occurring nucleic acid, alanine transfer RNA, was published in 1965, since when the technical difficulties of DNA sequencing have been greatly reduced. Cloning of DNA in bacteria has provided an easy and reliable method of purification. Restriction endonucieases are used not only to remove the sequence from the cloning plasmid but also to dissect it into a number of fragements of managebale size. DNA fragments are then isolated by gel electrophoresis and the order of bases in each short fragment determined directly by the selective parallel use of $^{32}P$-labelled nucleoside triphosphates.

***DNA shearing.*** Process whereby the extremely long molecules of high-molecular-weight DNA are reduced in size by mechanical tearing. Such shearing may be an accidental result of too vigorous stirring of a highly purified DNA sample by sharp blades, or may be international in order to reduce molecular weight to manageable proportions prior to cot plot experiments, using, for example, a waring blender.

***DNA splicing.*** Ligation of DNA in vitro by use of DNA ligases. The DNA must be double-stranded, but both blunt-end ligation and cohesive end ligation are possible.

***DNA vector.*** System, such as a plasmid or a virus, that is used as a vehicle to transfer DNA from one cell to another.

***Dollo's law of irreversibility.*** A principle formulated by the Belgian palaeontologist L. Dollo, stating that a structure once lost in evolution cannot be regained.

***Domain.*** Distinct region of a protein or segment of a polypeptide that can be recognized in the three-dimensional structure (as in dehydrogenases) or separated by chemical treatment (as in antibody domains). This has led to the domain hypothesis, which proposes that evolutionary generation of families of proteins has occurred by splicing the exon for one aspect of the protein fuction with a series of genes for other aspects (e.g., several dehydrogenases have very similar domains for NAD+ binding combined with varying structures for catalysis and binding the other substrate). This would be a very simple and powerful mechanism for the evolution of different enzymes and spreading adaptive advantages to different proteins.

***Dominance.*** 1. A genetic interaction where one allele of a gene masks the expression of an alternative allele in the heterozygote, so that the phenotype is of that form controlled by the dominant allele. For example, gene A has two alleles A1 and A2 :

A1/A2 = black phenotype
A2/A2 = white phenotype

but when heterozygous, A1/A2=black phenotype. Thus A1 is dominant to A2, with A2 'recessive' to A1. In molecular terms, the A1 allele is coding for a protein of such quality and quantity to allow the normal amount of black pigment to the produced, even though the A2 allele is not coding for a normal enzyme. 2. The preponderance of one species within an ecological community, for example, oaks in oak woods.

***Dominance hierarchy.*** A pehonomenon in animal societies where some members are subordinate to others, giving a reproductive advantage to the less subordinate members.

***Dominant.*** 1. (in genetics) Describing the allele that functions when two different alleles of a gene are present in the cells of an organism. For example, the height of garden peas is controlled by two alleles, 'tall' (T) and 'dwarf (t). When both are present (Tt), i.e. when the cells are heterozygous, the plant is tall since T is dominat and t is recessive. 2. (in ecology) Describing the most conspicously abundant and characterstic species in a community. The term is usually used of a plant species in plant ecology; for example, pine trees in a pine forest. 3. (in animal behaviour) Describing an animal that is allowed priority in access to food, mates, etc., by others of its species because of its success in previous aggressive encounters. Less dominant animals frequently show appeasement behaviour towards a more dominant individual, so overt aggression is minimized. In a stable group there may be a linear dominance hierachy or peck order (so called because it was first observed in domestic fowl), with each animal being subservient to those above it in the hierarchy and taking precedence over those below it.

***Dominant epistasis.*** A form of pistasis in which dominant allelles of one gene can cause a masking effect on the expression of alleles at another locus. Such an interaction would produce a dihybrid (1) ratio of 12:3:1 instead of the more normal 9:3:3:1.

***Dominant species.*** The commonest species in a community.

***Donor splicing site.*** Splicing site at the right-hand 3'-end of an exon in mRNA and the left-hand end of the next intron.

***DOPA decarboxylase.*** Enzyme that catalyses the decarboxylation of L-DOPA to dopamine.

***Dopamine.*** Catecholamine transmitter in the brain. Low levels of this neurotransmitter are associated with the neurological disorder Parkinson's disease, and overproduction is associated with psychological disorders such a schizophrenia. DOPA is also the biosynthetic precursor of noradrenaline (norepinephrine) and adrenaline (epinephrine).

***Dorsal.*** Situated at or near the back, or to that part of an animal which is normally directed upwards (backwards in the human).

***Dormacy.*** A state in which seeds and other structures (such as underground stems) reduce their metabolic activities to a minimum level during unfavourable conditions (e.g. low temperature, drought) so as to survive until conditions improve. In fungal spores dormancy can be exogenous, requiring an external stimulus for germination (e.g. presence of nutrients) or endogenous, where dormancy is controlled by an innate property of the spore and is unaffected by the ambient environment when in this state.

***Dormin.*** A growth-inhibiting substance found in buds of plants undergoing dormancy, with a chemical structure identical to abscisic acid.

***Dosage compensation.*** A genetical mechanism in which alleles of a gene automatically regulate the amount of a useful product produced, so that homozygous-dominant genotypes produce the same amount of gene product as heterozygotes. In this way the two genotypes cannot be distinguished. Dosage compensation occurs regularly in female mammals where one X-chromosome in each cell is thought to become inactivated, leading to equal amounts of gene products in males and females.

***Double cross.*** A method of plant breeding in which four different inbred lines are crossed together (A x B and C x D) and the progenies crossed again [(A x B) x (C x D)] to produce a four-way hybrid seed with good vigour.

***Double crossover.*** Two separate crossing-over events occurring between chromatids. In a test cross involving three genes, progeny that have carried out this process can be identified and usually from the least frequent type of offspring.

***Double fertilization.*** The situation in flowering plants where a male nucleus combines with the egg nucleus and another male nucleus combines with the primary endosperm to form an endosperm nucleus.

***Double recessive.*** Organism that is either homozygous for a recessive gene (or more correctly for a recessive allele of a gene) and therefore expresses the gene (or allele) in its phenotype. More frequently, the term refers to the presence of recessive alleles of two different genes simultaneously present.

***Double X.*** Double-length X chromosome in Drosophila that arises as a radiation-induced mutation. Unlike the commoner attached X chromosome, which have a medium centromere, double X chromosomes have a terminal centromere.

***Doubling dose.*** Amount of radiation necessary to increase the mutation rate to twice its original or background level.

***Double recessive.*** An organism that is homozygous for a recessive gene and therefore phenotypically shows the effect of this gene. It is only in double recessives that the effect of a recessive gene appears in the phenotype. Double recessives are important in back-cross breeding experiments.

***Doubling time.*** (in microbiology) the time in which the number of cells in a population doubles.

***Down.*** Describing a mutation in the promoter which decreases the frequency of transcriptional initiation.

***Down's syndrome or mongolism.*** A human abnormality caused by the presence of an extra autosome (number 21) in the chromosome complement of each cell. The main features of the syndrome are: mental retardation, short stature with stubby fingers, characteristic slanting eyes (hence 'mongolism') and heart defects. The abnormality arises in the mother's egg as a rule, with older mothers having a far higher chance of producing abnormal ova than younger mothers. This may be because the mother's eggs have.been part-way through Prophase 1 of meiosis since birth, so that eggs of older mothers have been at risk of nondisjunction much longer than those of younger mothers. Down's syndrome is the most common chromosomal abnormality in humans, with an incidence of 1 in 600 live births.

***Downstream.*** Further along a DNA sequence in the direction of sequence transcription or read out, that is, travelling in a 3'- to 5'-direction along the template strand of the DNA or 5'- to 3'- direction along the RNA transcript.

***DPN.*** Diphosphopyridine nucleotide.

***Driver DNA.*** Excess DNA used in a DNA driven reaction.

***Drosophila.*** Genus of some hundreds of species of two-winged flies, also called fruitflies, which have been extensively used in genetic experimentation. The most frequently used species is Drosophila melanogaster, Drosophila is easily cultured in the labouratory, has a short generation time, and has the unusual feature of possessing polytenee chromosomes in the nuclei of some larvel tissues (e.g., salivary glands). Such chromosomes permit microscopical visualization of many genetic conditions, including deletions and inversions, and greatly simplify the construction of linkage maps and assignment of gene loci.

***Dryopithecus.*** A genus of extinct apes, fossils of which have been found in India and dated as 30-40 million years old. Fossils of Dryopithecus and of the similar genus Proconsul are often referred to as dryopithecines. Dryopithecines are believed ot be either the ancestors of the fossil hominids or ancestral to both the human and ape lines.

***Duffy alleles.*** Alleles that determine erythrocyte antigen frequently used as a genetic marker in studies of human population genetics. These alleles are common in Chinese populations and are rate in those of black Africans.

***Duplex DNA.*** DNA in the double-stranded form, forming a double helix as described in the Watson-Crick model, that is with the two polynucleotide chains lying in opposite 3'- to 5'-polarities, intertwined and hydrogen-bonded together. Such DNA can be made single-stranded by dnnaturation or DNA melting.

***Duffy blood group.*** A red blood cell antigen found in certain human racial groups, controlled by a single autosomal gene on chromosome 1. Around 65% of Caucasians and 99% of Chinese are positive for the antigen being either homozygous or heterozygous for the allele $Fy^+$, while 92% of West Africans are not, being homozygous for $Fy^-$ alleles.

***Duplication, chromosomal.*** A type of chromosomal mutation in which part of a chromosome is replicated, so producing extra copies of those genes contained in the duplicated segement. For example, the 'Bareye' mutaiton in Drosophila is due to a duplication of a segment along the X-chromosome.

***Dynein.*** A group of at least four distinct proteins found in the flagella and microtubules of eukaryotic cells and possessing ATPase activity. Dynein occurs in the form of short arms projecting from the microtubule walls; its enzymatic activity is believed to be responsible for flagellar movement and microtubule contraction.

***Dysentery.*** A severe disorder of the ileum and colon caused by the bacterium Shigella dysenteriae (and several other species), resulting in abdominal cramps, diarrhoea and fever. The disease is spread by 'food, faces, fingers and flies', and can be controlled by sanitary precautions.

***Dysgenic.*** Of, or relating to a deleterious genetic change.

***Dyslexia or word blindness.*** Impairment of the ability to read, due to a brain disorder.

***Dystrophy.*** Defective nutrition, for example of muscles in muscular dystrophy, where muscle-wasting occurs.

# E

***E- or Ex-.*** Prefix denoting out of, without.

***Early Gene*** Genes contained in the circular genomes of viruses such as bacteriophage T4 and SV40. Early genes are transcribed early in the viral replicative cycle, and some of their products are necessary for the transcription or translation of other genes in the genome, termed late genes. In double-stranded DNA viruses, the early genes tend to be clustered on one DNA strand and late genes on the other; transcription involves both strands, each of which is read in an opposite direction.

***Ecad.*** A plant form that results from the habitat in which the plant occurs and is not brought about genetically.

***Ecdysis.*** The process of moulting the cuticle in insects, usually in the preadult stage. The old cuticle is split and cast off to reveal a new, soft cuticle underneath; the insect increases in size, often by intake of air, and the new cuticle hardens. Each larval stage is referred to as an instar, so that the first instar is terminated by the first ecdysis, the second instar by the second ecdysis. Ecdysis is initiated by the moulting hormone.

***Ecdysone (Moulting hormone).*** Steroid hormone, synthesized from cholesterol, which controls growth and ecdysis in Insecta and Crustacea. Ecdysone was important in first demonstrating hormonal action in stimulating messenger RNA synthesis by specific gene loci by puffing on insect salivary gland polytene chromosomes.

***Ecdysone.*** A steroid hormone, produced by insects and crustaceans, that stimulates moulting and metamorphosis. It acts on specific gene loci, stimulating the synthesis of proteins involved in these bodily changes.

***Eclipse.*** 1. n. The period during which a virus exists as a free nucleic acid in the host cell. 2. (of plumage in birds) occurring for a short time after the breeding plumage is moulted, particularly in ducks.

***Ecodeme.*** Local interbreeding population of organisms (deme) that is invariably associated with a specific habitat wherever it occurs. For example, an ecodeme could be restricted to bogs of sphagnum moss, mango swamps or the tops of alpine mountains.

***Ecological Equivalent.*** One of two species that have arisen from the same ancestral stock which have evolved in similar environments and have the same adaptive characters.

***Ecological Isolation.*** The separation of organisms (usually) within the same geographical region because of their preference for different habitat types. For example, the toads Bufo fowleri and B. americanus both live in the same areas but breed in different places, the former in large, still bodies of water such as ponds, the latter in puddles, or pools in brooks.

***Ecological Niche.*** 1. The physical space occupied by an organism.

2. The organism's functional role in the community (e.g. trophic level).

3. Other conditions of the organism's existence, such as preferred temperature, moisture and pH.

***Ecological Pyramid.*** A graphical means of illustrating the trophic structure of trophic function of communities. They are of three general types :

(a) The pyramid of numbers, which illustrates the numbers of organisms at each trophic level.

(b) The pyramid of biomass, based on dry weight (or occasionally live weight) at each level.

(c) The pyramid of energy which shows the energy flow between each level. See Figure E.1.

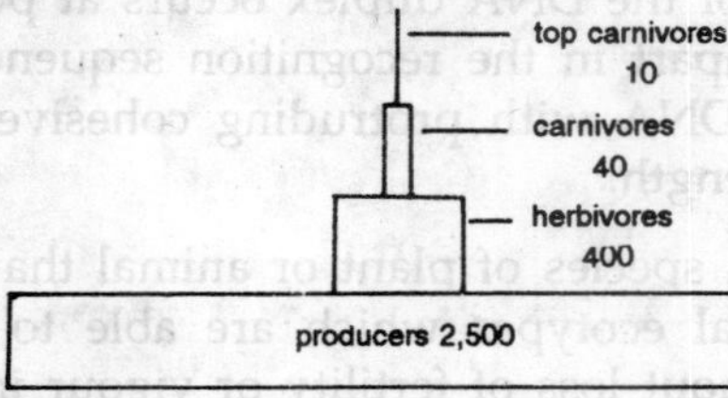


Figure E.1. Ecological pyramid. A hypothetical ecological pyramid for standing crop on tropical grassland. Figures in Kcal $m^{-2}$ $yr^{-1}$.

***Ecological Race.*** A localized form that has evolved characteristics as a result of the selective effect of a specific environment.

***Ecology.*** The study of the interrelationships between organisms and their natural environment, both living and non-living. For this purpose, ecologists study organisms in the context of the populations and communities in which they can be grouped and the ecosystems of which they form a part. The study of ecological interactions provides important information on the nature and mechanisms of evolutionary change. Advances made in ecology over the last 25 years have led to increased concerns about the effects of man's activities on the environment (notably the effects of "pollution), which has resulted in a greater awareness of the importance of "conservation.

***Ecophenotype.*** A modification of the phenotype of an organism, resulting from environmental influences, that is not heritable.

***Eco RI Restriction Enzyme.*** Type II restriction endonuclease (DNA retriction endonuclease) isolated from E. coli that recognizes the hexanucleotide target sequence

↓

5' ...GAATTC...3'

3' ,...CTTAAG...5'

↑

Cleavage of the DNA duplex occurs at positions four nucleotides apart in the recognition sequence to yield fragments of DNA with protruding cohesive 5' termini four bases in length.

***Ecospecies.*** A species of plant or animal that can be divided into several ecotypes which are able to exchange genes freely without loss of fertility or vigour in the offspring.

***Ecosphere.*** Those parts of the earth and its atmosphere where life can exist.

***Ecosystem.*** A biological community and the physical environment associated with it. Nutrients pass between the different organisms in an ecosystem in definite pathways; for example, nutrients in the soil are taken up by plants, which are then eaten by her bivores, which in turn may be eaten by carnivores. Organisms are classified on the basis of their position in an ecosystem into various "trophic levels. Nutrients and energy move round ecosystems in loops or cycles (in the case above, for example, nutrients are returned to the soil via animal wastes and decomposition).

***Ecotone.*** The transition zone between two major ecological communities where one does not merge gradually into the other, for example, that between grassland and woodland. Such steep gradients between communities are usually man-made.

***Ecotype.*** The product arising as a result of the response of the GENOTYPE of an organism to the particular habitat in which it lives, for example, Plantago maritima has a height of about 17.5 cm in waterlogged mud and 56 cm in fertile meadow.

***Eco-Or Ect-.*** Prefix, denoting outside.

***Ectoderm or Ectoblast.*** The germ layer lying on the outside of the developing embryo that eventually gives rise largely to the epidermis, but also to nervous tissue and, where present nephridia.

***Ectoenzymes.*** Enzymes secreted across the body wall of a saprophyte, into the materials which they have invaded, so facilitating absorption.

***Ectopic Expression.*** Expression of a molecule (e.g. a hormone) in an abnormal site. An example is the production of hormones by some tumours, including secondary tumours.

***Ectopic Pairing.*** Non-specific pairing of segments of heterochromatin in salivary gland chromosomes of Drosophila such that adjacent but non-homologous pieces of heterochromatin become aligned with one another and may become physically joined.

***Ectoplasm.*** The outer layer of cytoplasm as distinct from the endoplasm of a cell. It is often much more gel-like (plasma gel) than the liquid endoplasm, from which there is no clear line of distinction. It is important in the movement of unicellular animals such as Amoeba.

***Ectotroph.*** Any heterotroph that absorbs food materials directly from outside the body. Examples include bread mould and tapeworms. In contrast, an endotroph is a heterotroph that absorbs food material from a gut cavity. Examples include humans and Hydra.

***Ectotrophic Virus.*** Virus that can only replicate in host cells.

***Eczema.*** A blistery skin rash usually due to an allergy.

***Edaphic Factor.*** Any characteristic of the environment resulting from the physical, chemical or biotic components of the soil.

***Edaphic Race.*** An ecophenotype resulting from the properties of the substrate rather than other environmental factors.

***Editing Enzyme.*** Enzyme responsible for proof-reading the DNA and correcting errors in replication or following from mutation.

***Edwards' Syndrome.*** A human genetical abnormally in which there are multiple congenital, malformations: elongated skull, low-set ears, webbed neck, severe mental retardation. The condition is caused by trisomy of chromosome 18 and, like down's syndrome, is related to maternal age. 90% of cases die in the first six months after birth.

***EEG (Electroencephalogram).*** A recording of the electrical changes occurring in the brain, produced by placing electrodes on the scalp and amplifying the electrical potential developed. The EEG shows three main types of wave called alpha, beta and delta, that differ in their rates of production. Delta waves are the slowest and are found normally only during sleep.

***Effective Population Size.*** Size of the population of an organism that contributes genes to the succeeding generation. It differs from the absolute population size in that individuals lost by disease, predation or senility, for example, contribute to the annual total of the latter, but may not contribute to the former.

***Effector Molecules.*** Small molecules, most of which are hypothetical, but some are known in bacterial gene regulation, having a role of modifying the affinity of a repressor or activator molecule for a DNA sequence. Effectors act by combining with the regulatory molecule and thus altering its ability to bind to the DNA site.

***Egg Apparatus.*** Structure found in angiosperm ovules within the embryo sac. It consists of an egg cell, which produces the embryo after fertilization, with or without one or two synergidae (synergid cells) whose presence is believed to aid the fertilization process.

***Egg Membrane.*** Protective and/or nutritive membrane which, in addition to the plasma membrane, surrounds the oocyte or fertilized ovum of most animals. Egg membranes are divided into two groups depending upon their origin.

Primary egg membranes. These develop within the ovary and are derived from following cells that surround the oocyte or are also contributed to by the oocyte itself.

Examples are the vitelline membrane of amphibians, insects, molluscs and birds, the zona pellucida of mammals, the jelly coat and fertilization membrane of sea urchins, and the chorion of tunicates, bony fishes and insects.

Secondary egg membranes. These derive from secretions of the oviducts and other female accessory genital organs which are added to the egg during its expulsion. Examples are the jelly coat of amphibian eggs, the mermaids purse of dogfish, the albumen and shell of birds' egg and the horny shell of reptilian eggs.

***EGTA (Ethyleneglycoltetraacetic Acid).*** Chelating agent useful for the determination of calcium in the presence of magnesium.

***Ehlers-Danlos Syndrome.*** Disease in the human resulting from an autosomal dominant gene (although X-linked and recessive genes are known). It is characterized by hyperelastic skin, lax joints and poor wound healing.

***Elaioplast (Oleoplast, Lipidoplast).*** Type of plant plastid that stores lipids, either in the form of oil or fat. Since some algal chloroplasts store oil, they can also be classed as elaioplasts.

***Elastin.*** Structural protein found abundantly in the yellow fibres of connective tissue in animals. It is highly elastic and is predominant in such extensible tissues as long alveoli and the walls of large blood vessels.

***Elater.*** 1. A cell in which the wall is reinforced by spiral bands of thickening whose function is to assist in the discharge of spores in liverworts in response to high humidity. 2. An appendage of horsetail spores, whose function is similar to 1.

***Elaterid.*** Any coleopteran of the family Elateridae, including the click beetles, fireflies and wireworms.

***Electric Organ.*** An organ that is capable of giving an electric shock to any organism coming in contact with it, and occurring particularly in elasmobranch fish such as rays.

***Electromagnetic Spectrum.*** The entire range of wavelengths of electromagnetic radiation, most of which are not detectable by the human eye except in the visible spectrum from about 400-700 nm wavelength. Wavelengths shorter than the visible spectrum contain large quantities of energy which can be harmful to living material. See Figure E.2.

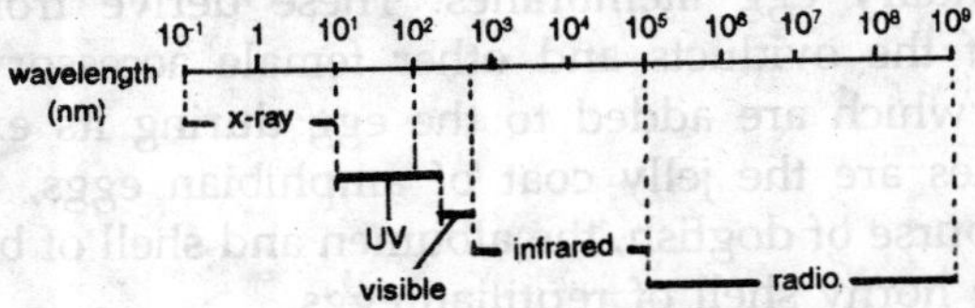


Figure E.2. Electromagnetic spectrum. The wavelength ranges of the electromagnetic spectrum.

***Electron Acceptor.*** Molecule within, for example, the electron transport chain of mitochondrial energy conversion, which takes up electrons. $NAD^+$ is a major electron acceptor.

***Electron-Dense.*** Descriptive of a region that is opaque to electrons in electron microscopy. It may be taken to imply that high concentrations of heavy metals are present or that the material in the area has bound heavy metal molecules used for fixation or staining (e.g. osmium, lead or uranium).

***Electron Donor.*** Molecule, such as that within the electron transport chains of mitochondrial energy conversion, which provides electrons.

***Electron Microscope (EM).*** A microscope that produces high-resolution images by the interaction of electrons with the specimen, the electrons being guided by electromagnetic lenses. There are two major types of EM :

(a) Transmission (TEM). The beam of electrons passes through the specimen (e.g. thinly-sectioned tissues) and is focused onto a fluorescent screen or a photographic film. Magnifications well in excess of × 250,000 are possible, with a resolution of less than 1 nm.

(b) Scanning (SEM). The specimen (which can be whole cells or tissues) is bombarded with high-energy electrons causing generation of low-power, secondary electrons from the specimen surface, which are collected to form an image of the surface. Magnifications in excess of × 100,000 are possible, with a resolution of about 5 nm. See Figure E.3.

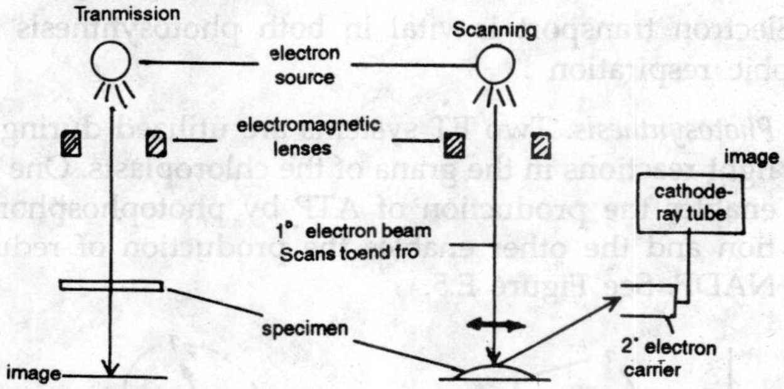


Figure E.3. Electron microscope. The movement of electrons through the transmission electron microscope (TEM) and the scanning electron microscope (SEM).

***Electron-Opaque Tracer.*** Compound (e.g. metal salt or ferritin), often in association with binding proteins such as antibodies, that is used to detect the presence of specific molecules or structures in the electron microscope or to indicate possible pathways of molecular transport.

***Electron Transport System (ETS).*** A series of biochemical steps by which energy is transferred in steps from a higher to a lower level. Each step involves a specific electron carrier which has a particular energy level (or redox potential), with the carriers organized in a sequence of decreasing energy. S5ee Figure E.4.

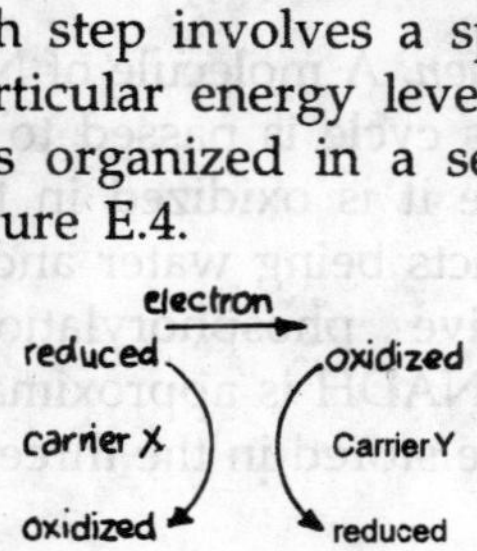


Figure F.4. Electron transport system. The role of electron carriers.

Thus the oxidation of X releases more energy than is required to reduce Y. The released energy can be used to produce ATP, in mitochondria and chloroplasts, probably by a process of chemiosmosis. This mechanism, proposed by P. Mitchell (b. 1920, Nobel prize-winner in 1978), involves hydrogen ions ($H^+$) being pumped in or out of the membranes containing the ETS, generating a proton motive force that enables ATP synthesis from ADP and P.

Electron transport is vital in both photosynthesis and aerobic respiration :

(a) *Photosynthesis.* Two ET systems are utilized during the light reactions in the grana of the chloroplasts. One ETS enables the production of ATP by photophosphorylation and the other enables the production of reduced NADP. See Figure E.5.

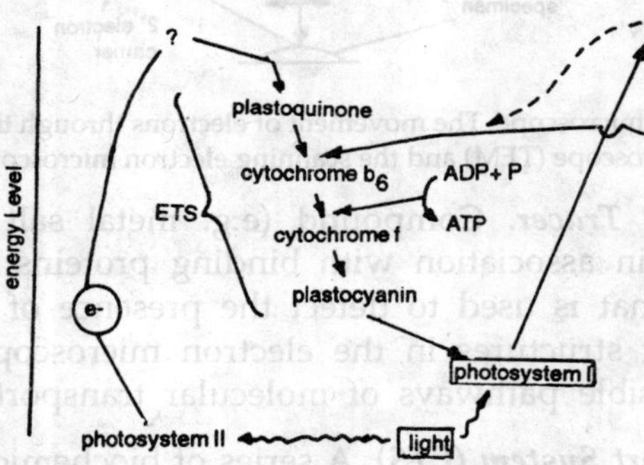


Figure E.5. Electron transport system. Photosynthesis.

(b) *Aerobic Respiration.* A molecule of NADH from glycolysis or the krebs cycle is passed to the cristae or mitochondria where it is oxidized in the respiratory ETS, the final products being water and three molecules of ATP (= oxidative phosphorylation). See Figure. The free energy of NADH is approximately 220 kJ. Of this, about 102 kJ are stored in the three ATP molecules (3 x

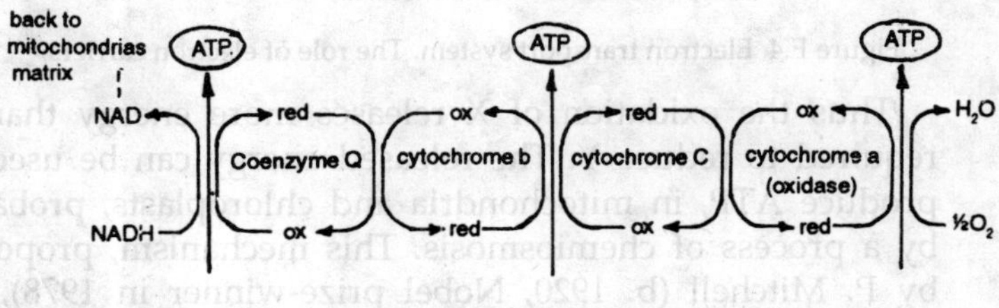


Figure E.6. Electron transport system. Aerobic respiration.

34 kJ) with the remaining energy being lost as heat a conversion efficiency of about 46%. FADH enters the ETS at a lower energy level than NADH, yielding only two ATP molecules, not three See Figure E.6.

***Electro-Osmosis.*** Type of osmosis in which the semipermeable membrane has a potential difference across it so that charged solvents move from the negative to the positive side.

***Electrophoresis.*** Method for separating particles with different electrical charges, for example, proteins. The apparatus consists of a supporting medium soaked in a suitable buffer with an electrical field set up across it. The mixture to be separated (e.g. blood proteins) is placed on the supporting medium. The components with different charges then separate from each other and their eventual position is compared with the position of known standards.

***Electrophoretic Transport Through Membranes.*** Movement of charged particles in solution through membranes such as the plasma membrane as a result of the existing electrical potential across the membrane.

***Elephantiasis.*** An abnormality of the human lymphatic system in which blockage of the lymph ducts causes gross swellings of the surrounding tissues, often resulting in limbs that appear like those of an elephant. The condition can be caused by bacterial infection, but in tropical regions is caused most often by nematode filarial worms, for example. Wucheria bancrofti.

***Elimination.*** The removal of waste and undigested materials from the body, defacation and exhalation of $CO_2$ during breathing.

***Elisa (Enzyme-Linked Immunosorbent Assay).*** Sensitive technique used to detect small quantities of specific proteins by antigenic means. A colorimetric reaction, often based on a peroxidase-conjugated antibody used to bind the protein, provides easy quantitation of the results.

***Elongation Factor.*** Protein which, following its binding to ribosomes, promotes elongation of the polypeptide chain during translation.

***Elution.*** Washing out or collection of liquid from a chromatography column. The liquid, which may contain the fractionated samples, is known as the eluate.

***Emasculation.*** 1. (In plants) the removal of stamens from hermaphrodite flowers before pollen is liberated, thus enabling artificial cross-pollination. 2. (In animals) also called castration or gelding, the removal of the testicles.

***Embedding.*** The process of sealing a specimen in wax which is to be sectioned, usually with a microtome.

***Embryo.*** 1. An animal in the earliest stages of its development, from the time when the fertilized ovum starts to divide, while it is contained within the egg or reproductive organs of the mother, until hatching or birth. A human embryo is called a "fetus after the first eight weeks of pregnancy. 2. The structure in bryophytes, pteridophytes, and seed plants that develops from the zygote prior to germination. In seed plants the zygote is situated in the embryo sac of the ovule. It divides by mitosis to form the embryonic cell and a structure called the suspensor, which embeds the embryo in the surrounding nutritive tissue. The embryonic cell

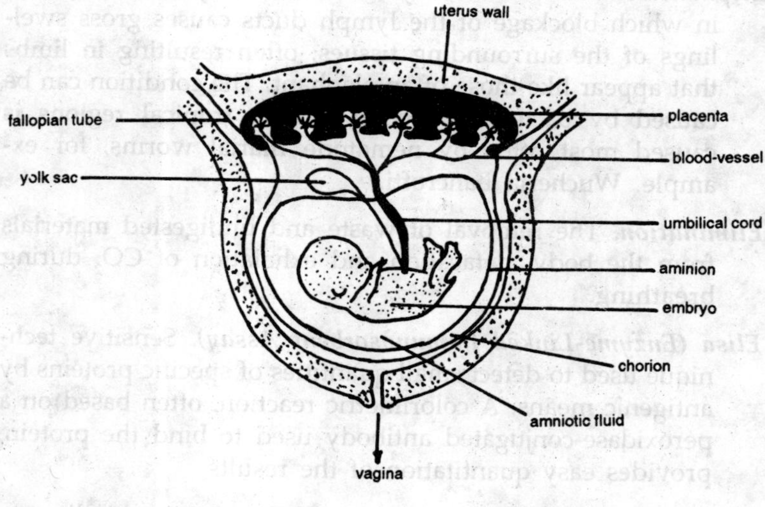


Figure E.7. A developing human embryo.

divides continuously and eventually gives rise to the radicle (young root), plumule (young shoot), and one or two cotyledons. (Seed leaves). Changes also take place in the surrounding tissues of the ovule, which becomes the "seed enclosing the embryo plant. See Figure E.7.

***Embryology.*** The study of the development of animals from the fertilized egg to the new adult organism. It is sometimes limited to the period between fertilization of the egg and hatching or birth.

***Embryo Culture.*** Artificial growth of embryos by fertilization in vitro and subsequent development in vitro or, in the more common use of the terminology, the excision of an embryo from its egg case or maternal environment, under aseptic conditions, and its maintenance in special nutrient medium.

***Embryogenesis.*** Development of a new individual organism from a fertilized egg. The term is equally applicable to plants and animals.

***Embryology.*** Study of embryos and their development; more frequently now termed developmental biology.

***Embryonal Carcinoma Cell.*** Cell from a teratocarcinoma. Many cell lines have been established in tissue culture from such tumours.

***Embryonic Fluid.*** Area of an embryo that, for some period of development, shows unitary characteristics. The distinctive nature of a field area has often been assumed to result from its common susceptibility to a single chemical or physical factor or force.

***Embryonic Induction.*** Determination of the developmental fate of a particular area of an embryo by a process at least partially external to the cells themselves. Embryonic cells that are induced must be competent to respond to the inducer. The nature of embryonic inducers remains unclear. Some may be simple molecules, or particular concentrations of molecules, others are suspected to be physical forces such as light or gravity. In some cases contact with another cell or tissue may be the effective stimulus, as in epithelial-mesenchymal interactions. In this situation, the underlying mesenchymal tissue instructs the epithelial cells above to differentiate in a particular way. Actual cell contact between the epithelial tissue and the mesenchyme has been proved to be essential in many such cases, and in the absence of the mesenchyme the epithelial cells simply fail to differentiate.

***Embryonic Membrane Or Extraembryonic Membrane.*** Any of the protective membranes surrounding the developing embryo in animals, that are involved in the respiration and nutrition of the developing organism. They derive from the zygote, lie outside the embryo proper, and form the chorion, allantois, amnion and yolk sac.

***Embryophyte.*** Any plant of the nontaxonomic group Embryophyta, possessing an embryo and multicellular sex organs. Examples, include mosses, liverworts, ferns and seed plants.

***Embryo Sac.*** The female gametophyte of flowering plants, consisting of a sac-like structure inside the ovule in which are found six haploid cells (without cell walls) and two haploid nuclei. See Figure E.8. The name 'embryo sac' comes from the fact that the plant embryo develops from within the sac. Two male gamete nuclei enter the embryo sac from the pollen tube and carry out a 'double fertilization. One male nucleus fuses with the egg cell to give a diploid zygote (the future plant), the other male nucleus fuses with two polar nuclei giving a triploid (3n) endosperm nucleus (the future food supply in some species).

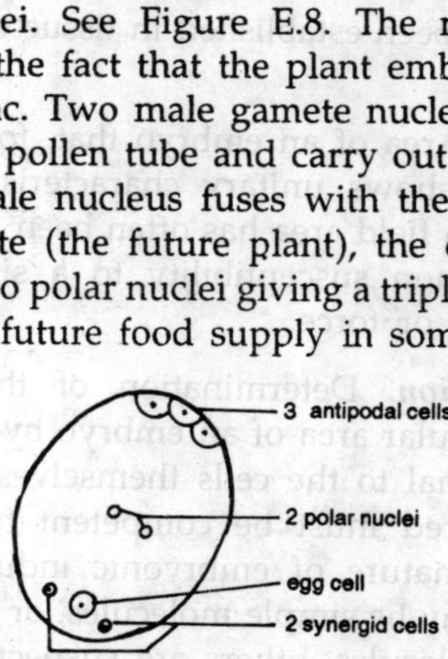


Figure E.8. Embryo sac. Vertical section.

***Emendation***. The correction of a previously published misspelt scientific name.

***Emigration***. The movement of animals away from a specific area.

***Emmer Wheat.*** Plant believed to be one of the origins of modern wheat and known to have been cultivated in neolithic times. It is a tetraploid wheat species, also called starch wheat or Triticum dicoccum.

***Emulsification***. A process in which an emulsion is formed, an emulsion being a liquid containing fine droplets of another liquid that do not together form a solution, for example, fats in milk. Bile is an important emulsifier in the mammalian digestive system.

***En-or Em-***. Prefix. Denoting in, into.

***Encystment***. A process found in the life stage of some organisms in which they surround themselves with a cyst. Encystment is usually a protective stage in the life history and occurs, for example, in Euglena and in a larval stage of flukes.

***Endangered Species.*** Any species at risk of extinction as a result of human activity.

***Endemic.*** (Of organisms or disease) occurrence limited to a particular geographical area such as an island.

***Endemism.*** Recouperative abundance or scarcity of endemic species in a confined geographical area.

***Endergonic Reaction Or Endothermic Reaction***. A reaction requiring free energy (e.g. heat) from an outside source to begin the reaction.

***Endo-***. Prefix. Denoting inside.

***Endocardium***. The inner lining of the heart.

***Endocrine Cell.*** Cell of an endocrine gland (e.g. the pituitary, adrenal, thyroid, parathyroid and pineal glands, and also the mammalian placenta, the gonads, the islets of Langerhans in the pancreas and parts of the alimentary tract).

Endocrine glands secrete their hormone products into the circulation, to be carried by the blood to their appropriate target organs.

*Endocytosis.* Process whereby extracellular materials are brought into cells within membrane-bound vesicles formed by extension or intucking of the plasma membrane. Phagocytosis, pinocytosis and receptormediated endocytosis are forms of endocytosis varying according to the nature of the ingested material, the size of the vesicle formed and the specificity of the process.

*Endoderm Or Endoblast.* The embryological germ layer in animals that gives rise to the gut system and its association organs. It arises initially as a result of gastrulation from cells which have moved in from the surface of the blastula.

*Endodermis.* A one-cell layer of tissue found outside the vascular areas in many angiosperms, which is particularly important in the roots where endodermal cells are thickened with casparian strips for control of water transport.

*Endogamy.* Pollination of a flower by another flower on the same plant.

*Endogenous.* (Of growth or production ) from within the body, for example, the development of new roots from the pericycle of the old root.

*Endometrium.* The lining of the uterus in female mammals, being a glandular mucus membrane that undergoes changes during the oestrus cycle during which it builds up in preparation to receive the fertilized egg. Where fertilization does not occur, it regresses, or in the case of humans, anthropoid apes and Old-World monkeys, suddenly breaks down, producing bleeding.

*Endomitosis.* Replication of chromosomes without nuclear division, and therefore resulting in some degree of polyploidy. In the giant polytene chromosomes found in the salivary glands of Drosophila larvae endomitosis occurs, but the replicate chromosome copies remain attached to one another to form a broad ribbon with homologous parts of the chromosome in register across the ribbon.

***Endonuclease.*** Enzyme that breaks the DNA molecule internally. The enzyme breaks an internal phosphodiester bond, either in one strand only to produce a nick or in both strands to break the DNA molecule into pieces. Some nucleases (e.g. restriction endonucleases of bacterial cells), which are now widely used in gene manipulation technology, make cuts only at specific short sequences of DNA bases.

***Endonuclease Restriction Enzymes.*** Bacterial enzymes capable of cleaving DNA at points where specific nucleotide sequences occur, a function thought to be important in defending an organism against invasion by foreign DNA. Such enzymes have been used extensively to map the base sequences of DNA controlling, for example, the structure of haemoglobin molecules.

***Endopeptidase or Proteinase.*** A type of protein-splitting enzyme that hydrolyses peptide bonds between amino acids located inside the chain, but not at the ends. There are three major endopeptidases in the mammalian gut : Pepsin (stomach); trypsin and chymotrypsin (pancreas). Such enzymes are responsible for the first stage of protein digestion; other proteases called exopeptidases complete the digestion of protein in the ileum.

***Endoplasm.*** Any cytoplasm present within the plasma membrane and ectoplasm of a cell. It is often more liquid than the ectoplasm and is important in locomotion of some protozoans. It contains more granules than the ectoplasm, from which it is difficult to distinguish, as there is no distinct boundary between the two.

***Endoplasmic Reticulum (ER).*** A system of membranes within the cytoplasm of plant and animal "cells. It forms a link between the cell and nuclear membranes and is the site of protein synthesis. It is also concerned with the transport of proteins and lipids within the cell. Rough, ER has "ribosomes attached to its surface; in smooth ER ribosomes are absent.

***Endopolyploidy.*** Condition in which a cell has an increased chromosome number as a result of endomitosis.

***Endoreduplication.*** Chromosome duplication without breakdown of the nuclear envelope, as occurs in the formation of some polyploid nuclei.

***Endorphins.*** Group of large polypeptides that have been isolated from the pituitary gland and are believed to have a morphine-like activity in binding to the surfaces of nerve cells in the brain and reducing pain sensation or altering mood. These so-called endogenous opiates are rapidly degraded after release, unlike morphine, which seems to owe its narcotic effects to binding to the same receptors for a more prolonged period. Other endogenous opiates are known; for example, the enkephalins which are of a much lower molecular weight than endorphins, but share the same four amino acid sequences which form the presumed binding site.

***Endosome.*** Large cytoplasmic vesicle resulting from fusion between coated vesicles prior to their association with lysosomes to form secondary lysosomes.

***Endosperm.*** Nutritive tissue that surrounds the embryo in seed plants and provides it with nourishment. Endosperm cells are commonly triploid.

***Endospore.*** Spore that forms as a single thick-walled cell within the vegetative cells of certain bacteria of the genera Clostridium and Bacillus. The endospore is very resistant to adverse conditions and may remain viable for many years. On the return of favourable conditions, the endospore germinates to yield a vegetative cell. Endospore production by a bacterial cell is a simple type of differentiation, since special genes are expressed at this time which are not active at other times in the life of the bacterium.

***Endosymbiont Theory.*** Theoretical evolution of mitochondria and chloroplast from endosymbiotic prokaryotes which originally existed within primitive eukaryotic cells.

***Endosymbiosis.*** Beneficial association between two different organisms in which one lives within the cell of the other. Thus some bacteria exist as endosymbionts in cells of Protozoa.

***Endothelium.*** Single layer of flattened, tile-like cells that line the inside of vertebrate blood and lymphatic vessels. Endothelium is derived from the embryonic mesoderm.

***Endothermy.*** The ability of an organism to produce sufficient metabolic heat to raise its core temperature above its surroundings. It may be maintained continually or for limited periods only, such as during activity.

***Endotoxin.*** Toxic substance, usually a macromolecular complex, that is produced by a bacterium but remains without the cell, usually within the cell wall. Bacteria such as Vibrio, Shigella and Salmonella, which all cause dysentery, contain endotoxins, and injections of cell wall material from these bacteria into mammals provokes an immunological response, chiefly against the endotoxin.

***End-Product Inhibition (feedback inhibition).*** Inhibition by the end-product of a multistep metabolic pathway of an enzyme catalysing an early step, usually the first, of the sequence. Alternatively, the susceptible reaction may be immediately after a branch point in metabolism. Control at an early stage adjusts the flow of metabolites through the entire pathway and helps to maintain a constant cellular concentration of the end-product. The control is particularly important if the cell is able to utilize an external supply of the end-product. Where an enzyme serves more than one pathway two or more end-products may inhibit in a concerted fashion. End-product inhibition has been demonstrated for most of the pathways leading to the biosynthesis of amino acids and nucleotides. A molecular explanation for end-product inhibition was first provided for the enzyme aspartate transcarbamylase which catalyses an early step in the biosynthesis of pyrimidine nucleotides. Binding of cytidine triphosphate (the end-product) at one site on the enzyme lowers the activity at the separate catalytic site through a conformational change in the protein.

***End-Product Repression.*** Decrease in the synthesis of the enzyme(s) of a metabolic pathway brought about by the addition of the end-product of the pathway. If the pathway involves more than one step the enzymes are repressed coordinately. End-product repression is observed for biosynthetic pathways (e.g. for amino acids and nucleotides) in microorganisms such as bacteria when end-products are added to the growth medium. Control is exerted at the level of transcription of the structural genes for the enzymes; these are often organized into operons. The end-product (e.g. tryptophan) binds to and activates a specific repressor protein which, in turn, binds to a site near the promoter for the genes, thus preventing transcription initiation. Enzyme repression may result also from attenuation. Branched pathways have special arrangements for regulating enzyme formation in order to avoid interference between the branches. An enzyme may be subject to multivalent repression by all the end-products acting together, or each enzyme of a parallel set (catalysing the same reaction) may be repressible by one of the end-products.

***Energy.*** The capacity of a body or system to do work. The most important energy forms, as far as living organisms are concerned, are heat, radiant, chemical and mechanical energy. Every units of important arc :

1 calorie = heat to raise 1 g of water through $1^0$C

$$1 \text{ erg} = \frac{\text{energy to raise 1 g through 1 cm against gravity}}{981}$$

1 joule = $10^7$ ergs

1 Calorie = 1 kcal (= 1000 cals)

1 calorie = $4.2 \times 10^7$ ergs

1 calorie = 4.2 joules

The quantity of solar energy entering the earth's atmosphere is $64.3 \times 10^8 Jm^{-2}yr^{-t}$. The amount of solar energy available to plants in Britain is $10.5 \times 10^8 Jm^{-2}yr^{-1}$. The SI unit of energy is the Joule (J). In plants and animals, energy is stored in ATP (short-term storage), and starch and fat (long-term storage).

***Energy Acceptor.*** A molecule (e.g. cytochrome) capable of receiving energy (usually in the form of electrons) and of passing it on to another acceptors, as in an electron transport system.

***Energy Donor.*** The molecules that give up the energy to drive an endergonic reaction.

***Energy Flow.*** The movement of energy through an ecosystem. The energy is usually first trapped as radiant energy (from the sum) by producers, which are then eaten by herbivores which, in turn, might be consumed by predators, with considerable loss of energy (both material energy and heat) back into the ecosystem (and out of it) at each level.

***Enhancer Element.*** Eukaryotic promoter element that increases the transcriptional efficiency of a nearby gene. The first enhancer element discovered was the 72-base pair tandem repeat of SV40 DNA. Deletion of this element, which is located upstream of the CAP site of the early viral genes, reduces early gene expression by a factor of at least 100. Enhancer elements have also been found in other DNA viruses (e.g. polyomavirus, bovine papillomaviruses and adenoviruses). Like the SV40 enhancer element, they are often present as short tandem repeats of 50-100 base pairs. It is also thought likely that certain cellular genes may possess their own less active enhancer-like elements. The molecular basis of enhancer activity is not understood.

***Enhancer Mutation.*** Attempts at investigating the function of enhancer elements have been made by producing enhancer mutation. Deletion and point mutation of the 72-base pair repeat SV40 enhancer element have been constructed to examine the effects of such changes on enhancer activity.

***Enkephalins.*** Low-molecular-weight pentapeptides (met-enkephalin and leuenkephalin) that can be recovered from preparations of mammalian brain. Like endorphins they are endogenous opiates, having a marked affinity for the same cell surface receptors on nerve cells as are recognized by morphine and other opiate drugs. They have been shown to have a morphine-like action of reducing pain sensation and enhancing mood, and, like endorphins, four of their amino acids are crucial for attachment to the appropriate nerve cell receptor. Unlike opiates, they are rapidly degraded, and there seems no natural addictive tendency involved in their activity.

***Enriched Medium.*** Culture medium supplemented (enriched) with blood serum, or a mixture of nutrients or growth factors suitable for the cultivation of fastidious bacteria and other microorganisms.

***Enrichment Culture.*** A technique for isolating an organism from a mixed culture by manipulating the growth conditions in its favour and to the detriment of other organisms.

***Ent-or Ento.*** Prefix. Denoting, within.

***Enteroviruses.*** Obsolete term for picornaviruses; a group of single-stranded RNA virus of small size. The virions have cubic symmetry. Because many picornaviruses, such as polio virus, were found in the intestine they were termed enteroviruses.

***Entoderm.*** Alternative and little used word for endoderm.

***Entomophily.*** The pollination of plants by insects. Such animal pollinators are one of the two main mechanisms for the transport of pollen to the stigma, the other being anemophily. In entomophilous flowers the colours are adapted to their pollinators, for example, moths are mainly active at dusk and at night and they visit flowers that are mostly white; bees cannot see red and will visit mainly blue or yellow flowers. Many flowers have patterns visible only with ultraviolet light which insects (but not mammals) can detect. Deep flowers are pollinated by insects with long mouthparts, and short flowers by insects with short mouthparts, an example of coevolution of plants and insects.

***Entropy.*** The amount of disorder or the degree of randomness of a system. For example, when a protein is denatured by heat, the molecule (which has a definite shape) uncoils and takes up a random shape, producing a large change in entropy.

***Enucleate.*** To remove the nucleus from a cell (e.g. by micromanipulation) although the term is sometimes used for cells that have been rendered anucleate by destruction of the nucleus through irradiation with ultraviolet light.

***Envelope.*** Any enclosing structure, such as a membrane or skin. In bacteria, it is the part of the cell enclosing the cytoplasm, i.e. the cytoplasmic membrane cell wall and capsule. In viruses, it is the outer lipid-containing layer of some virions.

***Environment.*** The surroundings of any organism, including the medium, substrate, climatic conditions, other organisms, light and pH.

***Environmental Resistance.*** The collective effect on populations growth of predators and competition for food and space.

***Environmental Temperature.*** The temperature at which an inanimate body of the same shape and size as a given organism will come to equilibrium with its surroundings when placed at the same point in space as the organism. The temperature includes radiative and convective influences on the organism.

***Enzyme.*** A protein molecule that catalyses a biochemical reaction by lowering the activation energy required for the reaction to proceed. Enzymes are usually specific to particular substrates and are sensitive to environmental conditions such as pH and temperature. (See Figure E.9) Allosteric enzymes exist in inactive and active forms, while

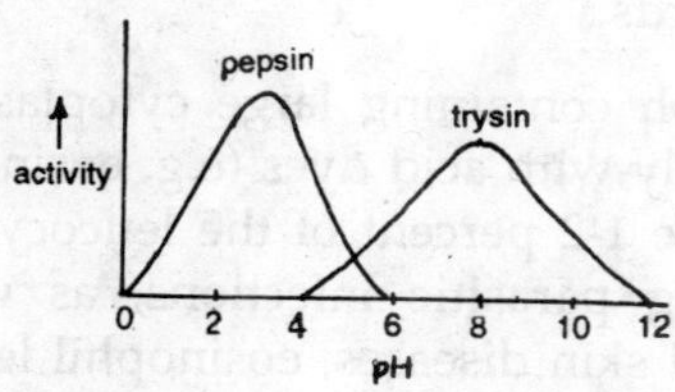


Figure E.9. Enzyme. The effect of pH activity.

others can be inhibited by nonsubstrate molecules. Protein-splitting enzymes (Proteases) are produced in nonactive forms in the mammalian digestive system to minimize the risk of self-digestion. For example, trypsin is produced as inactive trypsinogen.

***Enzyme Induction.*** The process in which a 'structural' gene is activated by a substrate binding with a repressor substance, thus enabling the production of an enzyme that will catalyse the metabolism of the substrate.

***Enzyme Inhibitor.*** A molecule that prevents an enzyme from catalysing a reaction. Such inhibitors can compete with the normal substrate or can block the active site, preventing entry of the substrate. Enzyme inhibitors often form part of a feedback mechanism to regulate a biochemical pathway.

***Enzyme Kinetics.*** Rate of a reaction controlled by an enzyme. At low substrate concentrations the reaction rate (V) is always proportional to the substrate concentration ([S]), but when the substrate is present at high concentration enzyme saturation will occur ($V_{max}$). The Michaelis-Menten equation expresses the rate of a reaction as $V = V_{max} [S]/(K_m + [S])$, where $K_m$ is the Michaelis constant and is equal to the concentration of the substrate when the speed on the reaction is half its maximum.

***Eobiont.*** A hypothetical chemical precursor of a living cell.

***Eocene.*** A geological epoch lasting from 54 to 38 million years ago; a subdivision of the tertiary period. During this time extensive planktonic populations of Foraminifera laid down rock beds (from which the pyramids of Egypt were built), and many groups of mammals appeared for the first time, for example, rodents, whales, carnivores. Britain was still moving northwards.

***Eosinophil.*** Polymorph containing large cytoplasmic granules that stain brilliantly with acid dyes (e.g. eosin). Eosinophils normally comprise 1-2 percent of the leucocytes in human blood, but during parasitic infections, as well as some allergic states and skin diseases, eosinophil levels increase. This condition is known as eosinophilia. Eosinophils may play a role in antibody-antigen reactions, possibly by releasing or absorbing histamine.

***Eosinophil Leucocyte.*** A type of white blood cell (of the granulocyte group) which takes up the stain of an acid dye. Eosinophils make up about 4% of the adult human leucocytes. They are produced in the bone marrow, and their function is probably connected with the immune response, particularly allergies.

***Ep-or-Epi-or Eph.*** Prefix. Denoting upon.

***Ephemeral.*** (Of organisms) having a very short life cycle. The term is used specifically to describe those plants that have more than one generation a year, as opposed to annual, biennial, perennial.

***Epiboly.*** Active spreading or expansion of superficial tissue layer(s) over the inert bulk of yolk during the initial stages of gastrulation in a meroblastic system (e.g. teleosts and birds) or over inert yolk-filled cells in yolk-rich, holoblastic systems (e.g. amphibia). This expansion positions the cells at a point where internalization will take place as a part of the gastrulation process. In all systems analysed, epibolic spreading seems to be driven by cell-autonomous changes in behaviour and shape, and not by cell division.

***Epidemic.*** The occurrence of many cases of a disease within an area.

***Epidemiology.*** The study of the incidence, distribution and control of an epidemic disease in a population.

***Epidermal Growth factor.*** Protein found in vertebrates, consisting of a polypeptide chain of 53 amino acids, that has the capacity to stimulate epidermal and some other cells to divide. Its site of synthesis is unknown.

***Epidermis.*** Outermost layer of cells covering an animal or plant. In many invertebrates it is one cell thick and secretes a protective, waterproof cuticle. In vertebrates the epidermis forms the outer layer of the skin and comprises several stratified layers of cells and is renewed continually. The stratum corneum, the outermost epidermal layers of land vertebrates, is composed of dead, cornified cells with cell contents being replaced by keratin. Nails, claws, hair and feathers are epidermal structures. Plant epidermis consists of a closely packed, single layer of cuboidal cells; it acts as a protective coat.

***Epifluorescence Microscopy.*** Light microscopy that depends on fluorescence emitted by cells, usually in the presence of ultraviolet light.

***Epigamic Character.*** Any secondary sexual character brought into existence by hormone action and used in courtship display.

***Epigenesis.*** Theory that a gradual process of growth and development, involving increasing complexity, accounts for the production of a newborn foetus from a fertilized egg. It was proposed in the 18th century in opposition to the theory of preformation, which proposed that the fertilized egg contained a miniature replica of the adult (the homunculus) and that growth in size alone was necessary to produce foetus or adult from the egg.

***Epigenetics.*** Study of the mechanism involved in producing phenotypic effects that result from gene action. All phenotypic characters involve, to some extent, an interplay of genetic and environment influences, but epigenetic studies concentrate on the former. One model, of gene action in development is that of the epigenetic landscape, proposed by Waddington in 1950s. In this model, the fate of a cell during development is likened to a stone tumbling down a hillside, falling as it will in a predictable way so long as a continuous valley is available, but occasionally forced to make choices of pathway where a valley bifurcates. Although these choices seem small at the time, their ultimate influence on the position of the stone (or the fate of the cell, as the model would propose) can be very considerable. This implies that genes that are active early in development, or mutants of these genes, will have greater effects on the adult than those that are active late in development.

***Epigenetic Landscape.*** A concept related to the developmental pathways along which a cell passes during differentiation.

***Epilepsy.*** A narrow condition due to abnormalities in the brain cortex that results in seizures ranging from a sense of numbness in certain body areas (petit mal) to extreme muscular convulsions and fits (grant mal). Epileptics exhibit large, abnormal brain waves, which can be detected on an EEG.

***Epimers.*** Pairs of monosaccharides that differ by dint of their three-dimensional configuration around one carbon atom. Thus D-mannose and D-glucose differ in the C-2 atom configuration and are therefore epimers.

***Epiphyte..*** A plant that grows upon another plant but is neither parasitic on it nor rooted in the ground. Epiphytes include many mosses and lichens and some tropical orchids.

***Epiphytotic.*** (of plant diseases and parasites) affecting plants over a wide geographical region.

***Episome.*** Genetic element or plasmid found in bacteria and perhaps also in eukaryotic cells such as yeast. Episomes are capable not only of autonomous replication independently of the host genome, but also at least under some circumstances of integration into the host genome and replication as part of the host chromosome. Thus only a proportion of plasmids can be correctly styled as episomes; the sex factor F in E. coli, and lambda phage are well-known examples. The term episome had tended to fall into disuse, and the word plasmid is often used for all classes of extrachromosomal genetic elements, whether or not they are capable of integration into the host genome.

***Epistasis..*** A form of genetic interaction in which one gene interferes with the expression of another gene, for example, if genes A and B code for enzymes active in the same pathway. See Figure E.10. If both alleles of gene A code for a nonfunctional version of enzyme A, then the pathway will shut down, irrespective of which B alleles are present, i.e. gene A is epistatic to gene B.

Figure. E.10 Epistasis. The interaction of genes A and B.

***Epizoite.*** Any animal that lives attached to another and uses it for protection or means of locomotion, there being no parasitic relationship.

***Epsilon-Globin Chain.*** Globin molecule synthesized in the human embryo and contributing to one of the human embryonic haemoglobins, which are composed of four globin chains — two alpha-chains and two epsilon-chains — each the product of a separate gene.

***Epstein-Barr Virus (EB Virus).*** DNA herpes-type virus that causes infectious mononucleosis (glandular fever) and is also causatively involved in Burkitt's lymphoma, a malignant tumour of lymph glands common in Central Africa.

***Equal Weighting..*** A taxonomic procedure where all characters are regarded as of equal importance. The procedure is commonly used in numerical taxonomy.

***Equatorial Plate.*** An arrangement of chromosomes lying in one plane at the equator of the spindle in metaphase of mitosis or meiosis.

***Equilibrium Centrifugation.*** A process of density-gradient centrifugation that continues until there is no net movement of the molecules, each molecule having come to rest when its density equals that of the solution.

***Eradicant.*** Any biocide (e.g. a fungicide) used to cure an established infection.

***Erection, Penis.*** The hardening and lengthening of the mammalian penis in order to bring it into condition for copulation. An erection is brought about by engorgement of blood in the corpus spongiosum and corpus cavernosum, causing them to become turgid.

***Erepsin.*** Mixture of proteolytic enzymes secreted by the small intestine of mammals.

***Ergonomics.*** The study of the engineering aspects of the relationship between workers and their working environment.

***Ergosome.*** Now obsolete term for a polysome, visualized in the electron microscope as a group of ribosomes associated together on the membrane of the rough endoplasmic reticulum.

***Ergosterol.*** Precursor of vitamin D in animals; natural plant sterol. It is converted to vitamin D by ultraviolet radiation.

***Ergot.*** A disease caused by the ascomycete Claviceps purpurea in cereals and grasses. 2. a sclerotium forming in place of grain in a diseased grain head. Ergots contain substances that are poisonous and sometimes used medicinally.

***Erose.*** (Of plant structures) having the appearance of being gnawed, with irregular notches.

***Erosion.*** The wearing away of geological formations such as rock, soil, etc. For example, deafforestation or the removal of hedges causes soil erosion.

***Error Catastrophe.*** Ageing theory which proposes that errors in the accuracy of DNA transcription and messenger. RNA translation, especially with respect to those molecules (e.g. RNA polymerases, transfer RNA synthetases) associated with further transcription and translation may lead by positive feedback to a 'catastrophe' with respect to cellular synthetic machinery and cell death. Error catastrophe in numerous cells could hasten an organism's senescence.

***Error-Prone Repair.*** Type of DNA repair in which DNA chain growth occurs across damaged DNA segments, but some of these new strands are themselves defective. Such error-prone repair appears to be the chief source of genetic mutation in the bacteria in which it occurs.

***Erythroblast.*** Nucleated cell found in small numbers in circulating blood and in larger numbers in erythropoietic organs, such as bone marrow. It is a precursor of the mature red blood cell which, although nucleated in lower vertebrates, is anucleate in mammals. Erythroblasts divided mitotically and, at least in mammals, produce reticulocytes which are the immediate precursors of the erythrocytes. Although early erythroblasts may lack haemoglobin, the more mature erythroblasts already possess some haemoglobin. In some diseases of the blood the normally small number of circulating erythroblasts is dramatically increased.

***Erythroblastosis.*** Release of erythroblasts from the erythropoietic tissues into the circulating blood. It is a clinical feature of several diseases of the blood cells.

***Erythroblastosis Foetalis.*** A haemolytic disease of newborn children brought about when a rhesus negative mother produces a rhesus negative child. In late pregnancy $Rh^-$ cells may pass into the mother who produces antigens which pass back across the placenta and adversely affect the child.

***Erythrocyte or Red Blood Cell (RBC).*** A vertebrate cell that carries some carbon dioxide as $HCO_{3^-}$ from tissues to lungs, and contains haemoglobin pigment for oxygen transport from lungs to tissues. Unlike other vertebrate cells, mammalian RBCs are non-nucleated and have definite biconcave shape. See Figure E.11.

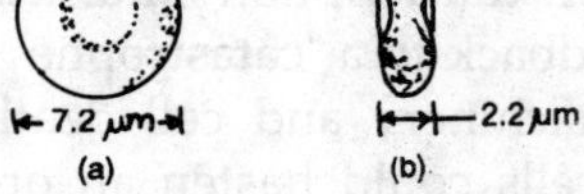


Figure E.11. Erythrocyte. (a) Surface view. (b) Vertical section.

***Erythrocyte Ghost.*** Empty, but relatively intact plasma membrane of an erythrocyte following its lysis and the release of its cytoplasmic contents. Erythrocyte ghosts have been greatly used for studies on cell membrane structure and permeability, since they may be readily obtained in bulk and at high purity.

***Erythromycin.*** An antibiotic produced by a strain of streptomycin that includes protein synthesis, particularly in organisms which are Gram-positive. See Figure E.12.

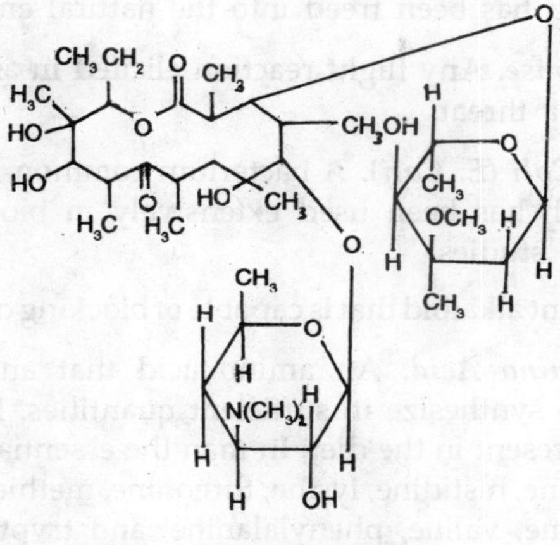

Figure E.12. Erythromycin.

***Erythropoiesis.*** Production of new red blood cells. It occurs substantially in the erythropoietic tissues and consists of the division of multipotential stem cells to produce erythroblasts (among many other blood cell types produced) which later divide to produce reticulocytes, the immediate precursors of the erythrocytes.

***Erythropoietic Tissue.*** Tissue responsible for erythropoiesis. Such tissue is concentrated in the bone marrow in mammals, but liver, spleen and kidney also constitute important locations in lower vertebrates and in mammalian embryos. The earliest blood cell formation in the vertebrate embryo occurs in blood islands of the yolk sac.

***Erythropoietin.*** Glycoprotein hormone ($M_r$ ~ 46 000) and produced chiefly in the kidney. The hormone is produced in response to reduced oxygen tension, and its production is enhanced by blood iron (which reduces oxygen-carrying capacity) and is depressed by erythrocyte excess. The hormone achieves an effect within a day or two or production and is thought to affect the speed of division and maturation of cells already committed to the erythrocyte line in differentiation.

***Escape.*** 1. Any cultivated plant growing in the wild that is not well naturalized. 2. Any organism that is normally captive but which has been freed into the natural environment.

***Escape Response.*** Any flight reaction elicited in an animal as a result of a threat.

***Escherichia Coli (E. Coli).*** A bacterium common in the human gut which has been used extensively in biochemical and genetical studies.

***Eserine.*** A plant alkaloid that is capable of blocking cholinesterase.

***Essential Amino Acid.*** An amino acid that an organism is unable to synthesize in sufficient quantities. It must therefore be present in the diet. In man the essential amino acids are arginine, histidine, lysine, threonine, methionine, isoleucine, leucine, valine, phenylalanine, and tryptophan. These are required for protein synthesis and deficiency leads to retarded growth and other symptoms. Most of the amino acids required by man are also essential for all other multicellular animals and for most protozoans.

***Essential Element.*** Any of a number of elements required by living organisms to ensure normal growth, development, and maintenance. Apart from the elements found in organic compounds (i.e. carbon, hydrogen, oxygen, and nitrogen), plants, animals, and microorganisms all require a range of elements in inorganic forms in varying amounts, depending on the type of organism. The major elements, present in tissues in relatively large amounts (greater than 0.005%), are calcium, phosphorus, potassium, sodium, chlorine, sulphur, and magnesium. The trace elements occur at much lower concentrations and thus requirements are much less. The most important are iron, manganese, zinc, copper, iodine, cobalt, selenium, molybdenum, chromium, and silicon. Each element may fulfil one or more of a variety of metabolic roles. Sodium, potassium, and chloride ions are the chief electrolytic components of cells and body fluids and thus determine their electrical and osmotic status. Calcium, phosphorus, and magnesium are all present in bone. Calcium is also essential to nerve and muscle activity, while phosphorus is a key constituent of the chemical energy carriers (e.g. ATP) and the nucleic acids. Sulphur is needed primarily for amino acid synthesis (in plants and microorganisms). The trace elements may serve as cofactors or as constituents of complex molecules, e.g. iron in haem and cobalt in vitamin $B_{12}$.

***Essential Fatty Acids.*** "Fatty acids that must normally be present in the diet of certain animals, including man. Essential fatty acids, which include linoleic and linolenic acids, all possess double bonds at the same two positions along their hydrocarbon chain and so can act as precursors of prostaglandins. Deficiency of essential fatty acids can cause dermatosis, weight loss, irregular oestrus, etc. An adult human requires 2-10g linoleic acid or its equivalent per day.

***Essential Oil.*** A natural oil with a distinctive scent secreted by the glands of certain aromatic plants. Terpenes are the main constituents. Essential oils are extracted from plants by steam distillation, extraction with cold neutral fats or solvents (e.g. alcohol), or pressing and used to perfumes, flavourings, and medicine. Example are citrus oils, flower oils (e.g. rose, jasmine), and oil of cloves.

***Established Cell Line.*** Cell line that demonstrates the potential to be subcultured indefinitely in vitro.

***Esterases.*** Large group of different enzymes that hydrolyse esters.

***Estuary.***The point at which a river meets the sea. There is thus a mixture of saline and freshwater conditions, often with areas of tidal mudflats and salt marsh. Because of the varying salinity and tidal cover there is often a specific flora and fauna associated with such areas.

***Ethology.*** The study of animal behaviour in the natural habitat of the animals concerned.

***Ethidium Bromide.*** Intercalating dye widely used to stain DNA in gels and gradients. The DNA can be visualized readily by irradiation with ultraviolet light, as little as 0.05 µg of

DNA being detectable by such methods. Ethidium bromide is also added to caesium chloride density gradients, since as an intercalating molecule it binds more readily to linear DNA than to closed colinear circles of DNA (such as plasmids). Binding of ethidium bromide reduces the density of DNA, thus covalent circles of DNA have higher densities at saturating concentrations of ethidium bromide, permitting the separation of plasmid DNA. See Figure E.13.

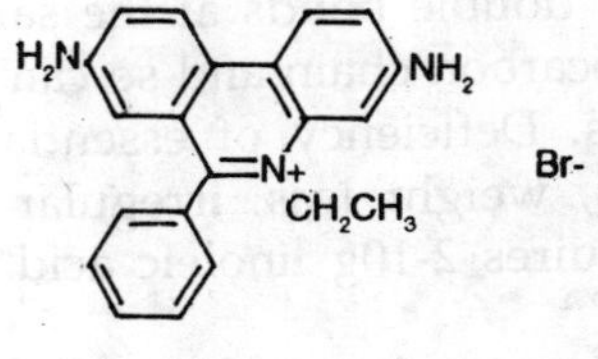


Figure E.13. Ethidium bromide.

***Ethylene or Ethene.*** A simple hydrocarbon with the formula $CH_2$=$CH_2$ that can act as a plant hormone even when present in very low concentrations (down to 1 ppm). Ethylene inhibits elongation in most growing tissues and promotes leaf abscission and fruit ripening in some plants. Plant cells produce ethylene from the amino acid methionine.

***Ethylene Glycol.*** Alcohol widely used as an antifreeze solution and also as a surface-active agent to promote cell fusion between plant protoplasts in vitro.

***Etiolation.*** The range of symptoms developed by plants when grown in the dark. Examples include: pale yellow or white colour due to lack of chlorophyll, long internodes, small and rudimentary leaves, poor development of lignified tissue.

***Etioplast.*** Type of chloroplast found in plant tissue kept in the dark, sometimes in roots and shoots but chiefly in etiolated leaves. Etioplasts contain a pseudocrystalline array of tubular and vesicular membranes called the prolamellar body. On exposure to light, this body rapidly forms a normal stack of chloroplast membranes.

***ETS.*** Electron Transport System.

***Eubacteria.*** The true bacteria, i.e. those typically having simple unbranched cells, rigid cell walls, and flagella for movement.

***Eucarpic.*** (Of an adult fungal thallus) having clear distinction between vegetative and reproductive parts.

***Eucaryote Or Eukaryote.*** Any member of a group of organisms that contains all plants and animals apart from bacteria and blue-green algae (which are procaryotes). Eucaryotes are distinguished by the fact that their cells possess a membrane-bound nucleus containing the genetic material, but there are also other differences from the procaryotes. See Table.

| *Procaryotes* | *Eucaryotes* |
|---|---|
| 1. No true nucleus. | Nucleus with nuclear membrane. |
| 2. Single chromosome made up of nucleic acid. | Several chromosomes with nucleic acid complexed with protein. |
| 3. Cell organelles absent. | Golgi apparatus, endoplasmic reticulum, lysosomes, mitochondria present. |
| 4. If present, chlorophyll not in chloroplasts. | If present, chlorophyll in chloroplasts. |
| 5. Flagella lack 9 + 2 structure. | Flagella with 9 + 2 structure. |
| 6. Cell division by binary fission. | Cell division by mitosis and meiosis. |

Table. Eucaryote. A comparison of procaryotes and eucaryotes.

***Euchromatin.*** A chromosome material that stains heavily in metaphase but hardly at all in interphase when it is relatively uncoiled and undergoes transcription.

***Eugenics.*** Study of human heredity as applied to the improvement of the human race. Practical eugenics involves promoting interbreeding between individuals having favourable genetic endowment and discouraging or preventing interbreeding of those with relatively unfavourable genetic endowment. Aside from the inherent ethical problems of deciding which genes are desirable, eugenics faces considerable, practical difficulties. These include the interplay of genetic expression and the environment in the determination of the phenotype with almost all genes, and the masking of undesirable alleles by other dominant alleles in the phenotype of all individuals. Only rarely it is possible to detect the individual who happens to be heterozygous for deleterious but recessive alleles. Genetic counselling as currently practised is a mild form of eugenics, attempting as it does to dissuade prospective parents from producing children if they have a high risk of begetting offspring suffering from thalassaemia or huntingdon's chorea, for example.

***Euglena.*** A genus of large, green flagellates (division Euglenophyta) that is common in both fresh and salt waters. Euglenoids produce a polysaccharide storage molecule called paramylum and, (unlike other flagellates), do not possess a cell wall, but produce a flexible pellicle instead.

***Eukaryote (Eucaryote).*** An organism consisting of cells in which the genetic material is contained within a distinct nucleus. All organisms, except bacteria and blue-green algae, are eukaryotes.

***Euphotic Zone or Photic Zone or Epipelagic Zone.*** The top 100 m of the sea into which light can penetrate and in which photosynthesis takes place.

***Euploidy.*** The condition of a cell, tissue or organism that has one or more multiples of a chromosome set, for example, a triploid (3n). Euploids with more than two sets of chromosomes are polyploids.

***Eupnaea or Eupnea.*** The normal, quiet breathing of an animal at rest.

***Euryhaline.*** (Of organisms) capable of tolerating a wide variety of salinity in the surrounding medium.

***Eurypterid.*** Any large extinct scorpion-like aquatic arthropod of the order Eurypterida, found in the silurian period.

***Eurythermous.*** (Of organisms) able to tolerate a wide range of environmental temperatures.

***Eusporangiate.*** (Of sporangia) arising from a group of parent cells and having a wall consisting of at least two layers of cells.

***Euthanasia.*** The act of painless killing to relative human suffering from an incurable disease.

***Eutrophic.*** (Of a body of water) being rich in organic and mineral nutrients, either naturally or by fertilization.

***Eutrophication.*** A process by which pollutants cause a body of water to become over-rich in organic and mineral nutrients, so that algae grow rapidly and deplete the oxygen supply.

***E Value.*** The solar energy present on other planets expressed as a percentage of the earth's solar energy.

***$E_0$ Values.*** A numerical series indicative of the redox potential of molecules. Protons are accepted by a molecule from any other molecule with a more positive $E_0$ value.

***Evaporation.*** The physical change when a liquid becomes a gas. Since such a change usually requires heat as an energy source, heat is drawn from the immediate environment, which produces a significant cooling effect. The size of the cooling effect depends on the latent heat of evaporation of the liquid. Evaporation of water is used by mammals in temperature regulation (sweat) and occurs in plants from the surface of the mesophyll cells during transpiration.

***Evocation.*** Induction of cellular differentiation or a pattern of development within an embryo by an evocator, deemed to be a molecular compound produced by the responding tissue. Evocators are more or less equivalent to the hypothetical substances more often referred to as morphogens or inductors.

***Evolution.*** An explanation of the way in which present-day organisms have been produced, involving changes taking place in the genetic make-up of populations that have been passed on to successive generations. According to darwinism, evolutionary mutations have given rise to changes that have, through natural selection, either survived in better adapted organisms, or died out. Evolution is now generally accepted as the means which gives rise to new species (as opposed to special creation)but there is still debate about exactly how it has taken place and how rapidly changes can take place.

***Evolution.*** It explains the development of relatively complex organisms from simple ones over the long periods of geological time. Although organic evolution was widely recognized as a more plausible alternative to special creation, even by Aristotle, it was not until Charles Darwin and Alfred Russell Wallace suggested evolution by natural selection in the early 19th century that a proper understanding of evolution began to emerge. It is now recognized that changes, both potentially beneficial and deleterious, are arising constantly in natural populations by random mutation, and that fortuitiously beneficial mutations may become selected for and established in a population by dint of the superior fitness (i.e. fertility and fecundity) of the individuals carrying such mutations. Present understanding of genetic drift and of mechanisms of genetic isolation have led to modification of existing evolutionary theory, but no fundamental change in understanding. Various theories including lamarckism and lysenkoism have provided temporary challenge to main stream evolutionary theory, but have proved either erroneous or of application only in very specialized situations. Lines of evidence that support the general tenet of organic evolution by natural selection include the following, stated only in the briefest terms (1) Mutations can be detected as occurring constantly in all populations at a measurable rate. (2) New species have arisen naturally in recent times (i.e. Spartina townsendii). (3) The fossil record presents evidence of many organisms no longer active and of an increase in the complexity of organisms with the passage of geological time. (4) The geographical distribution of related species is highly significant (e.g. the occurrence of indigenous marsupials in Australia and of penguins only at the South Pole). (5) Rapid mutation and evolution of certain pathogenic viruses and virulent strains of pathogenic bacteria are recognized in the constant need to change preventative vaccines.

***Evolutionary Clock.*** Time-scale of evolution determined by the rate at which mutations have accumulated in a given year.

***Evolutionary Rate.*** Rate at which changes can be detected in the characteristics of existing populations of organisms and, in particular, the rate at which any such changes become established or fixed. It is recognized that evolutionary rates vary greatly, and at certain cataclysmic times natural selection can operate very rapidly for certain species. Other species can remain essentially unaltered for many millions of years (e.g. Ginko tree, Ginko bilobe and the coelocanth fish).

***Evolutionary Tree.*** A diagram showing the relationships between a group of organisms and their evolution from an ancestral stock.

***Exchange Pairing.*** Pairing of chromosomes at meiosis such that recombination by crossing-over can occur between homologous chromosomes. The formation of the synaptonemal complex between the homologues facilitates DNA exchange between the paired chromosomes.

***Excision.*** Removal of damaged section of DNA strand, generally 10-100 nucleotides long prior to repair. Types of DNA damage include base modification by chemical mutagens, single-strand breaks and adjacent base dimerization through the action of ionizing or ultraviolet radiation. Excision is carried out by a number of specialized enzymes including DNA glycohydrolases and nucleases probably including (in bacteria) DNA polymerase I.

***Excision Repair.*** 1. Removal of damaged section of DNA strand and replacement by correct nucleotides. At least seven gene products in E. coli have been identified as components of the excision repair process, which is vital to the maintenance of genetic integrity in the living cell. The offending DNA is removed by specific enzymes, new nucleotides inserted and polymerized using the second strand as a template, and finally ligated together. The procedure can only work if one of the two strands remains undamaged to serve as a functional template for repair synthesis. Diseases involving lesions in DNA repair mechanisms are known, especially xeroderma pigmentosum.

2. The removal of damaged polynucleotide segments from DNA (e.g. thymidine dimers produced by ultraviolet light) and replacement with a correct segment using DNA polymerase and DNA ligase.

***Exclusion Principle.*** The principle that two species with the same ecological requirements cannot exist together.

***Excretion.*** Any elimination from an organism of unwanted materials, for example, carbon dioxide and nitrogenous substances produced in metabolism. It is worth nothing that excretory materials must be produced by the organism rather than just pass through it; thus faces in mammals contain a mixture of excreta (e.g. bile pigments) and undigested gut contents.

***Exergonic Reaction Or Exothermic Reaction.*** A reaction that releases free energy, as in a spontaneous change.

***Exogamy.*** The fusion of reproductive cells from distantly related or unrelated organism, i.e. outbreeding.

***Exogenote.*** Portion of the donor genome that is transferred into an intact recipient cell during gene transfer in bacteria.

***Exogenous.*** From the outside, as compared to endogenous, meaning native or internal. Thus molecules added to a cellular homogenate would be termed exogenous, those already present within it as endogenous.

***Exon or Extron.*** The DNA segments of a eucaryote gene that are transcribed into mRNA and then into protein. Exons occur along the length of the gene, and are separated by segments called introns whose sequences are also transcribed into m RNA. The intron m RNA segments are then excised, leaving behind the exon m RNA segment that join up to form a functional piece of m RNA, a process called RNA splicing.

*Exon Shuffle.* Recombination between two genes within their introns. Shuffling or juggling of exons has been suggested as a model for gene evolution. It has potential to generate rapidly new combinations of genetic material giving great selective advantage for the organism.

*Exonuclease.* An enzyme that removes a terminal nucleotide (3' or 5') in a polynucleotide chain. Exonucleases remove the nucleotides in a successive way, one by one, and are highly specific in their action.

*Exopeptidase.* A type of protein-splitting enzyme that hydrolyses the terminal peptide bonds rather than those bonds within the chain. There are three main types of exopeptidase in the mammalian gut, each attacking a particular area of the protein: carboxypeptidase attacks the carboxyl end of the chain; aminopeptidase attacks the amino end of the chain; dipeptidase breaks the bond between dipeptides. Such enzymes complete the digestion of protein prior to absorption into the blood stream.

*Exoscopic Development.* Development of the embryo of the sporophyte generation within the archegonium of the gametophyte plant. Following the first division of the zygote, the outer cell will subsequently give rise to the embryo and the inner cell, to the 'foot', a structure which grows into the body of the gametophyte obtaining nutrients for the growing embryo. It is applied to plant embryos of the Bryophyta, Psilopsida and Sphenopsida.

*Exotoxin.* Toxin produced by bacterial cells and excreted from the cells. Many bacterial exotoxins are extremely potent poisons and are important agents in diseases such as diphtheria, tetanus and botulism.

*Explant.* Tissue or group of cells isolated from the organism or embryo and subsequently cultured in vitro or on a host organism in such a way that normal tissue interactions are prevented. Frequently explants are used to assess whether or not embryonic cells have become determined, that is whether their developmental fate has been fixed. Cells that are determined before isolation from the surrounding tissue will undergo differentiation characteristic of their type; cells that are not determined will proliferate but not differentiate.

***Explantation.*** Preparation of an explant by isolating tissue or group of cells from an organism or embryo.

***Exponential Growth.*** A form of population growth in which the rate of growth is related to the number of individuals present. Increase is slow when numbers are low but rises sharply as number increase. If population number is plotted against time on a graph a characteristic J-shaped curve results. In animal and plant populations such factors as overcrowding, lack of nutrients, and disease limit population increase beyond a certain point and the J-shaped exponential curve tails off giving an S-shaped (sigmoid) curve. See Figure E.14.

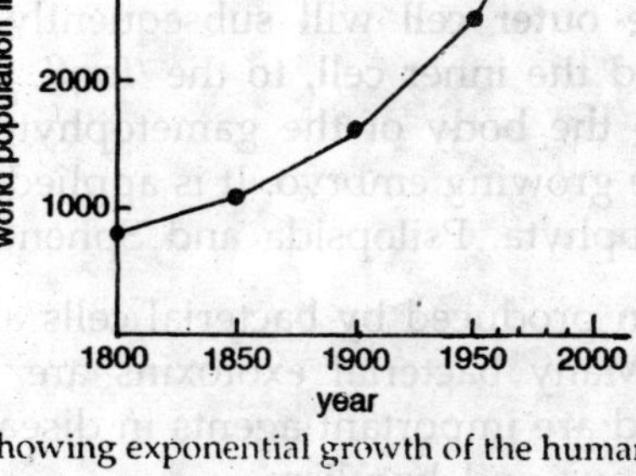


Figure E.14. Graph showing exponential growth of the human population.

***Explant.*** Any actively dividing plant tissue that can be induced to produce callus tissue in tissue culture.

***Exploitation.*** The situation in which one organism gains at the expense of another.

***Exponent.*** A number or quantity placed as a superscript to the right of another number or quantity, indicating how many times the number is to be multiplied by itself. For example, $10^6$.

***Expressivity.*** The degree to which a particular gene exhibits itself in the phenotype of an organism, once it has undergone penetrance. Thus, for example, a penetrant baldness gene in man can have a wide range of expressivity, from thinning hair to complete lack of hair.

***Extinct.*** (Of an animal or plant species)having died out, no longer present in the world population.

***Extinction.***1. The act of making extinct or the state of being extinct. 2. The elimination of an allele of a gene in a population, due to random genetic drift or to adverse selection pressures. 3. Any periodical, catastrophic event resulting in a species or larger taxonomic group dying out abruptly at a particular point in geological history. Such extinctions are thought to be cyclical, occurring every 28.4 million years, and have been attributed to cosmic activity such as showers or large asteroids or comets, though neither the periodically nor its causes are at present universally accepted.

***Extracellular Matrix.*** Formerly described as the ground substance of tissue, especially connective tissue. Extracellular matrices are complexes of interacting macro-molecules, secreted locally by the cells, and assembled (or, in part, self-assembled) to produce a semisolid meshwork which may not only hold the cells together in an organized fashion, but also impart a particular biomechanical property to that tissue (e.g. tensile strength in tendons, transparency in the cornea). Generally, extracellular matrices consist of hydrated polysaccharide gels within which fibrous proteins are embedded precise composition can vary enormously. It is now realized that virtually all tissues possess matrices, no matter how sparse, and that matrices serve a dynamic role, especially during development and differentiation. Cells not only synthesize matrix components, but also they respond constantly to local matrix composition, which helps maintain tissue organization. Breakdown of that feedback appears to underlie a number of disease states. Thus matrices regulate, or influence many aspects to cell behaviour (division, motility, shape) and metabolism.

Matrix composition has turned out to be far more complex than hitherto realized, is that most, if not all, tissues have a matrix of specific composition and display qualitative changes in matrix composition during differentiation. Consequently the range of matrix components identified is large (and constantly growing). The hydrated polysaccharide gel consists largely of glycosamino glycans which, with the exception of hyaluronic acid, are organized into proteoglycans. Because of their polyanionic character, they usually exist in a swollen hydrated state (the possibility of enormous tissue-specific diversity in proteoglycan core proteins is only just being appreciated). Within this gel are embedded a number of different fibrous proteins, primarily collagen and elastin, imparting tensile and elastic properties, respectively. Collagen displays considerable molecular polymorphism in that there are five major types and at least twice that number of minor types. This polymorphism is responsible for much of the qualitative difference between tissue-specific matrices. Cells also produce a number of pericellular glycoproteins, which enable them to attach to, and interact with, the immediate extracellular matrix. Thus, many mesenchymal cell types produce fibronectin, and epithelial cells laminin, multifunctional molecules with both cell-binding and collagen-binding domains.

The ability to produce an extracellular matrix is clearly very ancient; some colonial volvocine forms consist of cells embedded in gelatinous matrix of hydrated polysaccharides, and banded collagen is found in Porifera (sponges). It is likely that the acquisition of the ability to synthesize such molecules, and retain them all the cell surface, was one of the prerequisite steps in the evolution of multicellularity.

***Extraembryonic Membranes (Foetal Membranes).*** Four membranes that surround or are external to the embryo and/or foetus of certain vertebrates and that aid in its respiration, nutrition, excretion and protection during development.

Yolk Sac. Composed of endoderm and mesoderm, and vascularized. It grows so as to surround the yolk present in the egg and is connected ventrally to the gut of the embryo in most fish, birds and reptiles. As the yolk is absorbed in these species by endocytosis and breakdown in phagolysosomes in the yolk sac endoderm, the sac becomes drawn into the body of the embryo. A yolk sac also forms in mammals although the eggs are not yolky. In humans, sheep and cows it becomes an insignificant structure during development, whereas in rabbits, rats and mice what was the blastocoelic cavity becomes transformed into the yolk sac cavity by proliferation of 'parietal endoderm' and 'visceral endoderm'. Parietal endoderm together with trophoblast forms the outer wall (bilaminar omphalopleur) of the yolk sac; an inner, vascularized wall (yolk sac splanchnopleur) is formed from visceral endoderm and mesoderm. The bilaminar wall of the/yolk sac breaks down during development (in the guinea pig it never forms) and what was the yolk sac cavity becomes a new uterine lumen with visceral endoderm now exposed to proteinaceous uterine secretions. In these species the yolk sac splanchnopleur plays an important nutritive and transport role. Although many proteins are broken down within the visceral endoderm to provide essential amino acids, some maternal antibody molecules are transported intact to provide prenatal passive immunity.

Amnion. Membrane present only in amniotes (i.e. reptiles, birds and mammals). It arises in extraembryonic tissue usually as the inner membrane of the amnion fold created by formation of the exocoel (in a few mammals, including humans, simply by cavitation — not fold formation). It is composed of mesoderm on the outside and ectoderm on the inside facing the amniotic fluid and which the amnion encloses. Amniotic fluid provides hydrostatic support, lubrication, protection from mechanical shocks, contact with other tissues, and, in the case of reptilian and bird embryos, protection from desiccation since the eggs are laid on land. In humans the amnion becomes fused to the chorion by occlusion of the exocoel, and in ruminants and carnivores the amnion is secondary vascularized.

Allantois. Membrane present only in amniotes and composed of endoderm and mesoderm. It arises as a ventral outgrowth from what will become the hindgut region of the embryo. In reptiles and birds, the allantois is a sac that grows out across the exocoel between the amnion and yolk sac and acts as a repository for nitrogenous waste in the form of harmless uric acid. Eventually it fuses with the chorion (serosa), having become richly vascularized, and forms the chorioallantoic membrane which spreads underneath the shell membrane and functions in gaseous exchange. Fusion of the allantois with the chorion also occurs in mammals and is required in order to establish the chorioallantoic placenta, but the allantois although always vascularized may by a solid strand of cells with little or no endodermal component (human, rat, mouse), a relatively small sac lined with endoderm (rabbit) or a very large sac enclosing the amnion (pig, ruminants, carnivores) and serving as a receptacle for urine.

Chorion. In birds and reptiles also referred to as the 'serosa' to distinguish it from the chorion of mammals. It

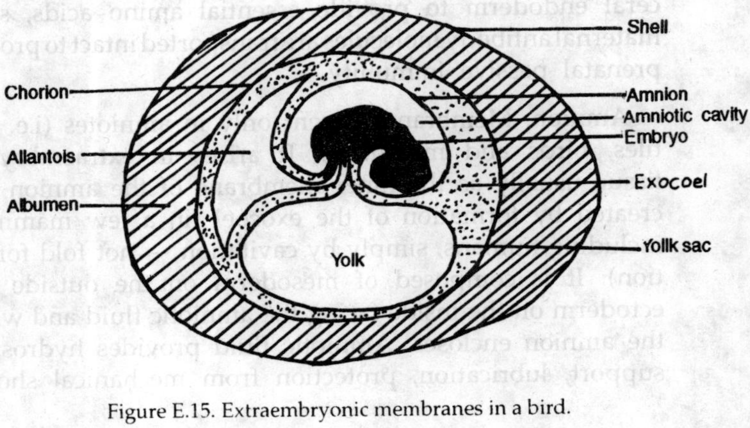


Figure E.15. Extraembryonic membranes in a bird.

arises as the outer wall of the amnion fold and consists of endoderm on the outside and mesoderm on the inside. In mammals chorionic ectoderm is derived from trophoblast. Depending upon the type of chorio-allantoic placenta that will be formed (epitheliochorial, syndesmochorial) following fusion with the allantois, trophoblast of the chorion either comes into close apposition with, or variously invades the maternal uterine tissues, effecting efficient exchange of gases, nutrients and waste products. See Figure E.15.

***Extraembryonic.*** Lying outside the embryo, e.g. embryonic membrane.

***Extrapolation.*** The estimation of a value beyond a given series, for example, the extension of the line of a graph beyond the calculated points.

# F

*$F_1$*. The first generation of filial offspring of a particular cross. The number can be changed to indicate the generation, for example, $F_3$ would be the great-grandchildren of a particular pair of individuals.

*$F_2$*. Second filial generation obtained when two organisms from an $F_1$ generation are mated. Progeny of the $F_2$ can be expected to provide phenotypic expression of recessive genes, since some will be homozygous for such genes. The ratios of phenotypic expression in the $F_2$ can be used to determine the true genotype of the parental generation.

***Fab Fragment.*** Part of an immunoglobulin molecule containing the antigen-binding site (Fragment antigen binding) and produced by treatment with the enzyme papain. It is composed of one light chain and part of one heavy chain joined by a disulphide bond.

***Facilitated Diffusion.*** The transport of molecules across the outer membrane of a living cell by a process that involves a specific carrier located within the cell membrane but does not require expenditure of energy by the cell. The carrier is believed to combine with a molecule on one side of the membrane, move through the membrane, and release the molecule on the other side.

***Factor, Genetical.*** An obsolete term that was used by early geneticists (e.g. R.C. Punnett) to describe an allele of a gene.

***Factorial Experiment.*** An experiment in which all treatments are varied together rather than one at a time, so the effect of each or combinations of several can be isolated and measured.

***Facultative.*** (Of an organism). Being capable of adopting an alternative life style from the nornal one. In this context, the word 'facultative' is followed by the unusual life style. Thus, a facultative parasite is one that is normally saprophytic but is occasionally parasitic; a facultative saprophyte is one that is normally parasitic but can become saprophytic; a facultative anaerobe is an organism that is normally aerobic but an exist in anaerobic conditions

***Facultative Heterochromatin.*** Highly condensed chromatin that only exists as heterochromatin in certain cells or at certain times. The heterochromatin of the inactive X chromosome (the barr body) of female mammals is said to be facultative.

***FAD (Flavin Adenine Dinucleotide).*** An electron carrier similar in action to NAD, picking up hydrogen from succinic acid in the krebs cycle. The hydrogen is transported to the mitochondrial lamellae where it enters an electron transport system at a lower point that NAD, with the release of only two molecules of ATP (rather than three ATP molecules when NAD is the carrier). See Figure F.1 on next page.

***Fallopian Tube.*** A tube forming part of the oviduct, present on either side of a female mammal, the transmits eggs from the peritoneal cavity to the uterus and is the usual site of fertilization. Ciliary action is involved in the egg movement, and muscular action facilitates the upward movement of sperms from the vaginal tract where they have been deposited after copulation.

***Familial.*** Trait that is transmitted in families (e.g. familial down's syndrome).

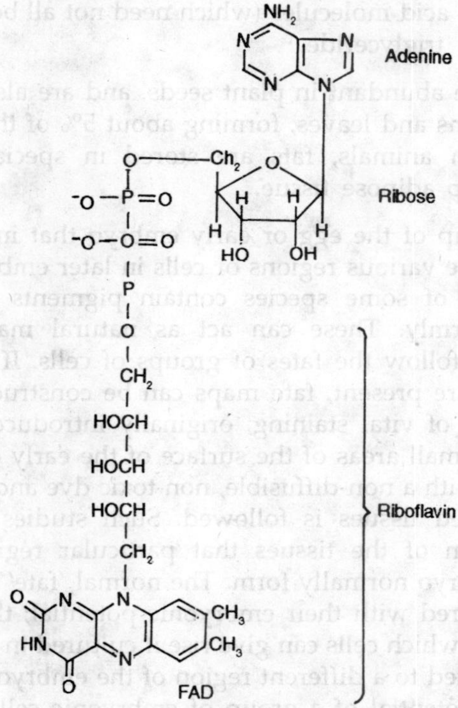


Figure F.1. FAD.

***Familial Hypercholesterolaemia (FHC).*** Human hereditary disease in which low-density lipoprotein is at an elevated level in the blood plasma. It is inherited as an autosomal dominant and leads to atherosclerosis.

***Farmer's Lung.*** A human disease in which lesions of minor blood vessles develop in the lungs. The disease is produced as a result of an immune response to the presence of fungal spores in hay. Similar symptoms have been recorded in other occupations, for example, malt workers, pigeon breeders, cheese washers.

***Fat.*** Type of simple lipid found in almost all organisms, which is an important energy-storage molecule (containing twice as much energy as carbohydrates per gram) that can also aid in heat insulation, cushioning and protection. Fats are produced by a combination of one glycerol molecule, and three fatty acid molecules (which need not all be the same) forming a triglyceride.

Fats are abundant in plant seeds, and are also found in roots, stems and leaves, forming about 5% of the total dry weight. In animals, fats are stored in specialized cells making up adipose tissue.

***Fate Map.*** Map of the egg or early embryo that indicates the fates of the various regions or cells in later embryogenesis. The eggs of some species contain pigments distributed non-uniformly. These can act as natural markers with which to follow the fates of groups of cells. If no natural markers are present, fate maps can be constructed by the technique of vital staining, originally introduced by Vogt in 1929. Small areas of the surface of the early embryo are marked with a non-diffusible, non-toxic dye and the fate of the marked tissues is followed. Such studies allowed a description of the tissues that particular regions of the early embryo normally form. The normal 'fate' of cells can be compared with their embryonic potential; the range of tissues to which cells can give rise if cultured in isolation or transplanted to a different region of the embryo. If the embryonic potential of a group of embryonic cells is greater than its fate, then factors must limit the differentiation of the cells in normal embryogenesis. See Figure F.2.

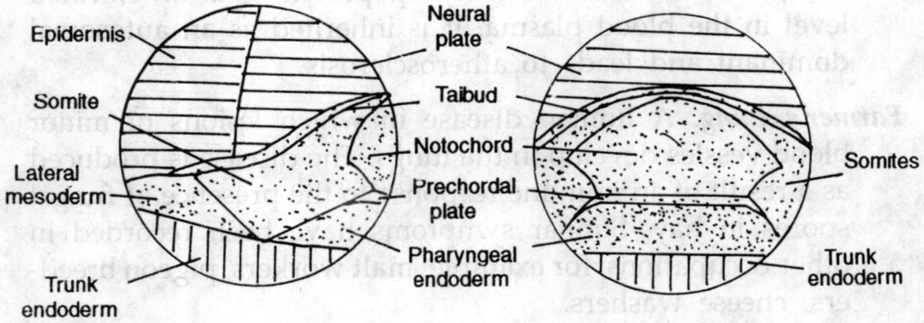


Figure F.2. Fate Map. Fate maps of the early amphibian embryo compiled from vital staining data.

***Fat Body.*** 1. (In amphibians and lizards) a structure in the form of finger-like growths immediately in front of the gonads.

The fat body stores fat as adipose tissue and is larger just before hibernation. It is of special importance in males where little or no food is taken in the breeding season, after which it is greatly reduced in size. 2. (In insects) a loose network of tissue in spaces between organs and around the gut, storing fat, proteins, glycogen and uric acid. It is found especially in juvenile insects before metamorphosis.

***Fat-Soluble Vitamin.*** Any of several vitamins, including A, D, E and K, that are soluble in organic solvents but insoluble in water.

***Fatty Acids.*** A range of molecules with the general formula $C_nH_{2n+1}COOH$ that occur naturally in many organisms, often combined with glycerol to form fats. Fatty acids are of two main types : unsaturated, with at least one carbon-to-carbon double bond, and saturated, with no such bonds. The greater the proportion of unsaturated fatty acids in a fat the lower its melting point, with many unsaturated fats being liquid oils at room temperature. There is evidence that excess consumption of saturated fats can lead to hardening of the arteries, but the facts are disputed, particularly by butter manufacturers.

***Fauna.*** The grouping of animals present in any one place or at any one time in geological history.

***Favism.*** A human disease characterized by the destruction of red blood cells, resulting in severe anaemia. The disease is triggered by the consumption of raw broad bean (Vicia faba), inhalation of broad bean, pollen or several other chemicals such as naphthalene (found in moth balls). The condition is due to a deficiency of the enzyme glucose-6-phosphate dehydrogenase found in red blood cells, the trait being controlled by an X-linked gene which is rare in most caucasian populations but more common in black populations. Since the condition is sex-linked it is more prevalent in males, although heterozygous females can be shown to have a deficiency of dehydrogenase enzyme.

***$F^+$Cell.*** A bacterial cell having an F factor.

***F-Cell.*** A bacterial cell that receive the F factor from an $F^+$ cell during conjugation, becoming $F^+$ in status.

***Fc Piece.*** Part of an immunoglobulin molecule produced by treatment with the papain and which is readily crystallizable (Fragment crystallizable). It comprises most of the constant regions of the two heavy chains joined together by a disulphide bond. Amino acid sequences determining class specificity, binding of complement and binding of antibody to certain cells are located in the Fc piece.

***Fc Receptor.*** Plasma membrane glycoprotein with high specificity for the Fc piece of particular immunoglobulin classes. Fc receptors for IgG are present on macrophages and polymorphs and effect phagocytosis of antibody-antigen complexes. Fc receptors for monomeric IgG (not complexed with antigen) are present on human syncytiotrophoblast, yolk sac endoderm of certain species and on gut epithelium of sucking rodents, where they effect transport of passive immunity. Fc receptors for IgE are present on mast cells and are involved in their degranulation following binding of reagins.

***F Duction (Sexduction).*** Transfer by bacterial conjugation of a limited segment of donor chromosome by an F′ factor. In the recipient cell the donor segment of the F′ factor (a plasmid) can recombine by a double cross-over with the homologous segment of the recipient chromosome, or the whole F′ can integrate into the chromosome by a single cross-over. The F′ plasmid replicates autonomously in recipients that are recombination deficient; this system has been used to bring alleles together in order to test for complementation and for chromosome mapping.

***Fecundity.*** The fertility of an organism (in higher animals, generally of the female of the species). Normally all organisms, assuming they reach reproductive age, are sufficiently fecund to replace themselves several times over. Darwin noted this, together with the fact that population numbers nevertheless tended to remain fairly constant : these observations led him to formulate his theory of evolution by "natural selection.

***Feeder Cell.*** Cell that when added to another cell population in tissue culture facilitates the growth of the latter. Frequently the feeder cells have been previously irradiated to prevent their division in the culture. The mechanism of their beneficial effect on the other cells results from the phenomenon of metabolic cooperation, a process by which nucleotides and other molecules pass from cell to cell via gap junctions. These cells may thus compensate for a genetic deficiency in the recipient cells (e.g. lack of an enzyme required for synthesis of an essential metabolite) and thus enable the deficient cells to survive and grow.

***Fehling's Test.*** A procedure used to detect the presence of reducing sugars in an unknown solution. Two solutions are mixed : Fehling's solution A containing copper tartrate (Cu(II)), and Fehling's solution B containing sodium hydroxide. The mixture is then added to the test solution and boiled. An orange-red precipitate of copper oxide (CU(I)) indicates the presence of a reducing sugar.

***Feline Leukaemia Virus.*** RNA virus associated with leukaemia in cats.

***Female Pronucleus.*** Haploid nucleus of an ovum. This nucleus results from meiotic divisions occurring during the formation of the egg; the other nuclei resulting from these divisions are eliminated or destroyed as polar bodies. Fusion of the female pronucleus with the sperm nucleus results in the formation of a fertilized egg.

***Feral.*** (Of plants and animals) existing in a wild state, outside human cultivation or habitation.

***Fermentation.*** Any industrial process involving the large-scale culturing of cells in either aerobic or anaerobic conditions using fermenters.

***Ferredoxin.*** An important iron-containing protein acting as an electron carrier in the electron transport system that operates in the light reactions of photosynthesis particularly in noncyclic photophosphorylation.

***Ferritin.*** A conjugated, electron-dense protein concerned in the absorption of iron through the intestinal mucosa. It serves as a storage protein for iron in the liver and spleen.

***Fertility.*** Measure of the ability of an organism to generate viable gametes capable of fertilizing gametes from the opposite sex to produce a zygote. Fertility is also used interchangeably with fecundity.

***Fertilization.*** Fusion of male and female gametes to form a zygote during sexual reproduction of both plants and animals. This event may take place internally or externally depending upon whether or not the female gamete, the egg or ovum, is retained within the maternal organism. In animals, an acrosome reaction ensures that the spermatozoon will penetrate the enveloping, non-cellular layer or egg coat (e.g. vitelline membrane, zona pellucida). In some systems, access to the egg can only take place at one or several points over the surface of the egg due to the existence of micropyles in an otherwise impenetrable egg coat. A cell recognition system, based on species-specific membrane proteins in the plasmalemmae in the gametes ensures that fertilization only takes place between gametes of the same species. The point of sperm entry will, in some systems, determine the future axes of the zygote and in turn of embryo.

Following fusion of the plasma membranes of the gametes, and the release of the male pronucleus into the cytoplasm of the egg or ovum, three events occur : (1) an immediate 'fast block to polyspermy' caused by a rapid depolarization of the egg plasma membrane, followed by a transformation of the enveloping layer/egg coat into a fertilization membrane, which constitutes a 'late block to polyspermy'; (2) the haploid male and female pronuclei will fuse to restore diploidy and combine, in a unique way, the genes from two individuals; (3) changes in intracellular ion concentrations, caused by ion fluxes at the cell surface, activate the developmental programme of the egg. Protein synthesis commences due to the unmasking of pre-existing, maternally derived messenger RNA, and DNA synthesis starts. Activation of the egg, and even very limited early development, may be initiated by non-specific experimental means (e.g., pricking amphibian eggs with a needle). All such techniques are thought to induce ion fluxes comparable to those normally triggered by fertilization.

***Fertilization Cone.*** Cone-shaped projection produced by certain eggs at the point of entry of a fertilizing sperm.

***Fertilization Membrane.*** A membrane that appears at the surface of the egg after fertilization. It is effectively a thickened vitelline membrane that may separate from the surface of the egg; it prevents the entry of additional sperms.

***Fertilizin.*** Substance secreted by some eggs. It has the property of attracting sperm of the same species.

***Feulgen-Positive.*** Characteristic of DNA and DNA-containing structures, indicating their positive response to staining with the feulgen stain procedure.

***Fetus (Foetus).***The embryo of a mammal, especially a human, when development has reached a stage at which the main features of the adult form are recognizable. In humans the embryo from eight weeks to birth is called a fetus.

***Feulgen, Robert (1884-1955).*** German physiologist and chemist best known for his discovery of a selective staining technique for DNA, the Feulgen reaction, which is based upon the reaction of an aldehyde group with leucofuchsin. The intensity of the purple colour in the cell nucleus is used as a measure for the quantitative estimation of nuclear DNA,

***Feulgen Reagent.*** A deep purple dye that stains the deoxyribose sugar of DNA in cell nuclei.

***Feulgen Stain.*** Important cytochemical test for DNA. It utilizes schiff's reagent and gives a purplish-pink colour when positive. Measurement of the intensity of the colour by microspectrophotometry or colorimetry can be used to measure the DNA content of tissues or solutions.

***Feulgen's Test.*** A histochemical test in which the distribution of DNA in the chromosomes of dividing cell nuclei can be observed. It was devised by the German chemist R. Feulgen (1884-1955). A tissue section is first treated with dilute hydrochloric acid to remove the purine bases of the DNA, thus exposing the aldehyde groups of the sugar deoxyribose. The section is then immersed in "Schiff's reagent, which combines with the aldehyde groups to form a magenta-coloured compound.

***F Factor or Fertility Factor or Sex Factor.*** An episome that confers donor status on an $F^+$ cell, so that the $F^+$ cell transfers a copy of the F factor and a small piece of bacterial DNA to an $F^-$ cell during conjugation, the recipient becoming $F^+$.

***F′ Factor.*** F factor carrying a limited segment of the bacterial chromosome produced by abnormal detachment of F from the chromosome. Although the primary F′ cell producing the plasmid is left with a defective chromosome, the F′ factor soon becomes stabilized by transfer to cells with normal chromosomes. F′ factors are used to create merozygotes in order to test for genetic complementation.

***Fibroin.*** Protein that is the major component of silk, a material used by spiders to build webs, and by insects to construct larval nests and cocoons. Silk is produced only by specialized cells within the silk glands, and is composed of long chains of the amino acids glycine and alanine, with occasional serine residues.

***Fibroin Gene.*** Gene coding for fibroin in the silk moth Bombyx moi. It has been studied extensively and also isolated and established in a bacterial clone. It is a large DNA sequence of about 15 kilobases in length, with a single intron of 970 base pairs near to the 5'-end of the gene. Only a single copy of this gene is present in the Bombyx genome, despite the massive amounts of silk made by the silk gland cells. To permit the enormous production of fibroin messenger RNA required, the entire genome is replicated some 17-18 times more than in a normal diploid cell. This entire polyploidization to achieve massive output of one gene sequence contrasts with the gene amplification mechanism found in genes coding for ribosomal RNA in Xenopus and egg chorion protein in Drosophila.

***Fibronectin.*** Group of large proteins secreted by many types of cells, and which form a fibrillar matrix linking cells to other extracellular proteins, such as collagen. Specific domains on the fibronectin molecule bind to the cell surface, collagen, proteoglycans, etc. At transformation cells fail either to secrete or to bind fibronectin, and this is thought to be responsible for some of the altered properties of transformed cells. Addition of fibronectin to transformed cells partially normalizes some of their properties. Fibronectin is thus also called LETS (large, external, transformation-sensitive) protein.

***Fibrous Protein.*** One of the basic architectural forms adopted by amino acid chains to construct proteins. Fibrous proteins consist most commonly of interlinked chains of polypeptides forming a rope, as in the molecule of collagen. Packing of the amino acid chain into a relatively tight three-dimensional form is the chief alternative to fibrous protein; such molecules are known as globular proteins.

***Ficoll.*** Synthetic sucrose polymer used widely in separation techniques and centrifugation in cellular biochemistry.

***Fight-or-Fight Reaction.*** A defence reaction or alerting response in higher animals, involving an increase in blood pressure and heart rate and a redistribution of the blood away from the viscera towards the striated muscle. These changes result from integrated nerve pathways in the brain known as defence centres, and from the secretion of adrenaline.

***Filamin.*** Long, flexible fibrous protein ($M_r$ ~ 250 000) that has a tendency to form dimers in solution. It is important in its role of forming cross-links between neighbouring actin molecules, thus changing a viscous fluid containing only actin molecules in solution, into a solid gel with the addition of filamin; another protein with a similar action to filamin is called α-actinin.

***Filopodium.*** Long, spike-like extension of cell surfaces that is larger than a microspike and is orientated in the same longitudinal direction. Filopodia may be up to 50 μm long and are characteristically found at the growing tip of developing nerve cell axons.

***Filter Hybridization.*** Exposure of DNA, bound as denatured single strands to an immobilizing filter material such as nitrocellulose paper, to a solution containing radioactivity labelled probe DNA or RNA. Subsequent washing leaves only base-paired double-stranded molecules and so identifies complementary sequences in the original sample.

***Fimbrin.*** Protein involved in cross-linking actin filaments in microvilli and other actin-containing extensions.

***Fine-Structure Genetic Mapping.*** Analysis of recombination within a gene sequence down to the level of the single nucleotide. Recombination occurs within gene sequences as well as between gene sequences, and the localization of particular base changes in mutant alleles can be determined by this means.

***Fingerprinting.*** Technique widely used to determine differences in amino acid sequence between proteins that are clearly related (e.g. products of mutant alleles). The technique involves the enzymic breakdown of the protein into peptides and separation of such peptides by electrophoresis or chromatography often two-dimensionally, permitting a comparison of the pattern obtained after migration of the peptides (i.e. the fingerprints).

***First-Division Segregation.*** The segregation of a pair of different alleles of a gene into different nuclei at the first division or meiosis. In tetrad analysis of an ascus such segregation would be detected by four adjacent ascospores carrying one allele type and other four ascospores carrying the other type.

***Fission.*** (1) Common method of asexual reproduction in bacteria and Protozoa, in which a single cell divides to produce two daughter cells that are identical to the parent cell. Fission usually involves division down through the middle of the parent cell. In a cell such as an Amoeba, nuclear division occurs first, followed by the cleavage of the cytoplasm. (2) Division of a eukaryotic cell nucleus is sometimes referred to as nuclear fission.

***Fission Yeast.*** Yeast that replicates by fission, with the formation of a cell plate in the middle of the rod-shaped cell. This is in contrast to propagation by bud formation in budding yeast. The best known fission yeast, widely used in studies on the cell cycle, is Schizosaccharomyces pombe.

***FITC (Fluorescein Isothiocyanate).*** Fluorescent dye, used in immunofluorescence and in fluorescence-activated cell, sorters.

***Fitness.*** The ability of an organism to transfer its genes to the next generation. Organisms favoured by selection (natural or artificial) have a high fitness, while those subjected to adverse selection pressure have a low fitness. Thus, under conditions of insecticide treatment, resistant members of an insect population will have a high fitness and produce more offspring as compared to susceptible individuals that have a low fitness.

***Fixation.*** A genetical situation where all members of a population are homozygous for one particular allele of a gene, so that no alternative alleles of that locus exist in the population. Fixation often occurs in small populations.

***Fixation of Alleles.*** State in which all members of a population are either homozygous or hemizygous for a particular allele, all other alleles at that locus having been lost in the course of evolution.

***Fixation Probability.*** Likelihood of an allele becoming fixed in a population. This probability is affected by a number of factors, including population size.

***Fixative.*** Solution used for the fixation of cells or tissues in the preliminary steps of their preparation for microscopy. Common fixatives include ethanol, acetic acid, formalin and osmium tetroxide. The last is most commonly used in the preparation of material for electron microscopy.

***Flagellin.*** Protein ($M_r$ = 20 000) that constitutes the chief constituent of a bacterial flagellum.

***Flagellum.*** Fine hair-like projection from the surfaces of some cells, with locomotory function or causing movement of the external medium relative to the cell surface. Flagella are found in some bacteria, many protozoa and algae, and also in sperm. The flagella of bacteria are structurally quite distinct from those of eukaryotic cells and have an exclusively locomotory function. They consist of hollow rods, the walls being composed of a helical array of spherical subunits of a single protein, flagellin. These flagella are based in a rotary motor device consisting of a protein disc, integrated into the plasma membrane but allowing turning of the flagellar filament. Eukaryotic flagella are larger than those of bacteria, being about 150 μm in length and with a structure identical to that of eukaryotic cilia. Eukaryotic flagella therefore are essentially large cilia, although because of their large size their motion is wave-like and propagated from base to tip or tip to base.

***Flame Cell (Solenocyte).*** Cell with an excretory function found in some lower animal phyla (e.g. Annelida and Rotifera). The cells absorb excretory products from surrounding tissues and, through the beating of cilia, propel these products down a protonephredial tube to the exterior.

***Flanking Sequence.*** Sequence that is either upstream or downstream, on the same DNA molecule, from a particular definitive sequence such as a gene. Enhancer sequences frequently flank gene-coding sequences.

***Flavin.*** Isoalloxazin ring of riboflavin, FAD and FMN.

***Flavoprotein.*** A protein that is combined with flavin prosthetic groups and acts as an intermediate carrier in respiratory chains between dehydrogenases and cytochromes.

***Fleming, Sir Alexander (1881-1955).*** Scottish bacteriologist and Nobel prizewinner (1945) who discovered the antibiotic penicillin (1928).

***Flightless.*** (Of certain birds and insects) unable to fly, having secondarily lost the ability. The term is usually applied to birds such as ratites and penguins.

***Flip-Flop Model.*** Model which proposes that a molecule that is part of a continuous layer would move head to tail within the layer so that its position relative to the two surfaces is reversed. Proteins in the cell plasma membrane, set within the more or less continuous lipid bilayer, are known to execute such movements very rarely, if at all.

***Floccose.*** (Of plant structures) covered in small hairs giving a down-like appearance.

***Flocking.*** The active coming together of animals to form a flock. In most organisms this usually takes place outside the breeding season. The term is normally limited to birds and mammals. Fish are usually described as schooling, and insects as swarming. Such grouping may serve as a defence against predators, or as a means of transferring information on food supplies, where one member of the group may follow another to a known good feeding area.

***Flora.*** 1. The plant life characteristic of a particular geographical area. 2. a botanical manual from which plants can be identified by the use of keys.

***Florigen.*** A hypothetical plant hormone that may be produced in leaves after suitable light treatment, and moves to the buds to stimulate flowering.

***Floristics.*** The branch of botany concerned with the study of vegetation in terms of the number of different species present in the flora.

***Fluctuation Test.*** Genetical test, originally devised by Luria and Delbruck in 1943. The test was devised to determine whether mutation in bacteria occurred randomly and non-adaptively, or in response to specific environmental demand. In the test these workers compared the numbers of a favourable mutation occurring in many small, parallel cultures of a bacterium with the numbers occurring in one large culture. Since the numbers in the small cultures were highly variable (hence the name fluctuation test) the test indicated that mutational events are random and non-adaptive.

***Fluid Mosaic Model.*** Model proposed by Singer and Nicholson, in 1972, to account for the observation on the structure of the plasma membrane that rendered the earlier davson and danielli model untenable. The Singer and Nicholson model proposes that the lipid bilayer of the membrane is essentially in a fluid state and that most of the proteins are located within this lipid layer in a discontinuous mosaic, either projecting on one surface of the membrane or, more commonly, set between the lipid so as to project on either side.

***Fluor.*** Compound that has the property of fluorescence.

***Fluorescence.*** The property of giving out light when molecules are excited by incident light. Emitted light is always of a shorter wavelength than the incident light.

***Fluorescent Antibody Technique or Immunofluorescence.*** A technique used to show up the presence of a particular antigen, in which an antibody is labelled with an ultraviolet fluorescent substance that combines with the antigen and is subsequently located by its fluorescence.

***Fluorescence-Activated Cell Sorter (FACS).*** Instrument that is able to separate cells that fluoresce from those that do not as they pass down through a narrow orifice for scanning. Cells may be conjugated with a specific fluorescein-conjugated antibody which binds only to a restricted population of a batch of cells. These will therefore be selected out by the cell sorter.

***Fluorescence Microscopy.*** Microscopy that allows the fluorescent components to be visualized and localized. When excited by ultraviolet light, certain chemicals fluoresce (i.e. emit light of visible wavelength). When preparations of biological material are viewed through a microscope using ultraviolet illumination, fluorescence can be seen where the fluorescing substances are located. Similarly, fluorescent stains and dyes (e.g. acridine orange, fluorescein) can be used to label biological components at the subcellular, cellular or tissue level.

***F-Mediated Transduction.*** Induction of a genetic change in a bacterial cell and its progeny by the introduction of novel genes from another bacterium through bacterial conjugation.

***FMN (Flavin Mononucleotide).*** Derivative of the B vitamin riboflavin. It is the prosthetic group of the membrane-bound NADH dehydrogenase, a complex flavoprotein which is the first complex involved in the electron transport chain for oxidation of NADH oxygen. The hydrogen atoms of $FMNH_2$ are released as protons, the electrons being transferred to the iron-sulphur centre of the enzyme complex. See Figure F.3.

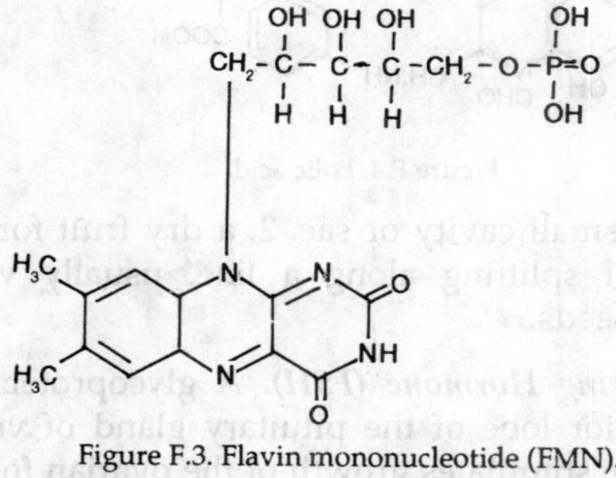

Figure F.3. Flavin mononucleotide (FMN).

***Focus or Primary Focus.*** An area containing a high concentration of diseased plants or animals and from which the disease probably spreads.

***Fodrin.*** Spectrin-like protein found in association with actin filaments in microvilli.

***Foetal Calf Serum.*** Extract from blood of foetal calves that is widely used to fortify tissue culture media for the growth of mammalian cells. The serum contains growth factors, some known, others unknown.

***Foetal membranes.*** The extraembryonic membranes of the mammalian foetus.

***Foetus.*** The embryo of mammals at the time when it achieves the main features of the adult form. This is usually at the time of the formation of the amnion which is after about eight weeks of pregnancy in women.

***Fold Back DNA (Snap back DNA).*** Short repeated sequences of the eukaryotic genome which can 'fold back' on themselves to form duplexes following denaturation. These sequences can be either dispersed or found in clusters.

***Folic Acid.*** Vitamin of the B complex; a precursor of tetrahydrofolic acid, a coenzyme with an important role in purine and pyrimidine synthesis and therefore in the synthesis of nucleic acids. Its deficiency is linked to the induction of megaloblastic anaemia in mammals. See Figure F.4.

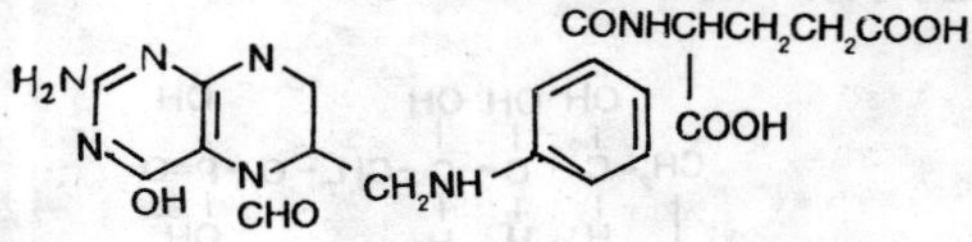


Figure F.4. Folic acid.

***Follicle.*** 1. Any small cavity or sac. 2. a dry fruit formed by a single carpel splitting along a line, usually ventral, to liberate its seeds.

***Follicle-Stimulating Hormone (FSH).*** A glycoprotein secreted by the anterior lobe of the pituitary gland of vertebrates. The hormone stimulates growth of the ovarian follicles and oocytes in the ovary, and spermatogenesis in the seminiferous tubules of the testis.

***Follicular Phase.*** That part of the oestrous cycle in which graafian follicles are formed and their secretions start.

***Fomite.*** Any inanimate object via which pathogenic organisms may be transferred, although it does not support their growth, for example, a book

***Food.*** A substance containing or consisting of chemicals which can be used in the body of an organism to build structures and provide energy to sustain life. Most plants are autotrophs and require only essential elements in their food, but animals are heterotrophs and their food must contain certain carbohydrates, fats and proteins as well as vitamins and essential elements.

***Food Chain.*** A sequence of organisms arranged in such a way that the second grouping, e.g. herbivores, feeds on the first, e.g. primary producers, and the third, e.g. carnivores, feeds on the second.

Each organism in the chain feeds and derives energy from its predecessor in the chain, the relative energy value at each trophic level often being assessed by the construction of ecological pyramids. In practice, such simple systems rarely exist and the nutritional relationships between organisms normally constitute a food web. See Figure F.5.

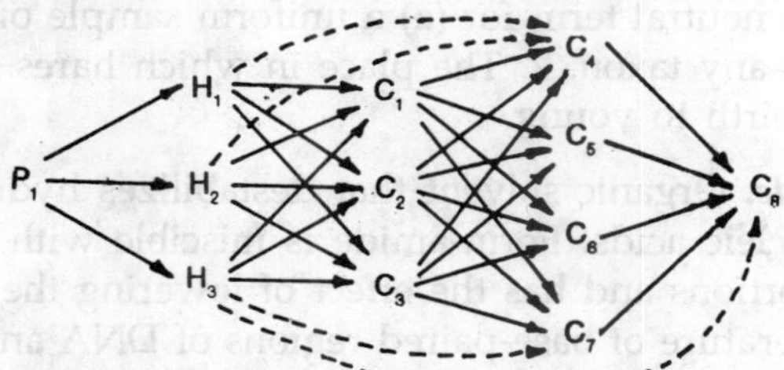


Figure F.5. Food Chain. A complex food web of producer (P), herbivore (H) and carnivore (C).

***Food Production.*** The growth of animal and plant material, and subsequent cropping for human consumption.

***Food Test.*** A method by which certain components of a food mixture can be detected. For example, fehlings tests for reducing sugars.

***Food Poisoning.*** An acute (2) disorder of the gut caused by food contaminated with bacteria or their toxins (e.g. botulism) or by some chemical.

***Footprinting.*** Technique used to detect regions of DNA which are conjugated to and thus protected by specific proteins. DNA with and without the protein conjugates is exposed to endonuclease, and the resulting fragments are run on electrophoretic gels. Comparison of the two gels reveals bands that resist attack only in the presence of the protein, and are thus selectively associated with such protein.

***Foramen Ovale.*** An embryonic opening in the septum that divides the left and right atria of the mammalian heart, providing a bypass to the lung circulation. Failure to close the aperture at birth can lead to a blue baby condition.

***Foraminifera.*** Amoeboid protozoans that possess chitinous, calcareous or siliceous shells that are usually many-chambered. Calcareous foraminifera are the main constituent of chalk.

***Ford, E.B. (1901-).*** English entomologist famous for his work on the genetics of lepidoptera and genetic polymorphism.

***Form.***1. A neutral term for (a) a uniform sample of individuals or (b) any taxon. 2. The place in which hares lie and may give birth to young.

***Formamide.*** Organic solvent that destabilizes hydrogen bonds in nucleic acids. Form-amide is miscible with water in all proportions and has the effect of lowering the melting-out temperature of base-paired regions of DNA and RNA. It is widely used in molecular hybridization and as a denaturant during RNA molecular weight estimations.

***Formaldehyde.*** Agent frequently used to preserve biological tissue, usually in the form of the aqueous solution, formalin. It is also used to denature DNA and RNA to single-stranded form by removal of intramolecular bonding.

***Formation.*** Any of the main natural vegetation types extending over a large area that is created by the nature of the climate. Examples include tundra, steppe, rainforest and coniferous forest.

***Formenkreiss.*** An aggregation of allopatric species or subspecies.

***N-Formylmethionine.*** Compound responsible for initiation of protein synthesis on bacterial ribosomes. It is brought to the ribosome by a novel species of transfer RNA (tRNA), the initiator tRNA.

***Forssman Antigen.*** Antigen, discovered by forssman in guinea pig tissue, capable of eliciting antibody production against cell proteins of many mammalian species.

***Forward Mutation:*** Mutation from wild-type of new form of a gene (i.e. the most usual form of mutation).

***Forward Mutation.*** A genetic change in which a wild type piece of DNA is altered to a mutant sequence.

***Fossa.*** A depression, pit or cavity.

***Fossil.*** The remains or traces of any organism that lived in the geological past. In general only the hard parts of organisms become fossilized (e.g. bones, teeth, shells, and wood) but under certain circumstances the entire organism is preserved. For example, virtually unaltered fossils of extinct mammals, such as the woolly mammoth and woolly rhinoceros, have been found preserved in ice in the Arctic. Small organisms or parts of organisms (e.g. insects, leaves, flowers) have been preserved in amber.

In the majority of fossils the organism has been turned to stone - a process known as petrification. This may take one of three forms. In permineralization, solutions originating underground fill the microscopic cavities in the organism. Minerals in these solutions (e.g. silica or calcite) may actually replace the original material of the organism so that even microscopic structure may be preserved; this process is known as replacement (or mineralization). A third form of petrification-carbonization (or distillation)- occurs in certain soft tissues that are composed chiefly of compounds of carbon, hydrogen, and oxygen (e.g., cellulose). After the organism has been buried, and in the absence of oxygen, carbon dioxide and water are liberated until only free carbon remains. This forms a black carbon film in the rock outlining the original organism. Moulds are formed when the original fossil is dissolved away leaving a mould of its outline in the solid rock. The deposition of mineral matter from underground solutions in a mould forms a cast. Palacontologists often produce casts from moulds using such substances as dental wax. Moulds of thin organisms (e.g. leaves) are commonly known as imprints. Trace fossils are the fossilized remnants of the evidence of animal life, such as tracks, trails, footprints, burrows, and coprolites (fossilized faces).

The ideal condition for the formation of fossils occur in areas of rapid sedimentation, especially those parts of the seabed that lie below the zone of wave disturbance.

***Fossil Record.*** The remains of organisms, or traces of their existence (such as footprints), present in the rock strata and forming a history of the development of life from its origins on earth. The record is very largely incomplete due to the comparative rarity with which fossils are formed, but provides evidence of evolution having taken place, particularly where long series of a particular form can be traced over an extended period of time.

***Founder Cell.*** Cell that becomes fixed in certain locations, and through division and differentiation gives rise to a tissue at that site. If only one founder cell is involved the tissue would be said to be monoclonal, but most tissues in higher eukaryotic animals are known to be polyclonal.

***Founder Effect.*** The result of starting a new population with a low number of individuals (founders), so that their gene pool may not contain the same proportions of alleles for a particular locus as in the original population. For example, instead of containing three alleles of the ABO blood group locus. Australian aborigines contain no B alleles and thus no group B or group AB individuals are produced, a situation probably caused by a 'founder effect.' Such small founder populations are subject to random genetic drift.

***F Pilus (Sex Pilus, Sex Fimbria).*** Long appendage extending from the surface of E. coli cells that carry an F Factor. F pili can act as conjugation tubes which allow transfer of the F factor from $F^+$ to $F^-$ cells. They also provide the attachment site for several bacteriophages (e.g. M13, Qβ, R17).

***Fragile X Syndrome (Martin Bell Syndrome).*** Human congenital syndrome characterized by mental retardation, enlarged testes and a fragile site on the x chromosome. After Down's syndrome, this is the commonest cause of moderate or severe mental retardation in males.

***Fragmentation.*** A type of asexual reproduction found in some lower plants (such as spirogyra or blue-green algae) where there is separation of the threadlike filaments (2), each segment of which is capable of growing into a mature organism. Fragmentation is caused by such mechanical forces as wind, wave action, rain, etc.

***Frameshift.*** An altered reading of the Generic code during the translation stage of protein synthesis caused by a change in the nucleotide base sequence of DNA and RNA due to an insertion or deletion in a point mutation. Figure F.6 shows an example of a DNA base insertion between bases 4' and 5'. When the sequence is read from left to right the first amino acid is unchanged, but the second and subsequent amino acids will be altered, producing a mutant protein.

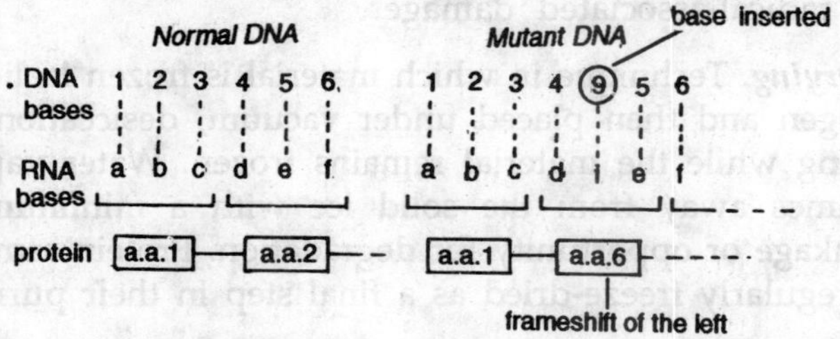


Figure F.6. Frameshift. The effect of inserting an extra DNA base into the nucleotide base sequence.

***Fraternal Twins (Dizygotic Twins).*** Two individuals that result from a single pregnancy, each having developed from a separate fertilized egg. The two egg cells contain different combinations of "alleles and so do the two sperm that fertilize them. The twins therefore have no more genetic similarity than brothers or sisters from single births.

***Freemartin.*** Sexually abnormal female member of a pair of dizygotic twins in which the other member is male. The condition arises in cows, sheep, pigs and goats, where twins frequently have anastomoses of blood vessels within their placentas (i.e. conjoined placentas). This results in transfer of blood stem cells, hormones and possibly some other inducing factor that in some way causes sex reversal of the ovaries, interference with the differentiation of the female reproductive tract and, consequently, sterility, in the female twin.

***Free Radical.*** Chemical species with an unpaired electron in its outer orbital. Generated as intermediates in metabolism (e.g. mitochondrial oxidative phosphorylation), these highly reactive entities may attack lipids, proteins and DNA, and it is suggested they may contribute to ageing. Free radicals formed by the ionization of water react with organic molecules and lead to peroxidation and polymerization, and cross-linking in or between molecules. membranes rich in unsaturated fatty acids are particularly prone to attack, and damage to mitochondria and lysosomes has been shown in old age. membrane damage due to free radical attack has been implicated in ageing fibroblast cultures. Antioxidant free radical scavengers (e.g. vitamin E) seem to ameliorate free radical-associated damage.

***Freeze-Drying.*** Technique in which material is frozen in liquid nitrogen and then placed under vacuum, desiccation occurring while the material remains frozen. Water vapour sublimes away from the solid ice with a minimum of shrinkage or opportunity for degradation. Protein samples are regularly freeze-dried as a final step in their purification.

***Freeze-Etching.*** Technique used in the preparation of biological material for electron microscopy. Specimens are frozen in a cold liquid such as liquid nitrogen or freon, fractured under vacuum, and exposed surfaces allowed to sublime so that surface irregularities become evident. A carbon replica is then made, stripped away, and examined in the electron microscope.

***Freeze-Fracturing.*** Technique used in the preparation of materials for electron microscopy. Following freezing, the specimen is fractured under vacuum or scratched so as to reveal particular surfaces or irregularities. The plane of fracture will often follow that of particular membranes or organelles within a cell. A carbon replica of the frozen surface is made and later examined. Since no chemical fixation or staining need be involved, surface structure is likely to resemble closely that present within living cells.

***Frequency-Dependent Selection.*** Any selection in which the fitness of genotypes is directly related to the proportions of the various phenotypes present in a population, so that the frequency of the more common types is decreased and the less common types is increased. Such selection pressure often produces a stable genetic polymorphism and when it involves predation is referred to as apostatic selection.

***Frequency Distribution.*** An arrangement of statistical data in order of the frequency of each size of the variable. For example, the numbers : 2, 3, 5, 3, 4, 2, 1, 3, 4, would have the frequency distribution shown in Figure F.7. Data from a large sample often produces a normal distribution curve.

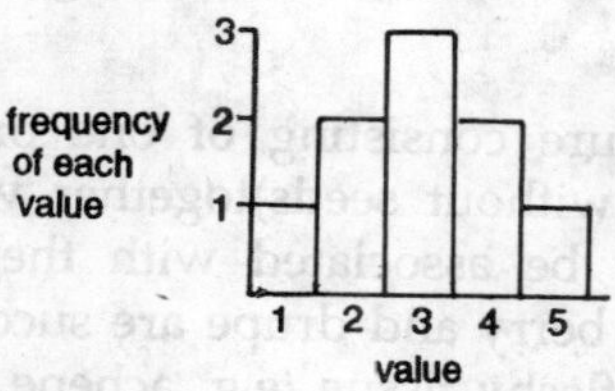


Figure F.7. Frequency distribution. Based on 9 numbers.

***Fresh Water.*** An aquatic environment such as streams, rivers, lakes, etc. where there is little dissolved mineral matter and which results directly from precipitation (rain), as opposed to saltwater (the seas and oceans).

***Freund's Adjuvant.*** (1) Complete Freund's adjuvant. Mineral oil mixed with an emulsifying agent and containing heat-killed tuberculin bacilli or related organisms. When a solution of antigen is added, a stable water-in-oil emulsion is created by vigorous mixing and antigen is distributed in the aqueous phase. (2) Incomplete Freund's adjuvant. As above, but without the addition of bacteria.

***Friend Cell*** (Mouse erythroleukaemia cell. MEL cell). Mouse haematopoietic stem cell that is infected by the friend leukaemia virus.

***Friend Leukaemia Virus.*** Virus that induces specific leukaemias in certain mouse strains, the cells of which can be readily maintained in culture. The cells are of an erythroid nature, and may be induced in culture to differentiate following treatment with dimethylsulphoxide, so making these cells a favoured material for studies on cell differentiation in vitro. The virus and its action on the mouse were originally discovered in the laboratory of Dr. Charlotte Friend.

***Frisch, Carl Von (1886-).*** Austrian behaviourist famous for his researches on the language, orientation and direction finding of bees. He also carried out extensive research on the colour sense of bees and fishes and their senses of hearing, smell and taste.

***Fructose.*** A carbohydrate that is considered to be an atypical ketose sugar because it acts as a reducting sugar in fehling's test.

***Fruit.*** A plant structure consisting of one or more ripened ovaries (with or without seeds)together with any flower parts which may be associated with the ovaries. Many fruits such as the berry and drupe are succulent, but often they contain no fleshy tissue (e.g. achene, nut).

***Fruitfly.*** Common name for flies in the genus Drosophila.

***F-Strain.*** Bacteria that do not harbour the F factor. They are nominally female and can therefore act as recipients during bacterial conjugation.

***$F^+$ Strain.*** Bacteria harbouring the F factor. They are nominally male and can act as donors of the F factor during bacterial conjugation. $F^-$ strains are recognized by the presence of surface pili which confer sensitivity to certain male-specific bacteriophages (e.g. M13, MS2, R17) and by surface exclusion, which prevents self-melting.

***Fucoxanthin.*** A brown carotenoid pigment found in brown algae and diatoms that is present together with chlorophyll o.

***Fucus.*** A genus of algae, typically having greenish-brown slimy fronds (2), such as Fucus vesiculosus, the bladderwrack.

***Fugacious.*** (Of plant organs) withering and falling quickly.

***Fungus.*** (Pl. fungi) an organism that may be unicellular or made up of tubular filaments (hyphae) and lacks chlorophyll. Fungi live entirely as saprophytes or parasites. There are two main divisions : the eumycota, the 'true fungi' and the myxomycota, the slime moulds, each of which is now given the status of division, though in older classifications both were grouped with algae in the Thallophyta.

***Furanose Ring.*** A monosaccharide having a five-membered ring structure.

***Fusiform.*** (Of plant structures) spindle-shaped.

***Fusion Gene.*** Gene derived from parts of two other genes, either by unequal crossing over or by deletion of part of the chromosome segment between two adjacent genes. Haemoglobin lepore is a fusion gene. In this haemoglobin, the 'beta-chains' of the tetrametric structure are abnormal and consist of a sequence from the left-hand end of a delta-chain gene joined to a sequence from the right-hand end of a beta-chain gene.

***Fusion Protein.*** Protein molecule produced by recombinant DNA technology, usually when a novel gene is inserted into a recipient plasmid vector in such a way that a terminal stop codon in a plasmid gene is deleted. Thus translational read-through occurs with the new fusion protein beginning with a plasmid sequence and continuing with the protein sequence of the inserted novel gene.

# ENCYCLOPAEDIC DICTIONARY
# OF
# GENETICS AND ORGANIC EVOLUTION

# Encyclopaedic Dictionary of Genetics and Organic Evolution

**Vol. 2**

[G — O]

*Editor*

**Kiran Narang**

**ANMOL PUBLICATIONS PVT LTD**

**New Delhi-110 002**

**ANMOL PUBLICATIONS PVT LTD**
4374/4B, Ansari Road
Daryaganj, New Delhi-110 002

*Encyclopaedic Dictionary of Genetics and Organic Evolution*

First Edition 1995
**ISBN 81-7488-044-5 (Set)**

**PRINTED IN INDIA**

Published by J.L. Kumar for Anmol Publications Pvt. Ltd. and
Printed at Mehra Offset Press, Delhi.

# Preface

This encyclopaedic dictionary has been essentially a compilation and editing of the terms and concepts taken from genetics and organic evolution. Many words borrowed from more general usage have been endowed with very special meaning, sometimes not obvious to the uninitiated.

The entries have been represented in a clear and explanatory style to provide both straight forward definitions and invaluable background informations. This approach combined with an extensive cross referencing system enables the reader to place each entry into a broader scientific context. Many diagrams have been incorporated whenever the meaning of a term can be best conveyed by means of a diagram.

Every effort has been made to include certain entries which take into account of recent developments and trends in genetics and organic evolution.

The terms included in this encyclopaedic dictionary have been presented in brief analytical phrases thereby avoiding the more comprehensive type of treatment appropriate to large reference works. The extent of each entry has been determined by the need for definition of meaning, function and agricultural relevance. Also, certain entries have been added to take into account of recent developments and trends in agriculture.

This encyclopaedic dictionary will be of immense value to the students of genetics and organic evolution, botany, ecology, biology, microbiology, anthropology, biochemistry, archaeology, geography, geology, agriculture and environmental science.

**Editor**

Vol. 2

# G

*G.* Symbol for guanine or guanosine in molecular biology.

*G.* Gravity; employed in the indication of centrifugal forces. Thus 10 000 x g implies that a force 10 000 times that of gravity has been applied as a centrifugal sedimentation force.

*G0.* Phase of the cell cycle entered by resting or quiescent cells such that division is suspended and normal metabolism drastically reduced. The suggestion that cells may be able to enter a resting or G0 phase stems from the observation that, at a crucial point in the G1 phase of the cell cycle, many cells display an enhanced resistance to adverse conditions as compared to other stages of the cycle. The point in G1 at which such cells can rest and opt out of the normal cycle is referred to as the R point, and the cells are then presumed to have entered G0.

*G1.* Phase of the cell cycle corresponding to the growth phase.

*G2.* Phase in the cell cycle between the S phase, when the DNA is replicated, and M phase, when the cell undergoes mitosis. Thus the nucleus of cells in the G2 phase contains twice the amount of DNA (4C, i.e., four time haploid) than is present in the G1.

***G6PD***. (Gamma-aminobutyric acid). Neurotransmitter, mainly found in the brain, formed by the decarboxylation of glutamic acid, used exclusively in inhibitory synapses. GABA increases the permeability of the postsynaptic membrane to chloride ions so that it becomes hyperpolarized.

***Gain.*** 1. (In physiological experiments) an increase in signal as a result of amplification. 2. A shift in the progeny mean relative to the mean of the original population brought about by directional selection. Gain is used to estimate the heritability of characters.

***Galactosaemia.*** A rare inborn error of metabolism in which the breast-fed human infant is literally poisoned by the mother's milk. The affected individuals are unable to metabolize the milk sugar galactose, which normally is converted to glucose ready for oxidation and the release of energy. Instead, affected infants store the galactose in various tissues including the brain, resulting in severe malnutrition along with mental retardation.

Galactosaemia is due to blockage of the step galactose-1-phosphate to glucose-1-phosphate because the enzyme uridyltransferase is absent or inactive. The condition is controlled by an autosomal gene probably on chromosome 9, affected individuals being homozygous for the recessive alleles. The transferase enzyme can be detected in foetal cells from amniocentesis before birth and, if newborn infants are given a special diet, development will be normal.

***Galactose.*** Monosaccharide carbohydrate that does not occur freely in nature, but is combined with glucose to form lactose, a disaccharide sugar found in milk.

***Galactosidase.*** Enzyme that hydrolyses galactosides to galactose plus a second molecule having a hydroxyl group. This is usually another monosaccharide (e.g. glucose, produced from lactose), but it may be methanol (from a methylgalactoside) or nitrophenol (from 0-nitrophenyl-galactoside). The β-galactosidase of E. coli has provided an important tool in microbial genetics and the study of the regulation of gene expression. Its synthesis is induced by the natural substrate (lactose) or by a range of β-galactosides. It is readily assayed in extracts or in whole bacteria by measuring hydrolysis of the artificial substrate 0-nitrophenylgalactoside to its coloured product (0-nitrophenol). The study of the regulation of synthesis of this enzyme laid one of the foundations of molecular biology—understanding of the lac operon of E. coli.

***Galactosyltransferase.*** Any one of a group of enzymes that help to make mature complex oligosaccharides from more simple sugars. Many of these complex sugars are finally attached to proteins, and much of this assembly occurs in vesicles of the golgi apparatus. Indeed these enzymes are used as specific markers for the golgi vesicles.

***Galapagos Islands.*** A group of 15 islands in the Pacific Ocean situated on the equator some 900 miles west of Ecuador. In 1835, Charles Darwin visited the islands during his voyage on the beagle and the fauna particularly influenced his views on evolution. According to his theory, geographical isolation has influenced divergence of different forms so that, for example, Darwin's finches have all probably evolved from a common ancestor, and now occupy numerous niches on the islands due to the absence of competition from other birds. Marine iguanas and giant tortoises are other interesting animals found there, and in the absence of palms and conifers, the normally small prickly-pear cactus has reached tree-like proportions.

***Gallus Domesticus.*** Domesticated chicken believed to be derived from a species of Indian jungle fowl.

***Galton's Apparatus.*** Piece of equipment in which marbles are dropped through a hole and then allowed to bounce randomly between pegs before falling into a series of basal slots. Most marbles end up in the central slot, but some marbles have been fed through the hole, piles of marbles in the basal slots reveal a bell-shaped distribution. This pattern represents the distribution probability curve for any such series of random events.

***Gametangium.*** The organ in which the gametes are produced in lower plants.

***Gamete or Germ Cell.*** A specialized haploid cell that fuses with a gamete from the opposite sex (or mating type) to form a diploid zygote. In simple organisms, the process is called isogamy, and oogamy in more complex organisms. In animals where oogamy occurs male gametes are called sperm, the female gametes eggs. The situation in higher plants is more complicated, but essentially the male gamete is the generative nucleus found in the pollen grain while the female gamete is the egg cell found within the embryo sac.

***Gametic Meiosis.*** Meiotic division that immediately precedes the formation of gametes. This type of meiosis is characteristic of higher organisms in which the organism is diploid for most of its life cycle, but does not typify organisms in which the organism is diploid for most of its life cycle, but does not typify organisms in which all or a substantial part of the life history is haploid.

***Gameto-or Gamo-.*** Denoting germ cells.

***Gametocyte.*** An animal or plant cell that develops into gametes by meiosis.

***Gametogenesis.*** The process in which haploid gametes are produced from diploid cells by meiotic divisions. See Figure G.1 for animal cells and Figure G.2 for plant cells.

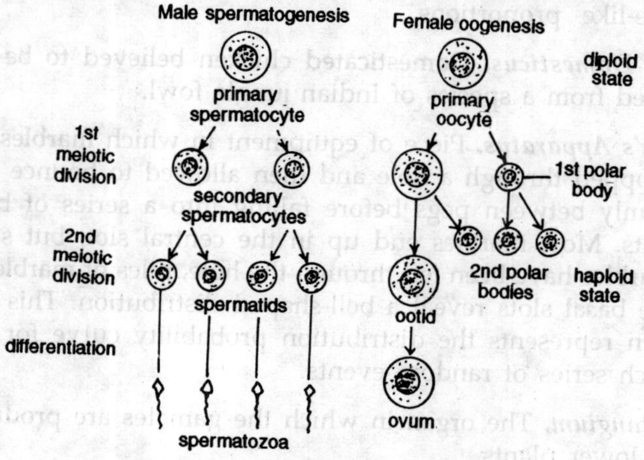


Figure G.1. Gametogenesis. In animals.

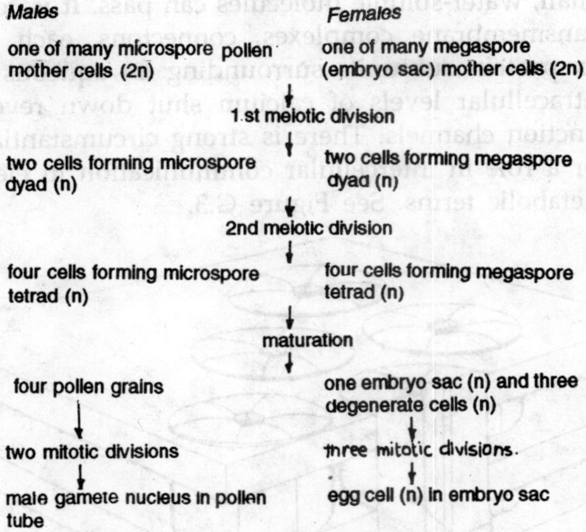


Figure G.2. Gamotogenesis. In plants.

*Gametophyte.* The generation in the life cycle of a plant that bears the gametes producing sex organs. The gametophyte is haploid. It is the dominant phase in the life cycle of mosses and other bryophytes, the sporophyte generation depending on it either partially or completely. In pteridophytes it is the prothallus. In seed plants it is very much reduced. For example, in angiosperms the pollen grain is the male gametophyte and the embryo sac is the female gametophyte.

*Gamma Globulin.* A member of a group of proteins found in blood plasma that may act as an antibody.

*Gamma-Radiation.* Electromagnetic radiation of short wavelength that is emitted during the radioactive decay of some atomic nuclei. Radioactive sources such as cobalt-60 are powerful emitters of gamma-radiation and as such may be used to induce cellular mutations or to kill cells.

*Gap.* Section on one strand of a DNA duplex in which some nucleotides are missing.

*Gap Junction.* Common type of intercellular junction creating aqueous channels between adjacent cells, through which small, water-soluble molecules can pass. It is composed of transmembrane complexes, connectons, each comprising six protein sub-units surrounding an aqueous core; high intracellular levels of calcium shut down reversibly gap junction channels. There is strong circumstantial evidence for a role in intercellular communication in electrical and metabolic terms. See Figure G.3.

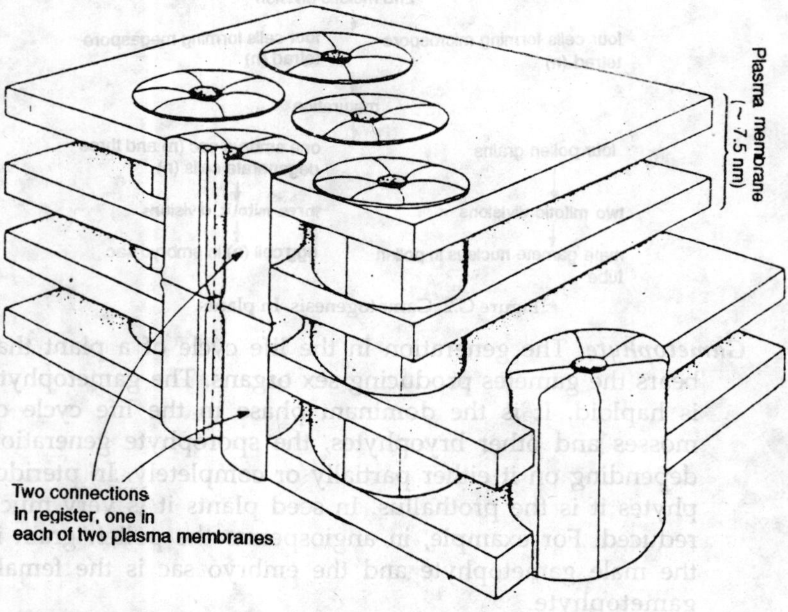


Figure G.3. Gap junction. Reconstruction of the organization of a gap junction.

***Gargoylism.*** Two distinct hereditary disease of the human-Hunter Syndrome and Hurler Syndrome. Both are connective tissue disorders involving storage of glycosaminoglycans, and result in facial and other deformities.

***Garrod, Archibald, E. (1857-1936).*** English hospital physician who between 1900 and 1910 described first demonstrable case of a human disease that is inherited according to the laws of mendelian genetics. The condition is alkaptonuria, which is controlled by a single autosomal recessive gene. Garrod proposed that the enzyme that catalyses the breakdown of homogentisic acid to acetoacetic acid is nonfunctional in alkaptonurics. This results in a build-up of the acid in the urine, which turns black on exposure to air, and is readily observed in infant's nappies. It was not, however, until 1958 that the absence of a functional homogentisic-acid oxidase enzyme was demonstrated in the liver of a patient with alkaptonuria. Garrod went on to explain several other human conditions such as albinism as inborn errors of metabolism.

***Gas-Liquid Chromatography.*** A technique for separating or analysing mixtures of gases by chromatography. The apparatus consists of a very long tube containing the stationary phase, a nonvolatile liquid, such as a hydrocarbon oil coated on a solid support. The sample is often a volatile liquid mixture (e.g. of fatty acids), which is vaporized and swept through the column by a carrier gas (e.g. hydrogen). The components of the mixture pass through the column at different rates and are detected as they leave, either by measuring the thermal conductivity of the gas or by a flame detector.

Gas chromatography is usually used for analysis; components can be identified by the time they take to pass through the column. It is sometimes also used for separating mixtures.

***Gastrula.*** Stage in development during which the embryo undergoes gastrulation. Gastrulation follows the rapid cleavage of the egg into many cells to form the blastula stage. The gastrula stage precedes, and is essential to, the formation of the nervous system of the embryo which is initiated in the neurula stage.

***Gastrula.*** A stage in embryonic development in which the blastula has invaginated, so giving rise to two-layered embryo by a process of gastrulation.

***Gastrulation.*** Formation of the gastrula in the development of the embryo. Gastrulation is the first and most major morphogenetic movement of tissues in embryogenesis. Before gastrulation the embryo has become multicellular, but the cells have not altered their position within the embryo.

During gastrulation, cells of the outer layer move into the embryo in an active and coordinated manner. This is achieved by the invagination of tissue at a particular site in the embryo, the blastopore. By the end of gastrulation cells are arranged in their germs layers — ectoderm, endoderm and mesoderm — and the basic body plan of the embryo has been established. Gastrulation also brings tissues into contact with each other in new ways, and allows novel tissue interactions. The most major of these-primary embryonic induction-results in the alteration of the fate of the dorsal ectoderm to form nervous tissue by its interaction with the newly underlying mesoderm tissue.

***Gastrulation.*** The process by which the blastula forms the gastrula.

***Gaucher Disease.*** Congenital disease of glycolipid metabolism with a high frequency among Ashkenazi jews. It is caused by an autosomal recessive gene and is typified by progressive neurological disease, splenomegaly, bone pain and lipid-filled cells.

***Gaussian Distribution.*** (Normal distribution). Pattern of distribution in which the frequency of occurrences of values becomes progressively rarer as the values deviate more from the commonest or mean value. Thus a gaussian distribution appears, when plotted, as a symmetrical, bell-shaped curve. Any gaussian distribution can be characterized by two parameters, the mean and the standard deviation — a measure of the spread of the data. Parametric methods of statistical analysis require that the data to be analysed are samples from a distribution which approximates to a gaussian distribution. If this requirement is not met, non-parametric statistical methods must be used.

***Gause's Law.*** A law stating that no two species with identical ecology can exist together in the same environment. Named after the German anatomist G.F. Gause.

***G. Banding.*** A method of treating chromosomes with Giemsa stain to show areas of the chromosomes with light and heavy staining. Such patterns are different for each chromosome type and thus are most useful when arranging chromosomes in karyotype analysis.

***Gel.*** A semi-rigid colloid as distinct from the more liquid sol.

***Gel Electrophoresis.*** Analytical and preparative technique used to separate proteins and nucleic acids. The rate of migration is proportional to net charge and inversely proportional to the effective size of individual molecules. Separations are carried out in slabs or cylinders of a porous, semi-solid supporting medium such as an agarose gel or a cross-linked polyacrylamide gel. The concentration of the gel used is varied according to the size range of the molecules being separated (for a fixed electric field a higher gel concentration lowers the mobility of a molecule). The best separations are achieved using gradient gels which have a continuously increasing gel concentration along their length. On completion of the separation the molecules can be visualized using a dye (e.g. Coomassie blue for proteins, ethidium bromide for DNA), and the gel sliced so that individual bands can be recovered. If the molecules are radiolabelled, they can be detected by autoradiography. A useful variation of polyacrylamide gel electrophoresis (page) involves denaturing the proteins by treating them with sodium dodecyl sulphate (SDS) and 2-mercaptoethanol. Disulphide linkages are cleaved, and the resulting unfolded protein is coated, through hydrophobic associations, with SDS molecules each contributing two negative charges to the complex. The result is that polypeptides of different sizes have the same (or nearly so) density of charge along their lengths (the acquired net negative charge being approximately proportional to molecular weight). Electrophoretic separation then depends solely on the sieving properties of the polyacrylamide gel, so that the smaller polypeptides move faster. As the gels can be calibrated with proteins of known molecular weight, SDS-PAGE provides a simple method for molecular weight determination.

***Gel Filtration.*** Chromatographic procedure used to separate molecules of different sizes. The insoluble gel is placed in the form of small hydrophilic beads in a glass column, and a solution containing the molecules to be separated is poured through the column. Large molecules move quickly through, but smaller molecules enter spaces between or within the beads and are therefore slowed in their progress through the gel. Different degrees of cross-linking between the polysaccharide dextran chains forming the beads provides for the variation in separation characteristics.

***Gel Staining.*** Procedure whereby proteins, nucleic acids or other molecules are visualized in an electrophoretic gel by staining. Stains such as coomassie blue are frequently used to stain proteins in gels, the initial staining procedure being followed by a regulated destaining until only the desired bands are left stained.

***Gene.*** The fundamental physical unit of heredity that transmits information from one cell to another and hence one generation to another. Genes consist of specific sequences of DNA nucleotides which can code for the structure of polypeptide chains, tRNA molecules and rRNA molecules. Individual genes can be recognized through the existence of variable forms, or alleles, that form the basis of genetic variability. Organisms can be considered as gene carriers, being controlled by genes in such a way as to maximize the changes of survival of the genetic material.

***Gene Amplification.*** A process in which many copies are made of some genes at one time, while other genes are not replicated. The replicated genes enable enhanced manufacture of product in a short time. For example, rRNA genes are amplified about 4,000 times in oocytes of the clawed toad Xenopus laevis to assist in protein production during egg development.

***Gene Bank.*** 1. A collection of clones containing all the genes of a particular organism, such as E. coli. 2. A collection of many lines of a particular crop plant, used as a genetic resource by plant breeders.

***Gene Bridge.*** The means by which a plant pathogen can survive between the main host-growing seasons by living on host plants grown out of the normal season. Thus, for example, a cereal pathogen can often transfer in September from a mature, spring-sown host to newly sown winter cereal plants.

***Gene Cloning.*** The technique of genetic engineering in which specific genes are excised from host DNA, inserted into a vector plasmid and introduced into a host cell, which then divides to produce many copies (clones) of the transferred gene.

***Genecology.*** The study of plant populations in relation to habitat and genetical structure.

***Gene Conversion.*** Phenomenon in which, following two rounds of meiotic division alleles are segregated in a 3:1 rather than a 2:2 ratio. It thus seems that the gene sequences of one allele of a gene has been converted to the sequence of the other allele present in the same cell. Gene conversion may be a result of the DNA polymerase suddenly switching templates to the other homologous sequence and then switching back. This was at one time referred to as the copy choice hypothesis.

***Gene Divergence.*** Process by which multiple copies of a gene sequence, presumed to have arisen from a single ancestral sequence, form a family of sequences with significant differences of base sequences between the multiple copies. For example, the human globin genes are presumed to have arisen in this way; the present gene family includes, alpha-, beta-, gamma-, delta-and other globin sequences, all having diverged to a greater or lesser extent from the ancestral gene.

***Gene Dosage.*** Frequency with which a particular gene is present in a cell or in the genome of an organism. Gene dosage varies from one, for single copy genes such as the fibroin gene in a sperm or egg cell, to the thousands of copies of some ribosomal RNA genes in organisms such as amphibians.

***Gene Exchange.*** New combinations of genes in offspring resulting from normal sexual reproduction within a breeding population where genes are contributed by both parents.

***Gene Flow.*** Movement of alleles from one population of an organism to another by interbreeding of individuals in the two populations. Genetic variation within the recipient population is thus increased by the new alleles contributing to the range of the gene pool of the population.

***Gene-For-Gene Concept.*** The theory that genes for pathogen resistance in a host plant are matched by corresponding virulence genes in the attacking pathogen.

***Gene Frequency.*** (allelic frequency). Frequency with which a particular allelic form of a gene occurs in a population. Frequencies of recessive alleles are often much higher than might be assumed from the number of individuals expressing the trait in the homozygous condition. For example, caucasians in the USA show a prevalence of cystic fibrosis of one in 2000 individuals but in fact one in 20 of this population carries the allele.

***Gene Induction.*** The activation of an inactive gene so that it can carry out transcription.

***Gene Library***(gene bank). Collection of cloned genes, frequently comprising most or all of the genes from a particular species. Such libraries may consist of genomic sequences or cDNA sequences, the latter having been made from messenger RNA and lacking intron sequences. Libraries are made by cutting purified DNA with selected restriction endonucleases, followed by the cloning of the fragments into viral or bacterial plasmid vectors. Gene libraries can be searched using a homologous sequence from a related organism in order to identify the clone within the library which represents the desired gene.

***Gene Locus*** (genetic locus). Position on a particular chromosome on which a specific gene is located. Locus is expressed as a map position, either relative to other genes which are adjacent on the same chromosome, or in terms of a particular mapping distance from the centromere of the particular chromosome. Thus, a gene might be described as being located on the long arm of chromosome 14 at so many map units from the centromere. Chromosome banding techniques have proved extremely useful in the assignment of genes to particular loci.

***Gene Magnification.*** Phenomenon in which the number of copies of the ribosomal genes is increased in mutants of Drosophila. Such mutants are termed bobbed, since they also have reduced numbers of bristles.

***Gene Map*** (genetic map). Order of nucleotides and genes that is deduced from genetic recombination experiments. Individual genes can be assigned to specific loci within a genome or a chromosome as a result of gene mapping.

***Gene Mutation.*** Change in the base sequence of a specific gene.

***Gene Pool.*** The sum total of all the genes of all breeding individuals in a population at a particular time, represented by their gametes. Note that those individuals which are too young to breed (juveniles) or those that have undergone genetic death do not contribute to the gene pool.

***General Recombination.*** One aspect of genetic recombination; in the genetic exchange that occurs between homologous DNA sequences, most commonly between the two homologous copies of the same chromosome. Although the results of recombination are evident as chiasma during meiotic division, the recombination event is believed to precede chiasma formation, but it also depends on the close association of the tetrad of the homologous chromosome copies during meiotic division.

***Generation.*** 1. A group of organisms of approximately the same age, usually derived from the same parents, referred to as the first filial generation ($F_1$). 2. the act of propagating a species or bringing about the formation of new individuals.

***Generation Times 1.*** Also called division time, the time required for a population of cells to double in number. 2. the time required for a generation of individuals to be born, reach sexual maturity and reproduce. The generation time is a critical factor in population growth rates and efforts are being made (particularly in China) to extend the human generation time so as to slow down the rate of population increase.

*Gene Redundancy.* Presence of multiple copies of the same gene on a chromosome; for example, the genes for ribosomal RNA occur as tandem repeat copies. The term should not be taken to imply that the extra copies are in any way useless or unnecessary.

*Gene Regulatory Protein.* Protein that functions by altering the transcriptional state of a specific gene. The repressor protein that regulates the activity of the lac operon in E. coli is one such protein, and they are widely believed to be an important aspect of eukaryotic gene regulation also.

*Gene Therapy.* The application of genetic engineering techniques to alter or replace defective genes. The techniques are still at the experimental stage but the eventual aim is to prevent such genetic diseases as sickle cell anaemia and thalassaemia.

*Gene Repression.* The deactivation of an active gene that causes a shut-down of transcription.

*Generic.* Of or belonging to a genus.

*Gene Switching.* The process in which genes are activated or deactivated during development, so that there is a sequential output of gene products, some taking part in current biochemical pathways others acting as inducers and/or repressors of other genes.

*Genetic.* Of or relating to genes.

*Genetic Assimilation.* Process by which a phenotypic character becomes genetically fixed in a population. Initially the trait would have appeared in response to particular environmental factors in a few individuals, but as these individuals proved successful at least one of them would, by chance, become endowed with a gene sequence that would produce the advantageous trait even in the absence of the environmental cues. With time the gene would spread through the population by the positive selection of the individuals possessing it and their contribution of the common pool of surviving progeny.

***Genetic Background.*** 1. Any genes other than those of special interest·in a study. 2. any effects in an experimental which can alter the main results in different crosses.

***Genetic Block.*** Break in a biochemical pathway such as that involved in the synthesis of a specific enzyme, resulting from a mutation in the enzyme-coding sequence or in an appropriate regulatory gene.

***Genetic Code.*** A collection of codons of DNA and RNA that contains information about polypeptide chain sequencing during translation, each triplet usually coding for one amino acid. A triplet code with four letters (Cytosine, Guanine, Adenine and Thymine bases) gives $4^3 = 64$ combinations. Each codon has been shown to have a specific function. See Figure G.4. Note that the code shows degeneracy, and that there is one triplet for initiating polypeptide chain production (AUG) and there is one triplets for terminating production (UUA, UAG and UGA). The code is more or less universal the same proteins being produced from a particular base sequence in both E. coli and mammals.

| First base (5'end) | Second base: U | C | A | G | Third base (3' end) |
|---|---|---|---|---|---|
| U | UUU, UUC } Phe<br>UUA, UUG } Leu | UCU, UCC, UCA, CUG } Ser | UAU, UAC } Tyr<br>UAA, UAG } Stop | UGU, UGC } Cys<br>UGA Stop<br>UGG Trp | U<br>C<br>A<br>G |
| C | CUU, CUC, CUA, CUG } Leu | CCU, CCC, CCA, CCG } Pro | CAU, CAC } His<br>CAA, CAG } Gin | CGU, CGC, CGA, CGG } Arg | U<br>C<br>A<br>G |
| A | AUU, AUC, AUA } Lieu<br>AUG Met (start) | ACU, ACC, ACA, ACG } Thr | AAU, AAC } Asn<br>AAA, AAG } Lys | AGU, AGC } Ser<br>AGA, AGG } Arg | U<br>C<br>A<br>G |
| G | GUU, GUC, GUA, GUG } Vai | GCU, GCC, GCA, GCG } Ala | GAU, GAC } Asp<br>GAA, GAG } Glu | GGU, GGC, GGA, GGG } Gly | U<br>C<br>A<br>G |

Figure G.4. Genetic code. The mRNA codons of the genetic code arranged in a genetic dictionary.

***Genetic Death.*** A sexually mature individual that is alive but unable (or unwilling) to breed and thus transmit his or her genes to the next generation via the gene pool. Genetic death is fairly rare in most populations of plants and animals, but in developed countries the amount of genetic death amongst humans is increasing, not only in terms of individuals surviving to old age but because of those who opt to practice birth control.

***Genetic Dictionary.*** A construction showing the relationship between the triplets in messenger RNA and each amino acid.

***Genetic Drift.*** Random changes in gene frequencies in small samples or populations. Although it theoretically occurs in all populations, its effects are only significant in small ones.

***Genetic Engineering.*** The modification of the genetic complement of an organism to the benefit of man. The term applies to a wide range of genetical techniques, for example, plant and animal breeding, to improve physiological performance by selection, but recently the term has become associated with the deliberate transfer to genetic material from one organism to another where it is not normally found. For example, a gene can be removed from human cells and transferred to microbial cells (using bacteriophage or plasmid vectors) where the 'foreign' gene can control the formation of useful products. Industrial production of insulin and interferon is now possible using such methods. In the near future it may be possible to transfer pieces of microbial genetic material to higher organisms. For example, genes from nitrogen-fixing bacteria could be introduced into the genomes of nonleguminous crop plants to supplement their nutrition.

***Genetic Equilibrium or Equilibrium of Population.*** A state that occurs when gene frequencies are constant in a population for several generations. Such equilibrium may also be found where selection is operating to produce a stable genetic polymorphism.

***Genetic Fine Structure.*** Consideration of genes at the level of nucleotide sequences, and the molecular events that are relevant to them.

***Genetic Homeostasis.*** The property possessed by a population for resisting sudden change and maintaining a steady genetic composition.

***Genetic Induction.*** Stimulation of a specific gene by an inducer molecule. In bacterial operons more than one gene may be induced simultaneously by the same inducer. Inducers may act directly or indirectly, usually through an effect on the RNA polymerase or on the promoter region upstream from the gene-coding sequence.

***Genetic Information.*** Store of information encoded in the nucleotide sequence of an RNA or DNA molecule.

***Genetic Isolation.*** A form of reproductive isolation in which hybrids from two different species are unable to produce fertile gametes and thus are sterile. For example, a horse crossed with a donkey produces a sterile mule.

***Genetic Linkage.*** The association between genes located (linked) on the same chromosome, thus producing proportions of gametes that are not those expected by independent assortment although, unless there is very close linkage, the same types of gamete will be produced. Instead, there tends to be association to particular alleles together in the gametes (the 'parental' types, in the same combination as the parent), with other combinations being less frequent.

By convention the amount of recombination between linked genes is a direct measure of their distance apart along the chromosome, 1% recombination being equivalent to the map unit. The amount of recombination occuring is best measured in testcross calculated from the total number of recombinant types in the testcross progeny as a proportion of the total progeny. For example, a testcross with genes in coupling produced the phenotypes, where the amount of recombination would be :

$$\frac{33 + 42}{280} \times 100 = 26.8\%$$

and the genes A and B could be represented on a genetic map as :

A ——————————— B
26.8

Had the two genes been independently assorting (i.e. on different chromosomes) roughly equal numbers of each phenotype would have been expected in the progeny (about 70). Similarly, since the maximum expected amount of recombination between two genes is 50%, if two genes are located more than 50 map units apart on the same chromosome they will appear to be independent of each other.

***Genetic Load.*** A measurement of the amount of deleterious genes in a population, calculated as the average number of lethal equivalents per individual

***Genetic Polymorphism or Polymorphism.*** The presence in a population of two or more morphs, produced when different alleles of a gene occur in the same population and the rarest allele is not maintained merely be repeated mutation (i.e. has a frequency higher than, say, 0.05%). Such a definition excludes continuously variable characters such as height or skin colour in humans, but the human blood groups are classic examples, where single genes have two or more alleles, producing different antigenic phenotypes. A genetic polymorphism can be maintained by several mechanisms such as heterozygous advantage or frequency-dependent selection, and can be stable over several generations (a balanced polymorphism) or may become 'transient' as when the environment changes.

***Genetics.*** The branch of biology concerned with the study of heredity and variation. Classical genetics is based on the work of Gregor Mendel. During the 20th century genetics has expanded to over lap with the fields of ecology and animal behaviour, and important advances in biochemistry and microbiology have led to clarification of the chemical nature of genes and the ways in which they can replicate and be transmitted.

***Genetic Variability.*** A range of phenotypes for a particular character produced by alternative alleles of one or more genes, the range containing discrete groups or a continuous spectrum of types. Genetic variability arises initially by mutation and is maintained by sexual reproduction involving crossing over in meiosis. Such variation is the raw material for natural selection to act upon, ensuring that the best-adapted variants are most likely to reproduce.

***Genetic Variance.*** Variance of a phenotypic trait in a population which is attributable to genetic heterogeneity.

***Genital Disc.*** Type of imaginal disc. During the early development of some insects, small groups of cell are set aside. After hatching these cells proliferate to form imaginal discs. The cells of the imaginal discs proliferate at each molt, and at metamorphosis they differentiate into specific adult structures such as leg, wing or genitalia. Transplantation of the genital discs to a different position in the larva or to a different larva shows that the imaginal disc cells are highly determined; a genital disc will nearly always differentiate into genital structures in whatever position it has been placed. Furthermore, the parts of the genital disc are determined.

***Genital Ridge*** (germinal ridge). Thickened, longitudinal strips of mesodermal epithelium tissue lateral to the dorsal mesentary in the posterior half of vertebrate embryos from which the gonads will form. Originally the genital ridge tissue is composed of somatic cells; these cells differentiate to form the structural and endocrine cells of the mature gonad. During development the genital ridge becomes populated with the primordial germ cells. These cells will differentiate to form the gametes. The primordial germ cells do not originate in the genital ridge, but migrate to the developing gonads from the site of their origin outside the gonad (in amphibian embryos) or even outside the embryo (in avian and reptile embryos).

***Genome.*** Entire set of genes carried by a gamete or present in the haploid cell of a particular organism.

***Genomic Clone.*** Clone of a genomic DNA sequence, held in a cloning vector.

***Genomic Exclusion.*** Abnormal form of sexual conjugation in the ciliate Tetrahymena in which the progeny are heterokaryons, having a macronucleus from one parent cell and a micronucleus from the other.

***Genomic Library.*** Library of DNA sequences of genomic origin, held in cloning Vectors. It contrasts with a cDNA library, which consists of sequences complementary to mRNA, and therefore contain only DNA coding sequences without introns or regulatory regions.

***Genotype.*** The genetic constitution of an individual, usually referring to specific characters under consideration. Thus, the two alleles of the human albino gene can be written A and a, with three possible genotypes : a/a and A/A.

***Genotype Frequency.*** The proportion of a particular genotype amongst all the individuals in a population. Thus, if population sample contained 5 albinos and 95 normally-pigmented individuals, the genotype frequency or albinos (a/a) would be 0.05 or 5%. Note, however, that it is not possible to be certain of the frequency of A/a and A/A genotypes among the normal individuals, since both genotypes have the same phenotype due to dominance, although their frequencies can be predicted using the hardy-weinberg law.

***Genus.*** A taxon immediately above that of a species and containing usually a group of closely related species. The name of genus (generic name) is written or printed with an initial capital letter and in binomial nomenclature precedes the specific name, which invariably has a small initial letter.

***Geobotany.*** The part of botany related to ecology and the geography of plants.

***Geoffroyism.*** The belief that there is an adaptive response of the genotype to the demands of the environment, i.e. an environmental induction of appropriate genetic, changes. Named after the French naturalist Hilaire Geoffroy (1772-1844).

***Geographical Isolation.*** The effective isolation of a gene pool by geographical barriers. For example, oceanic islands are isolated because of the difficulty of the sea-crossing for many organisms. The evolution of new species takes place through the prevention or limitation of gene flow and various isolating mechanisms may play a part in this, one of the most important being geographical isolation.

***Geographical Race.*** Phenotypically distinctive population of organisms inhabiting a defined geographical area and with characteristic gene frequencies that distinguish it from other such groups. It is normally assumed that the distinct genetic constitution of the race has resulted from its geographical isolation. Thus, in prehistorical times, it is assumed that separate races of humans evolved their separate traits of colour and physical form.

***Geographical Variation.*** Any variation that occurs in spatially separated populations of species.

***Geological Time.*** The period beginning with the formation of the earth and ending in the present day. It is often tabulated beginning with the Cambrian period, since the majority of fossil forms date from then. Precambrian time began with the formation of the earth about 4.600 million years ago. During of rocks is usually carried out by the measurement of radioactive decay. The older the rock the less radioactive it is. Organic remains are dated by carbon dating.

***German Measles Or Rubella.*** A mild human disease whose main feature is a rash on the body occuring about 18 days after infection. Caused by the rubella virus, the condition is highly contagious, being spread by direct contact via nasal secretions. The virus can be transmitted from mother to foetus and may cause serious damage in many foetal tissues and even death. The major period of risk to the child is the first 3 months of pregnancy when there is least a 30% risk of abnormality. For this reason many Western countries have a routine immunization programme for young female, either as babies or between the ages of 10-14 years.

***Germ Cell.*** Gamete, or any 'sex cell' capable of giving rise to a gamete, in multicellular animals. Germ cells are usually segregated from somatic cells very early in development and become associated with the developing ovary or testis where they become definitive germ cells comprising oogonia and spermatogonia. Progeny of definitive germ cells undergo meiosis to become eggs and sperm.

***Germinal Vesicle.*** Nucleus of a primary oocyte, often arrested in a postsynaptic stage of the first meiotic prophase. These nuclei are extremely large and produce the eventual female pronucleus by two separate divisions. As a result the other three nuclei resulting from the divisions are ejected or destroyed as the polar bodies.

***Genes Layers.*** The layers of cells in an animal embryo at the "gastrula stage, from which are derived the various organs of the animal's body. There are two or three germs layers; an outer layer, an inner layer, and in most animal groups a middle layer.

***Germ Line.*** A group of cells that give rise to the gonads, becoming differentiated from the 'somatic' cells early in embryonic development. Only germ-line cells have the potential to undergo meiosis, and a mutation event in these cells may well be transmitted to the offspring, unlike genetic change in somatic cells.

***Germ Plasm*** (germinal Plasm, germinal cytoplasm). Special region of cytoplasm, distinguished by its location, inclusions and staining properties, in the oocytes of insects and amphibians. During cleavages of the egg the germ plasm is segregated into certain cells. The progeny of these cells become the primordial germ cells which, in turn, populate the genital ridge or developing gonad. In the gonad, the primordial germ cells differentiate to form the germ cells. Experimental manipulations involving transplantation of the germ plasm have shown that it is the germ plasm that causes the cells that contain it to become germ cells. This is thus an example of cytoplasmic determinants dictating the differentiation of the cell.

***Germ Plasm Theory.*** A concept put forward by August Weismann (1834-1914) who suggested that the sex cells are produced by the 'germ plasm', which is passed on intact from generation to generation and gives rise to body cells in each individual. Nowadays we consider DNA to be the molecular equivalent of the germ plasm.

***Gestation.*** The development of the embryo in the uterus of mammals. The gestation period is the time elapsing from fertilization and the implantation of the embryo of birth. This takes 60 days in the domestic cat, 9 months in humans and 18 months in the Indian elephant.

***Gibberellic Acid.*** A crystalline acid that occurs in plants having similar growth-promoting effects to gibberellins.

***Gibberellin.*** One of a range of growth regulators in plants that stimulate stem elongation but, unlike auxins, do not inhibit root growth. Gibberellins can be used to induce bolting in immature plants and to remove dwarfness in mature plants. Unlike auxins, gibberellins can move freely around the plant.

***Gigantism.*** A rare human condition in which excess production of growth hormone by the anterior pituitary gland during childhood and adolescence causes over-elongation of bones, producing a pituitary giant.

***Glabrous.*** (Of plant structures) without hairs.

***Glaciation.*** One of the so-called ice ages; a period of ice cover.

***Gland.*** An organ producing substances which are then secreted to the outside of the gland, sometimes by means of a duct, as in the exocrine glands, for example, the salivary, mammary, lachrymal glands, but also.

***Glandular Fever or Infective Mononucleosis.*** An acute infectious disease, probably caused by the Epstein-Barr virus, that affects primarily the lymphoid tissue throughout the body, resulting in abnormal blood lymphocytes (the 'mononucleosis' of the title), enlarged lymph nodes and spleen, and sometimes fever and sore throat. The disease affects mainly teenagers from an affluent background and is prevalent therefore amongst students. No control measure is available at present.

***Glaucous.*** (Of plant structures) bluish.

***Globin Gene.*** Any one of a small family of genes in the eukaryotic genome. The genes are developmentally regulated during embryonic, foetal and adult life. Disturbances of the regulation of the globin genes result in some forms of the complex of human disease, the thalassaemias. The genes coding for alpha-globins are clustered on chromosome 16 (in the human and most vertebrates), whereas the beta-globin genes are clustered on chromosome 11. A number of pseudogenes have been identified in the globin gene family. A typical globin gene, the rabbit beta-globin gene, is approximately 1.35 kilobases long, with two introns, one of 53 bases and one of 660 bases.

***Globins.*** Polypeptide chains that form the protein components of haemoglobin, myoglobin and chlorocruorin. In humans several globin types with different primary amino acid sequences are known. Adult haemoglobin (HbA) has two alpha-and two beta-globin chains, adult delta-haemoglobin has two alpha-and two delta-globin chains. in the foetus, HbF has two alpha-and two delta-globins. Several embryonic haemoglobins with alpha-, gamma-and epsilon-chains exist. The genetics of globin synthesis and its control have been extensively studied. Numerous abnormal globins have been described.

***Globular Protein.*** Protein with a globular rather than a filamentous or sheeted conformation.

***Glucagon.*** A polypeptide of 29 amino acids produced by the cells in the islets of langerhans of the pancreas of vertebrates. Glucagon acts as a hormone, having the opposite effect to insulin, in causing the breakdown of liver glycogen and the release of glucose into the blood.

***Glucocorticoid.*** A steroid endocrine secretion produced by the adrenal cortex, influencing the metabolism of carbohydrates and proteins, e.g. cortisol (Hydrocortisone), corticosterone.

***Gluconeogenesis.*** The formation of glucose of glycogen in the liver from noncarbohydrate precursors such as certain amino acids, glycerol and lactic acid.

***Glucose or Dextrose.*** An important hexose sugar with an aldose structure that occurs in two forms, alpha and beta; it has the general formula $C_6H_{12}O_6$ and is found in sweet fruits, especially ripe grapes. Glucose is formed in the calvin cycle of photosynthesis and acts as a primary energy supply for both plant and animal cells, although usually it is converted to an insoluble form for long-term storage; starch in plants, glycogen in animals.

***Glucose-6-Phosphate Dehydrogenase (G-6-P.D.).*** An important enzyme in the pentose phosphate pathway for carbohydrate metabolism, catalysing the oxidation of glucose 6-phosphate in the presence of NADP coenzyme, giving 6-phosphogluconolactone and NADPH. G-6-P.D. of blood erythrocytes is of particular interest because a decrease in its activity can lead to the condition called favism.

***Glume.*** The chaffy scale that encloses the spikelets of grass or the flowers of sedges.

***Glutamate.*** The dissociated form of the amino acid Glutamic Acid.

***Glutamic Acid.*** One of 20 Amino Acids common in proteins that has an extra carboxyl group and is acidic in solution. See Figure G.5. The isoelectric point of glutamic acid is 3.2.

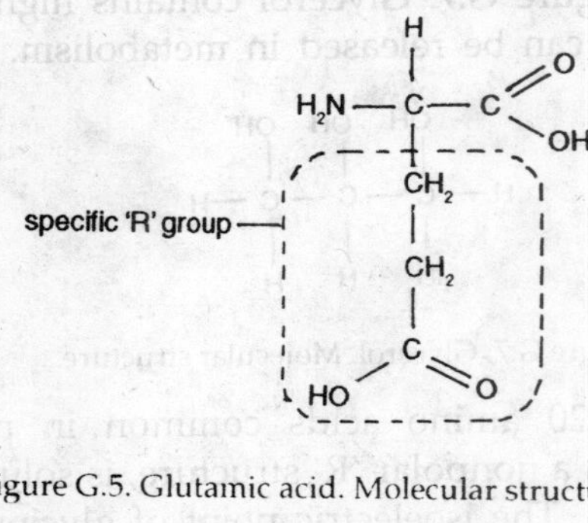


Figure G.5. Glutamic acid. Molecular structure.

***Glutamine.*** One of 20 amino acids common in proteins that has a polar 'R' structure and is soluble in water. See Figure G.6.

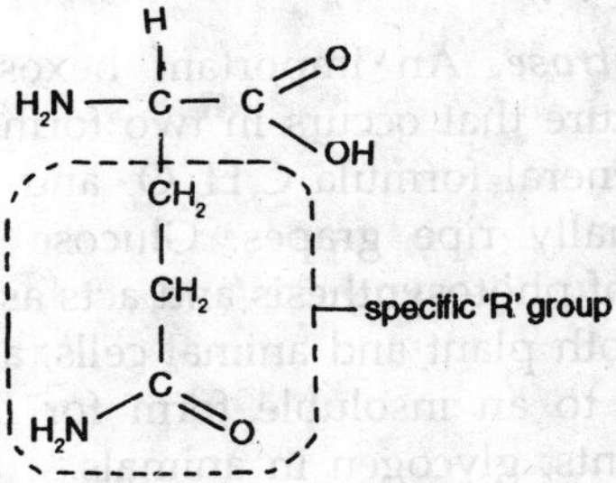


Figure G.6. Glutamine. Molecular structure.

***Glutathione.*** A "peptide comprising the amino acids glutamic acid, cysteine, and glycine. It occurs widely in plants, animals, and microorganisms, serving chiefly as an anti-oxidant. Reduced glutathione reacts with potentially harmful oxidizing agents and is itself oxidized. This is important in ensuring the proper functioning of proteins, haemoglobin, membrane lipids, etc. Glutathione is also involved in amino acid transport across cell membranes.

***Gluten.*** Plant storage protein, containing glutenin, found in cereal grains. Sensitivity to gluten in children leads to coeliac disease, with accompanying fat absorption abnormalities. Affected children must eat a gluten-free-diet.

***Glycerol or Glycerin.*** A simple lipid that is a basic component of fats. See Figure G.7. Glycerol contains high amounts of energy which can be released in metabolism.

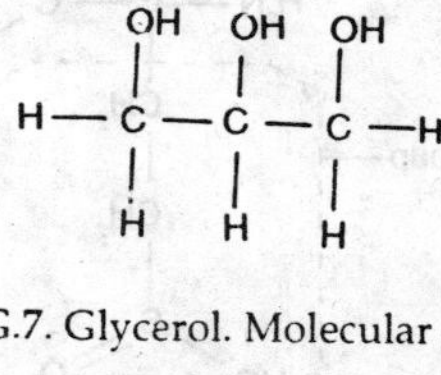


Figure G.7. Glycerol. Molecular structure.

***Glycine.*** One of 20 amino acids common in proteins that although it has a nonpolar 'R' structure, is soluble in water. See Figure G.8. The isoelectric point of glycine is 6.0.

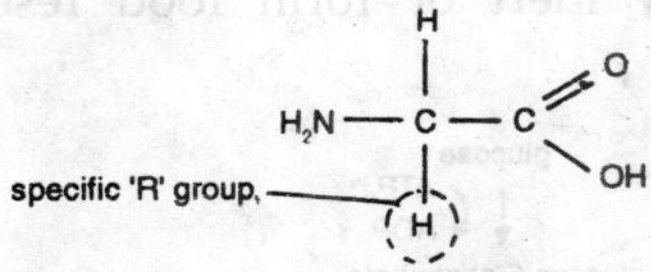


Figure. Glycine. Molecular structure.

***Glycocalyx.*** A mass of filaments up to 3 μm thick produced by the membrane of intestinal brush-border microvilli, consisting of acid mucopolysaccharide and glycorprotein, and thought to be associated with the digestion of small food molecules. Other animal cells also have a glycocalyx, on their cell coat, providing a mechanism that enables cells to recognise each other, an important process in embryonic development.

***Glycogen.*** The principal carbohydrate storage molecule of animals, being produced from glucose in the mammalian liver and muscles when blood sugar levels are too high, a process called glycogenesis which is under the influence of insulin. Glycogen in the liver can be broken down to glucose when blood sugar levels are low, a process called glycogenolysis which is under the influence of glucagon. Glycogen in the muscle, however, is broken down to lactic acid (not glucose) in glycolysis.

***Glycolipid.*** Any of the group of lipids containing a carbohydrate.

***Glycolysis.*** The first stage of cellular respiration, occurring with or without the presence of oxygen, in which glucose is converted to two molecules or pyruvic acid. See Figure G.9 on next page.

***Glycophorin.*** A glycopolypeptide found in human erythrocytes.

***Glycoprotein.*** Any protein that contains sugars as part of the molecule.

***Glycoside.*** An acetal derivative of a sugar that, on hydrolysis by enzymes or acids, gives rise to a sugar. Glycosides containing glucose are called glucosides, those with galactose are called galactosides. They render unwanted substances chemically inert or form food reserves, for example, glycogen.

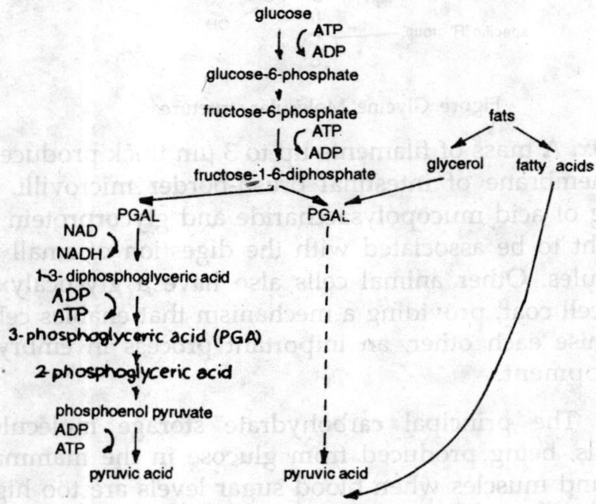


Figure G.9. Glycolysis. The individual steps of glycolysis.

***Glycosidic Bond or Glycosidic Link.*** A bond between the anomeric carbon of a carbohydrate and another group or molecule.

***Glycosuria.*** The condition where glucose is excreted in the urine because the blood sugar level exceeds the normal (hyperglycemia). Glycosuria is one of the symptoms of diabetes.

***Glycosylation.*** The addition of a carbohydrate to an organic molecule such as a protein.

***Gnotobiology.*** Biology of animals kept in germ-free, and often bacteria-free, conditions.

***Gnotobiosis.*** Maintenance of animals in bacteria-free conditions, or more rarely, in conditions in which the identity of all microorganisms present is known.

***Goblet Cell.*** Pear-shaped epithelial cell that secretes mucus glycoproteins. Goblet cells are found in the respiratory tract and gut of vertebrates, and in the skin of fishes and amphibians. They are rich in vesicles containing glycoproteins, and characteristically the nucleus lies in the base of the cell.

***Golgi Apparatus (Golgi Body, Golgi Complex).*** Cellular organelle consisting of tightly packed cisternae and vesicles of the endoplasmic reticulum. It is thus a modified area of smooth endoplasmic reticulum (i.e. it lacks ribosomes) and functions in packaging proteins synthesized on the endoplasmic reticulum into membrane-bound vesicles. Thence many are transported to the cell surface for secretion.

***Golgi Stain.*** Silver impregnation technique used chiefly to stain golgi apparatus of neurones.

***Gonad.*** Any of the usually paired organs in animals that produce reproductive cells (gametes). The most important gonads are the male testis, which produces spermatozoa, and the female ovary, which produces ova (egg cells). The gonads also produce hormones that control secondary sexual characteristics.

***Gonadotrophin (Gonadotrophic Hormone).*** Any of several hormones, secreted by the mammalian anterior pituitary gland, that stimulate reproductive activity of the testes or ovaries (the gonads). Gonadotrophins include follicle-stimulating hormone, luteinizing hormone, and a hormone produced by the placenta (chorionic gonadotrophin) that suppresses the menstrual cycle and whose presence in urine in large amounts is an indication of pregnancy.

***Gonadotrophin or Gonadotrophic Hormones.*** Hormones secreted by the anterior lobe of the pituitary gland and in some mammals, once pregnancy is under way by the placenta. FSH and LH are produced by all tetrapods though FSH appears to be absent in fish. LTH (Luteotrophin) is present in rats and maintains the corpus luteum though it is absent in other mammals. Prolactin is present in some vertebrates and controls milk production (LTH is a form of prolactin). Pituitary output is controlled by the hypothalamus. Gonadotrophins influence other glands connected with reproduction, controlling the activity of the gonads, the onset of sexual maturity, oestrous cycles, breeding rhythms and lactation.

***Gondwanaland.*** The southern group of continents at the end of the triassic period which had split from the northern group (laurasia). It consisted of South America, Africa, India, Australia and Antarctica.

***Gonochorism.*** The possession of gonads of only one sex, either male or female, in an individual.

***Gonophore.*** Any structure bearing gonads but particularly the specialized polyp of colonial coelenterates which bears the gonads and is shaped like a sessile medusa - a form of gonozooid.

***Gonorrhoea.*** A contagious inflammation of the mucus membranes in human reproductive organs, characterized by the discharge of mucus and pus from the urethra or vagina and caused by the gonococcal bacterium Neisseria gonorrhoeae. Gonorrhoea is probably the most prevalent communicable bacterial disease in man today and, although a venereal disease, is a distinct condition from syphilis.

***Graafian Follicle.*** Terminal stage in the differentiation of follicles within the mammalian ovary; first adequately described by Regnier de Graaf (1641-73). It consists of a spherical ball of cells that blisters out onto the surface of the ovary and whose wall is composed of outer thecal and granulosa cells enclosing a fluid-filled space—the antrum—with the oocyte, also surrounded by cells called the cumulus oophorus at one side. At ovulation, the protruding wall

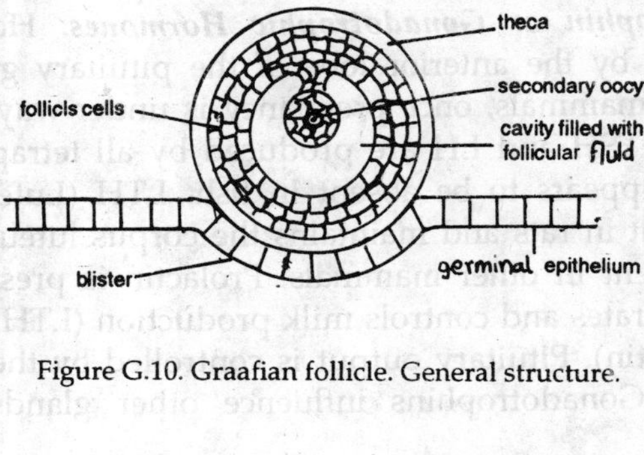


Figure G.10. Graafian follicle. General structure.

of the graafian follicle breaks down, and the oocyte whose cumulus cells had previously detached from the wall, together with antral fluid, is shed into the oviduct. The thecal and granulosa cells transform into the corpus luteum which secretes progesterone. See Figure G.10.

***Grade.*** A group of organisms having a similar level of organisation.

***Graded Response.*** A response that increases with the amount of energy supplied as opposed to the reaction brought about by the all-or-none law.

***Gradualism.*** View that evolution advanced by a great number of very small changes which gradually accumulate, as compared to the possibility of sudden abrupt change which often appears to be the easiest interpretation of cladogenesis.

***Graft.*** The transfer of a small part of an organism to a relatively larger part where it is transplanted. This may take place from one part of an organism to another part, or from one organism to another. Many embryological studies have involved grafting, and from a medical point of view, skin grafting, particularly after serious burns, is commonplace. Organ grafts such as heart transplants are now much more common, though rejection by an animal of the tissues of another is still a serious problem. In animals the graft comes from a 'donor' and is transferred to the recipient. In plants, grafts are used often in horticulture, where a scion, the plant to be cultivated, is attached onto a stock (1), the rooting portion.

***Graft Hybrid.*** 1. A type of plant chimaera that may be produced when a part of one plant (the scion) is grafted onto another plant of a different genetic constitution (the stock). Shoots growing from the point of union of the graft contain tissues from both the stock and the scion.

2. Plant that is permanently composed of two separate tissues, one from the original stock and one from the graft. Such plants may have the separate cell lines forming distinct leaves or flowers.

***Graft-Versus-Host Reaction.*** Reaction resulting from the transfer of histoincompatible immunologically competent cells derived from, for example, spleen, bone marrow or thymus, from a donor to a recipient that is incapable of rejecting the cells (graft) (i.e. instead of the host rejecting the graft as in an allograft, the graft rejects the host). In newborn rodents, which are immunologically immature, this manifests itself as runting, with inhibition of growth and splenomegaly (spleen enlargement). It occurs also in humans that have been immunosuppressed through X-radiation or drug treatment and have received bone marrow transplants. The greater the difference in major histocompatibility complex antigens of the donor and recipient the stronger is the graft-versus-host reaction.

***Gram's Stain.*** A stain taken up by the Gram-positive bacteria that differentiates these from bacteria which fail to take up the stain (Gram negative types). The initial stain is crystal violet/iodine complex, and Gram-negative bacteria are decolourized with alcohol whilst Gram-positive bacteria retain a blue/purple colour.

***Grandfather Method.*** A procedure for estimating the amount of recombination between X-linked genes in an individual that depends on the arrangement of genes in the maternal grandfather. For example, if a mother is known to be heterozygous her genes could be in coupling or in repulsion. However, this uncertainty can be removed if the phenotype of her father is known since he has only one X-chromosome. Thus if he was Ab, his heterozygous daughter must be Ab/aB, so ensuring that her children are properly identified as parental or recombinant type.

***Granulocyte.*** A type of white blood cell (leucocyte) that possesses granules in the cytoplasm and is formed in the bone marrow. Granulocytes form about 70% of all leucocytes and are of three types : eosinophils, basophils and neutrophils.

***Graptolite.*** Any extinct Palaeozoic colonial pelagic animal of the class Graptolithina. Branching forms are found in later strata and up to Carboniferous times.

***Green Gland.*** One of a pair of excretory organs of crustaceans with openings at the antennal base.

***Greenhouse Effect.*** 1. An effect occurring in greenhouses in which the glass transmits short wavelengths but absorbs and re-radiates longer wavelengths, thus heating the interior. 2. The application of this effect to the earth's atmosphere. Infrared radiation tends to be trapped by carbon dioxide and water vapour in the earth's atmosphere and some of it is re-radiated back to the earth's surface.

***Green-Island Effect.*** A localized increase of photosynthesis in plant tissues immediately surrounding a lesion caused by a biotrophic pathogen.

***Green Revolution.*** The process by which humans have exploited new hybrid varieties of food crops such as barley, rice, maize and wheat to meet their requirements. New varieties have been produced by crossing and selection. The green revolution has had particularly dramatic effects on developing countries. For example, wheat yields in Mexico have increased by about 300% since the introduction of a new dwarf variety in 1960. However, the attempts at plant improvements have not always been of benefit to the peasant farmer.

***Greeting Display.*** A form of behaviour in animals, particularly indulged in by some birds, where display arises on the arrival of the mate, say, at a nest site with food.

***Grey Crescent.*** Band of light pigmentation that appears shortly after fertilization in the amphibian egg. It forms opposite to the site of sperm entry and reflects a reorganization of cytoskeleton by the centriole which has been introduced by the sperm.

***Griffith, Frederick.*** English medical bacteriologist who, in 1928, published a paper showing that is was possible to convert one type of Streptococcus pneumoniae bacterium into a new type. More specifically, Griffith worked with two strains of bacterium :

| Type R | Type S |
|---|---|
| rough outer coat, nonvirulant in mice | smooth outer coat virulent in mice |

Griffith proposed that in experiment 4 the heat-killed 'S' type somehow converted the living 'R' type to virulent 'S' types, in a process he called transformation. Later it was shown that the transforming 'principle' was DNA.

***Griseofulvin***: Antibiotic synthesized by certain species of mould and used as a fungicide (e.g. in the treatment of the human skin disease ringworm).

***Ground State.*** The condition of a molecule when at its lowest energy level.

***Group.*** A collection of closely related taxa, particularly an assemblage of closely related species.

***Group Selection.*** Process in which natural selection acts upon a few individuals in a group to select characteristics that are beneficial to the group rather than the individual.

***Group-Specific Antigen (GAG).*** Core protein of retrovirus that confers on the virus its antigenic specificity. The GAG gene, together with other genes for envelope protein, polymerase and the protooncogene, if present, make up the main part of the retroviral genome.

***Growth.*** An increase in the dry weight or volume of an organism through cell division and cell enlargement. Growth may continue throughout the life of the organism, as occurs in woody plants, or it may cease at maturity, as in man, and other mammals.

***Growth Hormone or Somatotrophic Hormone (STH).*** A hormone secreted by the anterior pituitary gland mainly in the growth period, where it stimulates the lengthening of the long bones in tetrapods, induces protein synthesis and inhibits insulin, thus raising the level of blood sugar. Oversecretion during development produces gigantism but excess later in life gives rise to acromegaly where a massive forehead, nose and lower jaw are produced. Deficiency of the hormone results in dwarfism.

***GT-AG Rule.*** Observation that these dinucleotides occur on the first two and last two positions of intron sequences in eukaryotic DNA.

***GTP (Guanosine Triphosphate).*** Energy rich molecule required for the formation of peptide bonds between amino acids.

***Guanine.*** One of four types of nitrogenous bases found in DNA, having the double-ring structure of a class known as purines. Guanine forms part of a DNA unit called a nucleotide and always forms complementary pairs with a DNA pyrimidine base called cytosine. Guanine also occurs in RNA molecules. See Figure G.11.

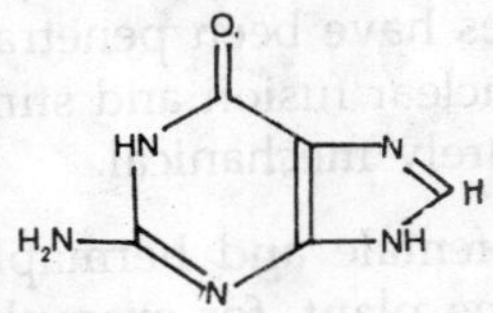


Figure G.11. Guanine. Molecular structure.

***Guano.*** The white nitrogenous dried excrement, high in uric acid content, that is produced by birds and reptiles. Guano is a valuable fertilizer and has been extensively harvested from guano bird (cormorant) colonies in South America.

***Guard Cells.*** One of a pair of specialized epidermal cells forming a pore (stoma) at the leaf surface.

***Guild.*** A group of species that exploits the same class of environmental resources in similar way.

***Gum.*** Plant-derived substance that swells when in contact with water to form a sticky solution. Slimy gum is termed mucilage. Most gums are large, flexible polysaccharides and are released in response to injury forming a hard exudate over the wound (e.g. gum arabic in acacia).

***Gurdon, J.B., (1933-).*** British experimental embryologist who demonstrated that a nucleus taken from the differentiated gut cell of a clawed toad, injected into an enucleated egg, could produce a normal adult. In other words, he demonstrated that a fully differentiated cell still contains the genetic information to direct the development of the cells in the entire animal.

***Gustation.*** The act of tasting or the faculty of taste. This is brought about by the effect of ions and molecules in solution, stimulating specialized sensory epithelial receptors.

***Gynandromorph.*** Any animal exhibiting both male and female features, often with the body divided into equal portions of the two sexes. For example, the left-hand side male, the right-hand side female.

***Gynogenesis.*** The parthenogenetic development of an egg after the egg membranes have been penetrated by a male gamete. There is no nuclear fusion and stimulation of development might be purely mechanical.

***Gynomonoecious.*** (of female and hermaphrodite flowers) occurring on the same plant, for example, the daisy.

# H

**_H-2 Antigen._** Antigens of the Major Histocompatibility complex (MHC) of the mouse. In humans they are termed HLA antigens.

**_H-2 Complex._** Mouse Major Histocompatibility Complex, which contains immune response and transplantation antigen genes. It is located on chromosome 17.

**_Habitat Selection._** The selection by a dispersing organism of a suitable habitat.

**_Habitable Zone._** The area around a star (such as the sun) in which there is sufficient energy present to sustain life.

**_Habituated Culture_** (Anergized Culture). Epigenetic change undergone by plant cells in vitro (in suspension or callus culture) that results in simplified requirements for growth. Usually the dependency upon exogenous Auxins and/or cytokinins ceases as the cells commence synthesis of their own endogenous supplies.

**_Habituation._** The progressive loss of a behavioural response as a result of continued stimulation.

**_Haekel's Law of Recapitulation or Palingenesis or Von Baer's Law._** A law stating that ontogeny recapitulates phylogeny. This means that an organism will go through embryonic stages similar to those gone through during its evolutionary development. For example, mammals have a fish-like stage in their embryology. The law was formulated by the German biologist Ernst Haekel (1834-1919).

***Haem- or Haemo- or Haemato-.*** Denoting blood.

***Haem or Heme.*** A ring-like chemical structure containing an atom of ferrous iron that is bound as a prosthetic group to each polypeptide chain within haemoglobin and myoglobin, giving blood and muscle their characteristic red colour.

***Haem.*** Chemical structure of the haem group associated with each Hb polypeptide chain (subunit), illustrating the state of the unit in deoxyhaemoglobin. See Figure H.1.

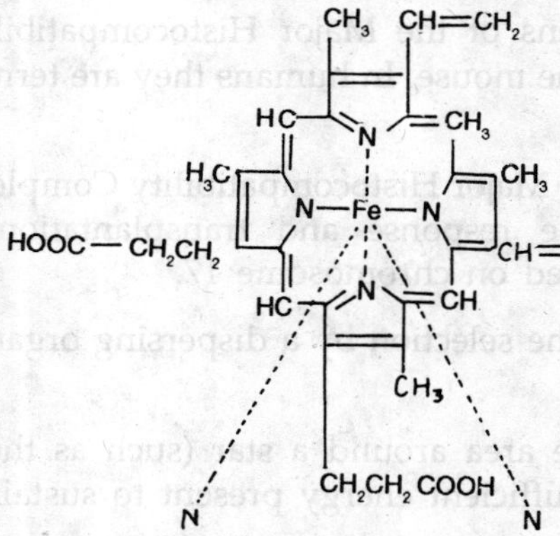


Figure H.1. Chemical structure of the haem group associated with each Hb polypepeptide chain (subunit), illustrating the state of the unit in deoxyhaemoglobin.

***Haemagglutinin.*** Substance capable of agglutinating erythrocytes. Invertebrates contain a number of such protein haemagglutinins in their body fluids. In vertebrates haemagglutinins are usually antibodies of the 1gm class; among these are the natural isohaemagglutinins of the human ABO blood group system.

***Haemalum.*** Water-soluble stain used in light microscope studies on cells and tissues.

***Haematin.*** An iron-containing pigment that is derived from the breakdown of Haemaglobin.

***Haematoblast.*** The parent cell of red blood corpuscles.

***Haematocrit.*** The percentage of the blood volume occupied by red blood cells. The percentage is 40.5% in man.

***Haematocyte.*** A blood corpuscle.

***Haematopoiesis Or Haemopoiesis.*** The process leading to red blood cell production.

***Haemerythrin.*** An iron-containing proteinaceous red pigment found in the blood plasma of some annelids and several minor invertebrate groups. Like haemoglobin, the pigment can become oxygenated, but in this case oxygen uptake involves a change in valency from Fe(II) to Fe(III).

***Haemin (Hemin).*** Oxidized form of haem in which trivalent iron replaces the divalent iron atom at the centre of the porphyrin ring.

***Haemocyanin.*** A respiratory pigment found in the blood plasma of many molluscs and crustaceans that performs the same function as haemoglobin in other animals. The metallic radicle of its prosthetic group, however, is copper rather than iron, giving the molecule a bluish colour.

***Haemocyte.*** Amoeboid blood cell found in insects and analogous to a mammalian leucocyte.

***Haemoglobin.*** A large protein molecule with a quaternary structure of four polypeptides chains, two alpha and two beta chains, each of which is complexed to a separate haem group. About 300 million molecules of haemoglobin occur in each red blood cell of the mammalian circulation, with each molecule binding to a maximum of four oxygen molecules, one per haem group (= oxygenation).

Haemoglobin is found in all vertebrates and many invertebrates. In mammals the foetal haemoglobin (HbF) has a different polypeptide combination from that in postnatal 'adult' haemoglobin (HbA), consisting of two alpha and two gamma chains, with different oxygen-carrying characteristics (up to 30% more at low oxygen tension). An altered beta chain in HbA produces sickle-cell anaemia.

***Haemolysis.*** The disintegration of red blood cells, with the release of haemoglobin. The process can occur (a) when the cells take in excess water by osmosis, (b) when there is an antigen-antibody reaction involving the cells, as in rhesus haemolytic antenna, (c) as a result of an abnormality such as favism. Addition of glacial acetic acid to a blood sample causes haemolysis of the red blood cells, thus making it easier to observe and count the white blood cells.

***Haemoglobin C.*** Type of haemoglobin with an abnormal beta-globin chain, in which lysine has replaced glutamic acid at position 6.

***Haemoglobin S.*** Type of haemoglobin with an abnormal beta-globin chain, in which valine replaces glutamic acid at position 6. Such beta-globin, when it replaces normal beta-globin, renders the molecule less soluble and the red blood cells containing the pigment tend to adopt a sickle shape. Haemoglobin S is the pigment present in the cells of individuals suffering from sickle cell anaemia.

***Haemoglobinuria.*** Excretion of hemoglobin in the urine, usually as a result of disease in the kidneys.

***Haemolysis.*** Lysis or rupture of erythrocytes. The empty red cells of mammals, following such lysis, are termed erythrocyte ghosts.

***Haemolytic Disease of The Newborn.*** Condition occurring in a rhesus-positive foetus with a rhesus-negative mother. Rhesus-negative mothers who have become immunized to rhesus factor (D antigen) make an IgG antibody to D which can cross the placenta. The maternal anti-D destroys the foetal erythrocytes by acting as an opsonin, as D is present on the foetal erythrocytes.

***Haemophilia.*** A rare human blood disorder in which blood clotting is deficient, resulting often in severe bleeding internally and externally. The condition is due to a lack of fibrin in the blood and is controlled by two closely linked genes on the X-chromosome that are responsible for production of different clotting factors. Haemophilia A individuals lack antihaemophilic globulin (AHG) while haemophilia B individuals lack plasma thromboplastin. Males carrying the mutant allele of either locus of (much more rarely)female homozygous for the recessive mutant alleles of either locus will be affected, although heterozygous females have normal blood. Haemophilia A is by far the most common form of the disease (about 80%) and can be treated by transfusions of AHG. See Figure H.2.

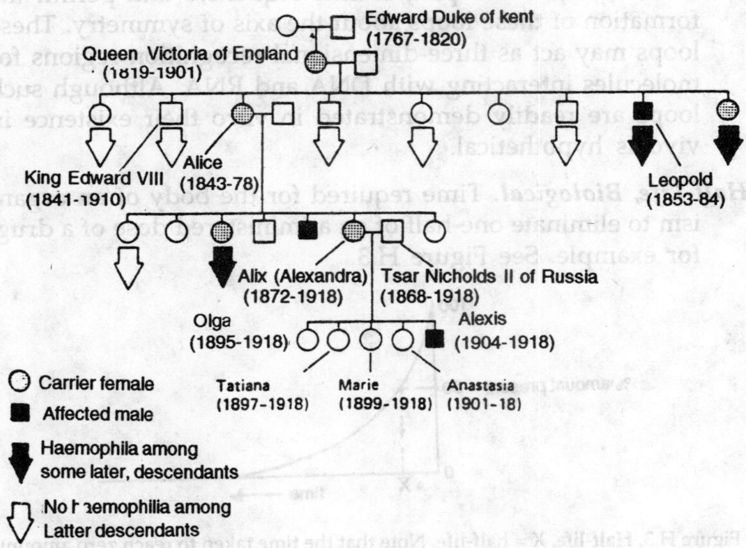


Figure H.2. Partial pedigree of haemophilia. A young descendents of Queen Victoria, including Alexandera, Empress of Russia, and her five children.

***Haemopoiesis*** (haematopoiesis). Process by which red and white blood cells are produced in the bone marrow and elsewhere by division and differentiation of multipotential stem cells. A hormone — erythropoietin — which is produced in the kidney in response to low oxygen tension in circulating blood stimulates the stem cells in the marrow to produce more erythrocytes.

***Haemostasis.*** Stopping of blood flow. The term is used : (1) with reference to the stagnation of blood within diseased, blocked or constricted blood vessels; (2) in connection with the prevention of blood loss from damaged or severed blood vessels by the contraction of muscles associated with the blood vessels and by the blood clotting processes.

***Hairpin Loop.*** Double-helical regions of DNA or RNA formed by hydrogen bonding between complementary base sequences present in the same strand. Such sequences exist as inverted repeats of palindromic sequences and permit the formation of these loops about the axis of symmetry. These loops may act as three-dimensional recognition regions for molecules interacting with DNA and RNA. Although such loops are readily demonstrated in vitro their existence in vivo is hypothetical.

***Half-Life, Biological.*** Time required for the body of an organism to eliminate one-half of an administered dose of a drug, for example. See Figure H.3.

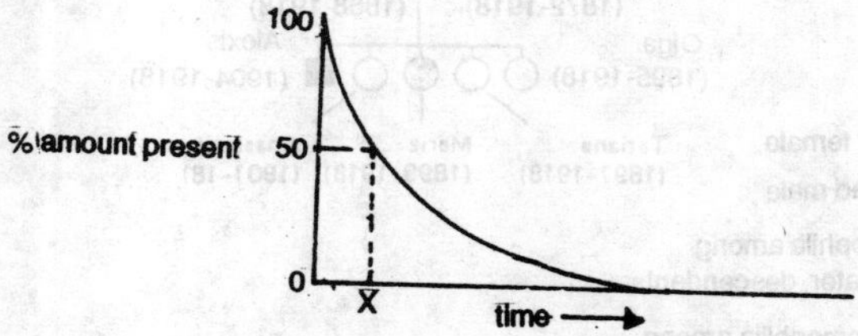


Figure H.3. Half-life. X = half-life. Note that the time taken to reach zero amount is not 2 × X.

***Half-Life, Radioactive.*** Time required for a unit mass of a radioisotope to lose one-half of its total original radioactivity due to decay into another non-radioactive isotope. Half-lives of radionuclides vary greatly, being a few days for $^{32}P$, over 12 years for $^{3}H$ and 5700 years for $^{14}C$.

***Half-Tetrad Analysis.*** Analysis of chromosome tetrads following recombination where only two out of the original four chromosomes of the tetrad can be analysed. The attached X chromosomes of Drosophila provide the best known example.

***Halobacteria.*** Bacteria capable of living in conditions of hign salt.

***Halophyte.*** A plant that is tolerant of high concentrations of salt in the soil and atmosphere and normally found close to the sea. For example, the marsh samphire, Salicornia europaea.

***Haplobiont.*** Organism in which all somatic cells are always in one somatic state (e.g. haploid or diploid).

***Haploid.*** 1. (of a cell nucleus) containing one of each type of chromosome. 2. A haploid organism in which the main life stage has cell nuclei with one of each type of chromosome, written as 'n'. Such organisms (e.g. fungi, many algae) usually have a brief diploid (2) phase (2n) returning to the haploid state via meiosis.

***Haploidiploidy.*** Genetic system found in some organisms such as bees, in which the males are haploid, developing from unfertilized eggs, whereas the females are diploid, developing from fertilized eggs.

***Haploidization.*** Process whereby what was originally a diploid nucleus becomes haploid, presumably by a progressive loss of one member of each chromosome pair.

***Haploid Number (n).*** Number of chromosomes in a gametic cell. Thus for the human n = 23. It is also the number of chromosomes in somatic cells of haploid organisms such as fungi.

***haploid Parthenogenesis.*** Situation found, for example, in the honey bee in which haploid cells — the eggs — develop without fertilization into haploid adults.

***Haplont.*** Organism in which the diploid phase of the life cycle is the zygote only, and meiosis yields the dominant phase of the life cycle which is haploid. This occurs in most algae, fungi and many protozoa.

***Haplotype.*** (1) Set of linked genes that tend to be inherited together (e.g. the A, B and C loci of the human HLA complex). (2) Set of isoantigens for which a single or a few closely linked genes are responsible.

***Hapten.*** A substance that is able to combine with specific antibodies but does not produce them unless attached to a large carrier molecule.

***Haptoglobin.*** Glycoprotein in plasma that binds to haemoglobin to ensure the recycling of the HAEM Group.

***Haptotactic.*** Describing a tropic response to contact with a solid object.

***Hardy-Weinberg Law.*** A law stating that in a randomly mating large population the frequency of alleles will remain constant from generation to generation. Proposed in 1908 by G.H. Hardy in England and W. Weinberg in Germany, the law explains how the various alleles of a gene could remain constant in a population and yet be inherited by the rules of mendelian genetics. The law shows why, for instance, dominant phenotypes are not necessarily in excess of recessive ones in a population. If a gene has two alleles, A and a, with a frequency of p and q respectively, the genotypic frequencies would have the proportions :

$$\begin{array}{ccccc} AA & & Aa & & aa \\ p^2 & + & 2pq & + & q_2 & = & 1.0 \end{array}$$

This equation is derived from the Binomial expansion $(p + q)^2 = 1.0$. Such Genetic equilibrium only occurs under conditions of zero selection and mutation, no emigration or immigration, random mating and a large population size. However, selection pressures can produce stability and selection and mutation effects might cancel each other out.

***Harlequin Chromosome.*** Chromosome from a cell treated with the thymidine analogue 5'-bromodeoxyuridine. This compound when incorporated into DNA leads to chromatin that stains less intensely than normal chromatin, and thus in cells that have been grown in the presence of the drug for at lest two replication cycles, chromatids stain differentially and following sister chromatid exchange show a harlequin pattern of alternating dark-and light-stained segments. This labelling technique and the detection of the resulting harlequin pattern of chromosomes can also be used to detect sister chromatid exchange in response to ultraviolet irradiation and other agents.

***Harvey Sarcoma Virus.*** Mouse retro-virus carrying the V-ras oncogene which is homologous to the cellular protooncogene C-ras, which is located on chromosome 11.

***Harvey, William (1578-1657).*** English physician who discovered the mechanism of the human blood circulation, in which blood flows away from the heart in arteries and towards the heart in veins.

***Hatch-Slack Pathway.*** An alternative pathway to the Calvin cycle of photosynthesis, thought to operate in some tropical grasses and some dicotyledons. Phosphoenolpyruvate is carboxylated to form oxalo-acetate as the first product.

***HAT-Selective Medium.*** Cell culture medium containing hypoxanthine, aminopterin and thymidine used to select hybridomas for the production of monoclonal antibodies. Myeloma cells used in the fusion process cannot grow in HAT medium unless fused with a splenocyte cell to provide salvage pathway enzyme for nucleotide biosynthesis. Such selective media select cells able to produce hgprt and thymidine kinase, and are also used to select other types of fused cell constructs besides hybridomas.

***Hayflick Phenomenon.*** Process in which there is a limit to the number of cell divisions that animals tissue cells will undergo when explanted into tissue culture. Any cells that grow after the initial 30-40 divisions are deemed to be transformed cells.

***Hb.*** Abbreviation for haemoglobin. HbA symbolizes normal adult haemoglobin. HbF is foetal haemoglobin, HbS sickle cell haemoglobin, and $HbA_2$ is the second, and rarer, form of adult haemoglobin.

***HbO.*** Oxyhaemoglobin, more correctly $HbO_2$.

***H Chain.*** Heavy chain.

***HCG (Human Chorionic Gonadotrophin).*** A hormone secreted by the trophoblast of the developing foetal tissues. It maintains the corpus luteum during the first three to four months in pregnancy, thus ensuring a supply of progesterone for maintaining the uterus lining and preventing menstruation. HCG begins to be secreted as soon as the trophoblast implants in the uterine wall and it is at its highest concentration between the 7th and 10th weeks of pregnancy. The urine of women in the first month of pregnancy contains enough HCG to be easily detected g chemical means. After reading its peak, falls to low concentrations and its only known function is to stimulate the production of testosterone by the testes of the male foetus. HCG has almost the same combined properties as LH and Luteotropic hormones

***Health Physics.*** The branch of medical physics concerned with the protection of medical, scientific, and industrial workers from the hazards of ionizing radiation and other dangers associated with atomic physics. Establishing the maximum permissible "dose of radiation, the disposal of radioactive waste, and the shielding of dangerous equipment are the principal activities in this field.

***Heat Exhaustion.*** The failure of cooling mechanisms resulting from an excessive rise in body temperature in warm-blooded animals, characterized by cramp and dizziness.

***Heat Gain.*** A rise in temperature of a body when obtaining heat by radiation of conduction from an outside source, leading to an increase in metabolic rate in all organs.

***Heat Shock Gene.*** Gene whose transcription is induced by heat shock and the products of which probably protect the cell against some effects of heat shock.

***Heat Shock Proteins.*** Group of proteins that are synthesized following heat shocking of a cell or tissue and probably help to protect the cell against some of the deleterious effects of heat shock. Although probably synthesized in all organisms, they are particularly studied in Drosophila where the genes responsible for their production can be seen to show puffing after heat shock.

***Heat Stock Puff.*** Gene activation in response to heat shock in Drosophila larvae leads to the appearance of these puffs in the polytene chromosomes. Such puffing represents the transcriptional activation of the heat shock genes in the larvae.

***Heavy Chain*** (H chain). Chain that makes up part of the structure of the molecule.

***Heavy Isotope.*** Stable (non-radioactive) form of an element with a nucleus of greater mass than that of the most abundant natural form. The most useful heavy isotopes for biological studies are hydrogen-2 (deuterium $^{2}H$), carbon-13($^{13}C$), nitrogen-15($^{15}N$) and oxygen-18($^{18}O$).

***Heavy Labelling.*** Introduction of a heavy isotope into a compound in order to more easily follow biochemical events involving the compound in whole cells or in cell-free preparations.

***Heavy Meromyosin.*** One of two active fragments cleaved from myosin by trypsin. It contains an ATPase active site and a binding site for actin, unlike the light meromyosin chain which is purely filamentous.

***Hedgerow.*** A row of shrubs that forms a habitat similar to a natural woodland edge, planted to form a division between two pieces of land.

***Heidelberg Man.*** Homo erectus heidelbergensis, who lived some 550,000 BP and became extinct some 400,000 BP. Heidelberg man, Java man (Pithecanthropus), Peking man (Sinanthropus) and Atlanthropus are usually all regarded as Homo erectus.

***Heinz Body.*** (inclusion body). Aggregated, precipitated globin molecules, found intracellularly and visible by light microscopy; they are the result of the dissociation of methaemoglobin.

***Hela Cell.*** A cell type used in tissue culture that is grown as a standard in research laboratories all over the world. The culture is derived from a cervical carcinoma obtained from Henrietta Lacks in 1951.

***Helicase.*** Enzyme that unwinds double-stranded helical DNA during replication.

***Helix.*** (Helixes or helices) a form of spiral in which any point is at the same distance from the central axis. RNA molecules have a single helix, DNA is a double helix.

***Helix-Destabilizing Proteins.*** Proteins that bind to single-stranded regions of duplex DNA and induce unwinding of further regions of the double helix. Helicase which unwinds bacterial DNA ahead of the DNA polymerase is one such enzyme.

***Helper T Cell.*** Type of T lymphocytes that functions as a helper cell to other T lymphocytes, B lymphocytes and macrophages, enhancing the normal activities of these cells.

***Helper Virus.*** Virus that enables a defective virus to replicate by providing, in the same cell, some component required for complete replication and lacking in the defective virus.

***Hemicellulose.*** Group of alkali-soluble polysaccharides that are important constituents to plant cell walls and also act as food reserves in some plants. They include mannans, glucans, xylans and galactans.

***Hemibiotroph.*** A pathogen (usually fungal) that has both a biotrophic and a necrotrophic phase in the course of one life cycle. Examples include scab and scald of barley (Rhynchosporium secalis).

***Hemichordate.*** Any small wormlike marine animal of the subphylum Hemichordata or Enteropneusta, a division of the protochordates that contains worm like forms such as Balanoglossus.

***Hemidesmosome.*** Cellular structure mor-phologically resembling half a desmosome, occurring on the basal aspect of epithelial cells and assumed to serve a comparable adhesive function, in this case, anchoring the cells to the basal lamina. Recent evidence indicates certain compositional differences from a true desmosome but these may turn out to be minor.

***Hemizygous.*** (of a diploid (2) organism) possessing only one allele of a gene, rather than the normal two. For example, male mammals have only one copy of each gene on the single X-chromosome.

***Hemizygous Gene.*** Gene present only as a single dose,usually as a gene on the sex chromosome in the heterogametic sex (e.g. and X chromosome in an XY male) or as a gene on a piece of chromosome where the homologous section of chromatin has been lost (i.e. a deficiency heterozygote).

***Henderson-Hasselback Equation.*** The formula for calculating the pH of a buffer solution, which states that :

$$\text{pH} = \text{pK} + \log \frac{(\text{H}^+ \text{ acceptor})}{(\text{H}^+ \text{ donor})}$$

where pK is the dissociation constant of an acid. The variable term is really a ratio of concentration values and can be taken as being proportional to the amount of acid and base added in the buffer. For example, when 30cm$^3$ of 0.1 M NaOH is added to 100 cm$^3$ of 0.1 M acetic acid and the pK for acetic acid is 4.73, we can estimate :

$$\begin{aligned} \text{pH} &= 4.73 + \log\,[30/(\,100\text{-}30)] \\ &= 4.73 + \log 0.429 \\ &= 4.36. \end{aligned}$$

***Heparin.*** A mucopolysaccharide molecule produced in the liver that acts as an anticogulant, inhibiting the transformation of prothrombin to thrombin, a vital stage in blood clotting.

***Hepatitis.*** A serious disorder of the liver that leads to severe jaundice, liver degeneration and even death. The condition is caused by two viruses : hepatitis A virus, which produces infective hepatitis transmitted by the intestinal-oral route, and hepatitis B virus, which produces serum hepatitis transmitted via infected blood or its products. Although these two viral types can be distinguishable in tests, the acute diseases caused by each may be clinically indistinguishable, the chief difference being that type A usually has a shorter incubation period than type B. No specific therapy is available for hepatitis, although vaccines are being developed.

***Heparin.*** Glycosaminoglycan that inhibits blood clotting. It allows the formation of complexes between antithrombin III and activated serine protease coagulation factors, thus irreversibly inactivating those factors. In clinical practice it is injected as an anticoagulant.

***Hepatocyte.*** Main cell type of the liver, derived from primitive gut epithelia. Hepatocytes are arranged in folded sheets facing the blood-filled sinusoids. They are responsible for synthesis, degradation and storage of a great range of different substances, including the production of bile.

***Hepes.*** (N-2- hydroxyethylpiperazine-N-2-ethanesulphonic acid). Compound used as a zwitterionic buffer. Use of this type of buffer avoids the presence of compounds, such as phosphate buffer which have high charge densities. It is particularly important in the preparation of media for studying active whole cells in tissue culture.

***Herbarium.*** A reference collection of preserved plants.

***Herbicide.*** Any chemical that kills plants. Herbicides can be highly selective. For example, 2,4,-D only kills dicotyledons (broad-leaved plants), leaving monocotyledons unharmed.

***Herbivore.*** Any animal feeding on plant matter.

***Hereditary Disease.*** Pathological condition resulting from the expression of a gene or genes, usually a mutant allele of a normal gene, or the lack of a gene or genes.

***Heredity.*** Phenomenon whereby characteristic traits are transmitted from one generation to another. It results from the transmission of genes from parents to offspring. Patterns of inheritance within a group of progeny result from the assortment of such genes in the gametes and zygotes.

***Heritability ($h^2$).*** The proportion of all phenotypic variance in a population that is due to genetic differences and which can be assessed in terms of two main ways, Broad-sense heritability and narrow-sense heritability. Heritability is thus a general measure of genetic variation without which selection (both natural and artificial), could not proceed, and is used widely by plant and animal breeders to predict the likely effect of selection. For example, if heritability values for a character are low this indicates high environmental variability, and suggests that the response to selection would not be very rapid.

***Hermaphrodite.***1. Any plant possessing stamens and carpels in the same flower. 2. Any animal possessing both male and female sex organs. The condition is usual in many plants and lower animals, but may occur in some unisexual organisms as an abnormality.

***Herpesvirus.*** One of a group complex DNA-containing viruses causing infections in man and most other vertebrates that tend to recur. The group includes herpes simplex, the agent of cold sores; herpes varicella/zoster, the virus causing chickenpox and shingles; Epstein-Barr (EB) virus, thought to be the causal agent of glandular fever and also implicated in the cancer Burkitt's lymphoma; and the cytomegalovirus.

***Hershey, Alfred (1908-).*** American scientist who in 1951 with his colleague Martha Chase showed, by means of differential radioactive labelling, that the DNA of $t_2$ Bacteriophages (rather than their protein) was necessary for the formation of new phages within the host bacterium, E. coli. The experimental results are taken as a demonstration that DNA functions as the genetic material.

***Heteroallelic.*** Describing an individual organism in which two homologous alleles are different, both carrying mutations but at differing sites. By applying the cis, trans test it may be found that intragenic recombination will result in a wild-type expression.

***Heteroblastic Development.*** Changes in the size and shape of an equivalent structure during development. Generally applied to plants, in which young leaves may have a strikingly different shape and form from leaves produced on a more mature plant.

***Heterochromatic.*** (Of chromosomal preparations) staining differently from the major chromosome parts.

***Heterochromatic.*** Any chromosomal segments or whole chromosomes that appear darkly stained during interphase of the cell cycle (as compared to euchromatin) due to tight condensation, which may indicate genetic inactivity. Heterochromatin may be condensed at all times (constitutive)or only at certain times (facultative).

***Heterochromosome.*** Chromosome entirely or largely composed of heterochromatin. These include the human Y chromosomes, and the supernumerarv B chromosomes.

***Heterocyst.*** Specialized cell of cyano-bacteria that is differentiated for vegetative reproduction.

***Heterodimer.*** Protein containing two subunits that differ in their amino acid sequences.

***Heteroduplex.*** (Of a molecule) possessing double-stranded nucleic acid in which the two polynucleotide chains come from a different source, either two different DNA strands or a DNA/RNA duplex, held together by complementary pairing.

***Heteroduplex Mapping.*** Accurate technique for the physical mapping of nucleic acids, and for determining the relatedness of two molecules, without knowledge of their sequences. An equal mixture of two DNA molecules is heat denatured followed by reannealing to create heteroduplexes which are then examined using an electron microscope. Single-stranded regions, prevented from collapsing by formamide, appear thinner than paired duplex regions. Consider, for example, the pairing of complementary strands from the DNA of a wild-type and of a mutant bacteriophage with a region of DNA deleted. The heteroduplex formed carries a single-stranded 'bubble' arising from the presence of a complete strand at the site of the missing DNA. A similar loop is generated if one DNA strand carries an insertion. Measurement of the structural modifications in the molecules are accurate to 50 base pairs if DNA molecules of known size are included on the grid as internal standards. A similar technique can be used to locate DNA sites that are complementary to RNA molecules and thus determine which regions of DNA are transcribed into RNA. Where RNA base pairs with one DNA strand the other DNA strand is displaced. Heteroduplexes made between functional mRNA molecules and their corresponding chromosomal genes first revealed the presence of introns in eukaryotic genes.

***Heterogametic Sex.*** The sex of a particular organism that contains within each nucleus one X-chromosome and one Y-chromosome (or just one X-chromosome), and therefore produces two different types of gamete with respect to the sex chromosomes. Usually the male is the heterogametic sex but in some organisms (e.g. birds), it is the female. Since the sex chromosomes usually are responsible for sex determination, it is the heterogametic parent that controls the sex of the offspring.

***Heterogamy.*** The alternation of forms of sexual reproduction.

***Heterogeneous Nuclear RNA.*** (hnRNA). Complex mixture of RNA molecules of varying sizes up to at least 30,000 nucleotides long found in the nuclei of eukaryotic cells, hnRNA molecules are synthesized at a rapid rate and have short half-lives, generally between 10 and 30 minutes in vivo. They include the largest types of RNA known in nature. Transcription of hnRNA is by RNA polymerase II, and the nascent transcripts are packaged with proteins and small nuclear RNA (snRNA) into ribonucleoprotein (RNP) particles as they are produced. A typical mammalian nucleus contains some 100 000 different hnRNA sequences at varying relative abundances. The only known function of hnRNA is as a precursor of messenger RNA (mRNA), hnRNA molecules are therefore transcripts of entire genes, including all introns and exons. Introns are removed by a processing stage within the RNP particle, and subsequently degraded, whereas the exons are spliced together and (usually) polyadenylated for transport to the cytoplasm as functional mRNA molecules.

***Heterogenote.*** Merozygote in which one or more pairs of corresponding alleles within the region of diploidy are non-identical. The term is also applied to the double lysogens formed as intermediates in the production of high-frequency transduction ($HF_R$) lysate.

***Heterograft*** (xenograft, heterologous graft). Graft taken from a donor of a species different to that of the recipient.

***Heterokaryon.*** A cell containing nuclei from two different sources, or in fungi a hyphal cell, spore, mycelium or organism that contains genetically different nuclei.

***Heterokaryosis.*** Situation that occurs in some fungal cells in which nuclei of differing genetic constitution occur in the same hyphal cell as a result of non-sexual cell fusion of two genetically differing types of hyphae.

***Heterokaryotypic.*** Describing an individual who carries a chromosome aberration in the heterozygous condition, thus having at least one pair of homologous chromosomes that are distinct from one another in some relatively major way.

***Heterokont.*** Describing a spore or cell that is flagellated, but in which the two flagella are of unequal lengths.

***Heterologous.*** Describing an antibody or antigen molecules that do not correspond, where it may be said that one is heterologous to the other. Serum or tissue may be described as heterologous if taken from a different organism, especially a different species, and the term may be used to describe relationships, for example, between DNA sequences, which is not one of homology.

***Heteromorphic.*** 1. (of an organism) having morphologically different forms in the life history, for example, where there is alternation of generations. 2. (Of pairs of homologous chromosomes) differing in size or form.

***Heteromorphic Chromosomes.*** Homologous chromosomes that differ in their morphologies.

***Heteromorphism.*** (1) Parts of organs of an organism that vary in their number or morphology at different stages in the life cycle. (2) Presence within a population of more than one type of individual (e.g. sexual dimorphism and polymorphism).

***Heteropolymer.*** Polymer that is made up of two or more different types of subunits.

***Heteropyknosis.*** Describing the state of chromatin which, by dint of its state of condensation, stains differently from the rest of the chromatin. Positively heteropyknotic chromatin stain more strongly and is more highly condensed than negatively heteropyknotic chromatin, which is relatively uncondensed and weakly staining. Chromatin regions such as centromeres and Y chromosomes are positively heteropyknotic and are referred to as heterochromatin.

***Heterosis (Hybrid Vigour).*** Increased vigour in terms of growth and fertility of hybrid organisms. Such hybrid vigour is most evident experimentally in crosses between individuals belonging to distinct inbred lines, and probably results entirely from the increased heterozygosity.

***Heterospory.*** The formation of more than one sort of spore, usually microspores and megaspores in ferns and seed plants, giving rise to distinct male and female gametophyte generations. The terms mega-and microspore were first used in connection with pteridophytes where differences in spore size occur. Later, because of how the structures are formed, these terms were used in reference to seed plants where such size differences are rarer. Here the microspore is the pollen, and the megaspore is the cell which gives rise to the embryo sac.

***Heterotroph.*** An organism dependent on obtaining organic food from the environment because it is unable to synthesize organic material. All animals, fungi, many bacteria and a few flowering plants such as insectivorous plants are heterotrophs, and they obtain almost all their organic material, either directly or indirectly, from the activity of autotrophs.

***Heterotroph Hypothesis.*** A hypothesis suggesting that the first organisms were heterotrophs.

***Heterozygosity.*** State of having one or more dissimilar pairs of alleles of particular genes. It is customary to use the term in reference to an individual, named gene locus, although it is legitimate to refer to increases or decreases in general heterozygosity. Thus inbred lines are relatively homozygous, and crosses between two such lines yield individuals that are broadly heterozygous.

***Heterozygote.*** An individual containing two different allelic forms of the same gene in all diploid (1) cells. Thus if gene A has two alleles, A1 and A2, the heterozygote would contain both alleles (A1/A2).

***Heterozygote Advantage.*** Increased heterosis or vigour that often characterizes individual that are broadly heterozygous at many loci, as compared with those that are broadly homozygous. It is normally assumed that the advantage follows from deleterious recessive genes being unexpressed, and also in the ability to produce progeny of varied genetic constitution, which, at least for the population of organisms, is usually advantageous in the long term.

***Heterozygous.*** Describing an organism that has two different "alleles controlling a particular feature. The aspect of the feature displayed by the organism will be that determined by the "dominant allele. Heterozygous organisms do not breed true.

***Hex-Or Hexa-,*** Denoting six.

***Hexose Sugar.*** A sugar containing six carbon atoms (e.g. glucose, $C_6H_{12}O_6$). Hexose sugars are the basic building blocks for more complex carbohydrates.

***Hfr Strain.*** A strain of E. coli bacteria that has the ability to transfer a chromosome to an $F^-$ cell and shows a high frequency of recombination. The F factor is integrated into the Hfr cell chromosome.

***HGPRT.*** (Hypoxanthine-guanine phosphoribosyl transferase). Enzyme that catalyses transfer of the phosphoribosyl moiety to hypoxanthine and guanine.

***Hha Restriction Enzyme.*** Type II restriction enzyme isolated from Haemophilus-haemolyticus that recognizes the tetranucleotide target sequence

↓
5'...G CGC...3'
3'...C GCG...5'
↑

Cleavage of the DNA duplex occurs at the positions arrowed to yield fragments of DNA with protruding cohesive ends two bases in length.

***High-Altitude Adjustment.*** The physiological adjustment to atmospheric pressure that occurs when an animal moves into high altitudes from a lower one, including changes in the respiratory and circulatory system, causing an increases in red blood cells and haemoglobin content of the blood.

***High-Energy Bond.*** A chemical bond containing several times more stored energy than is usual.

***Highly Repetitive DNA.*** Sequence of DNA that occurs repeatedly in a given genomic sample of DNA. Such DNA is chiefly centromeric and palindromic DNA. DNA reassociation and cot plot analysis reveal the respective amounts of repetitious DNA in a sample.

***Himalayan Rabbit.*** A strain of rabbit in which the coat colour is white but all body extremities are black (nose tip, paws, ears and tail). The condition is controlled by a single autosomal gene with multiple allelism, one for agouti, one for albinism and the third for Himalayan. The dominance relationship between the three alleles is : agouti > Himalayan > albino. The Himalayan allele is temperature-sensitive, coding for an enzyme that catalyses black pigment formation wherever the skin is cooler, the enzyme becoming inactive at higher temperatures.

***Hin dIII Restriction Enzyme.*** Restriction endonuclease extracted from the bacterium Haemophilus influenzae, with a recognition sequence of A↓AGGTT, which is cut between the two adenine bases.

***Hinge Region.*** Region of immunoglobulin structure involving only heavy chains, which have a distinct spatial angle in this region, allowing the open arms of the Y beyond the hinge to associate with the immunoglobulin light chains. The two heavy chains are joined in the hinge region by sulphur bridges.

***Hinny.*** Result of crossing a female donkey with a male horse; the mule is the result of a reciprocal cross. Since the horse diploid chromosome number is 64 and that of the donkey 62, both hybrids have 63 chromosomes and are sterile.

***Hirschsprung Disease.*** (Colonic Aganglionosis). Congenital malformation in the human; inherited as a multifactorial trait, with absence of ganglion cells in the rectal and colonic submucosa, leading to constipation and abdominal distension.

***His Operon.*** Genetic system, first described for Salmonella typhimurium, responsible for the synthesis of Histidine from its precursors ATP and phosphoribosyl pyrophosphate (PRPP). Studies were initiated in the late 1950s by Demerec, Hartman and Ames. over a thousand spontaneous and induced mutants of S. typhimurium, each requiring histidine as a growth factor were isolated. The mutations were mapped on the bacterial chromosome by two-factor crosses and by deletion mapping using transduction. Without exception the sites of mutation mapped in a linear sequence that represented about 0.26 percent of the total length of the chromosome. The histidine region was divided into nine contiguous functional subregions (A-1) by complementation tests based on abortive transduction. Each subregion (cistron) corresponds to the structural gene for a particular enzyme of the histidine pathway. (The most recent information indicates eight genes and 11 biochemical steps.) Three enzymes — the his D, his B and his I/E (one gene) products — are bifunctional proteins each with two distinct catalytic roles). Examples of interallelic complementation between mutations mapping within the same gene were also observed. Biochemical studies with the histidine auxotrophs allowed the assignment of enzymes to particular genes, and the ordering of the sequence of reactions in the pathway. Putative intermediates that were accumulated (and often excreted) by the mutants were checked for their ability to support the growth of other mutants (cross-feeding) and for their enzymic conversion to histidine by cell-free bacterial extracts. The metabolite accumulated by a double mutant (constructed by recombination) blocked in two separate reactions of the pathway was characteristic of the first blocked reaction; the metabolite normally accumulated as a result of the second block was not found, because the supply of its precursor had been shut off at the earlier step. The order of the genes does not correspond to the order of reactions in the biosynthetic pathway.

The gene cluster comprises a coordinated unit for controlling synthesis of the enzymes of the histidine pathway. Enzyme synthesis is sensitive to the presence of histidine in the growth medium, thus an auxotroph starved of histidine has 25 times more of the remaining active enzymes than the histidine operon is under negative control by a repressor protein with histidine acting as corepressor (i.e. an activator of the repressor). But no regulator gene nor repressor gene has been identified. Nevertheless derepressed (constitutive) mutants have been isolated by virtue of their resistance to the histidine analogue triazolealanine which acts a 'false corepressor' of enzyme synthesis, cis-Dominant constitutive mutations, mapping adjacent to the his structural genes, were assigned to a proposed his operator, but are now known to alter the his attenuator, trans-Dominant constitutive mutations, located at distinct chromosomal sites separate from the his operon, were designated his R, hisS, hisT, hisU, and hisW. These mutations alter either the synthesis (hisR), aminoacylation (hisS), modification (hisT), or maturation (hisU, hisW) of histidine-specific tRNA and in effect reduce the cellular concentration of histidyl-tRNA. In these strains there is an inverse correlation between the amount of his operon expression. These observations gave rise to the notion that histidyl-tRNA (rather than free histidine) is the repression signal.

The his operon is regulated solely by attenuation (note however that the first enzyme of the pathway is sensitive to end-product inhibition by histidine). The 5'- end of the his polycistronic message carries a 127-nucleotide leader sequence prior to hisG. The leader RNA carries a potential ribosome-binding site followed by coding sequence for a 16-amino acid leader peptide containing seven adjacent histidine residues. Beyond this is a GC-rich region with dyad symmetry (capable of forming a stem and loop 'attenuator') followed by a run of uracil residues within which rho-independent transcription termination can occur. Depending on the location of the ribosome translating the leader peptide coding region, the leader RNA transcript can form an alternative competing secondary structure that prevents formation of the attenuator (transcription termination signal). Ribosomes freely translate the leader peptide sequence when the supply of histidyl-tRNA is non-limiting; this allows formation of the attenuator and leads to termination of transcription before RNA polymerase enters the structural genes. During conditions of histidine starvation (or more specifically low endogenous levels of histidyl-tRNA) ribosomes stall at the histidine codons within the leader peptide coding region, prevent formation of the attenuator, and thus allow transcription to proceed into structural genes. The level of expression of the his operon, and hence the rate of histidine biosynthesis, is determined therefore by the availability of histidine for protein synthesis, the sensing mechanism being the protein-synthesizing machinery itself.

P L G D C B H A F I/E

(P = Promoter; L = leader sequence)

| Gene | Enzyme | Step catalyzed |
|---|---|---|
| hisG | ATP : phosphoribosyl transferase | 1 |
| hisD | Histidinol dehydrogenase | 10 |
| hisD | Histidinal dehydrogenase | 11 |
| hisC | Histidinol phosphate aminotransferase | 8 |
| hisB | Imidazoleglycerol phosphate dehydratase | 7 |
| hisB | Histidinol phosphate phosphatase | 9 |
| hisH | Glutamine amidotransferase | 5 |
| hisA | Phosphoribosyl formimino aminoimidazole carboxamide riboside isomerase | 4 |
| hisF | Cyclase | 6 |
| his/E | Phosphoribosyl-AMP cyclohydrolase/ phosphoribosyl-ATP pyrophosphohydrolase | 3<br>2 |

Table. His operon. Genes of the histidine operon.

***Histamine.*** A chemical ($C_5H_9N_3$) produced by leucocytes and other cells (e.g. mast cells) that causes blood capillaries to become more permeable and so lose fluids into the tissues, producing a local swelling. Histamines are released when foreign antigens are present.

***Histiocyte.*** Phagocyte found mainly in connective tissue. Although normally non-motile, it can become converted into a mobile, amoeboid macrophage. Histiocytes are large, irregularly shaped cells with granular, vacuolated cytoplasm. They are associated with inflammatory conditions, and are especially found near tissue haemorrhages.

***Histidine.*** One of the 20 amino acids common in proteins. It carries an extra basic group making it alkaline and is

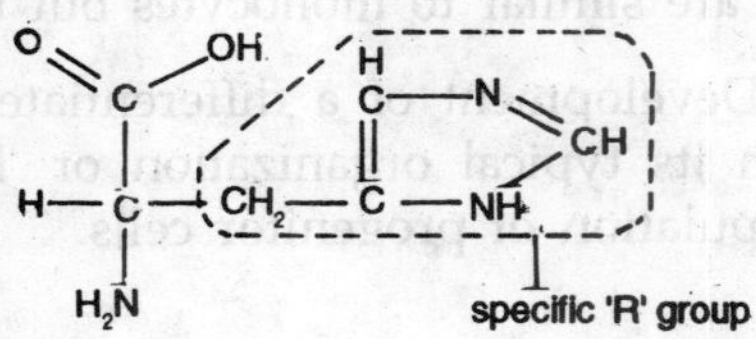


Figure H.4. Histidine. Molecular structure.

soluble in water. See Figure H.4. The isoelectric point of histide is 7.6.

***Histochemistry.*** The study of the distribution of substances in tissues by using staining methods on preparations such as sections or whole mounts.

***Histocompatibility.*** The acceptance by a. recipient of tissue transplanted from a donor, a state that is determined by histocompatability antigens.

***Histocompatibility Antigen*** (Transplantation antigen). Antigen responsible for evoking the immune reaction which is involved in recognition of foreign tissue and rejection of homografts. These antigens are glycoproteins of the cell surface, the most important of which are the HLA (human leucocyte antigen) proteins. These are analogous to H-2 antigens in mice. Although similar to antibodies in certain aspects of their structure, unlike antibody, all cells in the same organism have the same HLA antigens on their surfaces, but these will differ from those of other individuals of the same species and population. They therefore endow the individual with immunological uniqueness. Although not as great as the diversity of antibody structure, the structure of these proteins is highly varied, and this variation is generated in ways broadly similar to those employed in the production of antibody variability.

***Histocompatibility Genes.*** Genes belonging to the major histocompatibility system (MHC) and thus coding for HLA or to one of the minor groupings making similar antigens (e.g., H-2). The genes of the HLA complex are clustered on chromosome 6 in the human.

***Histocyte or Clasmatocyte.*** A large phagocyte of irregular shape that occurs in blood, lymph and connective tissue. Histocytes are similar to monocytes but take up stain.

***Histogenesis.*** Development of a differentiated and functional tissue with its typical organization or 'histoarchitecture,' from a population of progenitor cells.

***Histoincompatibility.*** Condition in which two individual vertebrates have different, genetically determined isoantigens on the surfaces of their cells. Tissue from one such animal grafted onto the other will be rejected by an immune reaction.

***Histology.*** Study of cells within tissues and the analysis of tissues by microscopy.

***Histone Acetylase.*** Enzyme responsible for histone acetylation.

***Histone.*** Any of a group of water-soluble proteins found in association with the "DNA of plant and animal chromosomes. They contain a large proportion of the basic (positively charged)amino acids lysine, arginine, and histidine. They are believed to be involved in the condensation and coiling of chromosomes during cell division and have also been implicated in nonspecific suppression of gene activity. Histones do not occur in vertebrate sperm cells or in bacteria and blue-green algae.

***Histone Acetylation.*** Attachment of an acetyl group ($CH_3CO$—) to some amino acids of certain histone molecules. Two distinct types of histone acetylation are known, each correlated with a different aspect of histone function. (1) Histones H1, H2A and H4 have the serine residues at their N-terminals irreversibly acetylated. This modification is associated with histone synthesis. (2) Reversible acetylation of N-terminal lysine residues of histones H2A, H2B, H3 and H4 may occur, and there is some evidence to support the view that genes which are being actively transcribed are associated in chromatin with histones which have highly acetylated lysines. This modification of histone molecules is rendered reversible by the activity of deacetylases in living cells.

***Histone Gene.*** One of a family of genes that code for histone proteins. They are distinguished by a complete absence of intron sequences. Genomes of different eukaryotes contain very different numbers of repeat copies of the five basic histone genes, yeast having two copies of each, the chicken

10 and some sea urchin species up to 600. Many of these repeats consist of similar tandem arrangements of the histone gene sequences each unit containing one copy of each histone gene in a standard sequence (e.g., H1-H4-H2B-H3-H2A-H1, etc.)

***Histone Modification.*** Following initial synthesis, histones may undergo various important modifications (e.g., methylation, acetylation, phosphorylation) within eukaryotic cells. Methylation is irreversible, affects only lysine and has little effect on the properties of this histone molecule. Acetylation is of two types, irreversible and reversible. The former affects only serine and is associated with histone synthesis, whereas the latter affects lysine residues and seems to be strongly correlated with transcriptional activity of chromatin. Phosphorylation affects mainly serine and threonine in H1 histone and is thought to help trigger and onset of chromatin condensation in preparation for mitosis.

***HIV (Human Immunodeficiency Virus).*** Accepted term for the causative agent of human AIDS, and previously known either as LAV or HTLVIII.

***HLA Complex (Human Leucocyte Antigen Complex).*** The human major his to compatibility complex (MHC).

***HLA (Human Leucocyte A) System.*** A major histocompatability complex of four genes (perhaps five) called HLA-A, HLA-B, HLA-C and HLA-D, with the D locus nearest to the centromere on the shorter arm of chromosome 6. Each gene has up to 35 alleles, the particular combination of alleles of the four genes on a chromosome being called the haplotype. Since humans are diploid organisms we have two haplotypes, these being determined by testing the individual's white blood cells for the specific HLA antigens.

Although these large numbers of alleles would appear to make the system a complex one in terms of possible combinations in each individual, in fact the situation is simpler than it seems. The four loci within the HLA system are so tightly linked together that there is very little crossing over between them. Thus each haplotype tends to be passed onto an offspring as a block rather than as four individual genes. Given no recombination between the four genes, four rearrangements would be expected to occur in the progeny of a mating. Thus any child of a cross has a one-in-four chance of inheriting precisely the same HLA combination as another sibling. Since the success of organ transplantation depends upon a close match of HLA alleles (even one allele difference can cause the foreign organ to be rejected), the chance of matching HLA types is highest within closely related individuals.

***HMG Proteins.*** (High-mobility group proteins). Group of non-histone proteins found in association with the DNA of eukaryotic chromosomes. HMGs are the most abundant of the many non-histone chromosomal proteins, with four types being especially common. At least two of the (HMG 14 and HMG 17) may have roles in the regulation of gene expression, although this has yet to be proven definitely. Their presence is generally associated with transcriptionally active chromatin.

***Holandric.*** (Of genes) carried on the Y-sex chromosome and transmitted via the heterogametic sex. In mammals, holandric genes are passed on from father to son.

***Holocene (Recent).*** The most recent geological epoch of the Quaternary period, comprising roughly the past 10 000 years since the end of the Pleistocene up to the present. It follows the final glacial of the Pleistocene and thus is sometimes known as the Postglacial epoch. Some geologists consider the Holocene to be an interglacial phase of the Pleistocene that will be followed by another glacial.

***Holliday Model.*** Model originally proposed by Holliday in 1964 to account for the DNA breakage and reunion events of chromosomal recombination. The model, which has now been broadly substantiated, implies that single-strand DNA breaks and rejoins between homologous chromosomes do not necessarily occur at the sites of visible crossing-over, but that, following the initial break and ligation, the chromosomes swivel about the branch point, forming in the process a configuration known as a Holliday intermediate. Molecular configurations resembling the predicted intermediates have been visualized in electron microscope-studies. Following formation of the intermediate, the model further proposes that cuts are made across the single strands at the branch point, followed by splicing of the strands across the branch to allow reformation of intact DNA duplexes. See Figure H.5.

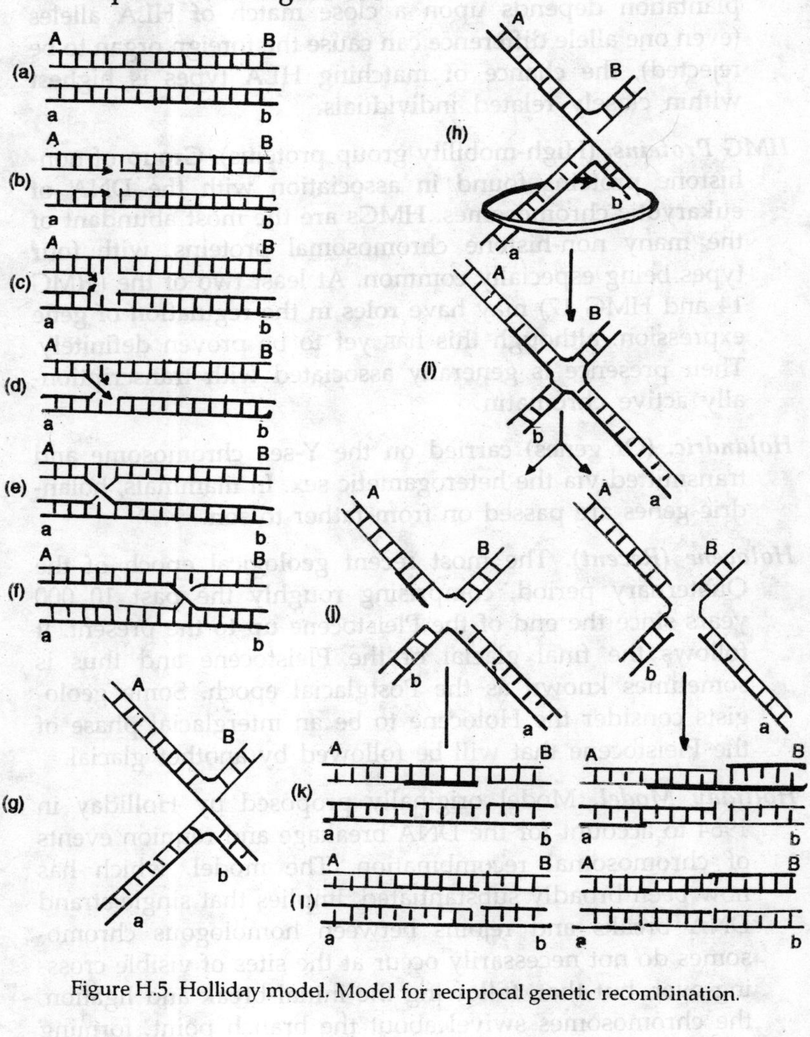


Figure H.5. Holliday model. Model for reciprocal genetic recombination.

***Holoblastic Cleavage.*** Pattern of division or cleavage of the egg into many cells shown by echinoderm, amphibian and mammalian embryos. In holoblastic or complete cleavage the cleavage planes pass right through the egg, and the contents of the egg, including the yolk, are retained within the embryonic cells. In contrast, in the meroblastic or incomplete cleavage planes do not pass right through the egg and the embryo forms as a layer of cells (the blastoderm) on top of the yolk.

***Holocentric.*** Describing chromosomes whose centromeres are diffuse rather than discretely located as they are in most chromosomes.

***Holoenzyme.*** An entire conjugated enzyme consisting of a protein component (an apoenzyme) and a nonprotein component (a coenzyme or an activator).

***Hologamete.*** A gamete formed by a full-sized ordinary individual protozoan that fuses with another similar individual to form a zygote.

***Holophytic.*** (Of plants) using the energy of the sun to synthesize organic compounds by means of chlorophyll.

***Holt-Oram Syndrome (Hand-heart syndrome).*** Human congenital disorder, caused by an autosomal dominant gene, in which variable arm malformations occur together with atrial septal defects in the heart.

***Homeo Box (Homoeo Box).*** Consensus sequence found in homeotic genes of Drosophila, but subsequently found to be present in a wide range of gene sequences in most eukaryotes. Genes that contain homeo box sequences frequently code for proteins that have a DNA-binding capacity, and this may explain the significance of the common sequence.

***Homeogenetic Induction.*** Process by which a differentiated cell can induce differentiation in an adjacent cell not previously so committed. The term is used chiefly in relation to plant cells.

***Homeosis (Homoeosis).*** Formation of an appendage or organ in one site that is inappropriate to that site, but entirely resembles an appendage or organ appropriate to another site. Thus the development of a leg in place of an antenna is an example of homeosis. It is a more widely accepted term than heteromorphosis.

***Homeostasis.*** The maintenance by an organism of a constant internal environment, such as the regulation of blood sugar levels by insulin. The process involves self-adjusting mechanisms in which the maintenance of a particular level is initiated by the substance to be regulated.

***Homeotic Mutant.*** The mutational change of one structure to another in insects, such as wing to haltere, arista to leg.

***Homeotic Mutation.*** Mutation producing a homeotic condition or aberration. Some remarkable homeotic mutations are known in Drosophila, such as aristapedia and bithorax. The genes involved in many of these homeotic mutations have now been cloned, and their precise effects studied. Many of these genes possess a common short sequence of DNA, known as the homeo box, and are found to be expressed for only short periods during development. They may well function as regulator genes, controlling the activities of other sets of genes during development.

***Home Range.*** The area in which an animal normally restricts its movements in search of food or a mate, and in which it cares for its young.

***Homing.*** (Modifier) relating to the ability to return to a place of origin.

***Homo.*** The genus of primates that includes modern man (H. sapiens, the only living representative) and various extinct species. The oldest Homo fossils are those of H. habilis, found in the Olduvai Gorge in Tanzania in 1960 and estimated to be about 1.75 million years old. The find was significant as it had been thought that man emerged in Asia rather than Africa H. habilis appears to have been 1-1.5 m tall and had more manlike features and a larger brain than Australopithecus. However, the direct ancestor of modern man is thought to be H. erectus, which includes Java man and Peking man and appeared about 1.5 million years ago. Fossils of H erectus, which are sometimes called Pithecanthropus (ape man), are similar to present-day man except that there was a prominent ridge above the eyes and no forehead or chin. They had crude stone tools and used fire H. sapiens appeared about 100 000 years ago as Neanderthal man and subsequently (about 35 000 years ago) as Cromagnon man.

***Homogametic Sex.*** The sex that contains in its nuclei similar sex chromosomes (e.g. XX) and produces gametes all with the same type of sex chromosome.

***Homogamy.*** The state of having anthers and stigmas maturing at the same time.

***Homograft or Allograft.*** A transplant from one individual to another individual that is of the same species but has a different genotype, and is therefore subject to rejection by the recipient as it contains foreign antigens.

***Homoiotherm or Homeotherm or Homotherm.*** Any warm blooded animal (mammal or bird). A homoiotherm can maintain its body temperature within a narrow range, usually above that of its surroundings despite large variation in environmental temperature. It may be maintained continually or for limited periods only.

***Homologous.*** (Of organs, or structures) deriving from the same evolutionary origins. For example, the forelimb of a quadruped, the human arm, the wing of a bird, are said to be homologous. Usually similarities are seen best in embryonic development, and are regarded by taxonomists as indications of relationships between present-day-organisms.

***Homologous Chromosomes.*** Those chromosomes containing identical genetic loci although possibly different allelic forms. In diploid organisms the chromosomes occur in homologous pairs, one member of each pair from a different parent, the pair becoming separated during meiosis and giving rise to genetic segregation.

***Homology.*** The condition of being homologous.

***Homoplasy.*** Convergent or parallel evolution, or similarity in organisms which is not directly a result of inheritance or development from common ancestry.

***Homopolymer.*** Polymer composed of a series of identical subunits.

***Homopolymer Tailing.*** Use of terminal transferase to add a series of identical bases of the 3'-end of a DNA molecule. In the test-tube it often involves the addition of a string of poly A to carrier DNA and a string of complementary poly T to the DNA to be carried following base pairing (or vice versa) or the use of the poly G and the poly C in a similar way.

***Homospory.*** The possession of only one form of spore. This gives rise to a single gametophyte generation carrying both male and female reproduction organs.

***Homothallism.*** The situation in algae and fungi where sexual reproduction occurs in a colony arising from a single spore, each thallus being self-fertile.

***Homozygosity.*** Condition in which both members of a pair of alleles are identical, or many pairs of alleles at different loci are identical.

***Homozygote.*** An individual containing two identical forms of the same gene in all diploid (1) cells that is capable of pure breeding. Thus if gene A has two alleles, A1 and A2 homozygous types are possible : A1/A1 and A2/A2.

***Homozygous.*** Describing an organism having two identical "alleles controlling a particular feature (these may be either dominant or recessive). Homozygous organisms breed true when crossed with genetically identical organisms.

***Homunculus.*** Minute, but fully formed human being that some 17th century microscopists believed they could see in the head of a spermatozoon and which was imagined simply to grow when nourished within the female uterus. Note that so-called ovists maintained the child was contained within the egg, not the sperm.

***Horizon.*** Any layer of soil that is distinguishable when soil is examined in vertical sections.

***Horizontal Transmission.*** Transfer of genetical material by infection-like processes; including transduction.

***Hormone.*** A chemical that is produced in the body of a plant or animal, sometimes in very small quantities, and which when transported (usually by the blood stream in animals) to another part of the organism, elicits a particular response. Hormones are thus chemical messengers. In animals the ductless glands that secrete hormones are called endocrine organs. Animal hormones that influence other endocrine glands are called trophins (or tropins) as in gonadotrophins.

***Horseradish Peroxidase.*** Enzyme used to identify endocytotic vesicles since the enzyme reacts with the contents of such vesicles and the products of the reaction are readily stained by osmium tetroxide for electron microscopy.

***Host.*** Organism that is either the recipient of a graft or is infected by parasites.

***Host Restriction.*** Bacteria of different species have a well-defined defence system against invading foreign DNA. The invaded cells have specific endonucleases which cleave this foreign DNA at specific target sequences, thereby making it susceptible to other non-specific nucleases. This phenomenon has been clearly demonstrated when coliphage, which has been grown on E. coli strain C is used to infect E. coli K-12. It grows only very poorly; the growth is therefore host-restricted.

***Hot Spot.*** Site at which the frequency of recombination or spontaneous mutation is high as compared to other sites in the same gene sequence. Hot spots were first noted by Benzer in his studies on the R11 region of the phage T4.

***Housekeeping Gene.*** Gene that is expressed in most or all cells of a complex multicellular organism; the products of such genes are essential enzymes or structural proteins in the basic form and general maintenance of the cell. Non-housekeeping genes are known as cell-specific genes or luxury genes.

***H-Substance Or H-Antigen.*** The carbohydrate precursor of the A and B antigens found in red blood cell and in various tissue fluids, recognized by an anti-H-reagent made from gorse seeds.

***Human Chorionic Gonadotrophin (HCG).*** A gonadotrophic hormone secreted by the Placenta (1) that has a similar effect to luteinizing hormone.

***Human Cytogenetics.*** Study of human chromosomes, chiefly by light microscopy, as a means of detecting chromosomal abnormalities and thus giving genetic counselling to prospective parents, or pregnant women following amniocentesis. Mitotic chromosomes are visualized by removing a sample of blood and incubating the leucocytes in the presence of colchicine. Microscope slides with squashes of the treated cells will have a large number of metaphase stage mitotic figures. Greater discrimination between chromosomes may be achieved through the use of chromosome banding involving quinacrine or giemsa strain.

Human mitotic chromosomes are grouped into seven classes (A-G), using criteria of size and centromeric position. Chromosomes 1-3 are group A, 4-5 are Group B,6-12 and X are Group C, 13-15 are Group D, 16-18 are Group E, 19-20 are Group F, and 21-22 and Y are Group G. Loci are assigned to chromosomes on the basis of quinacrine or Giemsa banding (bands that fluoresce with quinacrine are darkened by Giemsa).Thus the genes for colour blindness are assigned as q27-q ter on the X chromosome, meaning that they lie on the long arm of the X (the q arm) in the region 2 of this arm and between band 7 and the terminus of the arm.

***Human Karyotye.*** Chromosomal complement of the human. A visual montage or ideogram of human chromosomes can be readily prepared by cutting out the image of each metaphase chromosome from a photo micrograph and arranging the cut outs in a standard ordered sequence of matching pairs in order of size. There are 46 chromosomes in the human karyotype consisting of 22 pairs of autosomes and either two X chromosomes or an X and a Y chromosome, depending on whether the individual is female or male, respectively.

***Human T Cell Leukaemia Virus (HTLV).*** Any one of a group of retroviruses (HTLVI), HTLVII, etc.) of which one, now termed human immunodeficiency virus (HIV) and previously known as HTLVIII or LAV (lymphadenopathy virus), is the cause of acquired immune deficiency syndrome (AIDS).

***Humoral Immunity.*** One of the two systems of immunity in vertebrates (for the other), in which protection is provided by antibody molecules secreted into the lymph and blood by antigen-stimulated B Lymphocytes and their progeny. Humoral immunity is particularly effective against the extracellular phases of bacteria and viruses.

***Hunter Syndrome.*** One of a group of genetically inherited disorders of the human involving malfunction of mucopolysaccharide storage in connective tissue; a type of gargoylism. The gene of Hunter syndrome is X-linked.

***Huntington's Chorea.*** An incurable degeneration of the human nervous system characterized by involuntary movements of the head, face and/or limbs, leading to eventual death. The disorder is caused by a single autosomal dominant gene on chromosome 4 that shows delayed penetrance, fewer than 5% of cases being seen before the age of 25.Thus many individuals carrying the dominant allele have reproduced before their own gene shows itself; their progeny in turn may have to wait until middle age to discover if they have inherited the condition. Named after the American neurologist (1851-1916).

***Hurler Syndrome.*** Disease similar to hunter syndrome, but caused by an autosomal gene rather than an X-linked gene.

***Hyaluronidase.*** An enzyme present in snake venom and bacteria that catalyses the hydrolysis of hyaluronic acid, thus making it ineffective in stopping the spread of invading microorganisms and other toxic substances.

***Hybrid.*** An offspring of a cross between two genetically unlike individuals.

***Hybrid-Arrested Translation.*** Process by which a specific complementary DNA (cDNA) will hybridize with its specific messenger RNA (mRNA) and so prevent translation of the message. It may be used as a means of identifying the cDNA or mRNA.

***Hybrid Corn.*** Types of commercially grown maize. Zea mays, that are produced by a process of double-crossing from four inbred lines. They are characterized by good vigour and uniform growth.

***Hybrid DNA.*** A nucleic acid produced by joining together or 'annealing', polynucleotide chains of DNA from different sources

***Hybrid Dysgenesis.*** Syndrome of genetic abnormality that follows from mating particular strains of Drosophila. The condition is caused in many cases by a transposable element P, which is repressed in strains that normally carry it, but readily transposes when introduced into new strains, causing greatly increased mutation rates, chromosomal abnormalities and frequent sterility. The transposable element I also causes hybrid dysgenesis in Drosophila.

***Hybridization.*** (1) Crossing of inbred lines or individual organisms of differing genetic constitution or species. (2) The pairing of complementary strands of nucleic acid to form a duplex, especially of strands from differing original sources.

***Hybridoma.*** Hybrid cell resulting from the artificial fusion of an antibody-producing a lymphocyte and a myeloma cell from a lymphoid tumour. Such cells can produce a clone that may be maintained in tissue culture and used for the continuing production of monoclonal antibody.

***Hybrid-Released Translation (HRT).*** Method in which cloned DNA is bound to a cellulose nitrate filter and hybridized with a mixed population of mRNA or total cellular RNA. Hybridized message is then eluted and translated in a cell-free translation system.

***Hybrid Sterility.*** The inability of some hybrids to form functional gametes, due to chromosomes mispairing during meiosis. This is a form of reproductive isolation.

***Hybrid Swarm.*** A group of genetically variable organisms resulting from the hybridization of two previously distinct and separate populations. Subsequent crossing and back-crossing results in a very variable population as a result of segregation. often the genetical variability appears as morphological variability, such as different colour forms. Where different colour forms of an animal occur in different parts of the range, the hybrid swarm is characterized by the presence of all or a wide range of these forms.

***Hybrid Vigour (Heterosis).*** The increased vigour displayed by the offspring from a cross between genetically different parents. Hybrids from crosses between different crop varieties ($F_1$hybrids) are often stronger and produce better yields than the original varieties. Mules, the offspring of mares crossed with donkeys, have greater strength and resistance to disease and a longer lifespan than either parent.

***Hydantoin.*** Substance that is known to be a human teratogen. It is capable of inducing cleft palate and mental retardation.

***Hydatidiform Mole.*** Placental tumour resulting from excess growth of chorionic villi and with a significant incidence of malignancy.

***Hydrolases (Hydrolytic enzymes).*** Enzymes that catalyse the transfer of water molecules between receptor and donor molecules. Proteolytic enzymes (proteases) are a class of hydrolases.

***Hydrophilic.*** Having an affinity for water.

***Hydrophobic.*** Having an aversion for water.

***Hydrophyte.*** A plant that inhabits wet places and has its perennating buds lying in water.

***Hydroponics.*** The science of growing plants without soil, in which the roots are suspended in aerated water containing known quantities of chemicals that can be adjusted to suit changing conditions. The method is increasingly common in the glasshouse cultivation of, for example, tomatoes and cucumbers.

***Hydrops Foetalis (Alpha-thalassaemia major).*** Inherited condition that is lethal at or before birth, and results from absence or defects in the genes coding for alpha-globin. It is a homozygous conditions relative to the alpha-globin genes.

***Hydrosphere.*** The aqeuous envelope of the earth, including underground water and the atmospheric water vapour.

***Hydrostatic Skeleton.*** A liquid, usually water, that maintains the shape of an organism by filling internal spaces.

***Hydrotropism.*** The growth of plant roots in a particular orientation with respect to water,usually towards moisture.

***Hydroxyapatite.*** Calcium phosphate slurry or gel which can be used to bind specifically double-stranded DNA, and to separate it from single-stranded DNA in various kinds of column separations.

***Hydroxyurea.*** Compound commonly used in molecular biology to block DNA replication, but permitting repair synthesis to continue.

***Hydrozoan.*** Any colonial or solitary coelenterate of the class Hydrozoa, including most of the species that exhibit and alternation of generation between Hydroid and medusoid forms.

***Hypercholesterolaemia.*** Hereditary disease in humans in which the plasma concentration of low-density lipoprotein is elevated. It segregates as an autosomal dominant and is determined by an allele of a gene on chromosome 14. Although homozygotes are rare, heterozygotes occur in about one in 500 of the US and European populations. The symptoms of the disease result largely from the deposition of cholesterol on arterial walls and consequent formation of atherosclerosis.

***Hypertrophy.*** An increase in the size of a tissue or organ due to an increase in the size of its component cells. Hypertrophy often occurs in response to an increased work-load in an organ, which may result from malfunction or disease.

***Hyperparasite.*** An organism parasitic on another parasite.

***Hyperplasia.*** Increase in the size of an organ or tissue due to increase in the numbers of the component cells. It often implies a non-cancerous cell proliferation.

***Hyperpolarization.*** Increase in the electrical potential difference across a cell membrane.

***Hypersensitive Site.*** Short region of chromatin characterized by extreme sensitivity to digestion by DNase I and other nucleases. Such sites commonly appear in the promoter regions of active genes, are tissue-specific and may result from loss of, or conformational change in, the nucleosomes.

***Hypersensitivity.*** The process of localized plant cell death that occurs immediately after entry of a cell by a plant pathogen. Such a reaction can act as a host-resistance mechanism since the cell death often prevents further growth of biotrophic pathogens, e.g. powdery mildews or rusts.

***Hypostasis.*** A relationship between two genes whose products act in the same biochemical pathway, where the functional effect of one gene is masked by another. The enzyme coded by the hypostatic gene operates later in the pathway than the enzyme produced by the epistatic gene.

***Hypothalamus.*** The part of the sides and floor of the brain derived from the forebrain. Associated with the control of body temperature, it also partially controls the pituitary gland and contains centres controlling sleep and wakefulness, feeding, drinking, speech and osmoregulation, the last by secretion of ADH from neurosecretory cells. It is also associated with aspects of reproductive behaviour.

***Hypothermia.*** An abnormally low body temperature that reduce the metabolic rate to a dangerous level and can lead to death, often occurring in elderly people subjected to cold weather. Hypothermia is sometimes induced in medical treatment in order to reduce metabolic activity.

***Hypotonic.*** (Of a fluid) having a less-negative water potential or a lower solute concentration than another fluid, which is hypertonic to it.

***Hypoxanthine (6-Hydroxypurine).*** One of the rarer bases found in nucleic acids. It is a deamination product of adenine and is normally recognized as such by DNA repair enzymes and removed from the DNA sequence.

***H zone.*** The lightish area in the middle of a muscle sarcomere where myosin and actin filaments do not overlap.

# I

*$I_1, I_2, I_3$, etc.* First and succeeding generations obtained from outbreeding.

*IAA (Indole-3-Acetic Acid Or Indolacetic Acid).* The most thoroughly investigated type of Auxin, which has been extracted from various natural sources. See Figure I.1.

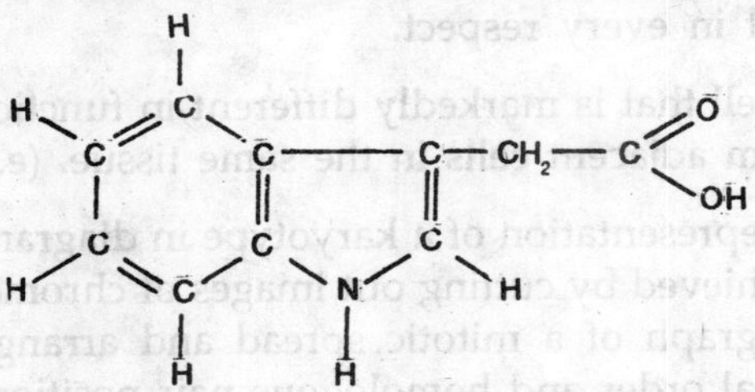

Figure I.1. IAA. Molecular structure.

*IAN (Indole-3-Aceto Nitrile).* A plant growth-regulating hormone.

*Ice Age.* A period in the earth's history during which ice advanced towards the equator and a general lowering of temperatures occurred. The last major ice age, that of the Pleistocene period (sometimes known as the Ice Age), ended about 10 000 years ago. At least four major ice advances (glacials) occurred during the Pleistocene period; these were separated by interglacials during which the ice retreated and temperatures rose. At present it is not known if the earth is between ice ages or is in an interglacial. It has been established that ice ages also occurred during the Precambrian (about 500 million years ago) and during the Permo-Carboniferous (about 250 million years ago).

***Ichthyosaur.*** A large extinct reptile that existed from the triassic period to the cretaceous period. It has paddle-shaped limbs, a head with long toothed jaws, and a fish-like tail.

***Ichthyosis.*** Extreme pilling up of the skin, which is commonly an X-linked recessive trait.

***Icosahedron.*** Polyhedron with 20 'triangular faces. The capsids of many phage and eukaroytic viruses are icosahedral.

***ICSH.*** Interstitial cell-stimulating hormone.

***Identical Twins (Monozygotic Twins).*** Two individuals that develop from a single fertilized egg cell by its division into two genetically identical parts. Each part eventually gives rise to a separate individual and these twins are therefore identical in every respect.

***Idioblast.*** Cell that is markedly different in function and structure from adjacent cells in the same tissue. (e.g. sclereids).

***Idiogram.*** Representation of a karyotype in diagrammatic form, often achieved by cutting out images of chromosomes from a photograph of a mitotic spread and arranging them in numerical order and homologous pair position. See Figure I.2 on next page.

***Idiotype.*** Collective antigenic determinants present in the variable regions of the light chains and heavy chains of antibody molecules. Anti-idiotypic antibodies (directed against the idiotype) can be produced by injecting specific antibodies from one animal into another animal of the same strain since the antigen binding sites of individual antibodies can create a unique protein structure.

***Idiotypic Variability.*** Antigenic variability of proteins, probably caused by variations in their encoding genes. Idiotypic

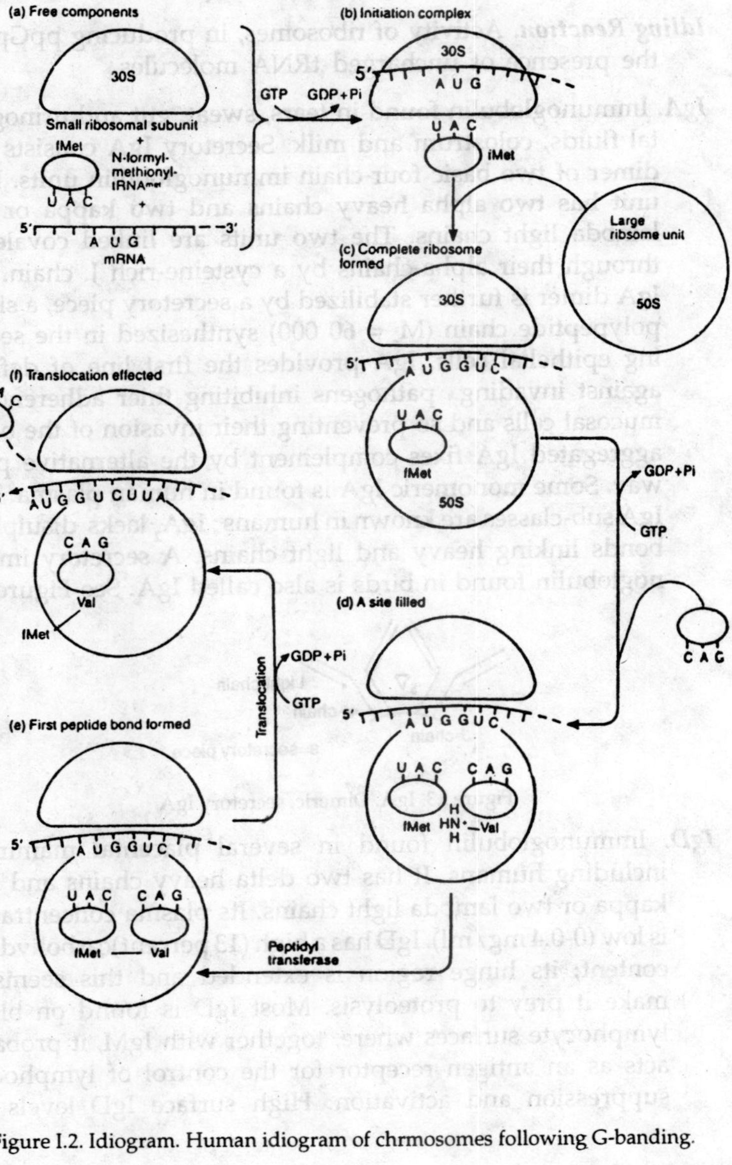


Figure I.2. Idiogram. Human idiogram of chrmosomes following G-banding.

variability is seen in the primary amino acid sequences in the variable regions of immunoglobulin molecules of the same allotype and isotype. Such variability confers antigenic specificity to a given molecule.

***Idling Reaction.*** Activity of ribosomes, in producing ppGpp in the presence of uncharged tRNA molecules.

***IgA.*** Immunoglobulin found in tears, sweat, gut and urinogenital fluids, colostrum and milk. Secretory IgA consists of a dimer of two basic four-chain immunoglobulin units. Each unit has two alpha heavy chains and two kappa or two lambda light chains. The two units are linked covalently through their alpha-chains by a cysteine-rich J. chain. The IgA dimer is further stabilized by a secretory piece, a single polypeptide chain ($M_r$ = 60 000) synthesized in the secreting epithelial cells. IgA provides the first line of defence against invading pathogens inhibiting thier adherence to mucosal cells and so preventing their invasion of the body; aggregated IgA fixes complement by the alternative pathway. Some monomeric IgA is found in human plasma: Two IgA sub-classes are known in humans : $IgA_2$ lacks disulphide bonds linking heavy and light chains. A secretory immunoglobulin found in birds is also called IgA. See Figure I.3.

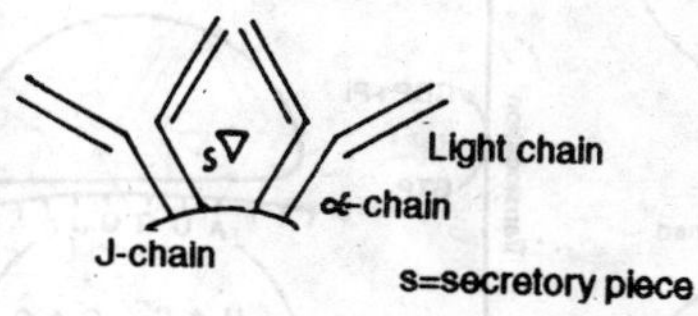


Figure I.3. IgA. Dimeric, secretory IgA.

***IgD.*** Immunoglobulin found in several placental mammals, including humans. It has two delta heavy chains and two kappa or two lambda light chains. Its plasma concentration is low (0-0.4 mg/ml). IgD has a high (13 percent)carbohydrate content; its hinge region is extended and this seems to make it prey to proteolysis. Most IgD is found on blood lymphocyte surfaces where, together with IgM, it probably acts as an antigen receptor for the control of lymphocyte suppression and activation. High surface IgD levels are found on foetal lymphocytes where its presence seems to be associated with antigen priming and increased resistance to the acquisition of tolerance.

***IgE.*** Immunoglobulin ($M_2$ = 200 000) found in mammals and possibly birds. It occurs at very low concentrations (17-450 ng/ml) in plasma; it is normally bound by its C-terminal end to mast cells (basophils). Contact with antigen at the N-terminal end of the IgE leads to mast cell degranulation and release of vasoactive amines (e.g. histamine). IgE is putatively a defence against helminth infection in the gut, but is principally known for its role in immediate, anaphylactic hypersensitivity, IgE has two epsilon heavy chains (each with five domains) and two kappa or two lambda light chains.

***IgG.*** Principal immunoglobulin ($M_r$ = 150 000) of the secondary immune reaction in mammals; its sedimentation co-efficient is 7S; at 3 percent, its carbohydrate content is low. IgG has two gamma heavy chains, each with four domains, three in the constant region and one in the variable region, and two kappa or two lambda light chains. IgG, found at a concentration of 8-16 mg/ml, comprise about 80 percent of the serum immunoglobulin. IgG is the only immunoglobulin capable of crossing the placenta; it is also found in colostrum and milk. IgG antibodies diffuse rapidly into extravascular body spaces where they neutralize bacterial toxins and opsonize (coat and make more palatable to phagocytes) particulate antigens. It fixes complement by the classical pathway, and potentiates antibody-dependent cellular cytotoxicity. Four IgG subclasses, designated $IgG_{1-4}$ each with slightly different biological properties, are found in humans. IgG is found in all mammals (including the egg-laying monotremes) but is absent in other vertebrates.

***IgM (Macroglobulin).*** Immunoglobulin of the primary immune reaction in mammals. ($M_r$~900 000, its sedimentation coefficient is 19S, and its carbohydrate content is 12 percent. IgM consists of a pentamer of five basic immunoglobulin units; each unit has two mu heavy chains (each with five domains, four in the constant region and one in the variable region) and two kappa or lambda light chains: The five units are linked covalently by a cysteine-rich J chain. In free solution IgM has a stellate configuration, but on combining with antigen it adopts a crab-like form. It has a valency of 10 (i.e. it can combine with 10 antigens), although antigen size and occlusion of binding sites mean that this valency is seldom achieved. IgM is an effective agglutinating antibody, and it fixes complement by the classical pathway. IgM is found in all vertebrates (usually as a pentamer, although monomeric, tetrameric and hexameric IgM are known) and considered to be evolutionarily the most primitive immunoglobulin. See Figure I.4.

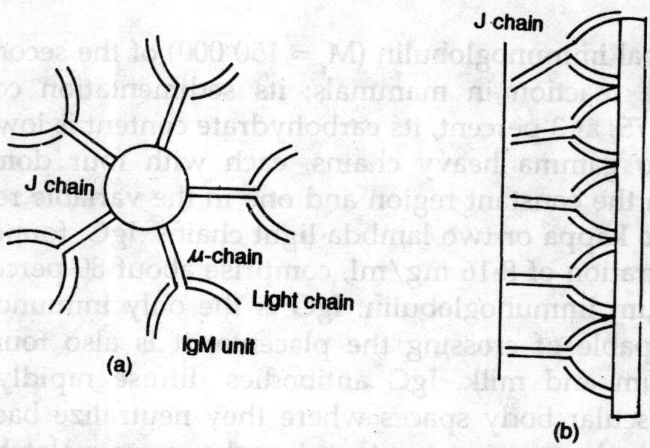


Figure I.4. IgM. (a) IgM pentamer in free solution (stellate configuration). (b) IgM in crab-like configuration when binding to antigen.

***IgY.*** Low-molecular-weight (sedimentation coefficient 7S) immunoglobulin of birds, reptiles and frogs and toads. Its function parallels that of IgG in mammals, although IgY has a Y heavy chain rather than a gamma chain.

***Imaginal Discs.*** Groups of cells found as single-cell layers of infolded tissue beneath the epidermis of holometabolous insects (insects having a series of distinct stages in their metamorphosis). Each disc represents the undifferentiated primordium of an adult organ, or appendage such as a leg or a wing, and becomes everted at the pupal stage to adopt the complex morphology of the adult structure. Imaginal discs, being dedicated to their individual fates without overt signs of differentiation, are described as being determined. They occasionally change their fate from the expected of them; a phenomenon known as transdetermination.

***Imago.*** Adult form; commonly applied to insects.

***Immediate Hypersensitivity.*** Reaction involving antibodies and occurring within a few minutes of exposure of the individual to the antigen or allergen. Individuals displaying such hypersensitivity have normally been previously sensitized to the antigen.

***Immortalized Cell.*** Cell which, by dint of transformation, perhaps by infection with virus, becomes capable of indefinite growth and division. Established cell lines in tissue culture are composed of immortalized cells.

***Immune Competent Cell (Immunocompotent cell).*** Cell that is capable of responding to an antigen, by division, transformation and production of antibodies or lymphokines or acquisition of other immunological effector function. Small lymphocytes are normally immunocompetent in vertebrates. When stimulated by antigen, B lymphocytes divide and transform into antibody-secreting plasma cells; T lymphocytes divide and transform into effector cells responsible for cell-mediated immunity and T-B cells cooperation.

***Immune Reaction.*** Measurable or observable reaction or response arising from antibody-antigen interaction, or from contact of immune competent cells with antigen. Responses and reactions (e.g., cell division, production of antibody, release of lymphokines and histamine, induction of immunological tolerance and allograft rejection) can occur in vitro and/or in vivo.

***Immune Response.*** An antagonistic host reaction in response to foreign antigens, involving the formation of antibodies by B-cells (or a cell-mediated response by T-cells). When such antibodies are present in the body, the individual is said to possess immunity against the specific antigen that stimulated the antibody production. The immune response is a vital defence mechanism but creates severe problems with, for example, kidney transplants from donors. In these cases the tissues are 'matched' for tissue compatibility and the recipient treated with chemicals that reduce the immune response.

***Immune Surveillance.*** Postulated mechanism whereby abnormal cells containing new antigens that have arisen through somatic mutation are removed from the body as a result of continuous monitoring of body cells by the immunological system. It is been suggested that potential cancer cells are removed in this way.

***Immune System.*** Complex of lymph nodes and lymphoid cells in the blood and tissues that gives an animal the capacity of an immune response.

***Immunization.*** Administration of an antigen or an antibody to a vertebrate animal so as to confer a state of active immunity or provide passive immunity against infectious organisms or their toxic products. (2) Administration of antigen so as to produce an immune response not necessarily for protective purposes (e.g., in order to raise specific antibodies for structural studies and for other in vitro investigations).

***Immunoelectrophoresis.*** Technique in which proteins are separated by gel electrophoresis and then challenged with specific antiserum. Arcs of precipitated protein form where antigen-antibody conjugation has occurred, and this can be used to identify the proteins and determine their electrophoretic mobilities.

***Immunofluorescence (Fluorescent antibody technique).*** Method whereby antigens can be localized microscopically in sectioned tissues or in isolated cells in smears and tissue culture. It involves the use of antibody labelled with a fluorochrome, usually fluorescein isothiocyanate (FITC) or tetramethyl rhodamine isothiocyanate (TRITC) which fluoresces apple green or orange-red, respectively, when exposed to ultraviolet light of the appropriate wavelength. The direct method of immunofluorescence involves applications of fluorochrome-labelled antibodies specific for the antigen under study, whereas the indirect method, which is more sensitive, utilizes a primary unlabelled antibody followed by a secondary labelled antibody directed against immunoglobulin. Double immunofluorescence enables two different antigens to be localized simultaneously by using FITC- and TRITC-labelled antibodies specific for one of the two antigens.

***Immunogenetics*** Study of the inheritance and genetic basis of the immune response, antibody structure and molecular aspects of antibody-antigen interactions.

***Immunity.*** The state of relative insusceptibility of an animal to infection by disease producing organisms or to the harmful effects of their poisons (toxins). Immunity depends on the presence in the blood of "antibodies and white blood cells ("lymphocytes), which produce an "immune response. Inherited (natural) immunity is that with which an individual is born. Acquired immunity is of two types : active immunity arises when the body produces antibodies against an invading foreign substance ("antigen), either through infection or "immunization; passive immunity is induced by injection of serum taken from an individual already immune to a particular antigen. Active immunity tends to be long-lasting passive immunity is short-lived.

***Immunization.*** The production of "immunity in an individual by artificial means. Active immunization (vaccination) involves the introduction, either orally or by injection (inoculation), of specially treated bacteria, viruses, or their toxins to stimulate the production of "antibodies. Passive immunization is induced by the injection of performed antibodies.

***Immunoglobulin.*** A protein (such as gamma globulin) made in B-cells that possesses antibody activity and is made up of four polypeptide chains, two identical light chains and two identical heavy chains joined by disulphide bonds. There are five main classes of human immunoglobins, differentiated principally by their heavy chains :

| Type | IgG | IgM | IgA | IgD | IgF |
|---|---|---|---|---|---|
| Heavy chain | gamma | mu | alpha | delta | epsilon |
| M.W. (x 1000) | 144 | 160 | 144 | 156 | 166 |

Each heavy and light chain consists of a constant region of amino acids that is virtually the same in all antibodies of that class and a variable region containing a sequence of amino acids that makes the antibody specific to a particular antigen. See Figure I.5.

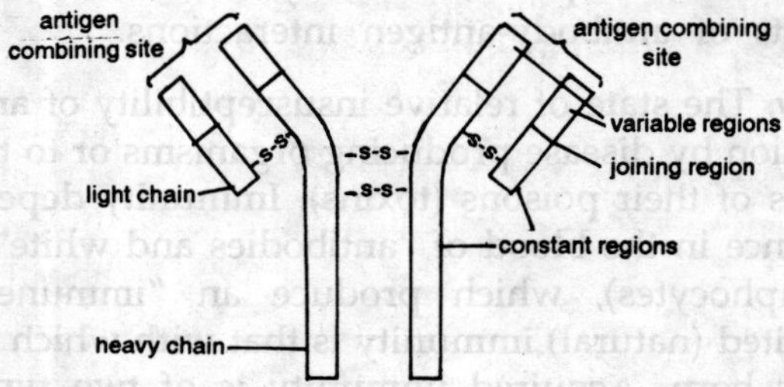


Figure I.5. Immunoglobin. Molecular structure. S = sulphur bonds.

***Immunoglobulin Gene.*** Gene that encodes the light chain and heavy chain of the immunoglobulin molecules. The great variability of antibody structure is achieved by a series of remarkable genetic mechanisms, which involve rearrangement of parts of the DNA sequence during the life of the B lymphocyte. The variable and constant regions are coded separately on the genome, but in a B lymphocyte they are made adjacent, with an additional J or joining sequence between. Both genetic rearrangement and somatic mutation are involved in increasing the sequence diversity of the V region genes.

***Immunological Tolerance.*** Failure of an animal to produce humoral immunity or cell-mediated immunity to a particular antigen, while at the same time being capable of responding normally in this way to other antigens. Immunological tolerance can be induced experimentally by injecting the antigen during foetal or early postnatal life, or by injecting adults with very high (high zone tolerance) doses of antigen.

***Immunosuppressive Drug.*** Drug that tends to suppress the immune response. Such drugs (e.g. cortisone) are given to patients after transplant surgery to prevent immune rejection of the transplanted tissue.

***Immunological Tolerance.*** The failure to respond to a potential antigen.

***Immunotoxin.*** An antibody attached to a specific toxic agent that is used to destroy specific cancer cells. Although experimental at present, these so-called 'magic bullets' hold out great hope as a new form of cancer chemotherapy.

***Implantation (Nidation).*** (In embryology) The embedding of a fertilized mammalian egg into the wall of the uterus (womb) where it will continue its development. After fertilization in the fallopian tube the egg passes into the womb in the form of a ball of cell (blastocyst). Its outer cells destroy cells of the uterine wall, forming a cavity into which the blastocyst sinks.

***Imprinting.*** An aspect of learning where there is a rapid development of a response to a particular stimulus at an early stage of development. Young animals 'recognize' the first object they see, such as a mother figure, and they can be 'imprinted' on objects other than their own species. For example, Konrad Lorenz 'imprinted' young greylag geese on himself as a mother figure. Imprinting also occurs in other areas of experience. For example, bird song, where young, inexperienced birds have adult calls 'imprinted' on them.

***Inactivation Centre.*** Region of an X chromosome that is responsible for ensuring the genetic inactivity of adjacent loci in the inactivated copy of the X chromosome. Other autosomal genes can be translocated to the X chromosome, and their active or inactive state can be used to determine the location of X chromosome inactivation centres in such mammals as mice.

***Inactive-X Hypothesis Or Lyon Hypothesis.*** An explanation for dosage compensation in the X-chromosomes of mammals including humans, proposed by Marry Lyon. The main features of the hypothesis are that only one x-chromosome in active in a mature mammalian cell, all other X-chromosomes present having been inactivated during embryological development. Difference X-chromosomes are thought to be inactivated in different cells, which may produce a mosaic phenotype in heterozygous individuals. Bare bodies are thought to indicate the presence of inactive X-chromosomes.

***Inborn Error Of Metabolism.*** An inherited biochemical abnormality in humans due to enzymic deficiencies. The term was coined by Archibald Garrod in the early 1900s, who theorized that various conditions he had studied in hospital cases were due to defective enzymes, causing the breakdown of biochemical pathways and the build-up of intermediate chemicals in the body. Garrod's work was not recognized as important until the one gene/one enzyme hypothesis was proposed in the 1940s.

***Inbreeding.*** Any mating between relatives, which can lead to a general lowering of viability due to a accumulation of deleterious genes passed on through both parents from a common ancestor.

***Inbreeding Depression.*** A reduction in viability resulting from increased homozygosity through inbreeding.

***Inclusion Body.*** A body present in the nuclei or cytoplasm of cells infected by viruses or other intracellular parasites.

***Incompatibility.*** 1. Differences between tissues that result in immunological rejection due to one or both tissues producing antibodies against certain antigens in the other.

2. The condition that exists when foreign grafts or blood transfusions evoke a marked immune response and are rejected. 3. The phenomenon in which pollen from one flower fails to fertilize other flowers on the same plant (self-incompatibility) or on other genetically similar plants. This genetically determined mechanism prevents self-fertilization (breeding between likes) and promotes cross-fertilization (breeding between individuals with different genetic compositions.

***Incomplete Dominance.*** A pattern of inheritance in which a cross between two phenotypically different parents produces an offspring different from either parent but containing partial features of both. The classic example is in flower colour where, for example, crossing white and red parents produce a pink offspring.

***Incomplete Penetrance.*** Situation in which only a proportion of individuals with a specific genotype express the appropriate characters in the phenotype, usually due to variation in the interaction between the individuals and the environment. If all individuals with a dominant mutant gene show the appropriate mutant phenotype, penetrance is said to be complete.

***Inbreeding.*** Mating between closely related individuals, the extreme condition being self-fertilization, which occurs in many plants and some primitive animals. A population of inbreeding individuals generally shows less variations than an outbreeding population. Continued inbreeding among a normally outbreeding population leads to inbreeding depression (the opposite of hybrid vigour) and an increased incidence of harmful characteristics. For example, in humans, certain mental and other defects tend to occur more often in families with a history of cousin marriages.

***Independent Assortment.*** The random arrangement and separation of chromosomes during meiosis, giving all possible combinations in equal frequency, unlike the situation with genetic linkage. The process is important in understanding mendelian genetics linkage. The process is important in understanding mendelian genetics and explains the random distribution in the gametes of genes or nonhomologous chromosomes. For example, take two pairs of homologous chromosomes in a diploid (1) cell. During anaphase I there are two ways in which the chromosomes can become separated (see Figure I.6). Independent assortment of the chromosomes in the Figure gives four types of possible gamete (1 + 3), (2 + 4), (1 + 4) and (2 + 3). In fact, the number of combination is 2 to the power of the number of pairs of chromosomes, $2^2=4$ in the above example. A human with 23 pairs of chromosomes would produce $2^{23}$ = 8,388608 combinations by independent assortment alone.

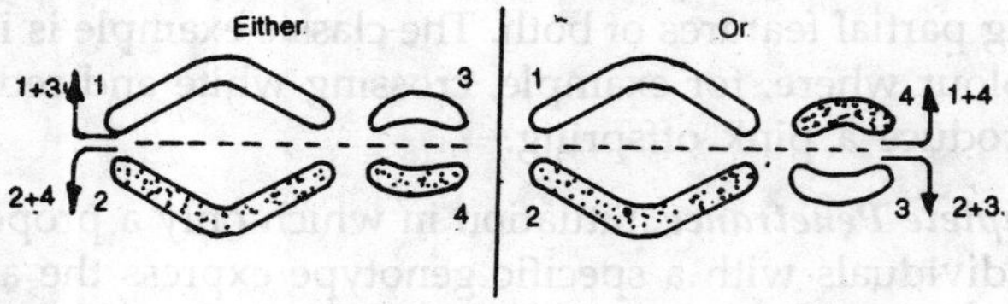


Figure I.6. Independent assortment. Separation of chromosomes.

***Index Fossil (Zone Fossil).*** An animal "fossil of a group that existed continuously during a particular span of geological time and can therefore be used to date the rock in which it is found. Index fossils are found chiefly in sedimentary rocks. They are an essential tool in stratigraphy for comparing the geological ages of sedimentary rock formations. Examples are ammonites and graptolites.

***Indicator Community.*** An association of species characteristic of particular conditions, or habitats. For example, a range of calcicole plants indicates a base rich soil.

***Indicator Species.*** Any species that is indicative of particular conditions or habitats. For example, the leech Erpobdella testacea is found only in alkaline or polluted waters, the arrowworm Sagitta setosa is characteristic of continental shelf water, whereas S. elegans is characteristic of oceanic water.

***Indigenous.*** Native, not introduced by man.

***Indirect Selection.*** The selection of mutant organisms (microorganisms) by determining those that do not grow on particular media.

***Individual Variation.*** The variation found in a population of the same species.

***Indoleacetic Acid. (IAA).*** Principal naturally occurring Auxin and one found in a wide range of plants. Substances other than IAA have been found in plants that have auxin-like activity. In many cases these substances are indoles, chemically related to IAA. Indoleacetonitrile (IAN) is known to be present in a number of plant species particularly members of the Cruciferae, whereas, in pea plants 4-chloroindoleacetic acid appears to be present as a natural auxin.

***Indoleacetonitrile (IAN).*** One of a range of naturally occurring Auxins.

***Inducer.*** A small molecule that inactivates the repressor of an operon, usually binding to the repressor and so preventing the repressor binding with the operator of the operon.

***Inducible Enzyme.*** An enzyme that is produced in response to the presence of its substrate (the inducer).

***Induction.*** 1. (In biochemistry) the synthesis of new enzyme molecules in response to a stimulus, usually another chemical. 2. (In embryology) the formation of an alternative cell type during cell differentiation under the influence of an 'inducer' molecule. 3. (In microbial genetics) the release of a prophage for the bacterial chromosome, initiated by, for example, ultraviolet light.

***Industrial Melanism.*** A phenomenon found in several groups, notably moths, in which a heavily pigmented variant (a morph) becomes the most frequent type in an area with heavy, man-made atmospheric pollution. Melanism is an excellent example of microevolution, in that rapid evolutionary change has been brought about by strong forces of natural selection acting in favour of a dominant allele for melanism. The agents of selection against moths (such as the peppered moth Biston betularia) are birds, which predate more heavily those types resting against an inappropriate background : poorly pigmented forms resting on sooty tree trunks, for example. The proportion of melanics to nonmelanics in an area is correlated with the level of pollution, although neither type appears to be completely absent in any environment, creating a genetic polymorphism.

***Infection.*** Invasion or contamination of an organism by bacteria, viruses or other microorganisms from the surrounding environment or other organisms.

***Influenza.*** An acute respiratory disease affecting the upper respiratory tract, with symptoms of fever, chills are generalized aching, cause by a number of influenza, viruses, particularly types A and B. Influenza outbreaks occur frequently and can have a world wide distribution, often being associated with secondary bacterial complications. Over 20 million people died in the pandemic outbreak 0f. 1918-1919, principally young adults who may have been previously exposed to an unusually virulent form of virus.

***Influenza Viruses.*** Group of viruses known as orthomyxoviruses. They are enveloped, single-stranded RNA viruses with a genome consisting of several fragments of RNA (a so-called segmented genome).

***Informosome.*** Type of ribonucleoprotein found by sucrose gradient centrifugation to be present in the cytoplasm of the eggs of certain species of echinoderms and fish. In eukaryote cells messenger RNA (mRNA) is usually associated with proteins to form an RNP. Informosomes may represent a category of RNP in which the mRNA is masked. Although present in the egg, the RNA of informosomes may not be translated until later in development. Thus the spectrum of proteins synthesized by the early embryo may be controlled at the translational as well as the transcriptional level.

***Infraspecific.*** Within a species.

***Infrasubspecific.*** Within a subspecies.

***Inheritance.*** 1. The acquisition of characteristics by the transfer of genetic material from ancestor to descendant. 2. The total of characters in the fertilized ovum.

***Inheritance of Acquired Characters.*** Tenet of genetics proposed in 1809 by Lamarck (lamarckism) in which characteristics acquired by an organism during its life (following from its interaction with the environment) are supposed to become genetic and thus would be transmitted to offspring. All experimental evidence contradicts the proposition, with the possible exception of infection of germ line cells of animals by integrated virus.

***Inherited Abnormality.*** Any genetically determined malfunction. These fall into two main types :

(a) Those controlled by single genes where, for example, a biochemical process is disrupted by faulty enzymes coded by abnormal alleles such as those causing albinism. In other cases, such as sickle-cell anaemia, a molecule is produced that does not function in the normal way.

(b) Those produced by chromosomal changes. Here, loss or addition of parts or of whole chromosomes can have serious effects.

Changes to autosomal chromosomes often produce more severe effects than to sex chromosomes.

***Inhibition.*** A state in which an enzyme is unable to catalyse reactions.

***Initiation codon.*** A triplet of bases in mRNA with the sequence AUG that acts as a 'start' signal for translation, specifying the first amino acid at the N-terminus of the polypeptide chain.

***Initiation Factor.*** Molecule that is necessary for correct initiation of protein synthesis on ribosomes. The factors help both to complex the mRNA molecule with the 30S particle of the ribosome and to enable the aminoacyl-tRNA (methionine) to engage with this complex. The molecules so far identified are themselves proteins.

***Initiator.*** Molecule that initiates DNA replication on a replicon.

***Innate Behaviour.*** An inherited pattern of behaviour that appears in a similar form in all normally reared individuals of the same sex and species.

***Inoculation.*** The introduction of biological material (the inoculum) into a medium such as a living organism, synthetic substrate or soil.

***Input Load.*** The quantity of inferior alleles in the gene pool resulting from mutation and immigration.

***Insecticide.*** Any substance such as DDT or malathion, that is used to kill insects.

***Insecticide Resistance.*** The ability of a member of an insect population to withstand the toxic effects of an insecticide to the point that it now resists control with that chemical. The genes controlling resistance are thought to be present in low frequencies within a generally susceptible population before application of the chemical. After treatment, susceptible members of the population are removed and the survivors thrive, becoming common in the population which is then described as 'resistant'.

***Insemination.*** Any means by which male sperm are introduced to the female prior to fertilization.

***Insertional Activation.*** Activation and expression of a DNA sequence as a result of the insertion of another sequence into it or beside it. Some vector phage genes may be activated when chimaeric plasmids are constructed.

***Insertional Inactivation.*** Process by which a gene sequence is inactivated by the insertion of another sequence into it or beside it. Such inactivation is used to identify phage or plasmid vectors that have accepted copies of novel genes and so have become chimaeric.

***Insertion Element.*** (IS element, insertion sequence). DNA sequence that is itself a transposable element or is a short sequence at the ends of a transposable element. They normally consist of inverted repeat sequences, and this facilitates the promiscuous integration which is a feature of transposable elements.

***Insertion Mutation.*** A point mutation in which one or more bases is inserted into DNA, causing a frameshift reading error during translation.

***Insight Learning.*** The production of a new and adaptive response as a result of 'insight'. For example, presented with a bunch of bananas that is too high to reach, chimpanzees will pile up boxes, or fit two sticks together in order to get them.

***In Situ Hybridization.*** Molecular hybridization carried out using unfractionated cells or cell organelles. Radioactive or enzymically labelled probes are added to a cell squash on a microscope slide and allowed to hybridize to sequences in intact chromosomes. In this way the precise locations of genes and other DNA sequences in the genome can be determined.

***Instantaneous Speciation.*** The production of an individual (or individuals) that is reproductively isolated from its parent and is capable itself of reproduction and establishing a new population.

***Instar.*** A larval stage of insect development. The first instar hatches from the egg and after the first moult becomes the second instar. Thus a third instar larva is one which has completed two moults.

***Instinct.*** Aspects of behaviour that are not learned, but which appear to be inherited, i.e. innate behaviour. It is not now learned, but which appear to be inherited, i.e. innate behaviour. It is not now used commonly as a scientific term because of the difficulty of distinguishing between some aspects of learning and some aspects of so-called instinctive behaviour.

***Instinctive Behaviour.*** Any behaviour pattern that is inherited and not clearly learned.

***Instructive Theory.*** Proposal that the shape of an antibody, and its consequent specificity for antigen, was conferred on it by its encounter with antigen. They theory has been disproved and is replaced by the clonal selection theory.

***Insulin.*** The hormone controlling the amount of blood sugar, which is secreted by the beta cells of the islets of langerhans in the pancreas. Insulin has three targets : the liver, the muscles, and adipose tissue, where its action helps to reduce the blood sugar level in the following ways :

(a) It stimulates the absorption of more glucose from the blood into muscle and adipose cells, by altering cell-wall permeability.

(b) It stimulates the conversion of glucose into glycogen in the liver and muscles, reducing the supply of free glucose.

(c) It promotes the conversion of glucose into fats in the liver and adipose cells (Lipogenesis).

(d) It inhibits gluconeogenesis.

(e) It promotes glycolysis of glucose in all cells.

Underproduction of insulin causes diabetes, resulting in an increase in blood sugar (hyperglycaemia) and sugar appearing in the urine. The condition can be fatal it untreated, treatment being by injection of insulin into the blood stream. The hormone cannot be taken orally as, being a protein, it would be digested. Insulin was discovered by ranting and best in 1921. The control of blood sugar, where a change in its level automatically brings about the opposite effect, is a good example of a negative feedback mechanism.

***Insulin Gene.*** Coding sequence for the insulin molecule. The human insulin gene has been isolated and cloned in E. coli, and human insulin is now commercially available from that source.

***Integrated Control.*** The use of chemical, biological, cultural and legislative methods in a complementary way to control pests and pathogens.

***Integration.*** The insertion of DNA from one organism into the recipient chromosome of another.

***Integration Efficiency.*** Frequency with which a particular DNA, sequence in incorporated into the genome, of a recipient bacterium following transformation, or into a recipient animal or plant cell or ovum following its artificial introduction.

***Integrator Gene.*** Hypothetical type of DNA sequence that controls a subset of other genes following its own stimulation.

***Intelligence Quotient (IQ).*** Measure of intelligence based on certain standardized intelligence tests. The score in such a test is divided by the individual's chronological age and multiplied by 100 to give the IQ. The scores of IQ are commonly grouped as follows: genius, 140 and over; very superior 120.139; superior, 110-119; average, 90-109; dull, 80-89; borderline, 70-79; mild retardation, 50-69; moderate retardation (imbecile), 25-49; severe retardation (idiot), 0.24.

***Interband.*** Region of a polytene chromosome that lies between the bands. DNA in the interbands is not in the form of condensed chromatin, as occurs in the bands, and thus there is much less DNA in the interbands than in the bands per unit area.

***Intercalary Regeneration.*** Pattern of cell regeneration in situations such as the cockroach leg, such that new tissue will grow to fill in all the missing positional values of the omitted leg segments following grafting.

***Intercalation*** (1) Insertion of a molecule (e.g. acridine dye) between base pairs in a DNA molecule. It causes disruption of accurate base pairing and alignment in the DNA double helix. (2) Growth of tissue to fill in missing parts of appendages following incomplete grafting. Thus if a tibia is grafted onto the proximal part of a femur, intercalary growth will occur to make good the absent part of the femur. (3) Growth of meristematic tissue in plants between two other differentiated tissues.

***Interferon.*** A glycoprotein produced by cells in response to viral attack, whose function seems to be triggering viral interference defence mechanisms in uninfected cells of the same species in which it was produced. Since it has been suggested that interferon might prove effective against viral diseases by inhibiting viral multiplication, and even some forms of cancer, strenuous efforts have been made to isolate sufficient quantities with which to run clinical trials. The problem of production has now been solved by genetic engineering but the results of trials are inconclusive, so far.

***Interkinesis.*** Short interphase that occurs between the first and second meiotic divisions. Unlike a premitotic interphase, no DNA replication occurs in interkinesis.

***Interleukins.*** Substances released by lymphocytes that activate other lymphocytes to respond to antigen. Lymphokines fulfil the same role, but need not be produced by lymphocytes.

***Intermediary Metabolism.*** Aspects of metabolism that are mainly concerned with the flow of carbon compounds; it excludes aspects that deal with synthesis and organization of macromolecules such as proteins, DNA or cell membranes.

***Intermediate Filament.*** Heterogeneous class of cytoplasmic skeletal protein filaments (8-12 nanometres in diameter). Many different cell types have characteristic intermediate filaments (e.g. the neurofilaments of neurones, desmin filaments of glial cells, keratin filaments of epithelial cells).

***Internal Environment.*** The conditions that prevail within the body of an organism, particularly with respect to the composition of the intercellular fluid. Selective absorption of materials across cell membranes plays a large part in controlling the internal environment of both animals and plants. Animals in addition can regulate their body fluids by the action of hormones and the nervous system.

***Interphase.*** Period between mitosis. Although at one time referred to as a resting phase, it is now clear that most protein synthesis and all DNA synthesis occurs during interphase.

***Interrupted Gene.*** A eucaryote gene (or one of its viruses) consisting of sequences of intron and exon segments.

***Intersex.*** An organism displaying characteristics that are intermediate between those of the typical male and typical female of its species. For example, a human intersex may have testes that fail to develop, so that although he is technically a man he has the external appearance of a woman. Intersexes may be produced in various ways; for example by malfunctioning of the sex hormones.

***Interrupted Mating Experiment.*** Technique devised by Wollman and Jacob in 1955 for studying chromosome transfer in E. coli during bacterial conjugation, which provides a method for mapping the bacterial chromosome independent of recombination frequency. Hfr donor and F recipient strains are mixed, and at regular intervals small samples are removed from the mixture, agitated vigorously to separate the mating pairs, and diluted to prevent further pairing. The bacteria are then plated onto media that prevent.growth of the two parental strains but select certain recombinants. Recombinants appear about eight minutes after the initial mixing. For a particular Hfr a given donor gene appears after a characteristic time interval : this depends on the distance between the gene and the leading end of the donor chromosome. Accordingly, as chromosomes transfer proceeds at a constant rate, map distances can be directly measured in units of time. Genes remote from the origin are transferred less frequently because of spontaneous strand breakage, but to accomplish complete chromosome transfer requires about 100 minutes. Different regions of the chromosome are mapped using different Hfr strains.

***Interspecific Behaviour.*** Any act of behaviour occurring between species.

***Interspecific Competition.*** Any limited competition between two or more different species populations for a resource such as food. All populations involved are negatively affected by the competition, and may exhibit increased mortality or decreased birthrate.

***Interspersion Pattern of DNA.*** Pattern of distribution of coding and non-coding sequences within a genome. In many genomes, especially of higher eukaryotes, there is a tendency for coding sequences of structural genes to be interspersed with long lengths of DNA that are not transcribed. Such DNA is partly regulatory, but much may be redundant.

***Intrachromosomal Recombination.*** Recombination of DNA between chromatids of the same chromosome rather than between the chromatids of homologous chromosomes (as occurs in crossing-over). Recombination between sister chromatids has no genetic consequences since the reciprocal exchange is between identical material, but it can be detected by cytological techniques such as the preparation of harlequin chromosomes following incorporation of BuDR.

***Intrademic Selection.*** Evolutionary selection within a deme of group. This is believed to be important in the selection for such features as altruism.

***Intragenic Recombination.*** Recombination of DNA within a gene.

***Intragenic Suppressor.*** Mutation that acts by suppressing the effect of another mutation within the gene. Intragenic suppressor mutations act by restoring the original reading frame following an earlier frame shift mutation.

***Intrallelic Complementation.*** Synergistic effect measurable in some proteins that are mixed polymers, having subunits coded by more than one allele or more than one gene. Thus mixed tetramers of haemoglobin and lactate dehydrogenase are more efficient in some situations than are the homopolymers.

***Intraspecific.*** Within the species.

***Intraspecific Competition.*** Any limited competition within the same species population for a resource such as food. Not all members of the population may be negatively affected by the competition, resulting in differential ability to survive and reproduce.

***Introduced Species.*** One that does not naturally occur in the area and has been brought in accidentally or intentionally by man, for example, rabbits in Australia (introduced originally to the British Isles from Spain).

***Introgressive Hybridization.*** The spread of genes of one species into the germ plasma of another species as a result of hybridization.

***Intron.*** A segment of DNA from eucaryotes that is transcribed into mRNA but is then excised from the RNA, leaving behind the exon sequences to be translated into polypeptide.

***Inulin.*** A complex polymer of fructose that is soluble in water and occurs in the cell sap of storage organs such as dahlia tubers and dandelion tap roots.

***Invariant Amino Acid Site.*** Amino acid residue, within the primary structure of proteins belonging to a family with similar or identical biological function, which is preserved in the proteins from different organisms. For example, the cytochromes c from organisms as diverse as mammals and green plants have invariant residues associated with haem interactions. Likewise the oxygen-binding globins share seven invariant residues involved with essential haem binding and protein folding. The serine proteases (trypsin, chymotrypsin and elastase) have invariant amino acids associated with catalysis at the active site of the enzymes.

***Inversion.*** Chromosome mutation in which an entire sequence has been rotated through 180°. Thus the sequence ABCFEDGH has had inversion of the DEF sequence. In the polytene chromosomes of Drosophila, inversion may be visualized by the appearance of inversion loops where the two homologous chromosomes are normally lying in precise register.

***Inversion Heterozygote.*** Individual in which one homologue of a pair of chromosomes carries an inversion and the other does not.

***Inversion Loop.*** Loop seen in the polytene chromosomes of Drosophila as a result of an inversion in one of the two homologous chromosomes lying in register.

***In Vitro.*** (Of biological processes or reactions) made to occur outside the body of an organism in an artificial environment (vitro - glass). For example, in-vitro fertilization of human eggs in the laboratory prior to reimplantation in the mother.

***In Vitro Complementation.*** Complementation of allellic sequences demonstrated in the test-tube.

***In Vitro Fertilization.*** Fertilization of an egg outside the body of the female and 'in the test-tube', using sperm already obtain from the male of the same species. Such fertilization is widely used to overcome human infertility due to blockage of the fallopian tubes, the resulting embryo being subsequently introduced into the uterus of its original donor.

***In Vitro Marker.*** Mutation that allows identification in vitro of a cell line possessing the marker. Such mutations are commonly expressed in culture as virus or drug resistance mutations.

***In Vitro Mutagenesis.*** Localized mutation induction in defined DNA sequences followed by assay of the activity and replication of the affected molecules, spliced into plasmid vectors, in cell-free systems or in vivo.

***In Vitro Packaging.*** Technique that allows the assembly of mature bacteriophage particles in vitro by mixing DNA with separated bacteriophage heads and tails.

***In Vivo.*** (Of biological processes or experiments) occurring in the living organism.

***In Vitro Culturing of Imaginal Discs.*** Procedure in which the imaginal discs of Drosophila larvae may be cultured by injection into the abdomen of a host larva or adult. This has permitted the distinction to be drawn between the stages of determination and differentiation in such tissues.

***In Vivo Marker.*** Mutation that occurs in the organism, but also allows detection in tissue culture; for example, genes causing galactosaemia, being detectable both in the phenotype of an individual and in vitro in tissue cells derived from such individuals.

***Involution.*** 1. A decrease in the size of an organ or the body. It may be associated with functional decline, as occurs in the ageing process, or follow enlargement, as when the uterus returns to its normal size after pregnancy. 2. The turning or rolling inwards of cells that occurs during the development of some vertebrate embryos.

***Ionizing Radiation.*** A beam of short-wavelength electromagnetic energy that can penetrate deeply into tissues, leaving a track of unstable atoms which have lost electrons (ions). Such radiations, X-rays and gamma rays, are powerful mutagens.

***Iridium Anomaly.*** The occurrence of unusually high concentrations of the relatively scarce metal iridium at the boundaries of certain geological strata. Two such layers have been discovered, one at the end of the Cretaceous, 65 million years ago, and the second at the end of the Eocene, 34 million years ago. One theory to account for these suggests that on each occasion a huge iridium-containing meteorite may have collided with the earth, producing a cloud of dust that settled out to form an iridium-rich layer. The environmental consequences of such an impact, notably in causing a general warming of the earth by the "greenhouse effects, may have led to the extinction of the dinosaurs at the end of the Cretaceous and the extinction of many radiolarians at the end of the Eocene.

***Iso-.*** Denoting equal.

***Isoacceptor Transfer RNA.*** Transfer RNA molecule that accepts the same amino acid although having a distinct anticodon base triplet. Such tRNAs explain the operation of the degeneracy of the genetic code.

***Isoagglutinin.*** Antibody elicited by an antigen present on cells of a genetically different individual of the same species (isoantigen), and which causes such cells to agglutinate. Naturally occurring antibodies to A.B. Antigens and rhesus antigens present on erythrocytes are isoagglutinins (isohaemagglutinins); they also arise to histocompatibility antigens present on leucocytes and are then called isoleucoagglutinins.

***Iso-Alleles.*** Alleles with so little phenotypic expression that special techniques are necessary to demonstrate their presence.

***Isoantibody.*** Antibody raised in an animal following its exposure to antigen derived from another animal of the same species.

***Isoantigen (Alloantigen).*** Antigen carried by an individual animal and capable of eliciting an immune reaction in another, genetically different animal of the same species. The two animals show histoincompatibility. Such isoantigens are different allelic forms of an antigen encoded at the same gene locus in all animals of the species.

***Isobilateral.*** Having a similar structure on each side, as in the leaf of a monocotyledon.

***Isochromosome.*** Chromosome with two arms of equal length and identical sequence. Such chromosomes result from splitting of centromeric regions in transverse direction during mitosis or meiosis.

***Isoelectric Focusing.*** The separation of molecules by differences in their charge, each molecule migrating to the point in a PH gradient where it has no net charge.

***Isoelectric Point.*** The PH of an amphoteric solution when at electrical neutrality, the ionic state of an amino acid at the isoelectric point being a zwitterion.

***Isoenzyme (Isozyme).*** One of the multiple forms of a given enzyme that occurs in a given organism. Isoenzymes are demonstrated by separation by electrophoresis. They are usually made up of at least two types of genetically distinct polypeptide chains. These may occur in various proportions thus giving rise to enzymes differing in affinity for substrates, inhibitors, etc. For example tetrameric mammalian lactate dehydrogenase is composed of various proportions of M and H polypeptide chains. There are therefore five isoenzymes ($M_4$, $M_3H$, $M_2H_2$, $MH_3$, $H_4$). The relative amounts of these isoenzymes differ from tissue to tissue and also at different stages of embryological development. In the case of lactate dehydrogenase, the presence of isoenzymes is related to two of its main functions : as the last enzyme in anaerobic glycolysis in skeletal muscle; as the first enzyme involved in the aerobic oxidation of lactate by heart muscle. The study of isoenzymes is of fundamental significance in studying the molecular basis of differentiation and morphogenesis.

***Isoform.*** One of a group of proteins of related function but slightly differing amino acid sequence. Many isoforms are a result of differential exon splicing.

***Isogamete.*** A gamete that is usually motile and appears similar to the gamete with which it unites at fertilization. Such sexual reproduction is called isogamy and occurs in several primitive plant groups such as many algae.

***Isogamy.*** Sexual reproduction involving the production and fusion of gametes that are similar in size and structure. It occurs only in some lower animals and plants, e.g. certain protozoans and algae.

***Isolating Mechanism.*** Any of the factors that prevent interbreeding (and therefore exchange of genes) between all the members of a species. Probably the most important isolating mechanism is geographical isolation, when different populations of the same species occupy different habitats and therefore never come into contact with each other. Ultimately this may lead to the populations becoming separate species by means of "adaptive radiation.

***Isogenic.*** Having an identical set of genes.

***Isograft.*** A transplant from one individual to a closely related individual of the same genotype, such as those between monozygotic twins, or between members of the same inbred line, as in rodents.

***Isolation.*** 1. Any geographical separation from other populations of the same organism. 2. A form of genetic isolation, where gene transfer is limited or entirely prevented by geographical separation. Such isolation can be termed behavioural, ecological, seasonal (different breeding seasons) and physiological. The prevention of gene transfer results in new lines of evolution.

***Isolating Barrier.*** Any structure that limits the movement of organisms to the extent of preventing gene flow. Examples include oceans, deserts, mountain ranges, salinity, temperature, etc.

***Isolating Mechanism.*** Any mechanism preventing successful breeding between two populations.

***Isoleucine.*** One of 20 amino acids common in proteins, that is nonpolar in structure and insoluble in water. The iseoelectric point of isoleucine is 6.0. See Figure I.7.

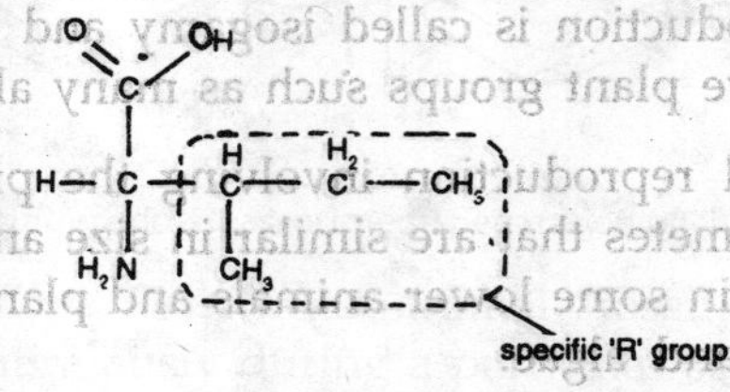


Figure I.7. Isoleucine. Molecular structure.

***Isomerase.*** A group of enzymes that converts organic compounds from D- to L-, or L- to D-forms.

***Isomerism.*** The phenomenon of two chemical compounds having the same formula but a different arrangement of atoms.

***Isomerous.*** (Of plants) having the same number of parts in different floral whorls, such as a plant possessing five stamens and five carpels.

***Isomorphic.*** (Of organisms, usually plants) having morphologically similar forms in different parts of the life history. For example, where there is alternation of generations in which the generations are similar.

***Isophene.*** A line connecting parts of equal character expression, i.e. one at right angles to a cline.

***Isopycnotic.*** Chromosomes or regions of chromosomes that stain similarly and are not highly condensed.

***Isoschizomers.*** Restriction endonucleases that, although distinct, cut the same target sequence. Some particularly useful pairs of such isoschizomers will cut a particular DNA sequence, but one is independent of the methylation of one of the bases, whereas the other is unable to cut when this base is methylated.

***Isosmotic.*** (Of two solutions) having the same osmotic pressure.

***Isostatic.*** (Of the earth's crust) movements resulting in sea level changes caused by ice-loading from glacier formation during the ice age.

***Isotonic.*** (Of a liquid) having a fluid state with the same water potential as another liquid.

***Isotope.*** Any of the forms of an element having the same number of protons (atomic number) but a different number of neutrons (atomic mass). Some isotopes of an element may be radioisotopes (e.g. $^{12}C$ is not radioactive while $^{14}C$ is) and yet can function normally in biological material. Isotopes can thus be 'tagged' (using suitable detection devices such as geiger counters) as biochemical processes occur.

***Isotypic Variability.*** Antigenic variability in antigens that is found in all members of a given species (e.g. the five immunoglobulin classes of humans, or the two immunoglobulin light chains classes).

***Isozyme or isoenzyme.*** One of several forms of an enzyme found in an individual or a population, each form coded by a different allele of a gene. An isozyme is a type of allozyme.

***IUD (Intrauterine Device).*** Any device such as a coil that is introduced into the female uterus as a means of preventing either fertilization of the egg or implantation of the embryo.

# J

***Java man.*** A primitive form of human-Homo erectus.

***J Chain.*** Polypeptide chain ($M_r$ = 35,000) linking, by means of disuphide bonds, the mu chains of the pentameric IgM molecule or the alpha chains of the dimeric secretory IgA molecule. It has a high cysteine content.

***Jenner, Edward (1741-1823).*** English physician who discovered that cowpox lymph matter could be safely used as an innoculum (a vaccine) to prevent smallpox. The first vaccination was carried out in 1796.

***Johannsen, Wilhelm (1857-1927).*** Danish botanist who, in the early 1900s, carried out selection experiments with beans (Phaseolus vulgaris) which showed that selection is a passive process that eliminates, but does not produce, variations. Johannsen is, however, chiefly remembered for having coined the terms gene, genotype and phenotype.

***Johnston's Organ.*** An organ situated at the base of the insect antenna consisting of a group of chordotonal receptors, probably associated with movement of the antenna.

***J Segment of Immunoglobulin Genes.*** One of three distinct gene segments encoding immunoglobulin light chain (the others are V and C) and of four gene segments encoding heavy chain (the others are V. D and C). The J (joining) segments encode the last 10 amino acids of the variable region of light and heavy chains. Random genetic rearrangement between light chain V, J and C, and between heavy chain V, D, J, and C, helps to create diversity in antibody specificity.

***Jumping Gene.*** Transposon that carries genetic information coding for an controlling its own transposition.

***Junctional Complex.*** Assemblage of specialized intercellular intercellular adhesions found on the lateral surface of epithelial cells towards the apical/lumenal end and responsible for :(1) sealing the epithelium against leakage of fluids from the lumen; and (2) maintenance of the structural integrity of the epithelial sheet. Typically it comprises tight junctions (zonula occludens), intermediate junction (zonula adherens) and desmosomes (macula adherens).

***Junctional Proteins.*** Proteins specifically associated with cell junctions.

***Junk DNA.*** DNA that has no genetic or structural function but persists within the genome since there may be no positive selection against it.

***Jurassic.*** The second geological period of the Mesozoic era. It followed the Triassic, which ended about 190 million years ago, and extended until the beginning of the Cretaceous period, about 139 million years ago. It was named in 1829 by A. Brongniart after the Jura Mountains on the borders of France and Switzerland. Jurassic rocks include clays and limestones in which fossil flora and fauna are abundant. Plants included ferns, cycads, ginkgos, rushes, and conifers. Important invertebrates includes "ammonites (on which the Jurassic is zoned), corals, brachiopods, bivalves, and echinoids. Reptiles dominated the vertebrates and the first flying reptiles- the pterosaurs-appeared. The first primitive bird, Archaeopteryx, also made its appearance.

***Juvenile Hormone.*** A hormone present in juvenile insects and secreted by the corpus allatum of the brain. So long as it is produced, the cuticle maintains the characteristics of the nymphal or larval form at each moult. Only when it ceases to be present or the level falls below a threshold value does the insect moult to the adult form. Juvenile hormones have been used as an effective means of controlling insects, for example, in preventing the development of adult ants during hospital infestations.

***Juxta-Glomerular Complex.*** A group of cells lining the efferent glomerular vessels of the kidney, that detect changes in blood volume. The cells secrete the enzyme renin when blood volume decreases, with subsequent release of aldosterone from the adrenal cortex, resulting in increased sodium retention. When the blood osmotic concentration increases, release of ADH occurs, and both these factors reverse the decrease in blood volume, an example of a feedback mechanism.

# K

***K.*** A symbol indicating the maximum number of individuals in the lotka-Volterra equations.

***Kanomycin.*** Antibiotic that operates through its ability to bind to bacterial ribosomes and cause misreading of the message.

***K. Selection.*** Selection proceeding in such a way as to maximize K and reduce R, so optimizing the use of environmental resources without expending excess energy in converting food into offspring.

***Kappa Chain (K chain).*** One of two types of light chain found in immunoglobulins (which differ by about 60 percent in their constant region amino acid sequences. In any one immunoglobulin molecule (for structure), both light chains are either kappa-or lambda-type.

***Kappa Particles.*** The bacteria that inhabit the cytoplasm of the ciliate Paramecium aurelia. Kappa-free Paramecia are sensitive to toxins produced by the particles, dying when exposed to them, after conjugation. Kappa carries (called killer stocks) are immune to the toxin.

***Karyogamy.*** Fusion of two nuclei, normally of gametic nuclei as in sexual reproduction. Fusion of dissimilar nuclei in fungal heterokaryons also falls within the meaning of the word.

***Karyological.*** Of or relating to the structure or number of chromosomes.

***Karyoplast.*** A nucleus surrounded by a thin layer of cytoplasm and membrane.

***Karyosome.*** A chromatin aggregation in the resting nucleus.

***Karyotype.*** The chromosome complement of a cell or organism, characterized by the number, size and configuration of the chromosomes as seen during metaphase of mitosis.

***KB Cells.*** Cultured cell line derived from neoplastic epidermal cells from the nasopharynx of humans; they were first propagated in a fluid medium by Eagle in 1955.

***Kbp.*** Kilobase pair.

***K Cell (Killer Cell).*** Weakly glass-adherent cell with an FC receptor that potentiates antibody-dependent cellular cytotoxicity (ADCC). K cells may play a role in immune surveillance against tumours, and are arguably the same cells as NK Cells.

***Katadromous.*** (Of fish) moving from freshwater to the sea in order to breed.

***Kelvin Scale.*** An absolute scale to temperature where a range of 1° kelvin (K) is equal to a range of 1°C.0°K= 273.15°C or-459.67°F.

***Keratin.*** A hard, fibrous, sulphur-containing protein with an alpha-helix structure, found in the epidermis of vertebrates, mainly in the outermost layers of skin. Keratin can have several forms : in scales, feathers, hooves, horns, claws and nails it is hard, while wool air hair are made up of a soft and flexible form.

***Keratin Gene.*** Since keratins are next to immunoglobulins, the most diverse proteins, the keratin gene family is very large. The genes range in size from 300 to 3000 bases, and some of the smaller ones have no intron. There is a tendency for some internal sequence repetition with some keratin genes, and some of these internal repetitious sequences consist of inverted repeats.

***Keratin Sulphate.*** Type of glycosaminoglycan found in the cartilage of cornea and the intervertebral discs.

***Ketogenesis.*** Production of ketone bodies.

***Ketone Bodies.*** Compounds formed by the condensation of acetyl CoA which result from fatty acid oxidation. They include such substances as b-hyroxybutyrate and acetone. They are synthesized in the liver and released into circulation. Overproduction, known as ketosis, occurs in diabetes and starvation and leads to acidosis and eventual coma.

***Ketose.*** Monosaccharide that contains a ketone group. The simplest example is dihydroxyacetone (a triose having three carbon atoms) and one of the most abundant in nature is fructose (a hexulose having six carbon atoms). The C-2 ketone in hexuloses can react rapidly and reversibly with the C-5 hydroxyl group to form an intramolecular ring structure consisting of four carbon atoms and an oxygen atom (furanose); it is the predominant form of hexuloses in solutions.

***Kettlewell, H.B.D.*** British biologist who in the mid-1950s carried out a series of elegant field and laboratory experiments using light-coloured and melanic forms of the peppered moth Biston betularia. He was able to show that the selective forces operating against the moths were due to visual predation by birds, which attacked preferentially those forms resting on a noncryptic background.

***Key.*** A character of special significance in an organism. Such characters are used in a system for determining the identity of characters. Usually such keys are dichotomous (2); that is to say, at each step there is a choice between two possibilities. Keys, however, may have more than two characters at each step and there is a gradual elimination of absent characters until identification is made.

***Killer Strain.*** Strain of Paramecium containing kappa particles.

***Killer Yeast.*** Yeast cells containing a double-stranded RNA plasmid that encodes genes responsible for production of a killer substance which is lethal to other cells. The substance is closely similar in its action and synthesis to a bacterial colicin.

***Kilobase (kb).*** Unit of DNA length representing 1000 nucleotides.

***Kinase.*** An enzyme that catalyses the transfer of a phosphoryl group from ATP to another compound.

***Kinesis.*** Any orientation behaviour in which the organism does not move in a particular direction relative to the stimulus, but instead simply moves at an increasing or decreasing rate until it ends up nearer or further from the stimulus. For example, when a woodlouse finds itself drying out it simply begins to move around a great deal until encountering a moist spot where it may settle.

***Kinetic Complexity.*** Complexity of a sample of DNA as determined by its reassociation kinetics in a renaturation experiment.

***Kinetosome.*** Basal body of various cellular organelles, especially of eukaryotic cilia and flagella. It is homologous with the centriole.

***Kinety.*** Row of ciliary basal bodies. The kineties are composed of linked kinetosomes and may be visualized by a silver staining procedure. Kinety pattern is independently inherited, and when artificially altered by surgery is passed on in modified form of progeny.

***Kinins.*** (1) Group of blood-borne polypeptides that cause smooth muscle contraction and blood vessel dilation, the best known is bradykinin. (2) Class of purine derivaties that act as plant growth substances, and include zeatin and cytokinin. Synthetic kinins include kinetin.

***Kinomere.*** Spindle attachment in the region of a chromosome that attaches it to a spindle.

***Kin Selection.*** A form of selection favouring altruistic (self-sacrificing) behaviour towards, relative. Such a process ensures that even if the chances of an individual surviying are reduced, some of his or here genes will survive in the relative.

***Kirsten Sarcoma Virus.*** Retrovirus, originally derived from mice, but subsequently passaged through rats. It contains the oncogene sequence (v-Ki-ras). The human proto-oncogene sequence has not been definitely identified.

***Kleinschmidt Spreading Technique.*** Technique developed by A.K. Kleinschmidt in which nucleic acids are spread, in the presence of small amounts of protein, as extremely thin films on cleaned water surfaces. Such spreads may be picked up on copper grids (precoated) and subsequently examined by electron microscopy.

***Klinefelter's Syndrome.*** A human chromosomal abnormality in which there is an extra X-chromosome making a complement of 44 autosomes plus XXY (47 in all). The affected individuals are male (showing the sex determination role of the Y-chromosomes) but with much reduced fertility, and a number of female secondary sexual characteristics,such as breasts, often occur. About 1 in 1,000 liveborn males are affected by this condition, which arises from nondisjunction in one or other parent, more probably the female where there is a distinct positive age effect (as in down's syndrome).

***Klenow Fragment.*** Part of the bacterial DNA polymerase I that lacks the exonuclease activity of the complete enzyme.

***Klinefelder Syndrome.*** Inherited human disease resulting from an XXY karyotype for the sex chromosomes. Affected individuals are phenotypically male, but have small testes and suffer from mental retardation.

***Knockdown.*** A measure of biocide effect that is used when it is difficult to assess actual mortality. The measure is used particularly in biocide tests on insects, and has been shown to produce similar results to actual mortality scores. Knockdown is often measured as the inability to respond to a stimulus such as light or touch.

***Knockdown Line.*** A graphical representation of the rate of response to a biocide as measured by knockdown (y-axis) against time or dose (x-axis). Strains of organisms such as insects are characterized by the slope and position of their knockdown lines relative to other strains.

***Koch, Robert (1843-1910).*** German bacteriologist who first introduced the method of making bacterial smears and fixing them with heat. He worked on bubonic plague and sleeping sickness and discovered how they are transmitted. He also developed means of culturing bacteria and rules for property identifying the agents of various diseases. He is most famous for establishing a series of criteria necessary to establish whether a specific microorganism causes a specific disease. These criteria are known as Koch's Postulates :

(a) The microorganisms must be present in every case of the disease.

(b) The microorganisms must be isolated from the diseased organism and grown in culture.

(c) The disease must be reproduced when a pure culture is reintroduced to a nondiseased, susceptible host.

(d) The microorganism must be recoverable from the experimentally infected host.

***Kornberg Enzyme.*** (DNA polymerase I. pol I). DNA polymerase,discovered in 1956 by A. Kornberg and coworkers in cells of E. coli. It catalyses the addition of mononucleotides to the 3'-end of a growing DNA chain provided in vitro with a DNA template, the four deoxyribonucleoside tripophates and $Mg^{2+}$. The nucleotides added are determined by the sequence of bases on the complementary template strand. Kornberg enzyme also has an associated 3'- to 5'-exonuclease activity, removing 5'- nucleotides from the 3'-end of a double-stranded DNA molecule (i.e. reversal of polymerization). The rate of polymerization normally exceeds that of depolymerization except when a mismatched base is accidentally inserted into the growing chain. Two activities provide a proof-reading (error-repairing) mechanism in DNA synthesis. The enzyme has a second exonuclease action catalysing 5' - to 3'- degradation of DNA (a path-clearing function). Subtilisin (a protease) cleaves the

Kornberg enzyme into two unequal fragments. The smaller fragment ($M_r$=34,000) retains the 5'- to 3'- exonuclease activity, the larger ($M_r$= 76,000), called the Klenow fragment, possesses the 3'- to 5'- exonuclease and polymerization activities. The activity of Kornberg enzyme to degrade DNA in either direction as well as to catalyse the polymerization reaction suggests functions in gap-filling and the repair of damaged DNA rather than it being the major DNA-synthesizing enzyme ( a role now attributed in E. coli to DNA polymerase III, pol III). Indeed bacterial mutants lacking pol I activity remain viable but have an increased mutation rate.

***Kupffer Cells.*** The phagocytic cells that form part of the reticulo—endothelial system, destroying old red blood cells and remove foreign particles from blood flowing through the liver. Named after the German anatomist K. Kupffer.

***Kuru.*** Degenerative disease of the central nervous system occurring in a restricted area of New Guinea. It is thought to be caused by an infectious agent, perhaps a protein, acquired by eating the brains of infected individuals. It is in some ways similar to the scrapie disease of sheep.

***Kwashiorkor.*** The most widespread and serious human nutritional disease, brought on by acute protein starvation. The condition is characterized by apathy, impaired growth, skin ulcers, swollen hands and feet and an enlarged liver. If untreated, it is fatal. Kwashiorkor typically affects children in the early stages after weaning.

# L

***Lac Operon*.** The sequence of DNA in the bacterium Escherichia coli that regulates and codes for three genes involved in the lactose pathway. β-galactosidase and two other enzymes in the pathway are synthesized coordinately when the operon is switched on. This activation is accomplished by a derepression process involving the effector molecule, usually allolactose, binding with the repressor protein and so permitting transcription of the operon.

Bacteria growing in a lactose-free medium contain about five molecules of β-galactosidase per cell. On adding lactose to the culture, a specific and rapid induction of the enzyme occurs (up to 5000 molecules per cell within five minutes). (In vivo the actual inducer is allolactose, a byproduct of β-galactosidase activity.) Experiments using radioactively labelled amino acids or specific antibodies against β-galactosidase indicate that induction involves synthesis of new enzyme molecules rather than conversion or activation of a pre-existing proenzyme. The appearance of β-galactosidase is coordinated with the production of permease and transacetylase because the structural genes are expressed via a common mRNA. On removing lactose from the medium enzyme synthesis stops as rapidly as it started because the mRNA decays with a very short half-life (about three minutes). Synthetic analogues of lactose that contain an intact unsubstituted galactosidic residue are also able to induce production of the enzymes. Isopropyl-β-D-thiogalactopyranoside (IPTG) is one of the most efficient inducers, although it is not a substrate for β-galactosidase (i.e. it is a gratuitous inducer). By contrast, phenyl-β-D-galactopyranoside can be hydrolysed by β-galactosidase, but is not an inducer. The system must therefore possess a component, distinct from β-galactosidase, that recognizes lactose and other potential inducers.

Jacob and Monod proposed a model for the genetic regulation of lactose metabolism based on studies using mutant strains of E. coli deranged for lactose utilization. The structural genes of the operon were defined by $lacZ^-$ mutations (no β-galactosidase activity; $Lac^-$ phenotype), $lacY^-$ mutations ('cryptic' mutants with defective permease, induced only at higher inducer concentrations), and $lacA^-$ mutations (strains without transacetylase that could still utilize lactose). Other mutants were control-deficient and carried pleiotrophic mutations in regulatory genes. Constitutive enzyme production was a feature of both the $lacI^-$ and $lacO^c$ mutations. The ratio of enzyme activities was the same in constitutive cells as in the induced wild-type strain, indicating a common mechanism for controlling enzyme production from the operon. The $lacI^s$ mutation resulted in permanent loss of all the enzymes, even in the presence of high concentrations of inducer. The lacI (regulator) and lacO (operator) genes were mapped close by the structural genes of the operon and their functions were determined by constructing partially diploid strains using f duction. The diploid strain $I^+O^+Z^+/I^-O^+Z^+$ had the wild-type (inducible) phenotype, hence $lacI^+$ is dominant to the mutant $lacI^-$ allele. The $lacI^+$ allele is dominant in the trans configuration (trans-dominant) as shown by the inducible phenotype of the diploid $I^+O^+Z^-/I^-O^+Z^+$. This indicates that the lacI+ allele, in the absence of lactose, prevents constitutive production of active enzyme from a lacZ gene on a separate chromosome. The diploid strain $I^+O^+Z^+/I^+O^cZ^+$ had the constitutive (mutant) phenotype, hence $lacO^c$ is dominant to the wild-type allele (note that this is opposite to the result with the lacI$^-$ recessive constitutive mutation; in fact lacO$^c$ mutations were originally isolated by selecting for constitutivity in cells diploid for the lac region). Dominance is observed only when lacO$^c$ is in the cis configuration to the expressed gene, hence the diploid $I^+O^+Z^+/I^+O^cZ^-$ is inducible for β-galactosidose. This indicates that the lacO$^c$ allele cannot cause constitutive production of enzyme from a separate chromosome but only from a lacZ gene to which it is adjacent on the same chromosome. Using these observations Jacob and Monod proposed that the lacI gene produces a trans-acting diffusible repressor protein which binds to the operator gene and thereby prevents expression of the adjacent structural genes of the operon. The lac operon is thus a system under negative control by the lac repressor. Repressor is lifted by removal of repressor from its operator binding site by lactose (or analogous inducer). Mutations that either cause production of inactive repressor or fail to produce a repressor (lacI$^-$), or are defective in repressor binding (lacO$^c$), are permanently derepressed (constitutive). In the lacI$^s$ mutants the repressor (called the superrepressor) is locked in the form that recognizes the operator; such mutations are trans-acting and are dominant to wild-type lacI$^+$. The lac repressor has been isolated using equilibrium dialysis based on its property of binding IPTG. It is a tetrameric protein. Each monomer binds one inducer molecule, but induction requires the binding of only two molecules of inducer per tetrameric repressor. There are about 10 molecules of repressor per cell, but none occurs free in the cytoplasm because of the repressor's high affinity for the operator (dissociation constant ~$10^{-13}$). However this binding to the operator occurs only in the absence of inducer. The lac repressor thus has the properties of a typical allosteric protein.

The lac operator region, which lies between the promotor and lacZ, has a feature common to many DNA recognition sites for proteins; it is a palindromic sequence with an axis of dyad symmetry.

5'...TGTGTGGAATTGTGAGCGGAT
3'...ACACACCTTAACACTCGCCTA
AACAATTTCACACA...3'
TTGTTAAAGTGTGT...5'

Binding of the repressor to the operator involves the N-terminal 60 amino acids of two repressor monomers. This binding does not inhibit the binding of RNA polymerase to the promotor, but impedes movement of the polymerase into the structural genes of the operon and thus prevents transcription of those genes. See Figure L.1.

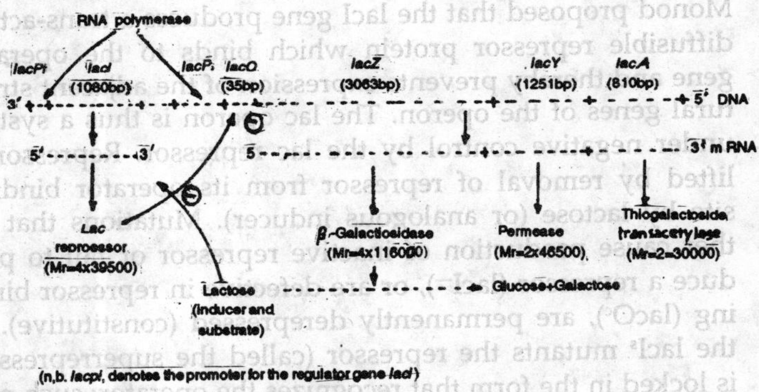


Figure L.1. Lac operon.

**β-*Lactamase*.** Enzyme that inactivates natural penicillins present in E. coli, the gene for which is carried on the plasmid pBR322. It is a periplasmic protein (i.e. it is secreted through the cell membrane and is normally found between the cell membrane and the cell wall). This property of being exported through the membrane results from a 23-amino acid leader sequence which is removed as the protein traverses the membrane.

***Lactate Dehydrogenase (LDH)*.** Enzyme that catalyses the interconversion of lactate and pyruvate in anaerobic glycolysis. Lactate dehydrogenase is a tetrameric molecule, each subunit of which can be of either the H (heart) or M (muscle) type. There are five isoenzymes of lactate dehydrogenase (i.e. four M-type subunits, three M-type subunits plus one H-type subunit, two M-type subunit plus two H-type subunits, etc.).

***Lactic Acid.*** An organic acid, $CH_3CHOHCOOH$, produced during the breakdown of glucose. Lactic acid is the major product of fermentation in certain bacteria.

***Lactic Acid Bacteria.*** A large group of rod-shaped or spherical Gram-positive anaerobic bacteria in which lactic acid is the major (and sometimes the only) end product of their fermentation. They have complex growth requirements, reflecting their limited biosynthetic abilities. The group includes the genera Streptococcus, Diplococcus, and Lactobacillus. Lactic acid bacteria are or economic importance in the production of cheese, yoghurt, etc., from milk.

***Lactose.*** Main sugar in milk; not found elsewhere in appreciable amounts. It is a disaccharide consisting of glucose joined to β-galactose by a galactosidic bond. The first step in its metabolism is by way of hydrolysis to the component monosaccharides. See Figure L.2.

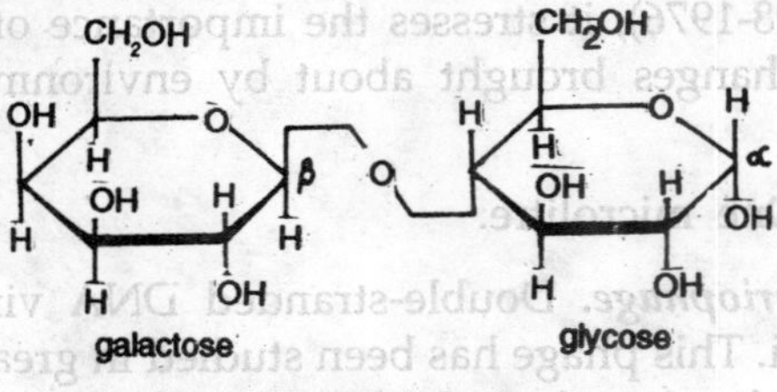


Figure L.2. Lactose.

***Lacuna.*** Space within a tissue or cell; for example, the spaces in bone matrix in which the bone cells reside, or, in plants, water-or gas-filled cavities that may provide buoyancy.

***Laemmli Loops.*** Loops of DNA visualized when chromosomes are viewed by electron microscopy following removal of histone; named after the originator of the technique, U.K. Laemmli. The loops all extend out from a central matrix or scaffold of non-histone protein, and each loop represents a distinct DNA domain.

***Lagging Strand.*** Strand of DNA that is synthesized discontinously during DNA replication, and consists of a series of okazaki fragments ligated together.

***Lag Phase.*** The initial phase in the growth of a cell culture, immediately after inoculation of the growth medium, during which there is no increase in cell numbers. During this time certain enzymes are induced and the cells adapt for growth in the new medium.

***Lamarckism.*** The theory of evolution put forward by Jean-Baptiste Lamarck (1744-1829) at the beginning of the 19th century. It proposes the origin of new species by the inheritance of acquired characteristics, i.e. characteristics developed during life by use and disuse are transmitted to the gametes and inherited by the offspring. This theory has lost support in the western world because it lacks definite proof and because a mechanism for the inheritance of acquired characteristics is difficult to postulate. However, in the Soviet Union a modern version of the theory has gained acceptance. Known as neo-Lamarckism (or Lysenkoism), its chief proponent being the Russian geneticist T. D. Lysenko (1898-1976), it stresses the importance of the inheritance of changes brought about by environmental influences.

***Lambda* (λ).** One microlitre.

***Lambda Bacteriophage.*** Double-stranded DNA virus that infects E. coli. This phage has been studied in great detail and has been developed as a vector for molecular cloning. Lambda DNA consists of 48,502 base pairs and codes for about 60 proteins. In the viral particle, the DNA is a linear duplex with single-stranded complementary ends of 12 nucleotides (cohesive ends). After entering the bacterial host, the DNA circularizes through pairing of the cohesive ends. Lambda can replicate lytically or as part of the E. coli chromosome. In the lytic cycle, the circular DNA is replicated many times and a larger number of bacteriophage gene products are synthesized. The DNA is packaged into mature phage particles, which are released upon lysis of the cell; the released phage can then infect other cells. In the lysogenic state, the lytic functions are repressed and the phage genome is integrated into the bacterial chromosome (it is then called a prophage) and is replicated and transmitted to progeny like any other gene on the chromosome. The host cells are not lysed. However, with a low frequency, lysogenic cells (i.e., those carrying a prophage, can spontaneously enter the lytic life cycle. Certain agents i.e., ultraviolet light) can induce this event in virtually all of the lysogenic cells. Most laboratory stains of lambda contain a mutant repressor, which is thermolabile, so that the prophage can be induced by heat.

Lambda bacteriophage has served as the basis for the construction of a large number of cloning vectors that can accept foreign DNA inserted into a variety of restriction sites. These vectors are of two types : (1) those with a single target site into which foreign DNA is inserted (insertion vectors); (2) those with a pair of sites spanning a nonessential segment of vector DNA that can be removed and replaced with foreign DNA (replacement vectors). Since there is an upper limit on the total amount of DNA that can be packaged, insertion vectors can accommodate less foreign DNA and are used for cloning cDNA or small restriction fragments; replacement vectors are used for cloning larger pieces of DNA.

***Lambda Chain*** (λ Chain). One of two types of light chain found in immunoglobulins which differ by about 60 percent in their constant region amino acid sequence.

***Lambda Phage.*** Double-stranded DNA phage that infects E. coli and is widely used as a cloning vector. Lambda phage may enter either a lytic growth or lysogenic growth cycle depending on a balance of genetic and molecular factors within the cell.

***Lamella.*** (1) Layer/sheet of calcified extracellular matrix contributing to the appositional growth of bone; lamellae are deposited either irregularly in woven/cancellous bone, or in concentric layers around haversian canals in compact bone. (2) Alternative term for one of the spore-bearing 'gills' of the sporophore of a basidiomycete fungus (e.g. an agaric). (3) Pectin-rich layer between the apposed cell walls of two adjacent plant cells.

***Lamellipodium.*** Cell surface extension in the form of a flattened sheet which is characteristic of cells such as fibroblasts, especially when motile on a surface under in vitro culture conditions.

***Lamina.*** Flattened portion of a leaf supported by the petiole. In animal cells the basal lamina is an extracellular matrix secreted by many cells and forming sheets between cell layers or tissues.

***Laminin.*** Glycoprotein found as a major component for the basal lamina, which forms the extracellular matrix of many cells.

***Lampbrush Chromosome.*** A type of chromosome, found in the oocytes of many vertebrates, that is much larger and less condensed than normal chromosomes. The long axis of the chromosome bears large numbers of paired loops, each loop arising from a chromomere, giving the chromosome a structure resembling a Victorian lampbrush. Lampbrush chromosomes persist for many months throughout the long diplotene stage of meiosis and, unlike other chromosomes (except the giant polytene chromosomes of Diptera) remain active in transcription. See Figure L.3.

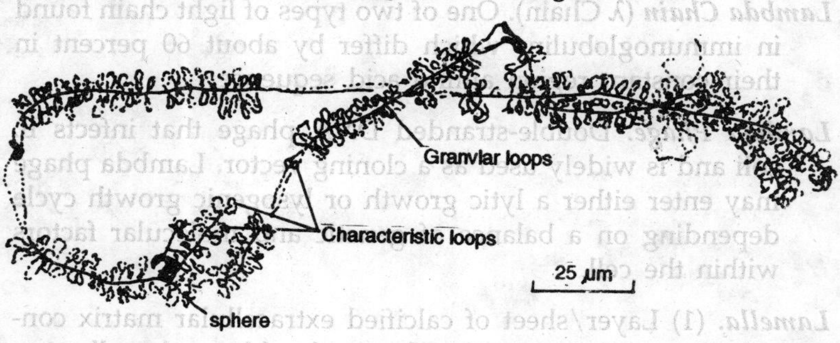


Figure L.3. Lampbrush chromosome. Structure of lampbrush chromosome from the oocyte of Triturus.

***Langerhans Cell (LC).*** Cell of the skin and lymphoid organs (where it is called a dendritic cell) characterized by multiple thin cytoplasmic processes that extend between neighboring cells. LC have a high density of class I and class II histocompatibility molecules and are active in antigen presentation. LCs in the skin have variable amounts of CD1, Fcy receptors and complement receptors 1 and 3. Many LCs have a characteristic cytoplasmic structure, the birbeck granule, which is a small round or rectangular vacuole of 10 nm, containing a central, irregular electron-dense mass. LCs are derived from bone marrow stem cells, migrate to the epidermis and then, by way of the lymphatic circulation, into lymph nodes where they localize in the deep cortex or via the blood to the spleen. Dendritic cells do not express CD1 and most have no Fcy receptors. LCs appear to be highly active in delayed-type hypersensitivity reactions of the skin where they take up antigen and carry it to the lymph nodes. LCs appear to be identical to veiled cells isolated from lymph.

***Lanthanum.*** Element used, usually as its hydroxide, as an electron-dense tracer in electron microscopy. The small size of the molecule allows it to be used to indicate sites of membrane permeability.

***Larva.*** The immature form in which many animals exist after hatching from the egg and before undergoing metamorphosis to the adult form. The larva is self-supporting and differs from the adult in structure and mode of life; it is usually incapable of sexual reproduction. Larval stages occur in anamniote vertebrates, e.g. the tadpole of frogs, and in most invertebrates, e.g. the caterpillar of butterflies and the ciliated planktonic larvae of many marine phyla.

***Late Genes.*** Genes that are expressed late in the life cycle of a virus. These genes usually code for proteins such as capsid subunits.

***Latent Allotype.*** Allotype that is not expected based on the genetic constitution of the animal, i.e. an allotype different from the expected or 'Nominal' allotype. This phenomenon has been described for the a (heavy chain variable region), b (kappa light chain), and d and e (gamma heavy chain constant region) allotypes of rabbit immunoglobulins. For example, an $F_1$ rabbit produced by mating a homozygous a1 rabbit with a homozygous a2 rabbit would be expected to produce heavy chains of allotypes a1 or a2. Occasionally, especially after suitable stimulation, such rabbits also produce heavy chains expressing the a3 allotypic determinants. Such an unexpected allotype is designated a 'latent allotype'. Latent allotypes are usually expressed at very low levels, although high levels have also been reported.

***Latent Virus.*** A virus that can remain in the host organism for long periods without any observable effect. It may be induced (by 'helper' viruses, a chemical, or radiation) to multiply and produce disease symptoms long after the initial invasion of the host. Probably only the genomes are retained, untranscribed, during the latent period. Latent viruses include herpes simplex, which causes cold sores, and chickenpox virus (varicella), which can become latent and recur later as shingles (herpes zoster).

***Late-Replicating X Chromosome (Barr Body).*** Condensed copy of the X chromosome of mammals. As compared with the non-condensed copy of the X, this condensed copy, which is composed of facultative heterochromatin, is replicated late in the S phase of the cell cycle.

***LAV (Lymphadenopathy Virus).*** Causative agent of human AIDS, and now more properly known as HIV (human immuno-deficiency virus).

***Lattice Theory.*** Idea that antigen-antibody precipitation results from the formation of large complexes (i.e. lattices) of antigens and antibodies. To form lattices, both the antigen and the antibody must have two or more binding sites (i.e. be bivalent or multivalent). Complex formation is particularly efficient if a variety of antibodies recognizing different determinants of the antigen are present.

***L-Cell Conditioned Medium.*** Medium from cultures of L cells (a long-term fibroblast line) that contains a potent growth factor for macrophages (M-CSF).

***L Cells.*** Cultured cell line, originally described by Earle in 1943. He took normal subcutaneous connective tissue cells from healthy C3H mice and treated them with 20-methylcholanthrene. The L cells thus produced could be cultured and yielded sarcomas when injected into healthy C3H mice.

***$LD_{50}$*.** Lethal dose 50; the dose of a drug, radiation treatment, or titre of a virus at which 50% of the organisms exposed to it are killed. It is used as a standard measure of toxicity.

***L-DOPA (L-Dihydroxyphenylalanine).*** An amino acid intermediate in the synthesis of the catecholamines dopamine, noradrenaline, and adrenaline. L-DOPA is administered therapeutically in the treatment of Parkinson's disease in order to raise the levels of brain dopamine, which are deficient in this condition.

***Lead Citrate.*** Heavy metal salt used as a stain in the preparation of specimens for transmission electron microscopy.

***Leader Sequence.*** Region at the 5'-end of a messenger RNA that is normally untranslated but contains regulatory signals involved in such processes as ribosome binding.

***Leader Sequence Peptide.*** Short length of amino acid sequence at the amino end of some protein molecules, which, as a result of hydrophobic amino acids, carries the protein through the membrane of the endoplasmic reticulum and so ensures its eventual secretion. The leader sequence peptide is commonly removed before the protein becomes active.

***Leading Strand.*** Strand of DNA that is synthesized continuously during DNA replication. The leading strand is synthesized towards the replication fork in a 5'- to 3'-direction.

***Leaky Mutant.*** Mutant gene that shows some residual activity.

***LE Cell (lupus erythematosus Cell).*** Neutrophil that has ingested insoluble complexes of nucleoproteins and antibodies. The complexes appear as large homogeneously staining cytoplasmic masses. The presence of these cells, after incubation of blood for one hour at 37°C, was used as a diagnostic test for systemic lupus erythematosus.

***Lectin.*** Protein that recognizes specific carbohydrate residues and binds to cell surface glycoproteins or glycolipids. Lectins were originally isolated from plants (especially seeds), but have subsequently been found in a variety of other organisms. Lectins can be soluble or membrane-bound; they are bivalent or polyvalent and often agglutinate cells (e.g. erythrocytes). Lectins interact with specific regions of relatively complex oligosaccharides; in some cases, their reactivity is directed to a particular monosaccharide constituent, and such lactins can be inhibited by low concentrations of the appropriate free sugar; other lectins can be inhibited only by oligosaccharides. Certain lectins (e.g. pokeweed and concanavalin A) are mitogens and stimulate the transformation of small, resting lymphocytes into large blast cells that may undergo mitotic division.

***Lectins.*** Highly specific carbohydrate-binding proteins or glycoproteins that will agglutinate cells and/or precipitate complex carbohydrates. Lectins are naturally occurring compounds isolated particularly from higher plants and seeds, but also from fungi, bacteria, sea-weeds, sponges, molluscs, fish eggs, body fluids of invertebrates and lower vertebrates and from mammalian cell membranes. Although their precise physiological role is uncertain, lectins have proved useful in a wide variety of applications in vitro, particularly in blood grouping and erythrocyte polyagglutination studies, stimulation of lymphocytes to divide, fractionation of cells, and the isolation and purification of carbohydrate-containing molecules.

***Leghaemoglobin.*** Haemoglobin-like iron-containing protein found only in root nodules of leguminous plants. These nodules are caused by infection with the nitrogen-fixing bacterium Rhizobium. Although Rhizobium respires aerobically and requires oxygen, the presence of oxygen destroys the nitrogenase and consequently the nitrogen-fixing capability. Oxygen bound to the leghaemoglobin is made available to the bacteria while keeping the oxygen tension of the nodule tissue very low. Leghaemoglobin is coded for by a legume gene, but its synthesis only occurs in the presence of the bacterium.

***Leishman's Stain.*** Dye, used in a solution of methanol, to give a blue colour to cell nuclei. It is used most frequently to stain the nuclei of leucocytes.

***Lepidosauria.*** A subclass of reptiles characterized by a diapsid skull, a median eye, and a body covering of overlapping horny scales. They first appeared in the Upper Permian and are divided into three orders; the extinct Eosuchia, the Rhynchocephalia (tuatara), and the Squamata (lizards and snakes).

***Lepospondyli.*** A subclass of extinct Amphibia of the Carboniferous and Permian, characterized by vertebrae with a single spool-shaped centrum surrounding the notochord, as in modern forms. Some members of the order Microsauria, e.g. Cardiocephalus of the Lower Permian, had well-developed limbs and are thought to have been possible ancestors of the modern Urodela.

***Leptocaul.*** Designating angiosperms that have a small primary structure, providing many small easily replaced buds and leaves.

***Leptocephalus.*** The marine larva of the eel. It has a small thin transparent leaf-like body with a small head and long fragile teeth for feeding on plankton. Leptocephali hatch in the Sargasso Sea in the west Atlantic and migrate eastwards, taking about 2.5 years, to European waters, where they undergo metamorphosis into elvers (young eels).

***Leptonema.*** Little-used term for leptotene stage of meiotic division.

***Leptotene (Leptonema).*** First stage of meiotic prophase. During this stage the chromosomes appear as thin threads with clearly demarcated chromomeres.

***Lethal Mutation.*** Mutation that induces the death of the organism prematurely. If the mutation is recessive, only organisms that are homozygous will be killed, but if dominant, heterozygous individuals will also be killed. Some lethal mutants die early in embryonic life and so are detected by aberrant ratios in mendelian crosses.

***Leu 7.*** Surface antigenic determinant of human natural killer cells, detected with a mouse monoclonal antibody.

***Leu 11.*** Surface antigenic determinant of fcy receptor III on human natural killer cells, detected with a mouse monoclonal antibody.

***Leucine (Leu).*** One of the 20 common amino acids. It carries a non-polar side-chain.

***Leucocytes.*** (white blood cells, white blood corpuscles). Generic name for a heterogeneous group of blood cell types which, in effect, includes everything other than erythrocytes and blood platelets. Principally leucocytes function as part of the body's defence mechanism by : (1) non-specific means (i.e. destruction and phagocytosis of foreign matter); (2) specific means (i.e. production of specific antibodies as part of the immune system). Leucocytes include granulocytes (basophil, eosinophil and neutrophil). Lymphocytes and monocytes (macrophage precursors).

***Leucopenia.*** Reduction in the number of leucocytes.

***Leucoplast.*** Colourless proplastid, common in non-photosynthetic plant tissues and from which other forms of plastid may develop.

***Leucosin.*** Polysaccharide food reserve of the algal group of Chrysophyta.

***Leucoviruses.*** Now little used name for retroviruses.

***Leukaemia.*** A malignant disease characterized by a high proportion of abnormal white cells in the blood. The disease is sometimes associated with a leukaemia virus. Certain chemical and physical agents, such as high doses of X-rays, can sometimes induce leukaemia, possibly by causing activation of a latent leukaemia virus already present.

***Leukoagglutinin.*** Substance (e.g. specific antibody) that agglutinates white blood cells.

***Leukocyte.*** White blood cell. The major classes of leukocytes are : granulocytes, lymphocytes, monocytes.

***Leukocyte Adhesion Deficiency (LAD).*** Defect in adhesion and mobility of phagocytes and lymphocytes, resulting from a deficiency of the membrane proteins p150,95, LFA-1 and complement receptor 3 (CR3) and leading to recurrent pyogenic infections. These three proteins are not expressed on the cell surface due to defective biosynthesis of the beta chain ($M_r$ 95,000), a subunit shared by all three proteins. Phagocytes are defective in random migration, chemotaxis and spreading on charged surfaces. C3-coasted particles do not induce a respiratory burst or degranulation of phagocytes and are not ingested. These defects of phagocytes have been ascribed to the deficiency of CR3 and p150,95. T lymphocytes of patients do not proliferate normally in response to stimulation by mitogens, antigens or alloantigens. They also do not provide adequate help for immunoglobulin production by B lymphocytes, do not secrete interferon-gamma and are defective in killing target cells. These defects of lymphocytes have been ascribed to the deficiency of LFA-1. Natural killer cells are also defective in killing target cells, and this has been ascribed to the deficiency of LFA-1. Patients with LAD deficiency have symptoms resulting from defects in phagocytes function (e.g., abscesses and periodontitis), but they have no clinical problems associated with the T lymphocyte deficiency. The defect is inherited as an autosomal recessive. Heterozygotes can be easily detected by their half-normal amounts of CR3 on phagocyte membranes but are clinically normal.

***Leukocyte Common Antigen (L-CA or T200).*** Family of major cell surface glycoproteins ($M_r$ 180,000-220,000) found on most leukocytes, but not on other cell types. These antigens are rich in carbohydrate and comprise up to 10 percent of the total membrane proteins. Rat thymocyte L-CA ($M_r$ 180,000) contains 1118 amino acid residues. The amino-terminal 391 residues are extra cellular. There is a transmembrane segment of 22 amino acid residues and a cytoplasmic portion of 705 residues. The cytoplasmic domain includes possible phosphorylation sites and two regions of internal homology. The function of this protein is unknown, but the large intracellular segment suggests a role in interaction with the cytoskeleton. In mice, L-CA is identified by antibodies to the Ly5 alloantigen. L-CA molecules show heterogeneity in size and antigenicity and different forms are specific to different lymphocyte types. Antigenic determinants include : (1) those common to all L-CA molecules; (2) those specific to B lymphocyte L-CA; and (3) those found on L-CA of B lymphocytes, CD8 + T lymphocytes and 70 percent of CD4+ T lymphocytes.

The gene encoding members of the L-Ca family consists of approximately 30 exons. The heterogeneity of L-CA molecules results from variable splicing between exons 3 and 7. Removing exons 4, 5 and 6 results in the lowest molecular weight form, found on thymocytes, whereas transcription of all the exons results in the highest molecular weight form, consisting of 1281 amino acid found on B lymphocytes. Of eight forms of L-CA, which could result from variable splicing of exons 4, 5 and/or 6, six have been identified.

***Leukocyte Inhibitory Factor (LIF).*** Lymphokine found in cultures of activated T lymphocytes that inhibits the migration of blood leukocytes, mainly neutrophils, from a capillary tube. LIF differs from migration inhibiting factor (MIF) in that LIF can be inhibited by serine esterase inhibitors, whereas MIF cannot be so inhibited.

***Leukotriene (LT).*** Molecule derived from arachidonic acid by the action of enzymes called lipooxygenases . LTs are released from mast cells following IgE-mediated reactions. Other cells (e.g. neutrophils) can also release LT. Slow reacting substance of anaphylaxis has been shown to be a mixture of $LTC_4$, $LTD_4$ and $LTE_4$. These three molecules are potent constrictors of smooth muscle, particularly of the small bronchi and bronchioles (about one hundred times more potent than histamine) and may be responsible for the bronchoconstriction in anaphylaxis of guinea-pigs and in asthma. $LTC_4$ and $LTD_4$ also increase vascular permeability. Another leukotriene, $LTV_4$, is a potent chemotactic factor for neutrophils; $LTB_4$ also cause aggregation and degranulation of neutrophils.

Arachidonic acid is converted to $LTA_4$ by a 5-lipooxygenase and a dehydrase; $LTA_4$ has no biological activity. It can be hydrolyzed to $LTB_4$ or converted to $LTC_4$ by addition of glutathione. Removal of glutamic acid by a transpeptidase reaction generates $LTD_4$. Further removal of a glycine by a dipeptidase results in the formation of $LTE_4$. Leukotrienes were so named because they were first isolated from leukocytes and contained a structure with three unsaturated carbon bonds (triene). See Figure L.4.

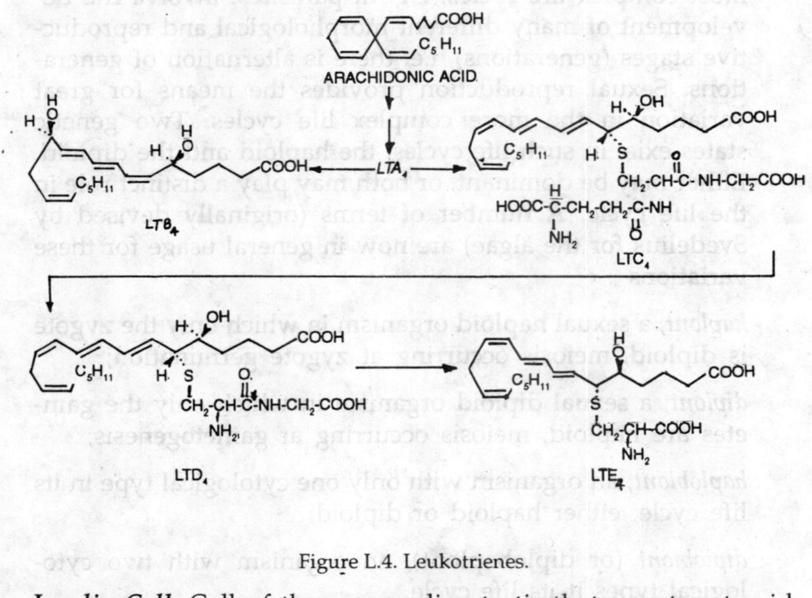


Figure L.4. Leukotrienes.

*Leydig Cell.* Cell of the mammalian testis that secretes steroid hormones and is particularly rich in smooth endoplasmic reticulum.

*L-Forms.* Forms of certain bacteria (e.g. some streptococci) in which the cell wall has been lost. L-forms can multiply and give rise to L-form colonies in suitable media. Some can revert to normal cells but others are stable. Their importance in nature is unknown but it is thought that they may persist in tissues for long periods and be responsible for relapses in certain diseases.

***Life Cycle.*** The various stages of development through which organisms of a species may pass from the fertilized egg cell of one generation to the same stage in the next generation. These are often various alternatives by which the adult stage is reached, and the term therefore describes the reproductive potential of the species. The term is less commonly used for the various stages through which an individual organism may pass from birth to death.

In the simplest life cycles, an individual gives rise to offspring similar to itself, e.g. by asexual reproduction; the most complex life cycles, e.g. in parasites, involve the development of many different morphological and reproductive stages (generations), i.e. there is alternation of generations. Sexual reproduction provides the means for great variation in the more complex life cycles. Two genetic states exist in such life cycles; the haploid and the diploid. Either may be dominant, or both may play a distinct role in the life cycle. A number of terms (originally devised by Svedelius for the algae) are now in general usage for these variations :

*haplont*, a sexual haploid organism in which only the zygote is diploid, meiosis occurring at zygote germination;

*diplont*, a sexual diploid organism in which only the gametes are haploid, meiosis occurring at gametogenesis;

*haplobiont*, an organism with only one cytological type in its life cycle, either haploid or diploid;

*diplobiont* (or diplohaplont), an organism with two cytological types it its life cycle.

In many species the different cytological generations are represented by different morphological forms; in addition each cytological type may also exhibit more than one mor-

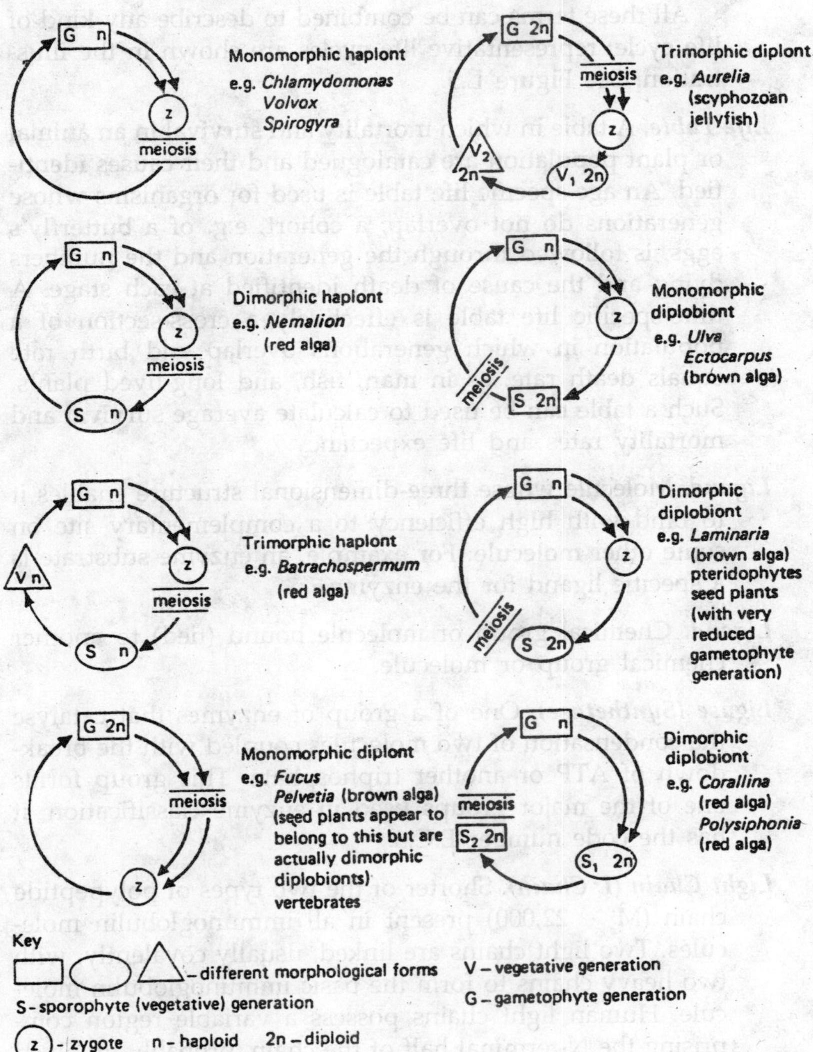


Figure L.5. Common types of life cycle.

phological form. These organisms are known as polymorphic, as distinct from monomorphic, i.e. having only one morphological type in the life cycle.

All these terms can be combined to describe any kind of life cycle; representative life cycles are shown in the illustration. See Figure L.5.

***Life Table.*** A table in which mortality and survival in an animal or plant population are catalogued and their causes identified. An age-specific life table is used for organisms whose generations do not overlap; a cohort, e.g. of a butterfly's eggs, is followed through the generation and the numbers dying and the cause of death identified at each stage. A time-specific life table is effectively a cross-section of a population in which generations overlap and birth rate equals death rate, as in man, fish, and long-lived plants. Such a table can be used to calculate average survival and mortality rates and life expectancy.

***Ligand.*** Molecule whose three-dimensional structure enables it to bind with high efficiency to a complementary site on some other molecule. For example, an enzyme substrate is a specific ligand for the enzyme.

***Ligand.*** Chemical group or molecule bound (tied) to another chemical group or molecule.

***Ligase (Synthetase).*** One of a group of enzymes that catalyse the condensation of two molecules coupled with the breakdown of ATP or another triphosphate. This group forms one of the major groups used in enzyme classification; it has the code number E.C.6.

***Light Chain (L Chain).*** Shorter of the two types of polypeptide chain ($M_r \sim 22{,}000$) present in all immunoglobulin molecules. Two light chains are linked, usually covalently, with two heavy chains to form the basic immunoglobulin molecule. Human light chains possess a variable region comprising the N-terminal half of the chain, probably involved in antigen-binding, and a constant region comprising the C-terminal half of the chain. Two classes of light chain are found in humans; kappa (60 percent of light chains) and lambda (40 percent of light chains). Kappa and lambda chains can be linked to any heavy chain class, but within a given immunoglobulin molecule only kappa or lambda chains will be present (i.e. not both).

***Light Chain.*** Smaller polypeptide chain in a heterodimer. As used by immunologists, the term light chain usually refers to the light chain of an immunoglobulin molecule.

***Light Green.*** Dye used in botanical histology to stain specifically cellulose (which is turned red by the stain). It is soluble in ethanol or clove oil.

***Light Meromyosin.*** Small molecular species of muscle myosin. Four molecules of two distinct types of light chain meromyosin associate with the heads of the two heavy meromyosin molecules to form the functional complex.

***Lignin.*** Common constituent of plant cell walls; major component of wood. It is a complex polymer of somewhat variable composition, made up from alcohols, sugars, aromatic amino acids and phenolic substances.

***Limiting dilution analysis.*** Method for estimating the frequency in a population, of responding cells of defined specificity and function, by application of the Poisson distribution. For example, to determine the frequency of a specific type of B lymphocyte frequency of a specific type of B lymphocyte in a suspension of spleen cells, aliquots in containing graded numbers of cells are cultured, in multiple replicas, under conditions designed to optimize the specific response. The B cells must be present in limited number (i.e. so that some cultures contain no B cells) and the cultures must be supplemented with an optimal number of any other type of cell (e.g. helper T lymphocytes) needed for the response. (In practice, T lymphocytes would be removed from the cell suspension that serves as the source of B cells so that the total number of T lymphocytes is limited to those that are added). At each cell dose, the fraction of nonresponding cultures (i.e. those containing no B cells) is determined and is plotted, on a logarithmic scale, against the number of cells. A linear relation should be obtained if the responsive B lymphocyte is limiting in number and if a single such cell is sufficient for the response. From the poisson distribution, it follows that the cell does (i.e. 2 x $10^5$ cells in the example shown) that yields a fraction of nonresponding cultures of $e^{-1}$ (i.e. 0.37) probably contains one specific B lymphocyte, a frequency of one per 2 x $10^5$ total cells. Such a frequency might be found in a primary response; the frequency of specific B lymphocytes in a secondary response is usually considerably higher. This type of analysis is also used to determine the frequency of helper T lymphocytes, T lymphocyte precursors, etc. See Figure L.6.

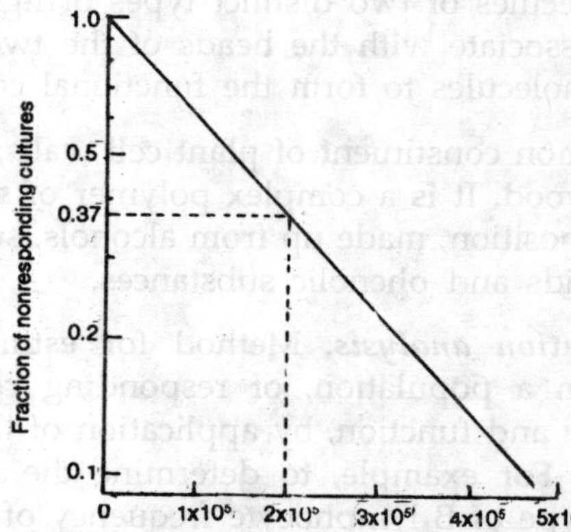


Figure L.6. Limiting dilution analysis.

***Line.*** Group of homozygous individuals that form a pure breeding population distinct from other individuals of the same species.

***Lineage.*** (1) Sequence of evolution from a particular ancestral species through intermediates to a more recent and distinct species.-

(2) Series of cells that are related by an uninterrupted sequence of cell divisions, and in which the cells at either end of the series may demonstrate distinct differentiative characteristics.

(3) The phenomenon of two or more genes being on the same chromosome. The genes are said to be linked, and the term linkage group is applied to all the genes on the same chromosome. The number of linkage groups in an organism is therefore equal to the haploid number of chromosomes. Linkage can be broken down by crossing over during meiosis. This leads to fresh linkage groups being formed in the gametes and therefore new combinations of genes in the progeny. Genes that are in the same linkage group do not show independent assortment.

***Linkage Disequilibrium.*** Occurrence on the same chromosome of alleles of two or more genes with greater or lesser frequency than would be expected from the frequencies of these alleles in the population. Genes may display linkage disequilibrium for two main reasons : (1) there has not been sufficient time to reach equilibrium; (2) a particular combination of alleles has a selective advantage. An example of linkage disequilibrium in human populations is the frequent occurrence on the same chromosome of HLA-A1 and HLA-B8 in populations of Northern European origin.

***Linkage Group.*** Group of genes located on the same chromosome.

***Linker DNA.*** (1) Segment of DNA between adjacent nucleosomes. Its length is variable, averaging about 50 base pairs, and it is a probable attachment site for histone H1. (2) DNA sequence used in recombinant DNA technology to join together two other DNA fragments or the ends of one fragment.

***Linking Number.*** Number of times that two strands of a double-helical closed-circular molecule cross one another. Molecules of DNA that are identical in all respects other than the linking number are termed topological isomers.

***Lipases.*** Enzymes that break down fats to yield acids and glycerol.

***Lipid Annulus.*** Ring of lipid molecules bonded by hydrophobic interactions around an intrinsic membrane protein. This lipid may have a different composition from the rest of the membrane lipid.

***Lipid Bilayer.*** All these classes of lipid found in biological membranes (phospholipids, glycolipids, cholesterol) comprise amphipathic molecules and, as a sequence, all biological membranes are basically lipid bilayers with associated protein molecules. In aqueous solutions such lipid molecules will self-assemble into energetically stable, bilayered configurations whereby the hydrophobic tails of the two layers of lipid molecule project inwards, sandwiched between the hydrophilic poles which face outwards on each aspect of the bilayer. In such a bilayer, lateral diffusion of individual molecules is extremely common and rapid (conferring fluidity within the plane of the bilayer) but flip-flop motion is extremely rare.

***Lipid Micelle.*** An aggregation of molecules of fatty-acid salts (soaps) or phospholipids in aqueous solution, the hydrophobic fatty acid chains orientated together at the centre of a sphere or oblong with the polar groups directed outwards (see Figure L.7(a)). Monolayers (one molecule thick) form on aqueous surfaces, the hydrocarbon chains pointing up into the air and the polar groups into the liquid (see

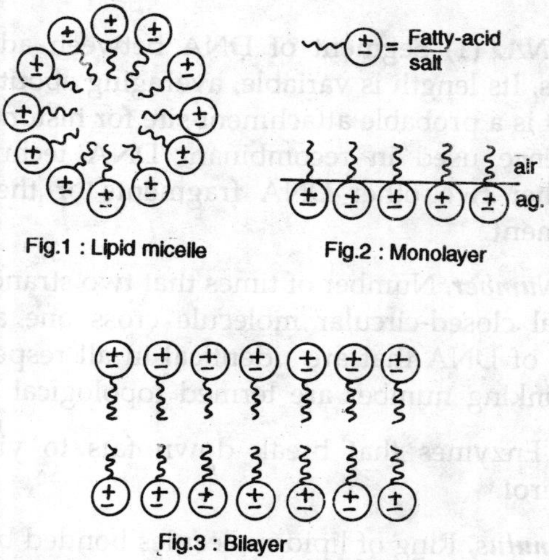


Figure L.7. Lipid micelle and associated forms. (a) Lipid micelle. (b) Figure. Monolayer. (c) Bilayers.

Figure L.7(b)). Similarly, at an aperture separating two aqueous compartments, bilayers 7 nm thick are spontaneously formed; due to their similarity to natural membranes bilayers are used experimentally as model membranes (see Figure L.7(c)).

*Lipids.* Large group of organic compounds found in living organisms, and distinguished by their solubility in non-polar solvents such as either and ethanol. They include fats, waxes, phospholipids, glycolipids and steroids, as well as simpler straight-chain hydrocarbons.

*Lipofuscin (Age Pigment).* Pigment that tends to accumulate as brown granules in the cytoplasm of long-lived, non-dividing cells; granules are often bounded by a single membrane. Lipofuscin, derived from the proteins, may be a residue from lysosome activity, particularly under hyperoxic conditions. Excessive accumulation of lipofuscin may impair cell function and contribute to cell ageing.

*Lipogenesis.* The biosynthesis of fatty acids. Substrates, such as glucose, that are able to yield acetyl CoA provide precursors for this process.

*Lipoic Acid.* A substance required for the growth of a number of microorganisms. It consists of a fatty-acid chain with a disulphide bridge and takes part in the enzyme sequences catalysing the oxidative decarboxylation of α-ketoglutarate and pyruvate in carbohydrate metabolism. See Figure L.8.

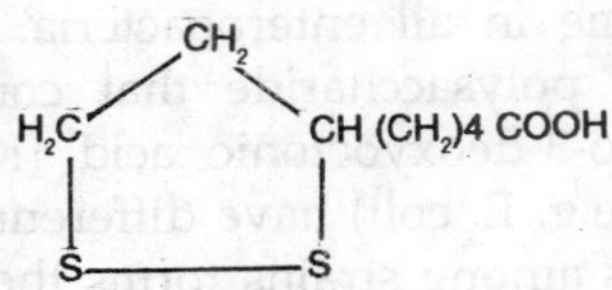


Figure L.8. Lipoic Acid.

*Lipolysis.* The hydrolysis of lipids, especially of the triglycerides in fat by lipases, to produce fatty acids for oxidative catabolism). Triglycerides, which are stored in adipose tissue, may be transported in the plasma to the liver where degradation occurs; alternatively they are first hydrolysed and the free fatty acids, noncovalently bound to albumin, are transported to the liver. Hormones such as adrenaline and ACTH increase adipose tissue lipolysis and hence increase the plasma levels of free fatty acids.

***Lipopolysaccharide.*** One of the main constituents, with lipoprotein, of the cell wall of Gram-negative bacteria; these two substances comprise 80% (dry weight) of the cell wall. The lipopolysaccharide is responsible for the antigenic specificity of the bacterium, the polysaccharide side-chains acting as the determinant sites. See Figure L.9.

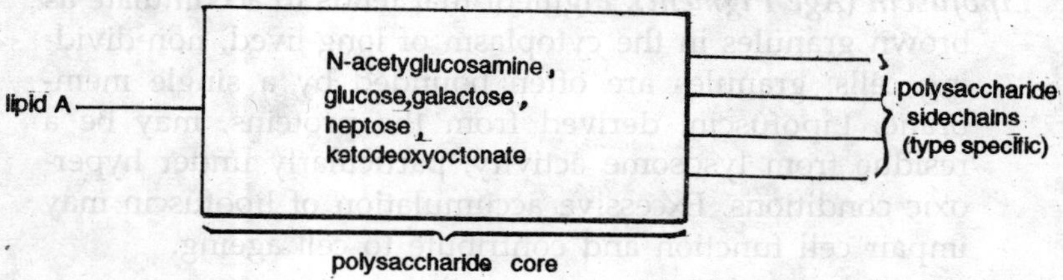


Figure L.9. Lipopolysaccharide.

***Lipopolysaccharide (LPS).*** Major constituent of the outer membrane of gram-negative bacteria (e.g. Escherichia, Salmonella, Bacteroides, Pseudomonas). LPS is a complex molecule composed of lipid A, a core polysaccharide, and a variable polysaccharide known as O antigen. Lipid A, which is buried in the membrane, consists of two phosphorylated glucosamine residues to which are linked six long-chain fatty acids. The structure of lipid A is practically the same in all enterobacteria. Salmonella have a common core polysaccharide that contains the unusual sugars 2-keto-3-deoxyoctonic acid (KDO) and heptose; other genera (e.g. E. coli) have different cores. Variation in the O antigens among strains forms the main basis for the classification of the salmonella in the Kauffmann-White scheme.

The introduction of gram-negative bacteria or of LPS lowers blood pressure, and can cause fever, neutropenia, blood clotting and shock, resulting in death. The lipid A moiety is responsible for the toxic activities of LPS. Many of these effects are indirect, i.e., LPS induces secretion of active agents by other cells, e.g. the production of interleukin-1 and tumor necrosis factor by macrophages. LPS can also activate the alternative pathway of complement, it can induce B lymphocytes of many species (but not of humans) to proliferate and differentiate into plasma cells.

***Lipoprotein.*** One of a group of conjugated proteins having polar lipids as the non-amino-acid group. They occur in the blood and lymph, where they function in the transport of lipids from the small intestine to the liver and from the liver to the site of fat deposition.

***Liposome.*** Artificial membranous vesicle made from lecithins and other lipids that is readily absorbed by living cells. Liposomes have been exploited for the delivery of novel genetic material to cells as an alternative to mechanical injection.

***Liposome.*** Synthetic lipid vesicle consisting of phospholipid bilayers (~5 nm thick) surrounding one or more aqueous compartments. Liposomes can be formed by : (1) suspending phospholipids (e.g. phosphatidylcholine (lecithin) in an aqueous medium (with or without sonication) or (2) dispersing phospholipids in aqueous medium with detergent, followed by dialysis to remove the detergent. Liposomes are spherical or slightly elongated in shape and may be up to 1-2 mm in diameter. Small (~25nm) liposomes are formed by sonication of larger ones and can be graded according to size by gel filtration. Liposomes may be simple unilamellar vesicles (single central aqueous compartment surrounded by a single bilayer) or they may be multilamellar (onion skin) with several shells of aqueous medium in addition to the central compartment, all separated by a series of concentric lipid bilayers. To mimic natural membranes, cholesterol and other membrane components (e.g. ionic channels) can be incorporated into the phospholipid bilayer. Solutes present in the aqueous phase when the liposome is formed become trapped inside the aqueous compartment(s).

Liposomes have been used as models for biological membranes (e.g., studies of membrane permeability or complement mediated lysis). Antigens can be embedded in liposome membranes for induction of immune responses. Liposomes can serve as vehicles for drug delivery. The latter application depends on the ability of liposomes to adsorb to virtually any type of cell and then to release their contents. Fusion of the liposome and cell membrane may or may not occur. Liposomes may be taken up by phagocytic cells. The efficacy of liposomes as therapeutic agents is, however, limited by their inability to leave the circulatory system and by their clearance by cells of the reticuloendothelial system.

***Lipotrophin (Lipolytic Hormone, LPH).*** One of at least two peptide factors (β– and α-LPH) produced by the pars distalis of the mammalian pituitary gland that are structurally related to β-melanocyte-stimulating hormone (β-MSH) stimulate and lipolysis. β-LPH, first isolated in 1964, may be the precursor of β-MSH but it may also function as a hormone since it has been found in the blood.

***Lipovitellin.*** Lipoprotein constituent of amphibian yolk platelets. Along with phosphovitin, it is a cleavage product of a large precursor protein vitellogenin.

***Living Fossil.*** Any organism alive today whose closest relatives are known only as fossils and which was formerly thought to be extinct itself. Latimeria (a coelacanth) is a well-known animal living fossil; Ginkgo is a notable plant example.

***Local Immunity.*** Immunological reactions that take place mainly in the gastrointestinal or respiratory tract due to antibodies that are present locally. For example, the gut-associated lymphoid tissue can mount a predominant IgA response to ingested antigens.

***Locus (Gene Locus).*** The region of a chromosome occupied by a particular gene and therefore determining a single biochemical function. The alleles of any one gene occupy the same loci on homologous chromosomes.

***Lod Score.*** Measure of the statistical significance of a departure from expected values; logarithm of the odds of such a departure on the basis of chance alone.

***Lomasome (Plasmalemmasome).*** Extracellular structure seen in some plant cells, and especially in fungal cells, consisting of membranous vesicles situated between the cell wall and the plasma membrane (or sometimes embedded in the wall itself). It is variously suggested that these structures may be fixation artefacts, or sites of enzyme activity involved in cell wall modification of synthesis.

***Long-Period Interspersion.*** Pattern of distribution of DNA sequences found in the genomes of some organisms such as Drosophila. It involves an alternative distribution of non-repetitive DNA sequences between long stretches of moderately repetitive DNA.

***Long Terminal Repeat (LTR).*** Sequence of several hundred bases found at either end of some DNA molecules, especially the genomic DNA of retroviruses. The sequences at either end are identical to one another or in at least some cases, are inverted repeats.

***Loop.*** Single-stranded region at the end of a nucleic and hairpin (in which the parallel portion will be hydrogen bonded as a duplex) and therefore represents the sequences between two terminal palindomic sequences.

***Low-Density Lipoprotein.*** Plasma lipoprotein fraction that is the chief source of cholesterol for cells outside the liver and intestine. Cells bind the lipoprotein by means of specialized receptors, and there is evidence that individuals suffering from the inherited disorder hypercholesterolaemia have absence or deficiency of these functional receptors. This deficiency produces abnormally high levels of circulating cholesterol and low-density lipoprotein, with consequent deposition of cholesterol in arterial plaques and greatly increased risk of heart disease.

***Low-Zone-Tolerance.*** Tolerance induced by very small amounts of protein antigens administered repeatedly.

***L Region.*** Region of the major histocompatibility complex (H-2 complex) of the mouse.

***LSD (Lysergic Acid Diethylamide).*** Hallucinogenic drug that acts by increasing the concentration of serotonin in the brain.

***Luciferase.*** Enzyme involved in biological photoluminescence.

***Luciferin.*** Compound responsible for the luminescent (light-emitting) properties of many organisms.

***Lucke Virus.*** Herpes virus that causes adenocarcinomas of the kidney in frogs.

***Luria and Delbruck Experiment.*** Experiment in genetics designed to show whether a specific mutation could be environmentally induced or occurred randomly. It involved the use of a fluctation test, in which numerous cultures of bacteria were simultaneously screened for resistance to lysis by bacteriophage. If mutation to phage resistance were random, then considerable fluctuation in the numbers of mutant bacteria would be expected in the parallel cultures, depending on precisely when the mutation had occurred (if it occurred early in the life of the culture, many progency would have accumulated). Since marked fluctuations in the numbers of surviving resistant colonies were obtained, it was concluded that mutation was occurring at a constant random rate and was not being induced by exposure to the phage or other environmental factors.

***Lutein.*** Xanthophyll, pigment active in photosynthesis.

***Luteinizing Hormone (Interstitial-Cell-Stimulating Hormone, LH, ICSH).*** A glycoprotein hormone secreted, with follicle-stimulating hormone, by the pars distalis of the pituitary gland under hypothalamic regulation. In female mammals LH promotes the maturation of Graafian follicles and stimulates them to produce oestrogens; its presence is also required for ovulation and the formation of corpora lutea. In males it stimulates the interstitial cells of the testis to produce androgens.

***Lutheran Blood Group.*** Antigenic determinants of human red blood cells detected by alloantibodies to the products of two alleles : $Lu^a$ and $Lu^b$. The lutheran antigens have not been biochemically characterized. Alloimmunization of mothers by Lutheran antigens during pregnancy can lead to hemolytic disease of the newborn.

***Luxury Gene (Tissue-Specific Gene).*** DNA sequence that is not expressed in all cells. Such genes include many which have been intensively researched, since luxury genes often code for products which are made in very large amounts in particular tissues. Globin genes, Fibroin genes, Insulin genes and Crystallin genes are examples of such genes which are active only in the specialized tissue of the erythroid cells of the blood, the silk glands of invertebrate animals, the pancreatic islets of Langerhans, and the lens tissues of the vertebrate eye, respectively. The products of luxury genes are sometimes referred to as luxury proteins. The non-luxury genes, the so-called house-keeping genes, include sequences coding for histone or lactate dehydrogenase, which occur in all cells.

***Ly Antigen.*** Alloantigen found on the surface of mouse lymphocytes. Ly antigens are expressed to variable degrees on T and B lymphocytes and thymocytes.

***Lyases.*** Group of enzymes that catalyse double bond formation or modification.

***Ly1 B Cell.*** Mouse B cell lymphocyte containing the Ly1 (CD5) antigen on its surface. Ly1 B cells comprise no more than 5-10 percent of all B lymphocytes in the spleen and lymph nodes. They are markedly increased in inbred strains of mice with autoimmune diseases (e.g., New Zealand Mice). The relationship between Ly1 B cells and the majority of B lymphocytes is not known.

***LyB.*** Alloantigen on the surface of mouse B lymphocytes. The structure and function of these alloantigens is not known.

***Lymph.*** Fluid of the lymphatic circulation which contains a variety of leukocytes. Most (80 percent) of the cells in lymph are small lymphocytes. There is less protein in lymph than in plasma.

***Lymph.*** Fluid found in the Lymphatic system of vertebrates. Although ionically similar to the blood plasma of the blood it lacks many of the plasma proteins. Most of the cells in the lymphoid vessels are lymphocytes.

***Lymph Node.*** Small (normally less than 0.5 cm) encapsulated, bean-shaped secondary lymphoid organ, containing a mixture of lymphocytes and accessory cells held together in a loose reticulum, that filters the lymph. Lymph nodes are distributed widely throughout the body, often in groups draining a particular anatomical location (e.g., axilla, neck, groin). Lymph enters the node via afferent lymphatics and exits at the hilus via efferent lymphatics to more central lymph nodes and eventually to the thoracic duct. Lymph nodes have an outer domain (cortex) and an inner domain (medulla). The cortex is subdivided into a superficial cortex composed of accumulations of B lymphocytes called follicles, and a deep cortex composed of T lymphocytes in no particular organized pattern of distribution. Antigen comes into the node through the afferent lymphatics and is trapped by phagocytic cells (e.g., macrophages and follicular dendritic cells) in the stroma. The stroma of the node is com-

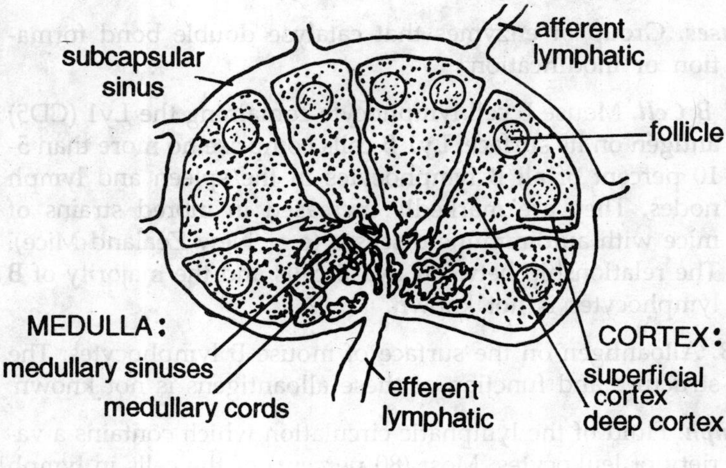


Figure L.10. Lymph node. Modified from Unanue, E.R., and Benacerraf, B. Textbook of Immunology, 2nd edition, 1984, William and Wilkins, Baltimore, MD.

posed of reticulum cells that, in the central portions, form medullary cords and sinuses. T lymphocytes continuously circulate through the nodes; they emerge from the blood at the post-capillary venules in the deep cortex, drain into the medullary sinuses and exit in the efferent lymphatics. Plasma cells are also found abundantly in the medulla. However, if T lymphocytes encounter antigen they are arrested in the lymph node. Immune responses can be initiated in lymph nodes.

True lymph nodes do not occur below the phylogenetic level of mammals. However, clusters of lymphoid cells (e.g. jugular bodies) that perform a similar function are found in some higher amphibians and birds. See Figure L.10.

***Lymphatic System.*** Extensive network of distensible vessels resembling veins (lymphatic vessels) arising from small, thin-walled lymphatic capillaries, which is found only in higher vertebrates. Its primary function is to recirculate interstitial fluid to the blood stream. This is effected by diffusion of interstitial fluid through the lymphatic capilaries to form lymph, and eventual passage from the largest lymphatic vessel, the thoracic duct, into the left subclavian vein. The lymphatic system also provides protection against disease by means of lymph nodes interspersed throughout the larger lymphatic vessels, serving to trap foreign antigens before they enter the blood stream.

***Lymph Node (Lymph Gland).*** Any one of a series of glandular structures of lymphoid tissue found in many situations around the vertebrate body, such as in the axillae, the neck (tonsils and adenoids) and they are particularly numerous in the peritoneal cavity around the gut (where they are known as Peyer's patches). The lymph nodes are interconnected by vessels of the Lymphatic system and the various types of lymphocytes which make up a large part of the lymph node tissue are able to move from node to node via the lymph. Lymph nodes are foci where invading bacteria and viruses are often concentrated by the defence system of the body, and inflammation of the lymph nodes is a frequent accompaniment to bacterial or viral infection.

***Lymphadenitis.*** Inflammation of lymph nodes, usually resulting from bacterial or viral infection.

***Lymphocyte.*** Spherical cell (6-12 μm in diameter) involved in immune responses, with a large, round, and deeply staining nucleus and very little cytoplasm. Small lymphocytes (6-8 μm in diameter) are extremely heterogeneous in function despite similar morphology.

***Lymphocyte.*** Cell that mediates the specificity of immune responses. Lymphocytes are spherical or ovoid cells, 8-12 μm in diameter. The nucleus is ovoid or indented into a kidney-shape; its chromatin is densely packed and stains intensely blue with most routinely used stains (e.g. Giemsa or Wright). The cytoplasm forms a thin rim around the nucleus and stains light blue; it contains few organelles. By scanning electron microscopy, lymphocytes are seen to have many surface villi covering 70-90 percent of the cell surface. Lymphocytes are divided into two major groups : B and T lymphocytes. These two groups of cells cannot be distinguished by routine staining or by morphological characteristics; the distinction between them is based on the presence of different surface molecules and on their different roles in immunological reactions. In addition to B and T lymphocytes, there is a small population of large lymphocytes (~15 μm in diameter) that have prominent granules in the cytoplasm - so called large granular lymphocytes or natural killer cells. Lymphocytes of the thymus are called thymocytes. Lymphocytes are the most numerous cell in the body.

***Lymphocyte Function Associated Antigen-1 (LFA-1, CD11a,18).*** Membrane glycoprotein of lymphocytes and phagocytes. LFA-1 participates in the adherence of cytotoxic T lymphocytes and natural killer cells to target cells and in other cell-cell interactions. The ligand for LFA-1 on target cells is called intercellular adhesion molecule-1 (ICAM-1). LFA-1 is composed of an alpha chain ($M_r$ 180,000) and a beta chain ($M_r$ 95,000), which is identical to the beta chain of p150,95 and complement receptor 3. The beta chain is composed of 769 amino acid residues including a signal sequence. There are six sites for N-linked oligosaccharides. The gene for the alpha chain is on chromosome 16 and the gene for the beta chain is on chromosome 21.

***Lymphocyte Function Associated Antigen-2 (LFA-2).*** Synonym for CD2.

***Lymphocyte Function Associated Antigen-3 (LFA-3).*** Cell surface antigen on all B and T lymphocytes as well as on monocytes, granulocytes, platelets, vascular endothelium and fibroblasts. LFA-3 ia a single polypeptide chain ($M_r$ 60,000). Mouse monoclonal antibodies to LFA-3, when bound to target cells, inhibit cytolysis by cytotoxic T lymphocytes. LFA-3 has been mapped to human chromosome 1. LFA-3 has recently been shown to be the ligand for CD2.

***Lymphocyte Recirculation.*** Continuous passage of lymphocytes from blood to lymph nodes and spleen and back to the blood via the lymphatics. Lymphocytes enter the nodes and spleen from the blood; they bind to and traverse the high endothelial cells of the post-capillary venules of lymph nodes or the marginal sinuses of the spleen, and after a day or two exit into the efferent lymph. From the lymph, they reenter the blood stream via the thoracic duct. This continuous process allows lymphocytes to sample the lymphoid tissues for antigen. The encounter of T lymphocytes with antigen interrupts the re-circulation; the T lymphocytes remain in the node, proliferate and later re-enter the circulating pool.

***Lymphocyte Transformation.*** Change from a small, resting lymphocyte into a large lymphocyte. This change may follow (1) stimulation by antigens or lectins or (2) viral infection (e.g. with Epstein-Barr virus, human T cell leukemia virus I).

***Lymphocytic Choriomeningitis (LCM).*** Infection caused by an arenavirus that is endemic in mice and occurs sporadically in humans and household pets. Infection of an immunocompetent host by LCM leads either to immunity or to death from the acute infection. The acute infection is characterized by enlargement of the spleen and lymph nodes and perivascular infiltration by T lymphocytes of all viscera, particularly the brain. Infection of a neonatal or immunosuppressed mouse results in a chronic carrier state. The carriers produce large amounts of anti-viral antibodies that do not eliminate the infection. These mice may develop immune complex disease of the renal glomeruli, arterial walls, lungs, liver and heart. Transfer of lymphocytes from an immune donor into a carrier causes death of the carrier. The transferred cytotoxic T lymphocytes recognize LCM viral antigens on the membranes of cells in the brain and meninges; this leads to severe inflammation and death. The phenomenon of MHC restriction of cytotoxic T lymphocyte cells was discovered in the LCM system.

***Lymphocytosis.*** Increased number of lymphocytes in the blood.

***Lymphocytotrople.*** Having an affinity for lymphocytes. For example, human immunodeficiency virus and human T cell leukemia virus are lymphocytotropic for CD4+ lymphocytes and epstein-barr virus is lymphocytotropic for b lymphocytes.

***Lymphoid.*** Referring to lymphocytes or to tissues that contain large accumulations of lymphocytes (e.g. spleen, lymph nodes, thymus).

***Lymphoid Tissue (Lymphatic Tissue).*** The vertebrate tissue that is responsible for the production of lymphocytes and occurs in the form of diffuse or dense aggregations of lymphocytes. In some parts of the body, lymphoid tissue exists as identifiable organs, e.g. the tonsils, spleen, thymus, and lymph nodes, although in other areas, especially in the respiratory and gastrointestinal tracts, diffuse lymphoid aggregations occurs that are not structurally separated from the surrounding connective tissue.

***Lymphokine.*** Polypeptide (but not an immunoglobulin) secreted by lymphocytes that affects the functions of other cells. There are many lymphokines and they have a wide range of biological activity. The first lymphokine to be studied was the migration inhibitory factor (MIF). Well-characterized lymphokines include interleukin-2, interleukin-3, interferon-gamma, interleukin-4 and interleukin-5.

***Lymphokines.*** Generic name for a heterogeneous group of soluble, physiologically active factors ($M_r$=20,000-80,000), released by effector T lymphocytes when in contact with specific antigen. They are important in cell-mediated immunity, Lymphokines include macrophage inhibition factor (MIF), lymphocyte inhibition factor (LIF), inter-leukins, Y-interferon, specific macrophage arming factor (SMAF), chemotactic factors and cytotoxic factors.

***Lymphoma.*** Neoplastic growth of the lymphatic tissue. One form of this tumour common in Central Africa is Burkitt's Lymphoma; it involves monoclonal proliferation of B lymphocytes which follows from infection with epstein-barr virus (probably mosquito-borne). A chromosomal translocation near to the locus of the mgc oncogene on chromosome 8 is a frequent symptom in Burkitt's lymphoma.

***Lymphoma.*** Malignant tumor of lymphocytes (e.g. Burkitt's lymphoma, Hodgkin's disease).

***Lymphomatoid Granulomatosis.*** Distinctive, usually fatal, vasculitis of the lung of unknown cause. All types of pulmonary blood vessels are infiltrated by atypical lymphocytes and plasma cells, which exhibit frequent mitoses. Cavities form in the lung. Nodular vasculitis occurs less frequently in the skin, kidneys and nervous system.

***Lymphomatosis.*** Multiple lymphomas in various parts of the body. Lymphomatosis occurs in hodgkin's disease, avian leukosis, etc.

***Lymphopenia.*** Decreased number of lymphocytes in the blood.

***Lymphotoxin (LT).*** Protein secreted by activated T lymphocytes or lymphoid cell lines that have cytolytic and/or cytostatic properties for susceptible tumor cells or tissue culture cell lines, particularly the mouse fibroblast line L-929. LT is secreted following stimulation of T lymphocytes by antigen or mitogen. It kills target cells more slowly than do intact cytotoxic T lymphocytes. Human LT is a protein of 205 amino acid residues, including a signal sequence of 34 residues; it has one site for an N-linked oligosaccharide (asparagine at position 62). Mouse LT is composed of 202 amino acid residues, including a signal sequence of 33 residues, it has one site for an N-linked oligosaccharide (asparagine at position 60). Human and mouse LT have 74 percent amino acid sequence identity.

It has been proposed that lymphotoxin has a role in target cell damage by cytotoxic T lymphocytes, but this has not been clearly established. Target cells, which are killed by LT, do not have pores in their membranes, such as those induced by perforin or complement. Susceptible target cells bind LT with high affinity ($K_d \sim 1.5 \times 10^{-10}$ M) and internalize it. Even though receptor binding of LT occurs at 4°C, LT kills target cells at 37°C by disrupting unknown metabolic processes.

LT is approximately 30 percent identical in amino acid sequence to tumor necrosis factor (TNF). The gene for LT has been mapped to the major histocompatibility complex of mouse chromosome 17 and human chromosome 6. The gene encoding LT is closely linked to the gene encoding TNF; they are separated by approximately 1,100 nucleotides. LT has also been called TNFβ while tumor necrosis factor has been called TNFα.

***Lyon Effect.*** Random inactivation, early in development, of most of the gene loci on one of the two X chromosomes in each somatic cell of female mammals. This inactivated state persists stably in all the cell's descendants and can lead to mosaicism of traits encoded by genes on the X chromosome; the inactive chromosome appears as heterochromatin (condensed chromatin) and this heterochromatin is known as a Barr body. The effect was discovered by and named after Mary lyon, a British cytogeneticist.

***Lyon Hypothesis (Inactive X Hypothesis).*** Proposal advanced by Mary Lyon, suggesting that random inactivation of all but one of the X chromosomes in somatic cells of the female is the mechanism that achieves dosage compensation of X chromosomes in the homogametic sex of the mammal. Inactivates copies of the X chromosome form the barr bodies of the female nucleus.

***Lyonization.*** Term bases on an interpretation of certain genetic traits expressed in the female as if she were carrying an X-linked recessive gene in a hemizygous condition (e.g. a woman who suffers from haemophilia yet carries this normally recessive allele on only one X chromosome). The phenomenon is described as lyonization on the assumption that one of the two X chromosomes is preferentially condensed in most or all somatic tissues.

***Lysate.*** Product of cell lysis; often used to refer to a suspension of phage particles released by the lysis of host bacteria, or to a cell-free homogenate following the action of detergent or mechanical means to break the cells.

***Lysenkoism.*** School of genetics, which gained acceptance in the Soviet Union between 1932 and 1960s, based on ideas advanced by T.D. Lysenko. Lysenko, arguing from his work on vernalization in barley and other seeds (a process of chilling seeds prior to sowing, which may be necessary to achieve cropping of normally biennial plants in the same year as sowing) proposed that acquired characters could be inherited, that is that modifications to the phenotype due to environmental effects could become permanently established in the genotype, Lysenko eventually largely discarded the classical concept of the gene. There is little doubt that what was little more than 'pseudo-science' flourished in the Soviet Union because it appeared to fall in line with the Marxist doctrine of improvement of the individual through training and the correct environment.

***Lysin.*** Substance (e.g. bacterial toxins, antibodies plus complement) that brings about cell lysis. At one time, it was thought that only a particular type of antibody had the capability of sensitizing cells for complement-dependent lysis, but it is now known that many antibodies have this capability, providing that they can fix complement.

***Lysine (Lys).*** An amino acid, $H_2NCH_2CH_2CH_2CH_2CH(NH_2)COOH$, one of the 20 common amino acids occurring in proteins and an essential amino acid for man. Lysine is a precursor of the polyamine cadaverine.

***Lysis.*** The destruction of a cell, usually by rupture of its membrane. Under normal conditions lysis of cellular constituents of the body may be initiated by the cell itself or by phagocytes, which also lyse invading cells. Most bacteriophages cause lysis of their bacterial host cells after infection.

***Lysis.*** Dissolution of cells. In immunology, lysis usually refers to destruction of cells by antibodies and complement or by cytotoxic T lymphocytes.

***Lysogen.*** Bacterium carrying, in stable form, a complete set of bacteriophage genes. The phage DNA in the bacterium is called a prophage. Usually; as in the case of Lambda bacteriophage, the prophage is integrated into the bacterial chromosome. Sometimes, However, as in E. coli phage P1, the phage genes are carried as a plasmid. In a lysogen, expression of most of the phage genes is prevented by a phage-specific repressor protein. When a lysogen carrying an integrated prophage is induced by various environmental changes, the repressor is inactivated and a lytic cycle is initiated. The prophage is excised as a single segment of DNA, which replicates and produces active phage particles.

***Lysogenic Bacterium.*** Bacterium carrying a temperate phage as a prophage. In this state, the state of lysogeny, the bacterium grows normally and no vegetative production of phage occurs, but under the influence of agents such as ultraviolet light the state of lysogeny can be broken, with consequent phage multiplication and eventual cell lysis of the host.

***Lysogenic Conversion (Phage Conversion).*** Any phenotypic changes in a host bacterium when it carries a prophage in the state of lysogeny. In some cases no changes are detectable, but in others the synthetic or morphological properties of the host cell may be slightly altered. See Figure L.11 on next page.

***Lysogenic Virus.*** Virus capable of becoming a prophage by entering into a stable relationship with a lysogenic bacterium lambda phage can occur in either a temperate or virulent state in host bacteria, and in the former case it acts as a lysogenic virus. It is preferable to refer to such viruses as temperate, however.

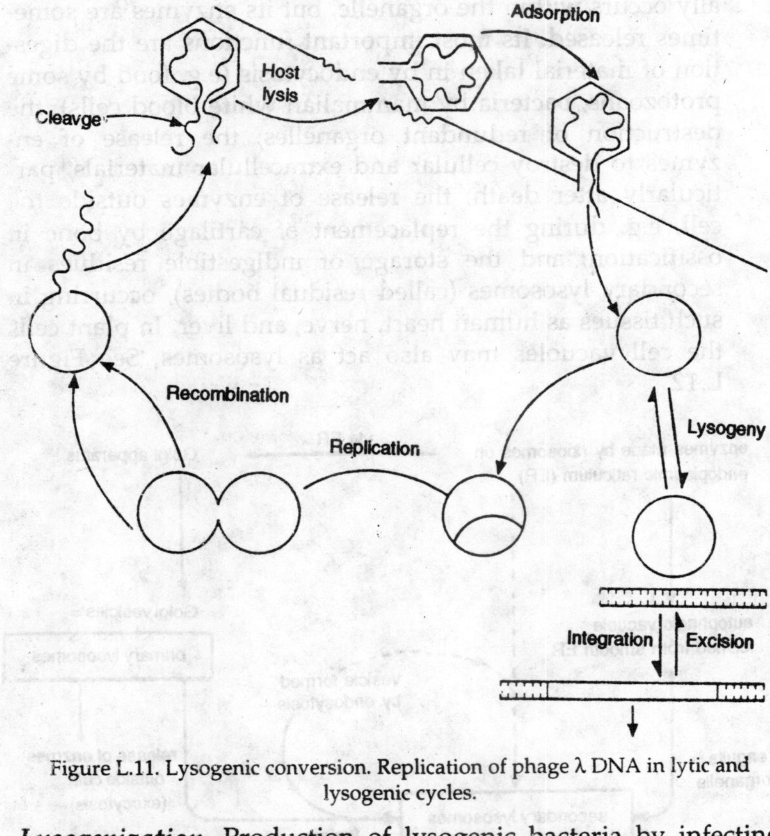


Figure L.11. Lysogenic conversion. Replication of phage λ DNA in lytic and lysogenic cycles.

***Lysogenization.*** Production of lysogenic bacteria by infecting them with a temperate phage.

***Lysogeny.*** Situation in which a temperate phage integrates into a bacterial genome as a prophage and thereby sets up a lysogenic state.

***Lysosome.*** An organelle of eukaryotes, bounded by a single membrane, that contains hydrolytic enzymes, such as acid phosphatases, proteases, nucleases, and lipases. In animal cells lysosomes are commonly 0.1-0.5 μm in diameter and have homogeneous contents. They are often derived from vesicles of the Golgi apparatus as shown in the diagrams. Lysosomes have many functions, mostly involving intracellular digestive (degradative) processes. Digestion usually occurs within the organelle, but its enzymes are sometimes released. Its most important functions are the digestion of material taken in by endocytosis (e.g. food by some protozoans, bacteria by mammalian white blood cells); the destruction of redundant organelles; the release of enzymes to destroy cellular and extracellular materials, particularly after death; the release of enzymes outside the cell, e.g. during the replacement of cartilage by bone in ossification; and the storage of indigestible residues in secondary lysosomes (called residual bodies), occurring in such tissues as human heart, nerve, and liver. In plant cells the cell vacuoles may also act as lysosomes. See Figure L.12.

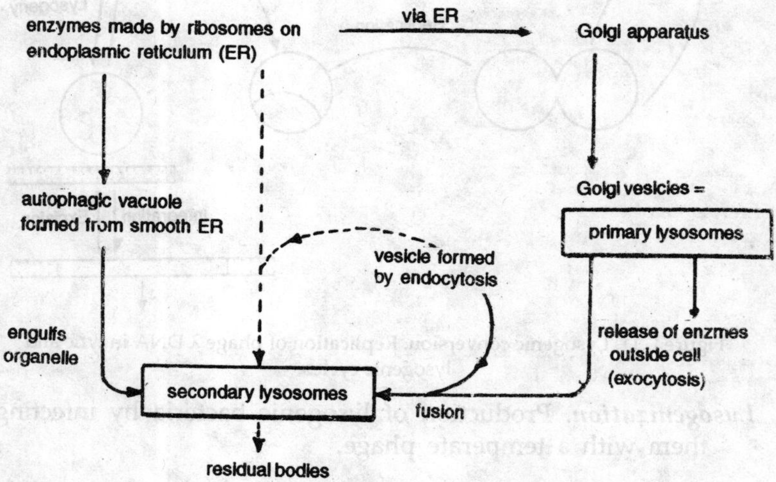


Figure L.12. Origin of lysosomes.

***Lysozyme (muramidase; peptidoglycan N-acetylmuramoylhydrolase; EC 3.2.1.17).*** Enzyme that hydrolyses the β-1,4 glycosidic bond between N-acetylmuramic acid and N-acetylglucosamine in the peptidoglycan (mucopeptide) of bacterial cell walls, leading to the osmotic lysis of bacteria. The usual turbidometric assay for lysozyme measures the decrease in absorbance of a suspension of Micrococcus luteus. With gram-negative bacteria, the outer membrane must be disrupted (e.g., by treatment with EDTA) to allow access of lysozyme to the underlying peptidoglycan layer. Lysozyme can potentiate the action of antibodies and complement on Gram-negative bacteria. It also enhances the phagocytic activity of mononuclear phagocytes and polymorphonuclear leukocytes.

Lysozyme is widely distributed, being found in bacteriophage, bacteria, fungi, plants, invertebrates and vertebrates. Four distinct classes of lysozyme have been described: (1) chicken-type lysozyme, typified by the enzyme from hen eggs (129 amino acids residues; $M_r$ 14,000); (2) goosetype lysozyme, found in nine different orders of birds (185 amino acid residues; $M_r$ 21,000); (3) phage-type lysozyme, described in T4, T2, and P22 bacteriophage (164 amino acid residues; $M_r$ 18,700); (4) a bacterial lysozyme produced by Streptomyces erythraeus. The amino acid sequences of lysozymes within one of these families are clearly related, but there is no significant overall homology among members of different families. However, similarities in the three-dimensional structure of the first three classes of lysozyme are consistent with the hypothesis that these enzymes have evolved from a common ancestor.

In vertebrates, lysozyme is found particularly in egg white, tears, saliva and mucus; it is also secreted by mononuclear phagocytes and is found in plasma. The mammalian lysozymes that have been characterized belong to the chicken-type lysozyme family. Lysozyme was the first protein to have both its amino acid sequence and three-dimensional structure determined. It has been used as a model antigen in many immunological studies.

*Lyt.* Alloantigen on the surface of mouse T lymphocytes. Since many Lyt antigens are found also on the surface of B lymphocytes, the term Ly is preferred for those also found on B lymphocytes. Lyt 2 and Lyt 3 are two polypeptide chains of mouse CD8.

***Lytic Growth.*** Development phase of a virulent phage during which the viruses multiply vegetatively and kill the host cells by lysis at the end of the growth cycle. Lytic growth occurs also following induction of a temperate phage.

***Lytic Response.*** Lysis of bacteria following their infection with virulent phage, in contrast to the lysogenic response.

***Lytic Virus.*** Virus that kills the host cells which it infects by causing cell lysis.

# M

***M13.*** Widely used cloning vector, single-stranded bacteriophage with a closed circular DNA genome. Since the product of replication of this phage, even when it carries an insert of some other gene, is a single-stranded DNA molecule, this implies that the molecules are readily used as a template for sequence analysis.

***Macroevolution.*** Evolutionary pathway or pattern viewed over a long geological time span. The evolutionary development of taxa above the species level are generally regarded as falling within this subject area.

***Macroglobulin.*** High molecules weight ($M_r$ >400,000) globulin (e.g., IgM, alpha-2 macroglobulin).

***Macroglobulinemia of Waldenstrom.*** Form of myelomatosis occurring mainly in elderly males and characterized by monoclonal IgM in the serum. In contrast to multiple myeloma, skeletal lesions do not occur. The bone marrow contains increased numbers of lymphoid cells and plasmacytoid lymphocytes, which contain cytoplasmic IgM. The elevated levels of IgM in blood increase its relative viscosity; symptoms of circulatory failure appear when the relative viscosity increases more than approximately fourfold. Anemia, cutaneous hemorrhages and diverse neurological symptoms are the most common manifestations of macroglobulinemia. Macroglobulinemia of waldenstrom is a more benign disease than multiple myeloma.

***Macromere.*** Group of large cells that are produced in unequal cell divisions during early embryogenesis in such animals as sea urchins and molluscs.

***Macromolecule.*** Molecule with a molecular weight upwards of a few thousand daltons. Most proteins and nucleic acids and many polysaccharides are macromolecules.

***Macronucleus (Meganucleus).*** Larger of two distinct sizes of nuclei occurring in ciliated protozoa. These nuclei are highly polyploid and are essentially responsible for vegetative growth, whereas the much smaller micronuclei (absent in the cells of some ciliate strains) have important sexual functions during conjugation.

***Macrophage.*** Highly differentiated mononuclear phagocyte found in various tissues. Macrophages are more mature than monocytes.

***Macrophages.*** Group of several cell types that together form the reticuloendothelial system of metazoan organisms. Cells of this system have the common property of.

***Macrophage.*** A motile phagocytic cell, found throughout vertebrate tissues, that can be identified by its ability to store certain vital dyes, e.g. trypan blue and Indian ink. Macrophages occur principally as resting cells in connective tissue, in the spleen and lymph nodes, in the endothelial lining of blood vessels and sinusoids of bone marrow, in the liver, adrenal glands, and the anterior lobe of the pituitary, and in the blood as monocytes.

***Macrophage-Activating Factor (MAF).*** Lymphokine that activates macrophages. The major MAF is interferon-gamma.

***Main Band.*** In density gradient separation of genomic DNA, a broad peak containing most of the DNA and excluding any visible satellite DNA bands.

***Major Histocompatibility Complex (MHC).*** Region of vertebrate chromosomes initially discovered through its control of immunological rejection of organ transplants and now known to mediate control of nearly all aspects of the immune response. The genes making up the MHC are present on chromosomes 6 and 17 in man and mouse, respectively, and code for glycoproteins present on surface of cells.

***Major Histocompatibility Complex (MHC).*** Chromosomal region containing genes that encode cell surface glycoproteins that regulate interactions among cells of the immune system. These genes were discovered because of their role in immunologic rejection of grafts. The MHC typically contains genes encoding class I histocompatibility molecules and class II histocompatibility molecules, which are important for the growth and differentiation of B and T lymphocytes, antigen presentation, cytotoxicity, graft rejection and mixed lymphocyte reactions. The genes encoding these molecules are the most highly polymorphic genes known. The MHC also contains genes encoding proteins that are not cell surface glycoproteins; class III molecules (components of the complement system (C2, C4 and factor B) and P-450 cytochrome 21-hydroxylase), tumor necrosis factor and lymphotoxin. An MHC has been identified in anuran amphibians, birds and mammals. The best studied MHCs are those of mice and humans. In mice the MHC consists of the H-2 complex and occupies 0.5-1 centiMorgan of chromosome 17. In humans the MHC consists of the HLA complex and occupies about 1.5-2.0 centiMorgans of the short arms of chromosome 6.

***Malaria.*** Disease caused by the single-celled parasite Plasmodium falciparum. Geographical areas of major incidence of the disease correspond closely with the distribution of sickle cell anaemia. It is believed that the prevalence of the latter disease may be explained because individuals who are heterozygous for the sickle cell allele are more resistant to malaria and are therefore selected for in the population.

***Malate.*** Carbon compound that is one of the final stages of the citric acid cycle.

***Male Gametophyte.*** In higher plants, the pollen grain plus the pollen tube, containing three haploid nuclei.

***Male Pronucleus.*** Nucleus of the male gamete.

***Malignancy.*** Attribute of cancerous neoplasms when they display characteristics of invasiveness and spread by metastasis. Neoplasms or tumours are not necessarily malignant and when not, they are termed benign.

***Maloney Leukaemia Virus.*** Mouse retrovirus that produces a lymphocytic leukaemia. Newborn mice can be infected with the virus via the milk from an infected female mouse.

***Malpighian Layer (stratum Malpighii).*** The layer of cells in the vertebrate epidermis that lies adjacent to the basement membrane. It consists of two distinct cell layers: (1) the lower stratum germinativum (stratum basale), whose cells are usually in active mitosis and are continually migrating towards the surface, and (2) the overlying stratum spinosum, whose cells contain fine keratin filaments. The cells of the Malpighian layer often contain granules of the pigment melanin, which is responsible for skin colour.

***Malpighian Tubules.*** Slender blind-ending excretory tubes opening into the alimentary canal near the junction of the midgut and hindgut in the Arachnida, Insecta, Chilopoda (centipedes), and Diplopoda (millipedes). They lie in the haemocoel and extract from the blood the excretory products (mainly uric acid) that pass into the hindgut and exit with the faeces. The number of Malpighian tubules varies from two to about 150.

***Malthus.*** English social economist who in 1798 published 'An Essay on the Principle of Population', in which he predicted wide-spread world famine as a result of suggested increases in the future world human population.

***Maltose.*** A disaccharide consisting of two glucose molecules in a glycosidic link. Maltose is formed in the enzymic degradation of starch and occurs in germinating cereal seeds, especially barley. See Figure M.1.

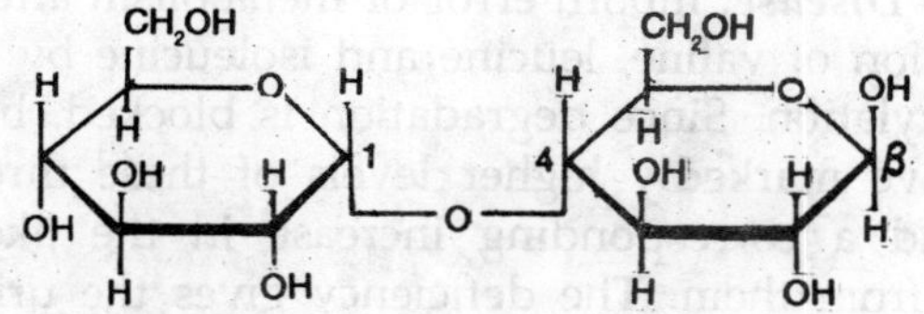


Figure M.1. β-maltose.

***Mammary Gland.*** The milk-producing gland that is characteristic of all female mammals. One or more pairs of these glands develop on the ventral surface of the body and are thought to have evolved from sweat glands. Although the state of the gland fluctuates during the oestrous cycle, its complete development and functioning generally occurs only after parturition, for the purpose of suckling the young. The mature gland consists of several lobes of multiple branching ducts embedded in fatty tissue. The ducts lead from numerous alveoli of milk-secreting cells and in most mammals drain into sinuses that open to the exterior via pores at the nipple. In the Monotremata nipples are absent and the milk is secreted directly from the sinuses onto the surface of the body.

***Mammary Tumour Virus.*** Retrovirus causing mammary tumours in mice and transmissable from mother to offspring via milk.

***Mannitol.*** Polyhydric alcohol derived from mannose of fructore. It is a white crystal line powder with a sweet taste and is widely distributed in plants and fungi.

***Mannose.*** Aldose; an epimer of glucose.

***Mantoux Text.*** Test for cell-mediated immunity to tuberculosis in which tuberculin is injected intradermally.

***MAP (Microtubule-Associated Proteins).*** Proteins ($M_r$=200,000-300,000); accessory proteins to tubulin and induce tubulin polymerization in microtubules.

***Map Distance.*** Distance between two gene loci expressed as morgan units or some other representation of a map unit.

***Maple Syrup Disease.*** Inborn error or metabolism affecting the degradation of valine, leucine and isoleucine by oxidative decarboxylation. Since degradation is blocked, blood and urine have markedly higher levels of these three amino acids and a corresponding increase in the βketo acids derived from them. The deficiency gives the urine of affected patients an odour of maple syrup. Unless affected individuals are placed on a diet low in these amino acids early in life the disease normally proves fatal.

***Map Unit.*** Measure of distance between the loci of two linked genes, that is two genes on the same chromosome. The map unit is generally regarded as being equivalent to 1 centimorgan (i.e. one-hundredth of a morgan unit) which corresponds to recombination frequency of 1 percent between the two genes.

***Marfan's Syndrome (Arachnodactylyl).*** Disorder of connective tissue in the human, inherited as an autosomal dominant. The disease is characterized by extremely long fingers and toes, and has a prevalence of approximately one in 20000.

***Marker.*** (1) Molecules of known size or identity that are run on electrophoretic gels to provide an indication of the expected position of other equivalent molecules of proteins or nucleic acid. (2) Molecules used to identify particular classes of lymphocytes by acting as specific antigenic conjugants. (3) Gene, with a characteristic phenotypic expression and a known chromosomal location, used to provide a point of reference in determining the mapping position of other genes. (4) Characteristic of a cell or cell line that enables separate cell identities to be established in mixed cell tissues. Particular staining properties, or nuclear or nucleolar characteristics, or ever an aberrant mitotic chromosome, may serve to identify the cells of a cell line. Thus, if marked quail cells are injected or transplanted into a chick embryo, the destiny of the implanted or injected cells may be followed in tissue sections if the quail cells carry a marker such as an enlarged nucleolus.

***Marker Rescue.*** Phenomenon in which a population of bacteria is infected with two distinct 'marked' phages (i.e. two types that can be genetically distinguished), but following the irradiation of one of the two phage strains. Because of recombination, some of the surviving page come to possess properties of the irradiated strain.

***Masked mRNA.*** Messenger RNA present in a cell, but not being actively translated into protein. Masked mRNA is associated with particular types of proteins as messenger ribonucleoprotein (mRNP) particles and can be activated to function in protein synthesis by specific physiological triggers (e.g. hormones).

***Mast Cell.*** Cell type found in connective tissue and characterized by basophilic cytoplasm and storage of compounds such as heparin and histamine. During inflammatory and immune responses, these substances may be released from mast cells in the form of secretory granules.

***Mast Cell.*** Cell found in connective tissues, especially around blood vessels and under mucosal surfaces, characterized by the presence of numerous basophilic granules. Mast cells are important in meditating immediate hypersensitivity reactions. Mast cells have Fc receptors for IgE. Cross-linking by antigen of IgE bound to Fe receptors triggers the release of granules from mast cells. Other methods of cross-linking the Fce receptors (e.g., by anti-IgE, anti-idiotype or antibody to the receptor) also trigger granule release. The granules contain preformed mediators of immediate hypersensitivity : Histamine and/or serotonin (depending on the species), several enzymes (e.g., hexosaminidase, aryl sulphatase, glucuronidase, chymotrypsin, trypsin-like protease) and chemotactic factors for eosinophils and neutrophils. Cross-linking of fce receptors also induces the synthesis and release of leukotrienes, prostaglandins and platelet-activating factor. The release of granules is an energy-dependent reaction that requires $Ca^{2+}$. Biochemical events that accompany mediator release include activation of adenylate cyclase, resulting in a rapid burst of cyclic AMP synthesis, activation of a protein kinase, methylation of phospholipids and activation of a serine esterase.

In addition, mast cells of the gastrointestinal and respiratory mucosa contain chondroitin sulfate; they synthesize and release mainly leukotriene $C_4$. Mast cells in connective tissue contain heparin; they synthesize and release mainly prostaglandin $D_2$.

***Mast Cell Growth Factor-1.*** Synonym for interleukin-3.

***Master Cell Growth Factor-2.*** Synonym for interleukin-4.

***Master Gene.*** Gene that controls other genes, particularly when the genes controlled are all expressed characteristically in a particular type of differentiated cell.

***Master-Slave Hypothesis.*** Proposal made by H.G. Callan that most eukaryotic genes existed in multiple identical copies (the slaves) and that the sequences were all kept identical by frequent correction, using a 'single master' copy of the gene as a template for correction of the 'slave' copies. Apart from possible correction mechanisms in ribosomal gene copies, the hypothesis has not been substantiated by the evidence.

***Mastigonemes.*** Short hairs that project laterally from some eukaryotic flagella, usually in one or two rows. Some mastigonemes are relatively stiff and hollow, others are flexible but solid, the two types occurring in different organisms.

***Masugi Nephritis.*** Glomerulonephritis induced in experimental animals by injection of antibodies to the glomerular basement membrane. Antibodies are produced in one species by immunization with basement membranes from kidneys of the species of the prospective recipient (e.g., rats develop glomerulonephritis when injected with rabbit antibodies to rat glomerular basement membrane). The antibodies circulate briefly, bind to the glomeruli and produce injury, with an increase in glomerular permeability and infiltration of neutrophils and monocytes. masugi nephritis has been used extensively to study the mechanism of tissue injury induced by antibodies. Good-pasture's syndrome, an autoimmune disease of humans, resembles Masugi nephritis.

***Mate Killer.*** Cell of paramecium aurelia that kills or seriously harms a non-killer (sensitive) cell with which it conjugates. The killing property derives from the presence of mu-particles within the cell.

***Maternal Effects.*** Effects of the phenotype or genotype of the mother on the phenotype of immediate offspring, generally of an impermanent nature. Thus maternally derived protein or messenger RNA stored in the egg leads to maternal effects in some early embryos.

***Maternal Immunity.*** Immunity acquired passively by a newborn from its mother (e.g., by ingestion of colostrum or transplacental passage of antibodies). Maternal immunity, is, in fact, passive immunity of the neonate and not immunity in mothers.

***Maternal Inheritance.*** Genetic effects that are transmitted via the maternal line. There are many such effects, some resulting from the purely maternal origin of mitochondria or chloroplasts, others from effects on the phenotype of the embryo by early development within the female, such as the maternal influence on coiling in snails. See Figure M.2 on next page.

***Mating.*** Sexual reproduction between pairs of organisms of two distinct sexual types.

***Mating System.*** Pattern of reproduction within a species, sometimes involving sex ratios different from 1:1, sometimes involving changes in individual sex with time or circumstance, sometimes involving total parthenogenesis and complete absence of mating for part or all of the annual cycle.

***Mating Type.*** Either of the two strains of a heterothallic fungus that are needed for fertilization to take place. Since the two mating types and their gametes are morphologically identical, they are designated plus and minus rather than male and female.

***Mating Type Gene.*** Sequence that controls the choice between two mating types known as α and a; best known in the yeast Sac-charomyces. Haploid yeast cells occasionally switch their mating type. At a genetic level such a switch has been shown to involve excision of a particular mating type gene sequence from the genome, with its replacement by a gene of the alternative mating type. This process has come to be referred to as a cassette mechanism.

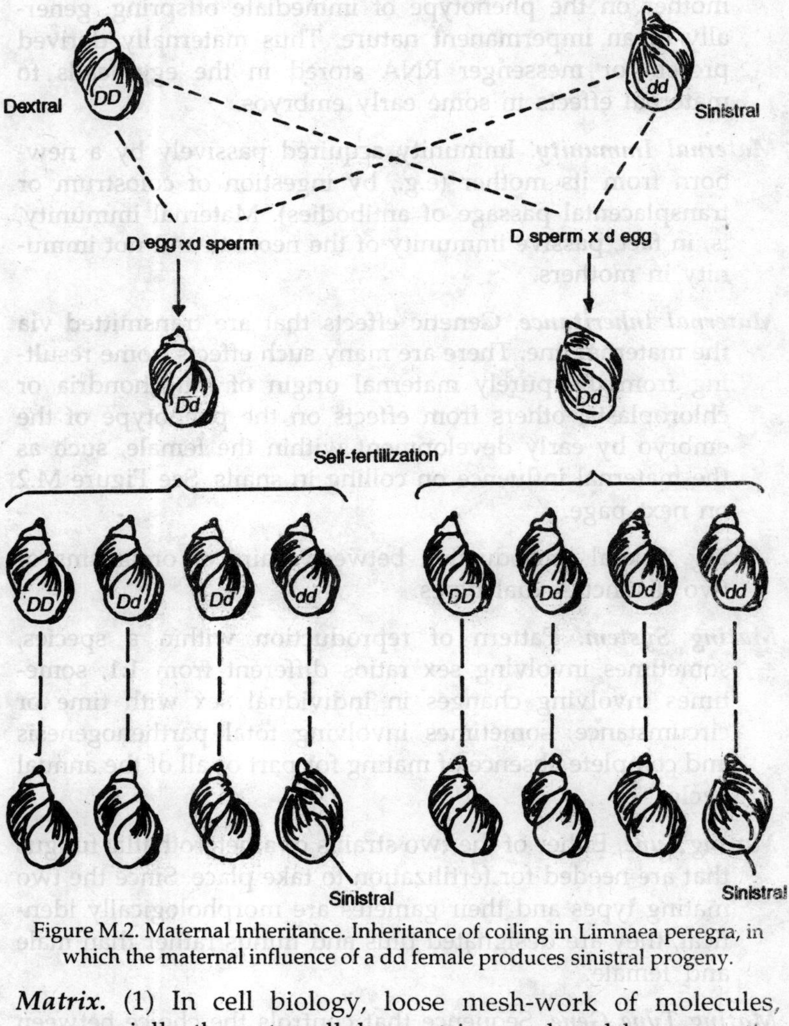


Figure M.2. Maternal Inheritance. Inheritance of coiling in Limnaea peregra, in which the maternal influence of a dd female produces sinistral progeny.

***Matrix.*** (1) In cell biology, loose mesh-work of molecules, especially the extracellular matrix, produced by many tissue cells. This complex of proteins and polysaccharides is especially important in connective tissue, which is the main constituent of skin and bone. Cell walls of bacteria, fungi and plants are also examples of extracellular matrices. (2) Filter or other absorbent material used as a sterile surface or three-dimensional area for cell growth in tissue culture.

***Matrocliny.*** Situation in which offspring resemble the female parent more closely than the male parent. In Drosophila, an example is afforded by daughters of attached X females.

***Maturase.*** Protein that catalyses the removal of introns. It is likely that such proteins are not enyzmes, but act as factors that modify the activity of the splicing enzymes. Many maturases are themselves products of the sequences whose correct splicing they help to control, and at least some are coded on introns (e.g., maturases found in yeast mitochondria).

***Maturation Division.*** Nuclear division during which the chromosomal complement of a nucleus is adjusted to some desired amount. Thus the divisions involved in meiotic divisions to produce haploid gametes are maturation divisions.

***Maturation of Affinity.*** Progressive increase in the affinity of antibodies that often occurs after immunization.

***Maxicell.*** Cell of E. coli or other bacteria that has been UV-irradiated, but still retains some genomic DNA. It has multiple copies of plasmids, thus facilitating studies on plasmid transcription.

***Maximum Permissible Dose.*** Maximum level of ionizing radiation that present safety standards permit over a unit period.

***M13 Bacteriophage.*** Filamentous bacterio-phage of E. coli containing a single-stranded circular DNA molecule 6,407 nucleotides in length. M 13 is a male-specific phage; only strains of bacteria harboring F pili are infected. When viral DNA enters the bacterial host cell, it is converted to a double-stranded replicative form (RF). The RF multiplies rapidly until there are about 100 Rf molecules per cell. Replication of the RF then becomes asymmetric; only one of the two DNA strands is produced in large amount and this becomes complexes to a single-strand-specific DNA binding protein. As the DNA single strands are released from the cell, the DNA binding protein is replaced by a capsid protein. Phage particles - as many as 1,000 per cell per generation-are extruded from infected cells into the medium. Replication of phage DNA does not result in lysis of the host cell. Instead, infected cells continue to grow and divide, although more slowly than uninfected cells. The inhibition in growth of infected cells leads to the appearance of tůrbid plaques on a bacterial lawn.

M13 bacteriophage have been widely used as cloning vectors. A major advantage is that the DNA can be obtained easily either in the single-stranded or double-stranded form. The double-stranded replicative form (isolated from the bacterial cell) can be used just like plasmid DNA to make recombinants in vitro; the single-stranded DNA (from phage particles) can be used directly as template for DNA sequencing by the dideoxy-chain termination method. Another advantage of filamentous phages like M 13 is that they are not fixed in length and can accommodate variable amounts of DNA; this flexibility is very useful in a cloning vector. A large number of vectors based on M 13 have been developed.

***McArdle Disease.*** Hereditary disease in the human resulting from a deficiency of glycogen phosphorylase in skeletal muscle, the gene for which is encoded on chromosome 11. The disease involves glycogen storage and has a frequency of about one in 500 000.

***M Cell.*** Epithelial cell of the gastrointêstinal tract that transports macromolecules and microorganisms (e.g., viruses) from the lumen to the underlying Peyer's patches. M cells have broad apical surfaces with short micro-villi. Macromolecules and microorganisms bind to the microvilli, are taken up into coated pits and are transported to the basolateral surface. The basolateral surfaces are deeply invaginated and the invaginations are filled with lymphocytes and mononuclear phagocytes. Substances, transported through M cells, are exposed on the basolateral surfaces, where they can be sampled by lymphoid cells, and presumably, initiate an immune response.

***Mcg Isotypic Determinant.*** Antigenic determinant of human immunoglobulin lambda chains, associated with asparagine at position 112, threonine at position 114, and lysine at position 163. This determinant is present on some of the lambda chains of every individual. It is, therefore, not the result of genetic polymorphism.

***McLeod Phenotype.*** Absence of Kell or Cellano antigens on red blood cells. The red blood cells appear under the microscope to have spikes or burrs (acanthocytes). The Xk, gene, which encodes a precursor of the Kell or Cellano antigens, is closely linked to the gene for chronic granulomatous disease on the short arm of the X chromosome. Hence, deletion in this chromosomal region (Xp21) may result in the McLeod phenotype and chronic-granulomatous disease.

***Megakaryocyte.*** Very large cells (35-160 μm in diameter) of the bone marrow, from which platelets are derived. The cytoplasm of megakaryocytes forms filamentous arms that break up into platelets.

***Megakaryocyte.*** Amoeboid giant cell found in the bone marrow. It contains a large, multinucleolate, polymorphous nucleus. Derived from haemocytoblasts, megakaryocytes probably give rise to blood platelets, the formation of which is seen in the megakaryocyte cytoplasm.

***Megaphyll (Macrophyll).*** One of two types of leaves found in pteridophytes (which includes plants such as ferns). Leaves of angiosperms and gymnosperms are sometimes also designated as megaphylles.

***Megaspore*** One of the four products of the meiotic division of the megasporocyte in angiosperm plants. Three out of the four haploid megaspores do not survive, whereas the fourth divides to form the female embryo sac or gametophyte.

***Megasporocyte.*** Megaspore mother cell of angiosperm plants. Meiotic division of this cell gives rise to the megaspores, one of which develops into the embryo sac.

***Meiosis (reduction division).*** The process by which a nucleus divides into four daughter nuclei, each containing half the number of chromosomes of the parent nucleus. Meiosis has two functions: firstly the reduction of the chromosome number from diploid to haploid, and secondly the exchange of genetic material by the process of .crossing over, allowing genetic diversity to be produced. There are two successive divisions, known as division I and division II. Each division may be divided into four stages, which are not distinct and grade into each other. The first stage (prophase) of the first divisions is subdivided into five phases. In the first phase, leptotene, the chromosomes appear as thin threads that are not divided into two chromatids and have a visible centromere. This is followed by zygotene, when homologous chromosomes are attracted to each other and come together. They pair, forming a bivalent, starting at one end and zipping up like a zip fastener, a process known as pairing (or synapsis). Zygotene is followed by pachytene, when the chromosomes become shorter and thicker by coiling; they also coil around each other and each divides into two chromatids. In diplotene crossing over occurs; breaks occurs in homologous chromatids due to the strain of their coiling; they then join up crosswise with the chromatid of the homologous chromosome. This grades into diakinesis, when the chromatids of homologous chromosomes, no longer attracted to each other, try to move apart but are held together at the point where they crosses over. This point, known as a chiasma, appears as a visible cross. By the end of prophase, the nucleolus and nuclear membrane have broken down and in animals and lower plants a spindle is organized in the cytoplasm by the centrioles. In the second stage (metaphase) of division I, the bivalents orientate themselves on the spindle. Their centromeres come to lie on either side of the equatorial plate and equidistant from it. The homologous chromosomes strain to separate but are held together by their chiasmata, which may begin to slip towards the ends of the chromosomes, a process known as terminalization. This stage is followed by anaphase, when the spindle contracts and elongates. The pairs of homologous centromeres finally separate and move towards their respective

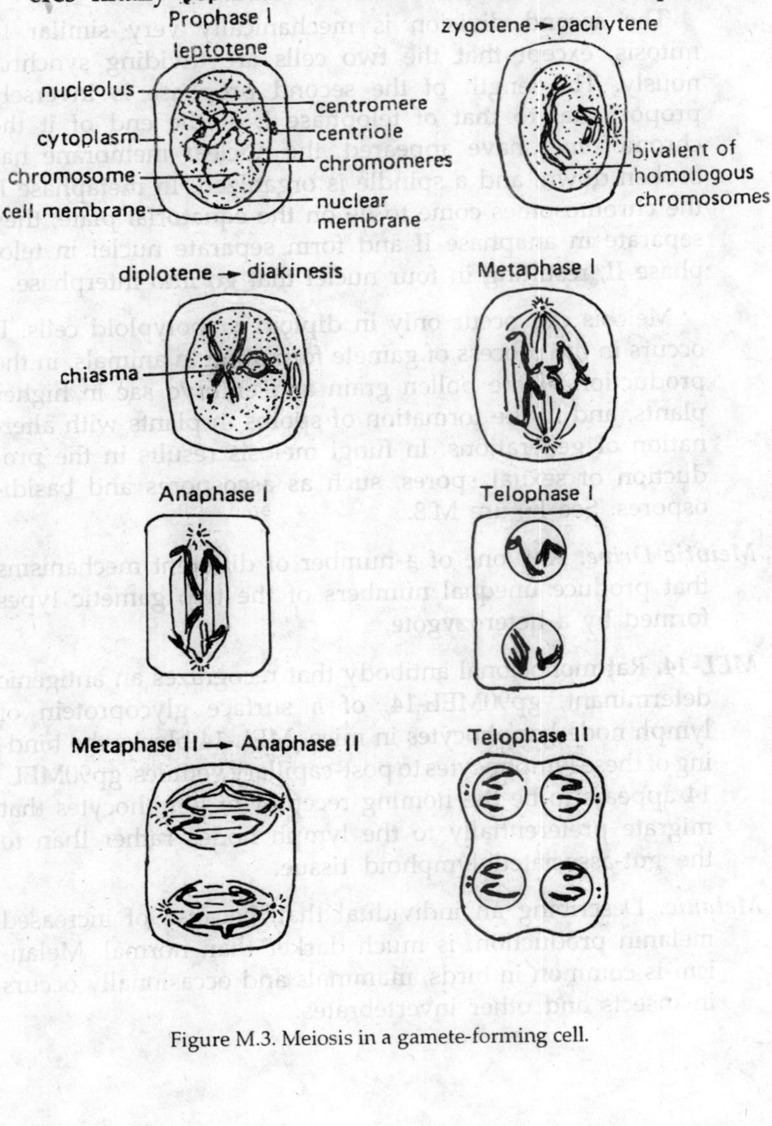


Figure M.3. Meiosis in a gamete-forming cell.

poles, pulling the rest of the chromosome after them. Telophase follows, during which the spindle disperses and a nuclear membrane usually forms around each group of half-bivalents. The length of telophase varies in different species: two complete interphase nuclei may form and cell division may occur, or telophase may be very short with only partial elongation of the chromosomes.

The second division is mechanically very similar to mitosis, except that the two cells are dividing synchronously. The length of the second prophase is inversely proportional to that of telophase I; at the end of it the chromosomes have appeared, the nuclear membrane has broken down, and a spindle is organized. In metaphase II the chromosomes come to lie on the equatorial plate; they separate in anaphase II and form separate nuclei in telophase II, resulting in four nuclei that go into interphase.

Meiosis can occur only in diploid or polyploid cells. It occurs in the process of gamete formation in animals, in the production of the pollen grain and embryo sac in higher plants, and in the formation of spores in plants with alternation of generations. In fungi meiosis results in the production of sexual spores, such as ascospores and basidiospores. See Figure M.3.

***Meiotic Drive.*** Any one of a number of different mechanisms that produce unequal numbers of the two gametic types formed by a heterozygote.

***MEL-14.*** Rat monoclonal antibody that recognizes an antigenic determinant, gp90MEL-14, of a surface glycoprotein of lymph node lymphocytes in mice. MEL-14 blocks the binding of these lymphocytes to post-capillary venules. gp90MEL-14 appears to be the homing receptor of lymphocytes that migrate preferentially to the lymph nodes rather than to the gut-associated lymphoid tissue.

***Melanic.*** Describing an individual that, because of increased melanin production, is much darker than normal. Melanism is common in birds, mammals and occasionally occurs in insects and other invertebrates.

***Melanin.*** One of the pigments occurring in the hair, skin, integument, etc., of many animals. It is contained in melanophores and consists of complex polymers of tyrosine derivatives and proteins, either eumelanins (brown or black) or phaeomelanins (yellow, orange, or red).

***Melanism.*** The existence, in a population of animals, of individuals that are black (melanic) due to excessive production of the pigment melanin. For example, the black panther is a melanic form of leopard. Several species of moths exist in a melanic form.

***Melanocyte.*** Pigment cell containing melanin granules.

***Melanocyte-Stimulating Hormone (MSH, Intermedin).*** One of several peptide hormones that stimulate pigment cells. They are secreted by the pars intermedia of the mammalian pituitary gland and by homologous structures in other vertebrates. Two types, structurally resembling the N-terminal portion of ACTH, have been isolated from a number of species, α-MSH (13 amino acid residues) is present in most mammals but is thought not to be secreted into the blood in significant amounts. Since the early 1960s various β-MSHs (18-22 amino acid residues) have been described and measured in the blood. The precise role of MSH in mammals remains to be established, but in lower vertebrates it regulates changes in skin colour by acting on the chromatophores, as was first shown in Amphibia by Hogben in 1922. The best-known action of MSH is on the dispersion of melanin in melanophores, an effect mediated by cyclic AMP. The production and secretion of MSH is under hypothalamic control.

***Melanoma.*** Tumour caused by excessive growth of melanocytes. Non-invasive tumours of melanocytes include moles, whereas malignant melanomas are noted for their efficient metastatic spread.

***Melanosome.*** Intracellular organelle of melanocytes containing melanin and tyrosinase aggregates.

***Melanotic Tumour.*** Tumour that contains melanin. One melanotic tumour in Drosophila consists of an aggregation of blackened cells at various developmental stages and results from melanization of haemocyte-encapsulated cells.

***Melatonin.*** A substance synthesized from serotonin and secreted mainly by the vertebrate pineal gland. It causes melanin to be less widely dispersed in dermal melanophores, as was first demonstrated in 1917, when pineal glands fed to tadpoles resulted in extreme lightening of the skin. It is also implicated in reproductive function and the photoperiodic regulation of the gonads. Melatonin was isolated and identified as the active principle of beef pineals in 1958. See Figure M.4.

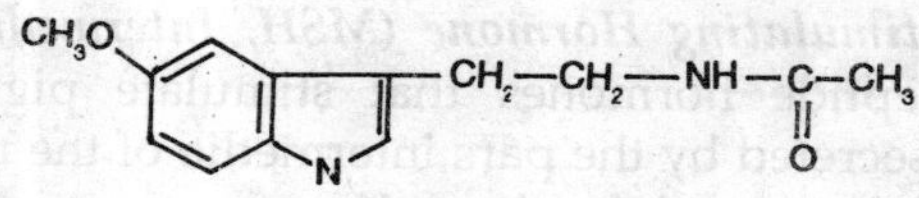


Figure M.4. Melatonin.

***Melphalan.*** (1-phenylalanine mustard). Nitrogen mustard used for the treatment of multiple myeloma. See Figure M.5.

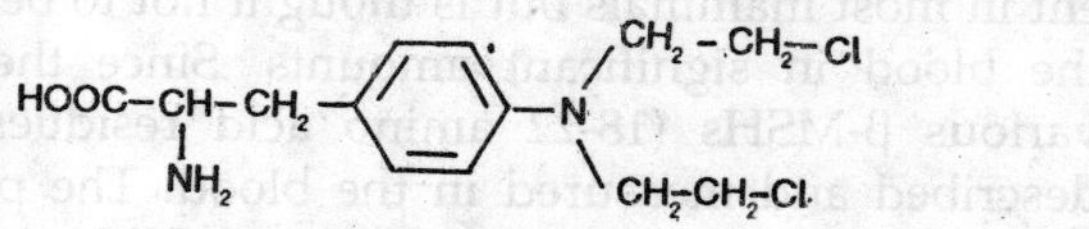


Figure M.5. Melphalan.

***Melting-Out Temperature.*** Temperature at which nuclei acid duplexes of DNA-DNA or DNA-RNA melt by breakage of the hydrogen bonds between the complementary molecules.

***Melting Profile.*** Profile, commonly represented on a graph, showing the percentage of a given sample of DNA that melts in a specific time on a gradually increasing temperature scale. Since some DNA, such as imprecisely base-paired sequences, low-molecular-weight material, and molecules rich in AT bases, will melt out at lower temperatures than other DNA, some useful information can be derived from melting profiles.

***Membrane.*** Biological membranes (the plasma membrane, mitochondrial membranes, the membranes of the endoplasmic reticulum and of the nucleus) show the same basic structure: a lipid bilayer with which proteins are associated. The lipid bilayer is formed by the orientation of the individual phospholipid molecules with their non-polar, hydrophobic, fatty acid chains towards the centre of the membrane and with their polar, hydrophilic sections towards the cytoplasm or extracellular compartment, both of which are aqueous. Proteins associated with the membrane have been classified as integral (intrinsic) or peripheral (extrinsic), according to the degree of their association with the membrane. Some proteins are distributed asymmetrically; some proteins span the membrane. Membrane proteins perform a variety of functions: hormone receptors; membrane-bound enzymes, membrane transport molecules. Some of the proteins which are associated with the membrane are not held rigidly in place and can move laterally within the membrane. Thus the membrane is described as having a fluid mosaic structure.

***Membrane Attack Complex (MAC).*** Amphiphilic macromolecular complex composed of one molecule each of C5b, C6, C7 and C8 and 12 or more molecules of C9. MAC formation is the end result of activation by the classical pathway or the alternative pathway of complement. The MAC inserts into the membrane of target cells and kills them.

When C5 is cleaved by C5 convertases, the C5b, which is formed, has a metastable binding site for C6 and C7. Complexes of C5b, C6 and C7 appear, under the electron microscope, like a leaf on a stalk, the leaf being composed of C5b and the stalk of C6 and C7. These complexes are embedded in the target cell membrane without inflicting any damage. C8 then binds to the C5b67 complex; a transmembrane channel (pore) is formed, 3 nm in diameter. The C5b678 complex can cause lysis of target cells, albeit very slowly. The process of lysis is rapidly accelerated, in the presence of $Ca^{2}+$, $Mg^{2+}$or $Zn^{2+}$, by the polymerization of C9 forms a cylindrical structure, 16nm in height, with an internal diameter of 10nm; the wall of the cylinder is 2nm thick. The top of the cylinder is hydrophilic and is capped by a ring or an annulus, which remains outside the target cells; the other end of the cylinder is lipophilic, becomes embedded in the target cells; and forms transmembrane channels. This causes a micellar rearrangement of the lipid bilayer; the pores coalesce into so-called 'leaky patches;. The target cell loses potassium, imbibes sodium and water, swells and bursts (lyses). The entire series of events leading to lysis is non-enzymatic. S protein inhibits MAC formation.

***Membrane Conductance.*** Transport of ions through proteins channels in the lipid bilayer of cell plasma membranes.

***Membrane Immunoglobulin.*** Immunoglobulin that is inserted into a cell membrane and that may function as a receptor for antigen. Membrane IgM and membrane IgD are expressed on unstimulated B lymphocytes. After the B cell interacts with antigen, the cell differentiates into a plasma cell, which actively secretes IgM. The switch from membrane to secreted IgM is accompanied by an increase in the synthesis of J chain. Secreted IgM is a pentamer (five four-chain units), whereas membrane-bound IgM is a monomer (a single four-chain unit). Presumably, all immunoglobulins exists in a membrane form (mIg) as well as a secreted form (sIg). Membrane immunoglobulins of the IgG and IgA classes are thought to function as antigen receptors on memory B lymphocytes. The portion of the immunoglobulin that is inserted into the membrane is a hydrophobic segment of the heavy chain near its carboxy-terminus; there is no known difference in the light chains of membrane and secreted immunoglobulins.

Information about the heavy chains of membrane immunoglobulins has been derived mainly by analysis of the genes encoding these chains. For a given isotype, the membrane form of the heavy chain is longer that the secreted form, the two differing at their carboxy-terminal ends. The two forms of heavy chain are encoded by different mRNA species that are derived from a single gene. It is thought that competition between splicing of the $CH_4MI$ intron and polyadenylation at a site within the inttron determines which of the two mRNAs is produced. The transcript for the membrane-bound chain is longer than that for the secreted chains and includes sequences from one or two exons that encode the carboxy-terminal portion that is specific for the membrane form. (Usually there are two such exons but, in the case of the mouse alpha chain, there is only one.) This longer transcript is processed so that the termination site of the mRNA for the secreted form is removed and the terminal $C_H$ exon is spliced to the first membrane exon.

Analysis of a number of genes encoding membrane-associated heavy chains has revealed that the carboxyl-terminal segments, which are unique to the membrane forms of the heavy chains range in length from 41 amino acid residues (mouse and human membrane mu chain to 72 residues (mouse membrane epsilon chain). These segments can be divided into three regions: (1) an acidic spacer (12-26 amino acid residues) at the amino-terminal end, which connects the terminal $C_H$ domain to the transmembrane segment; this spacer is thought to be external to the membrane; (2) a hydrophobic transmembrane segment consisting of 26 amino acid residues, which presumably spans the

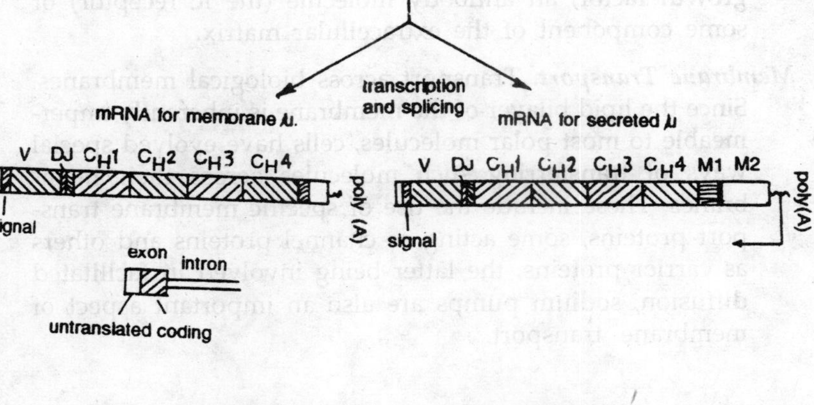


Figure M.6. Membrame immunogllobulin.

lipid bilayer; this segment is highly conserved in mouse and human membrane heavy chains; (3) a hydrophilic carboxy-terminal segment (3-28 residues), which is thought to lie in the cytoplasm and which may communicate external signals to intracellular structures. See Figure M.6.

***Membrane Potential.*** Potential difference across the cell membrane. The magnitude of the membrane potential is characteristic of cells of different types; it ranges from -20 to -100 mV. The membrane potential, conventionally written as negative to indicate that the inside of the membrane is negative with respect to the outside, is generated by a differential distribution of charged particles (e.g., ions) across the cell membrane. This distribution of ions (a concentration gradient) is created by active (energy-requiring) mechanisms, and by the differential passive (non-energy-requiring) permeability of the membrane to different ions. Changes in the permeability of the membrane lead to an alteration in the distribution of ions and thus to a change in membrane potential. In neurones a local reduction in membrane potential or depolarization of the membrane propagated along the axon is the basis of the conduction of a nerve impulse.

***Membrane Receptor.*** Integral membrane protein inserted into the plasma membrane and projecting at the cell surface where it functions as a specific receptor binding with high affinity a signal molecule, or ligand, such as a hormone or growth factor, an antibody molecule (the fc receptor) or some component of the extracellular matrix.

***Membrane Transport.*** Transport across biological membranes. Since the lipid bilayer of the membrane is inherently impermeable to most polar molecules, cells have evolved special ways of transferring such molecules across their membranes. These include the use of specific membrane transport proteins, some acting as channel proteins and others as carrier proteins, the latter being involved in facilitated diffusion, sodium pumps are also an important aspect of membrane transport.

***Membranoproliferative Glomerulonephritis (MPGN).*** Form of immune complex disease of the renal glomerulus that usually progresses to renal failure. Glomeruli have enlarged lobules due to an increase in the number of cells. Subendothelial deposits contain C3, IgG and to a lesser extent IgM and IgA as detected by immunofluorescence. In a variant of MPGN, electron-dense deposits are found in the basement membrane of the glomerulus, so-called dense deposit disease. MPGN is presumed to have an immunological cause.

***Meme.*** Term devised by R. Dawkins to indicate a pattern of information or transmissable idea that can spread from brain to brain, computer to computer, and therefore comes to acquire characteristics of a transmissable element.

***Memory Cell.*** Cell in the immune system that retains immunological memory and so enables an organism to mount a secondary immune response when challenged by an antigen for the second time.

***Mendelism.*** The branch of genetics concerned with the transmission of characteristics from parents to offspring, as studied in breeding experiments. The characteristics chosen for study must be produced by pairs of alleles, typically with one allele of each pair dominant to the other. The ratios of dominant to recessive characteristics observed in the progeny are used to deduce the genotypes of parents and progeny. This technique was elucidated by Gregor Mendel (1822-84) in the 1860s, who stated the principles governing the transmission of his alleles in two laws.

***Mendel's Laws.*** The two law proposed by Gregor Mendel (1822-84) to explain the behaviour of factors (now known as genes) that govern the transmission of inherited characters from generation to generation.

Mendel's first law, the Law of Segregation, states that factors are present in pairs in somatic cells. When an organism forms gametes, the pairs separate so that each gamete contains only one factor. It is now known that genes are arranged on chromosomes, which are present in homologous pairs in somatic diploid cells. When the haploid gametes are formed, homologous chromosomes are separated by meiosis so that each gamete contains one chrmomosomes of each pair. Thus genes presentt in pairs in somatic cells are present singly in gametes. To this extend Mendell's first law is always true. However, it implies that genes are entirely discrete particles, which do not blend with or modify each other, whereas in fact the action of genes can be modified in various ways.

Mendel's second law, the Law of Independent Assortment, states that when more than one pair of factors are considered, each pair segregates independently of every other pair. This law is not always true; it does apply to genes on different chromosomes but the segregation of genes on the same chromosome is affected by linkage.

***Menstrual Cycle.*** The type of oestrous cycle that occurs in higher primates (Old World monkeys, apes, and humans). It is characterized by a rapid breakdown of the uterine endometrium after metoestrus, which results in bleeding (menstruation). In addition, the animal remains sexually receptive throughout the cycle.

***6-Mercaptopurine (6-MP).*** Analogue of hypoxanthine in which the 6-hydroxyl group is replaced by 6-thiol. 6MP is a substrate for the enzyme hypoxanthine-guanine phosphoribosyl-transferase (HGPRT); it converts 6-MP to 6-thioinosine-5' phosphate, which inhibits several vital metabolic reactions of purines. In addition 6-MP is incorporated into DNA in the form of thioguanine. 6MP is used in cancer chemotherapy and for immunosuppression. See Figure M.7.

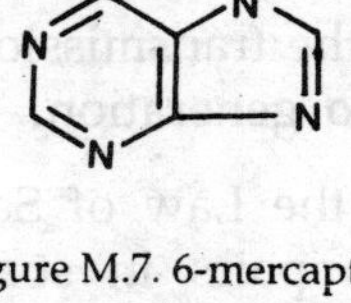


Figure M.7. 6-mercaptopurine.

***Mericlinal Chimaera.*** Organism or part of an organism, in which two genetically distinct cell lines are present, one being inside of the other, but only partly so. Such chimaera are well known in plants and provide two distinct varieties or even two distinct species, growing together.

***Meristem.*** A tissue responsible for plant growth whose cells divide mitotically, the derivatives differentiating into the new tissues of the plant body. Meristematic activity is generalized in the embryo but in vascular plants it becomes restricted principally to the apices of the shoots and roots and, later, to the lateral meristem. Meristematic tissue may be interspersed between more-or-less differentiated tissues, as in the internodes and leaf sheaths of many monocotyledons; this is termed intercalary meristem. In nonvascular plants the position of the meristem varies; for example it is apical in the bryophytes and intercalary in some large brown seaweeds, such as Laminaria.

The term primary meristem is used for tissue, such as apical meristem, that has at no stage undergone differentiation; the term secondary meristem is applied to meristems, such as the cambia, that occur on the older parts of the plant.

***Meristematic.*** Relating to meristems; of plant tissue that is relatively undifferentiated and capable of repeated mitotic division.

***Meroblastic Cleavage.*** Division of the egg cytoplasm that leads to unequal distribution of yolk between the resulting cells, so yielding an embryo with cells of markedly different sizes.

***Merogony.*** Development of part of an egg into a complete, but undersized embryo. The egg fragments that produce merogones are produced by microsurgery and are normally nucleated (although the nucleus may be haploid), but have a reduced amount of egg cytoplasm.

***Meromyxis.*** Process such as bacterial conjugation in which transfer of only some genes rather than an entire genome occurs.

***Merozygote.*** Partially diploid bacterium resulting from the transfer of a genome segment from a donor into an intact recipient cell. The transfer can be via bacterial conjugation, transduction or transformation.

***Meselson And Radding Model.*** Modification to the holliday model of chromosome recombination. A twisting and isomerization of strands in the cross-over intermediate is proposed, avoiding the requirements in the original Holiday model for nicking in both strands.

***Meselson And Stahl Experiment.*** Experiment in molecular genetics first published in 1958. It proves the semiconservative replication of DNA. The protocol used involved labelling E. coli DNA with $^{15}N$, then abruptly transferring the bacteria to a medium containing only $^{14}N$. The distribution of the DNA that had incorporated the two isotopes was followed by caesium chloride density centrifugation, and the appearance of a band partially labelled and therefore of intermediate density constituted the evidence for a semiconservative pattern of DNA replication.

***Mesenchyme.*** Type of connective tissue found abundantly in embryos, and consisting of amoeboid cells with numerous pseudopods. Mesenchyme is chiefly a derivative of mesoderm, and during development, gives rise to connective tissue and cells of the erythroid and lymphoid pathways, as well as cartilage. Many important embryonic tissue interactions are between mesenchymal tissue and epithelial tissue.

***Mesoderm.*** Middle of the three cell layers of triploblastic animal embryos. In coelomates (animals with a body cavity), the mesoderm grows as two distinct layers-an inner splanchnic mesoderm and an outer somatic mesoderm. In vertebrates, the former develops into visceral organs and the latter into somites, which form muscular and skeletal elements. So in toto the mesoderm is the progenitor tissue for blood, kidneys, gonads, lymph nodes, cartilage, bone and muscle.

***Mesoglea.*** Literally middle jelly; gelatinous layer that lies between the ectoderm and endoderm in Coelenterate (e.g. Hydra and jellyfishes). It does contain cells, but these have most commonly migrated from the inner or outer cell layers of the animal.

***Mesosome.*** A membranous structure found in the cells of some Gram-positive bacteria, such as Bacillus subtilis. The mesosome consists of whorled membranes infolded from the plasma membrane at the cell surface. It is rich in respiratory enzymes and often closely associated with a developing cross-septum of the cell wall, but its precise function remains unclear.

***Mesophilic.*** Describing microorganisms that have an optimal growth temperature of 30-40$^0$C.

***Mesophyll.*** Leaf tissue that lies between the two outer epidermal layers. Although composed mainly of parenchyma cells, it also contains collenchyma and sclerenchyma. In the leaves of many angiosperms, which are flattened in a dorsiventral plane, the mesophyll is sharply divided into an upper palisade layer of columnar cells very richly supplied with chloroplasts, and a lower, somewhat irregular layer of spongy mesophyll cells with numerous air spaces between the cells. These air spaces connect with stomata and facilitate gaseous exchange between the leaf tissue and the external atmosphere. The leaves of monocotyledons are not structured in quite the same way as described above.

***Mesosome.*** Intercellular inclusion in many gram-positive bacterial cells, consisting of a whorled membrane infolded from the surface plasma membrane. It is often closely associated with the developing septum of the cell wall and is rich in respiratory enzymes, but its precise function is unclear.

***Mesothelium.*** Certain types of epithelium derived embryonically from mesoderm or mesoblast; applied particularly to the epithelial lining of coelomic cavities and of the synovium of diarthrodial joints.

***Mesothelium.*** A sheet of cells that is derived from mesoderm and lines the coelom, synovial sac, etc.

***Mesozoic.*** The second era of the geological time scale, beginning with the Triassic period and ending with the Cretaceous and extending in time from 225 million to 70 million years ago.

***Messenger RNA (mRNA).*** A type of RNA, often between $10^3$ and $10^4$ nucleotides long, by which the coding information from the structural genes is conveyed to the site of protein synthesis, the ribosomes. A single strand of the DNA acts as a template for its synthesis. Although messenger RNA comprise a linear sequence of bases complementary to the DNA coding sequence, in eukaryotic cells the RNA sequence is not entirely colinear with the DNA sequence because the latter contains introns. The introns are transcribed along with the exon coding sequences to yield an intermediate product, HnRNA, from which the introns are removed to produce messenger RNA. On the ribosome the messenger RNA code is translated into the polypeptide sequence of a protein molecule by the action of transfer RNA.

***Metabolic Mutant.*** Mutant having a lesion in a gene coding for an enzyme involved in metabolism. Non-metabolic mutants might (For example) have alterations in parts of their DNA not expressed as enzyme proteins.

***Metabolic Pathway.*** Sequence of enzyme catalysed reactions by which compounds are interconverted in living organisms.

***Metabolism.*** Highly integrated network of enzyme-catalysed reactions that occurs in all living organisms. Although it includes all such reactions, the term is sometimes used more specifically to refer to those reactions involved in the degradation of a particular compound.

***Metabolite.*** Product of metabolism, particularly of degradative metabolism (catabolism).

***Metacentric.*** Describing a chromosome in which the centromere is more or less centrally placed.

***Metachromatic Stains.*** Stains that yield colours in cells or tissues which are different from that of the stain solution. For example, aqueous methyl violet, differentiated with acetic acid, stains amyloid pink/red.

***Metachronal Rhythm.*** Characteristic pattern of beating of groups of cilia in ciliated animal cells and surfaces, and also of parapodia in some marine worms. The wave-like progression of successive ciliary beats in thus smoothly coordinated and is exploited to move fluids relative to the ciliated surface. The apparently highly organized rhythm is known to result from simple physical coordination of closely packed cilia all engaged in a beating movement.

***Metagenesis.*** Alteration of generations in animals as, for example, in the medusoid and sedentary stages of the coelenterate life cycle. Unlike alternation of generations are diploid.

***Metalloenzyme.*** Enzyme consisting of a protein molecule complexed with one or more metal atoms. Carboxypeptidase A, for example, contains an atoms of zinc.

***Metallothionein.*** One of a group of proteins that bind heavy metals, especially copper, cadmium and zinc. They have two important functions: homeostasis, ensuring that metal-requiring enzymes are provided with these atoms; protection, binding excess heavy metal and thus, by the excretion of the complex, reducing the heavy metal content of the cell or tissue. These proteins are probably ubiquitous and are remarkable in that they are specifically inducible by the heavy metals which they bind. They are also characterized by their low molecular weight and high glycine content.

***Metallothionein Genes.*** Small gene family of some 11 separate sequences (in the mammal, including human); the number of copies in the family is less in lower eukaryotes. The genes code for the metal-binding protein metallothionein and are inducible by heavy metals such as cadmium and zinc, and corticosteroid hormones. The genes are some 900 bases in length, with two introns of 400 and 200 base pairs. Some of the genes in the family have been recognized as pseudogenes and lack intron sequences. Two particular features are of interest in relation to these sequences. They are subject to special amplification in the mouse when induced with heavy metals. Also the sequence involved in heavy metal induction, upstream from the coding sequence, shows evidence of being palindromic, thus having a dyad symmetry and capable of adopting a unique tertiary configuration.

***Metaphase.*** Stage of mitosis and meiosis in which the chromosomes are arranged on the nuclear spindle so that they are aligned across the spindle axis, thus forming a visible metaphase plate of chromosomes. In the first metaphase of meiosis, the bivalent groups of homologous chromosomes which have formed during prophase are also aligned as a plate, but the centromeres are conspicuously dissociated and drawn apart by attachment to the spindle fibres.

***Metaphase Plate.*** Plate-like appearance of the chromosomes aligned across the axis of the nuclear spindle during mitosis and meiosis. Chromosomes are attached to individual spindle fibres by their centromeres and, following metaphase, are drawn to either of these two spindle poles with the ensuing separation of the chromatid pairs.

***Metaplasia.*** The transformation of certain types of cell into others not normally associated with the same anatomical loci. It is essentially an abnormal process resulting from disease, e.g. tumour formation, or exposure to unusual conditions, e.g. epithelial metaplasia in the respiratory tract, which occurs in response to irritants such as smoke and sulphur dioxide.

***Metaproterenol*** ***(dl-β-[3,5-dihydroxyphenyl]-α-isopropylaminoethanol).*** Beta-adrenergic amine that relaxes smooth muscle, particularly of the bronchi. It is used in the treatment of asthma. See Figure M.8.

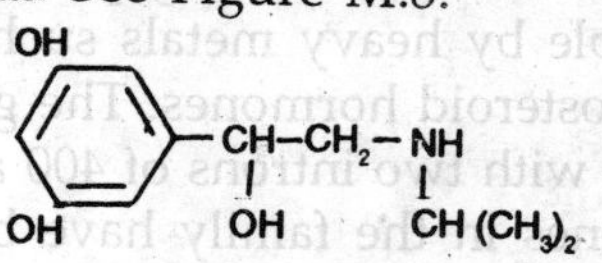


Figure M.8. Metaproterenol.

***Metastasis.*** Formation of secondary cancers at a distance from the primary one by a spreading process of malignant tumour cells. Frequently this is via the lymphatic system (lymphatic metastasis) and blood vessels (haematogenous metastasis).

***Metaxylem.*** The part of the primary xylem that is laid down after the axis or structure in which it occurs has finished elongating.

***Metazoa.*** A subkingdom of animals whose bodies are composed of many specialized cells grouped together to form tissues and that possess a coordinating nervous system. This subkingdom includes all animals except the Protozoa and Parazoa (sponges).

***Methaemoglobin.*** Oxidized haemoglobin, containing iron (m), and produced by oxidizing poisons (e.g., nitrite, chlorate(. If a cells' reductive capacity is exceeded, methaemoglobin builds up and dissociates into its haem and globin components. The latter denatures, aggregates and precipitates in the cell, binding to the cell membrane as heinz bodies. Deliberate production of methaemoglobin is induced in cases of cyanide poisoning by inhalation of amyl nitrite. The iron (m) binds cyanide to form non-toxic cyanomethaemoglobin.

***Methanogen (Methanogenic Bacterium).*** Chemolithotroph, assimilating cell carbon at the level of carbon dioxide and obtaining the energy for this process by the anaerobic reduction of carbon dioxide to methane, using hydrogen gas as electron donor. The electron transport chain involved in this process does not have the usual quinones, flavoproteins and cytochromes. Methanogens are very strict anaerobes and grow only at a redox potential below-0.33 V. They have unusual cell walls, do not have normal lipids (no glycerol esters) and have characteristic transfer RNAs and ribosomal RNA. These bacteria are so different from all other bacteria that they have been separated into a new 'primary kingdom'- the Archaebacteria.

***Methanol Dehydrogenase.*** Enzyme responsible for the oxidation of methanol to formaldehyde in methylotrophic bacteria. It has an unusual prosthetic group. Pyrroloquinoline quinone. It is also unusual in being a dehydrogenase that interacts with the electron transport chain at the level of cytochrome c, thus bypassing the quinones and b-type cytochromes which are usually involved in the oxidation of organic molecules. The result of this arrangement is that only one molecule of ATP is synthesized for every molecule of methanol oxidized to formaldehyde.

***Methionine (Met).*** An amino acid, $CH_3SCH_2CH_2CH(NH_2)COOH$, one of the 20 common amino acids occurring in proteins and an essential amino acid for man.

***Methotrexate ((+)-amethopterin, 4-amino-10-methylfolic acid).*** Cytotoxic drug used in clinical medicine and cell biology. It acts as a folic acid antagonist and affects the activity of dihydrofolate reductase. Exposure of tissue culture cells to gradually increasing concentrations of the drug results in selection for mutants with increased copy number of the dihydrofolate reductase gene, a process somewhat misleadingly referred to as gene amplification. This use of this term is confusing in that it has been otherwise used in the context of cell biology to refer to purely temporary increase in the copy number of an individual gene.

***Methotrexate (N-[p-[[(2,4-diamino-6-pteridinyl) methyl] methylamino] benzoyl] glutamic acid).*** Folic acid analogue that binds to folate reductase and competitively inhibits conversion of dihydrofolate to tetra-hydrofolate, thereby inhibiting thymidine synthesis. It is used in cancer chemotherapy and for immunosuppression, particularly for the suppression of graft-versus-host disease following bone marrow transplantation. See Figure M.9.

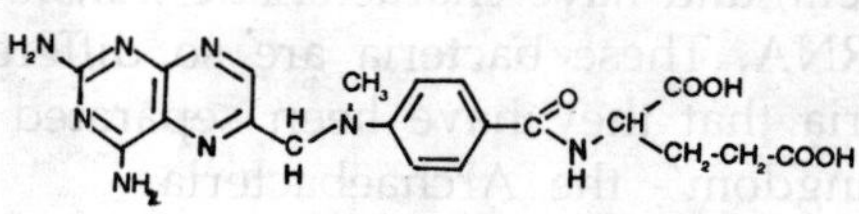

Figure M.9. Methotrexate.

***Methylated Cap.*** Methylated guanine nucleotide that is added to the 5' end of eukaryotic hnRNA and mRNA after transcription but prior to later processing and translation.

***Methylation.*** Attachment of a methyl group to some other molecule, such as a histone, RNA or DNA.

***Methyl Blue.*** Dye, normally dissolved in ethanol, that is used in histology for staining cell nuclei.

***Methylene Blue.*** Histological stain, distinct from methyl blue, but fulfilling a similar function.

***Methyl Green.*** Basic dye used in histo-chemistry to stain DNA. It is often used in conjunction with pyronin.

***Methylotroph.*** Microorganism able to grow at the expense of reduced carbon compounds containing one or more carbon atoms, but not carbon-carbon bonds. Obligate methylotrophs grow only on such compounds, whereas facultative methylotrophs are also able to grow on a variety of other organic multicarbon compounds. Examples of growth substrates used by methylotrophs are methane, methanol, formate carbon monoxide, methylamine, dimethylamine are trimethylamine. Methylotrophs occur in a wide range of different bacteria genera and yeasts. They are important in the natural carbon cycle and are important commercially as a source of single-cell protein.

***Methyl Violet.*** Histological stain, soluble in water or ethanol, that is used to stain cell nuclei.

***Micelle.*** Spherical aggregation of lipid molecules formed in an aqueous environment. Lipid molecules are amphipathic; one region of the molecule—the head—is hydrophilic and the other region of the molecule—the 'tail'—composed of fatty acid chains, is hydrophobic. Because of their amphipathic nature, lipid molecules assume an orientation in an aqueous medium with the heads exposed to the aqueous environment and with the tails directed towards the centre of the membrane. At one time it was suggested that the lipids of biological membranes were arranged in micelles, but it is now believed that they are arranged predominently as a bilayer.

***MHC Class I Deficiency.*** Form of severe combined immunodeficiency associated with absence of class II histocompatibility molecules on membranes of lymphocytes. The deficiency is inherited as an autosomal recessive trait. B lymphocytes from patients do express class I molecules when they are transformed.

***MHC Class II Deficiency.*** Form of combined immunodeficiency associated with absence of class I histocompatibility molecules on membranes of lymphocytes and monocytes. The deficiency has been observed mainly in children from North Africa. It is inherited as an autosomal recessive trait. It is inherited as an autosomal recessive trait. Transformed B lymphocytes from patients do not contain mRNA transcripts of any alpha or beta genes of the HLA-D region. Synthesis of beta-2 microglobulin and the I invariant chain is normal. The amount of class I expression on lymphocytes and monocytes is also decreased. patients have agammaglobulinemia, normal numbers of B and T lymphocytes in the circulation and a decrease in cell-mediated immunity. Diarrhea with intestinal malabsorption is the most prominent symptom observed in these patients.

The genetic defect does not map to the major histocompatibility locus. It may result from the failure of binding of a protein to the upstream promoter region of the class II histocompatibility genes.

***MHC Restriction.*** Phenomenon in which the interaction of T lymphocytes with antigen presenting cell or with target cells is restricted by histocompatibility molecules. CD4 + T lymphocytes proliferate when they recognize antigen presented by self class II histocompatibility molecules; CD8+ T lymphocytes kill target cells when they recognize antigen in association with self class I histocompatibility molecules. In an $F_1$ of two inbred strains, two distinct sets of T lymphocytes are found, each restricted by the histocompatibility molecules of one or the other parent. MHC restriction develops during maturation of lymphocytes in thymus where thymocytes first encounter histocompatibility molecules on the thymic stromal cells.

***Michaelis Constant*** ($K_m$)**.** Concentration of substrate that permits an enzyme reaction rate to be half-maximal, or at which half of the substrate molecules are engaged with enzyme molecules.

***Microbiology.*** Study of microorganisms, including the biochemistry, genetics, structure, taxonomy, ecology and pathogenesis of microbes, and their applications.

***Microbody.*** A small (0.3-1.5 μm) roughly spherical organelle of many plant and animal cells that is bounded by a single membrane and often has dense homogeneous contents, though crystalloids and filaments are sometimes present. Microbodies perform oxidation processes and are classified according to function. Peroxisomes produce hydrogen peroxide as a by-product and an enzyme, catalase, that breaks it down. In liver and kidney cells peroxisomes may be important in degrading purines. In higher plants they are functionally and spatially associated with chloroplasts and mitochondria, oxidizing excess glycollate produced in the chloroplasts during photorespiration and passing products to the mitochondria. In certain animals and higher plants fats may be converted to carbohydrates (gluconeogenesis) in peroxisomes. A special type of fat conversion to carbohydrate takes place during germination of many fat-storing seeds via the glyoxylate cycle in special peroxisomes called glyoxysomes.

***Microcarriers (Cytospheres).*** Small non-toxic plastic beads used for the culture of anchorage-dependent cell lines in suspension cultures. The beads are slightly denser than water, but remain in suspension when stirred; cells grow readily on their surfaces.

***Micrococcal Nuclease.*** Nuclease active only in the presence of calcium ions; its activity is terminated by addition of the chelating agent EDTA. Micrococcal nuclease is used to treat reticulocyte lysate destroying endogenous mRNAs so that translation activity is completely dependent on exogenously added mRNAs.

***Microevolution.*** Pattern of evolution viewed over a comparatively short time span, such as a few generations of an organism. Changes in gene frequency can often be noted in only a few generations, even with eukaryotic organisms, when the environment imposes a particularly strong selection pressure.

***Microfibril.*** Crystalline aggregate of hydrogen-bonded cellulose molecules, which constitute an important part of the cell wall matrix of plant cells.

***Microfilament.*** Intracellular fibre of polymerized actin, of between 5 and 7 nm in diameter. Many cellular extensions have cores of such cross-linked actin filaments, as for example the microvillus brush border of many intestinal cells, and the hair cells of the cochlea of the ear. Dynamic actin filament structures are also found on the surfaces of many cells, and appear to act as sensory devices, enabling the cell to detect particular features of its immediate environment.

Orientated arrays of microfilaments are not restricted to surface protrusions on cells, however, since all eukaryotic cells contain further bundles of these filaments running through the cytoplasm. For example, during cell division a belt-like contractile ring of microfilaments helps to contract the central section of the cell just below the plasma membrane. Belt desmosomes, the constituents of many epithelial cells, are also composed of microfilaments, as are the stress fibres. Actin filaments are often anchored in cell membranes, at least at one end, and these are known as adhesion plaques. The precise mechanism of this attachment is not understood.

***Micrograph.*** Photograph of an image produced by microscopy, either light microscopy or electron microscopy. In the latter case, the photograph is frequently termed an electron micrograph.

***Microglobulin.*** Small protein, with some homology to immunoglobulin, which binds to glycoproteins of the major histocompatibility complex.

***Microinjection of Cells.*** Procedure whereby molecules (e.g. antibody, mRNA, DNA) or organelles (e.g. nuclei, mitochondria) are introduced into cells by direct injection using ultrafine glass needles. Although relatively large tissue culture cells can be injected, favoured cells are the eggs of eukaryotic animals, since they are often very large; in some cases direct injection into the cell nucleus is possible. Injection of DNA may lead to permanent incorporation of some of the DNA into the nuclear genome of the cell. If the cell is a fertilized egg, this may achieve genetic transformation of the organism and its progeny.

***Micromanipulator.*** Mechanical device that reduces the scale of manual manipulation. Used in conjunction with a light microscope, it enables a microscopic level of manual dexterity to be achieved such that individual nuclei may be injected into single cells, microsurgery carried out on very small embryos, microelectrodes inserted into individual neurones, etc.

***Micromere.*** Small cell produced by unequal cell division in the developing embryos of animals such as molluscs and sea urchins. Such unequal divisions lead to a group of micromeres at the animal pole and a group of macromeres at the vegetal pole.

***Micrometre (μm; micron, μ).*** Unit of length equal to $1 \times 10^{-6}$ metres, or one-thousandth of a millimetre. Many bacteria are about 1 μm in cross-section and many eukaryotic cells are between 10 and 50 μm.

***Micronucleus.*** Smaller of the two types of nuclei found in cells of ciliated protozoa. Whereas the large macronucleus is polyploid and involved in vegetative growth, the micronucleus is diploid and, although transcriptionally inactive, is involved in meiosis and conjugation between cells.

***Microorganism (microbe).*** Living organism that requires a microscope for its observation. Microorganisms include bacteria, actinomycetes, cyanobacteria (all prokaryotes), yeasts, microfungi (e.g. Penicillium, Aspergillus), small algae (e.g. Chlorella) and protozoa. It should be noted that among the microbes are microfungi whose colonies grow to many centimetres in diameter, whereas some multicellular worms that are not visible to the naked eye would not be called microbes.

***Micropyle.*** (1) Pore in the chorion of certain types of eggs such as those of insects, through which the sperm enters. (2) Small hole in the outer coat of a seed or ovule that persists after integument formation. It allows water to enter the seed and is frequently the site of sperm entry.

***Microscope.*** An instrument used to magnify material for examination of structure invisible to the naked eye.

The light microscope uses light as a radiation source for viewing the specimen. The usual type is a compound microscope, i.e. one that possesses two (rather than one) short-focal-length converging lenses that combine to give high magnification (the product of the magnification of the two lenses). An enlarged image of the specimen is formed by an objective lens and this is magnified further by the second lens, the eyepiece lens. When the specimen is thin enough to be viewed by transmitted light, a condenser situated below the specimen focuses light through it. Resolution is the ability to distinguish (resolve) two adjacent and separate points or objects. Two objects lying closer together than the limit of resolution of a microscope cannot be distinguished as two separate objects. The theoretical limit of resolution of a microscope is about half the wavelength of the radiation used to view the specimen and resolution is therefore higher the shorter the wavelength. Magnification up to the limit of resolution reveals further detail but further magnification increases blurring as well as size of the image. The best light microscopes give a magnification of about x 1500 using green light (higher using ultraviolet light). Contrast of material examined can be improved by staining either of living material or of material preserved in its living state by appropriate fixation procedures. Examination of material, particularly living material (which often lacks contrast), can also be improved by the use of the following specialized forms of light microscope. The phase-contrast and interference microscopes make use of the fact that cells contain regions of different refractive index, which change the light path (refractive index x thickness) and hence retard light to varying degrees. These differences in refractive index are translated by special optical systems into differences in contrast (of brightness or colour). In phase-contrast microscopy, two light rays differing by a quarter of one wavelength in phase are added (made in phase so that they reinforce each other) to give a brighter image (bright contrast phase) or subtracted (made out of phase by half a wavelength so that they partially cancel each other) to give a darker image (dark contrast phase). In interference microscopy the relative phase of the two beams is continuously variable so that contrast of object can be heightened or reduced at will. Both phase-contrast and interference microscopy can be used for quantitative determinations of amounts of materials present in specific areas of cells as well as visualizing structures otherwise difficult or impossible to see, particularly in living cells, e.g. flagella, chromosome movements.

In the polarizing microscope plane-polarized light, produced by a polarizer, is passed through the specimen. Plane polarized light (in which the wavelike vibrations of light are confined to one direction only) can interact with areas of the specimen that are highly oriented e.g. crystalline areas) and the interaction can be translated into contrast by means of an analyser. Ordered (birefringent or anisotropic) areas can be made to look brighter or darker than surrounding material. Polarizing optics have been used in, for example, the study of biological membranes, fibrillar structures, and cell division.

The ultraviolet microscope uses ultraviolet (UV) radiation as a light source. It has the advantage of greater resolution since UV radiation has a shorter wavelength (as short as 220nm) than visible radiation (390-780 nm). The radiation is made visible by projecting it onto a fluorescent screen or is recorded photographically. UV radiation is damaging to living cells, so these can be studied only for a short time. An additional advantage is the visualization of certain biological molecules that strongly absorb UV light; areas in which these are concentrated (e.g. DNA in chromosomes) appear dark.

The dark-field microscope is fitted with a special condenser that passes an oblique beam of light through the specimen. This is not visible in the eyepiece (hence a dark field or background is seen) but light reflected or scattered from interfaces is visible. Thus cell outlines, organelles (such as nuclei and mitochondria), chromosomes and spindles in dividing cells, oil droplets, and other inclusions are visible as bright objects against a dark background. Dark field microscopy provides more contrast between unstained objects than is possible by normal light microscopy and sometimes allows detection (but not resolution) of objects too small to be seen by normal light microscopy.

The electron microscope (e.m.) uses electrons as a radiation source. Since the wavelength associated with a beam of electrons is much shorter than that of light, the e.m. has much greater resolution that the light microscope. It is operated under high vacuum to minimize electron scattering through collision with air molecules. In the transmission e.m. electrons pass through the specimen and are focused either onto a fluorescent screen for a visible image or onto a photographic plate or film for a permanent photograph (electron micrograph). Specimens are commonly ultrathin sections, larger macromolecules (e.g. DNA), small particles (e.g. viruses, ribosomes), fragments (e.g. membranes, cell walls), or thin replicas of the surface features of larger objects. Various techniques for providing contrast include heavy-metal staining, negative staining, and shadowing. High-voltage electron microscopes are a new generation of transmission e.ms. in which the electron beam is accelerated at very high voltage (e.g. 1000 kV, as compared to 40-80 kV in a conventional electron microscope). It can therefore penetrate thick sections and even whole cells or organelles to give information on three-dimensional structure. In the scanning e.m. a narrow beam of electrons scans to and fro across the specimen and reflected electrons control the production of a television-like image on a cathode-ray tube. Features are viewed with great depth of field, giving a three-dimensional effect. Resolution is, so far, lower than for the transmission e.m. (5-20nm) but specimens can be larger and thicker. It is particularly useful for studying surface features, for example of pollen grains, diatoms, and leaves and certain other structures, e.g. wood (including fossil woods).

***Microsome.*** A composite structure consisting of ribosomes associated with vesicular fragments of endoplasmic reticulum. The term was originally applied to small particles (microsomal fraction) isolated from tissue homogenates by differential centrifugation, which, under appropriate conditions, would synthesize proteins. This was later shown to be a property of the ribosomes alone, the microsomes being largely artefacts.

***Microspectrophotometer.*** Instrument that combines light microscopy of cells or tissues with spectrophotometry, and electronic method of measuring absorbance of light of any particular wavelength. This apparatus can be used to give readings in transects across a cell or in a given cytoplasmic or nuclear area, and concentrations of dye-binding or ultraviolet-absorbing materials estimated.

***Microspike.*** Thin spike-shaped projection of the cell surface, about 0.1 μm in diameter and between 5 and 10 μm long. Very long microspikes, called filopodia, develop at the growing tips of nerve axons. Microspikes form and retract with great speed and are characteristic of active cells in tissue culture. They are filled with actin filament bundles and are believed to act as cell sensory devices.

***Microsporangium.*** Sporangium produced from the microsporophyll, and responsible for producing the microsopores. In angiosperms, the former is the stamen, the latter the pollen grain, and the microsporangium is the anther.

***Microspore.*** Precursor of the pollen grain in angiosperms, and of the gametophyte prothallus in pteriodophytes. It is borne within the microsporangium (the pollen sacs or anthers of angiosperms).

***Microsporophyll.*** Sporophyll that produces the microsporangia or pollen sacs. In gymnosperms and pteridophytes, it is borne on a cone or strobilus, whereas in angiosperms the microsporophyll is the stamen, the microsporangium being the anther.

***Microtome.*** An instrument for cutting sections ( thin slices) of biological material for microscopic examination. For light microscopy, where sections of a few micrometres thick are required, a steel knife is used. The material is usually embedded in a medium such as paraffin wax for support; alternatively a freezing microtome is used, which keeps the specimen frozen, and thus rigid, while cutting.

The ultramicrotome is used for cutting extremely thin sections (20-100 nm) for electron microscopy. The material is embedded, usually in a hard resin, and cut with a glass or diamond knife.

***Microtomy.*** Technique in which a microtome is used to cut thin sections of biological material for microscopy.

***Microtrabeculae.*** Fine protein filaments of the cellular cytoskeleton that together form the microtrabecular network.

***Microtubule.*** A minute unbranched tubule occurring in groups in the cytoplasm of virtually all eukaryote cells. They usually have an external diameter about 24 nm and their walls, about 5 nm thick, are composed of globular protein subunits. At intervals cross-bridges (arms), probably involved in motility and in linking adjacent microtubules, project from the walls. Microtubules function passively in cell support and shape (cytoskeletal role), particularly in asymmetric cells, developing cells, and in elongate cell processes, e.g. axons of neurones. A layer of microtubules is commonly found in the outermost layers of the cytoplasm of plant cells. Microtubules are also associated with cellular motion: they form spindle fibres and are responsible for chromosome movements during nuclear division (in plants a band of microtubules also encircles the cell before prophase in the future plane of division); they are also found in cilia and flagella. Elsewhere they may have a role in orienting the movement of cytoplasmic constituents, as in phragmoplasts (where microtubules are involved in cell-plate formation) and in melanophores (where they are associated with movement of pigment granules). Microtubules are found in basal bodies and centrioles, often in close association with these structures (as in asters). They may sometimes define channels of cytoplasmic streaming.

***Microtubule-Organizing Centre.*** Region of the cell cytoplasm in which microtubules are chiefly synthesized or organized. Many microtubules continue to associate with these centres after growth, although some become linked to other cellular structures. The two types of organizing centres in the cell are the basal bodies of cilia, from which ciliary microtubules grow, and the cell centre, from which other cytoplasmic microtubules develop.

***Microvilli.*** Microscopic projections of cytoplasm, usually 2-4 μm high, that protrude above the free surface of epithelial cells and increase their absorptive area. Each cell usually has many regularly arranged microvilli. They are particularly prolific in the linings of the intestinal and respiratory tracts; such regions of dense regularly arranged microvilli are called brush borders.

***Mid Body.*** Centrally constricted region that forms across the central axis of a cell during cell division. It is constricted by a contractile ring of actin filaments until only a narrow bridge joins the cells prior to final separation.

***Middle Lamella.*** Intercellular layer occurring between adjacent plant cells. It is secreted outside the cell wall and is composed of magnesium and calcium pectates.

***Mid-Piece.*** Obsolete term for the complement components found in the euglobulin fraction of serum. It is now known that this fraction contains all of the C1, no C2, and some of the remaining complement components.

***Midwife Toad.*** Amphibian, so-called because of the behaviour of the male who carried the fertilized eggs and young tadpoles on his back and attached to his hind legs. In 1923, Kammerer claimed that he had carried out experiments in which the normally terrestrial animals were kept in water and, in breeding from such aquatically adapted stock, a change in the form of the foot pads in the male toads was acquired in the aquatic adaptation and passed on to their progeny. These experiments, which support lamarkism have never been successfully repeated and are now thought to be flawed in execution or interpretation.

***MIF (Migration Inhibition Factor).*** Lymphokine that inhibits macrophage migration and encourages localized phagocytosis.

***Migration.*** The periodic movement of populations of animals between one region and another, usually brought about by seasonal changes in the climate resulting in lower temperatures and a reduced food supply (in many species migration is the alternative to hibernation).

Migration occurs in many animal groups, including mammals (such as whales and caribou), fish (such as eels and salmon), a few reptiles, and some insects; it is especially prevalent in birds, whose migrations are spectacular. The longest migration is performed by a bird, the Arctic tern, which breeds in the circumpolar regions of the Arctic and a few months later migrates to the Antarctic; a distance of 17 600 km. Animals that migrate must have great powers of orientation in order to navigate, but their methods of orientation are poorly understood. In aquatic animals sea currents may be important. Various mechanisms have been suggested for land and aerial migrants, including orientation to the sun's rays. In some birds, following coastlines may be important for part of the route.

Migration is a very regular process; all members of the same species migrate at about the same time. Several stimuli have been suggested as causing the onset of migration. Seasonal changes in temperature and food supply are very variable; the more regular seasonal change of day length is a more likely stimulus. Several theories have been proposed to explain the evolution of migratory behaviour, especially in birds. One of the more recent is the continental drift theory, which suggests that birds originally undertook short flights between their breeding and winter feeding ranges. As the continents drifted apart, birds continued to fly from one range to the other, although these ranges had become widely separated.

***Migration Inhibitory Factor (MIF).*** Lymphokine that inhibits the movement of monocytes and macrophages. A test for MIF is carried out by placing a capillary tube containing macrophages, usually from peritoneal exudates, in a culture dish. During incubation, the macrophages move out of the tube, and the extent of migration can be estimated by measuring the area occupied by the cells. Addition of a culture supernatant from activated T lymphocytes, containing MIF, reduces the area of migration usually by 25-75 percent. Interferon-gamma has MIF activity, but it is not clear whether there are additional proteins with this property. The MIF test became popular as a test to measure cell mediated immunity, but it has largely been superseded by more direct and quantitative assays. The biological significance of MIF is not known; perhaps it serves to minimize the migration of cells out of areas of immune reactivity.

***Miller Spread.*** Preparation of chromatin prepared for electron microscopy by spreading on a surface, as first devised by

O.C. Miller and B.R. Beatty in 1969. Chromatin from nucleoli and composed of multiple tandem copies of genes coding for ribosomal RNA provides the familar pattern of christmas trees when spread and examined by this technique.

***Millicurie (mCi).*** One-thousandth of a curie; defined as the amount of radioactive material in which the number of disintegrations per second is $3.7 \times 10^7$.

***Millilitre (ml).*** One-thousandth of a litre; the volume contained in 1 cubic centimetre at 4°C. Thus 1 ml of water=1cc of water, and weighs 1 gram at 4°C.

***Millipore Filter.*** Synthetic filter bearing holes of a specific diameter penetrating through its surface, hole sizes varying between 0.005 and 8 μm. They are used in presterilized filtering equipment to render solutions free of microorganisms, especially when autoclaving might destroy some components in the solution. Viruses were originally termed filterable viruses because they will pass through filters that hold back bacteria. Other filters of similar construction are now offered under alternative names such as micropore filters.

***Millon's Test.*** A biochemical test for protein. The suspected protein is heated with Millon's reagent—a solution of mercuric nitrate and nitrous acid. The positive result is a pink or dark red precipitate of coagulated proteins; the negative result is a clear solution.

***Milt.*** Seminal fluid of fishes, consisting primarily of a dense concentration of sperm.

***Mimicry.*** The phenomenon of one species of animal (especially an insect) resembling another, sometimes to the benefit of both species and sometimes to the benefit of only. the mimic. In Mullerian mimicry, two or more predator-resistant species, e.g. species that are distasteful, poisonous, or stinging, have similar warning coloration. Thus when a predator has found a few individuals distasteful, it will leave all similarly coloured insects alone. Therefore fewer individuals of each species are taken before the bird learns to avoid all such insects. In Batesian mimicry, one palatable or harmless species resembles a predator-resistant one by mimicking its warning coloration. Once the predator has learnt to avoid the distasteful species, it also avoids the harmless one. Batesian mimicry can work only if the harmless species is less numerous than the predator-resistant one.

***Mineralocorticoid.*** Any of a group of corticosteroid hormones whose principal action is on electrolyte and water metabolism, chiefly involving the stimulation of sodium and water reabsorption by the distal tubules of the kidney. The most potent mineralocorticoid is aldosterone, but other corticosteroids that are secreted in larger amounts and contain no oxygen at C11 also show significant mineralocorticoid activity.

***Minicell.*** Small, spherical bacterial cell that is produced during the culture of some mutant strains of bacteria. These cells are easily separated from normal cells by sucrose gradient centrifigation. Although they contain RNA and protein, the cells lack genomic DNA. Depending on the strain from which they are derived, they may or may not contain plasmid DNA. Those from plasmid-bearing strains present an excellent situation in which to study the expression of genes carried by recombinant plasmids.

***Minichromosome.*** The chromatin structure within which the DNA of some eukaryotic viruses occurs. Viruses, such as SV40, that replicate within the nuclei of eukaryotic cells derive histone molecules from the host cell; these, together with their own DNA, form the viral nucleosomes. The minichromosome of SV40 occurs not only within infected cells but also persists within the free virus.

***Minimal Essential Medium (MEM).*** Medium that contains only the minimum ingredients to sustain growth of a particular cell line in culture.

***Minimal Medium.*** Medium for the cultivation of bacteria and other microorganisms of chemically defined composition and containing only those basic ingredients necessary for supporting growth of the organism. For example, a minimal medium for E. coli has the following composition (in g/l): $K_2HPO_4$ (7.0); $KH_2PO_4$(3.0); sodium citrate, $3H_2O$ (0.5) $MgSO_4.7H_20$ (0.1); $FeSO_4$ (0.01); $(NH_4)_2SO_4$ (1.0); glucose (2.0).

***Minor Histocompatibility Antigen.*** Transplantation antigen that is not encoded in the major histocompatibility locus. Each minor histocompatibility antigen plays a weak role in graft rejection, but since there are many such antigens (~50), their aggregate effect may be considerable.

***Minor Histocompatibility Locus.*** Genetic locus encoding an antigen that provokes a relatively weak immunological response to grafts. The response is weak compared to the response to antigens encoded by the major histocompatibility complex because there are fewer cytotoxic T lymphocyte precursors specific for the minor antigens. Typically, grafts transplanted across a single minor histocompatibility difference are rejected slowly, i.e., in more than three weeks, rather than one to two weeks for grafts transplanted across a single difference in the major histocompatibility complex. However, the effects of differences in minor antigens can be cumulative, so that many differences may result in rapid graft rejection. In contrast to products of the major histocompatibility complex, which can be recognized by T lymphocytes and serve as restricting elements in recognition of foreign antigens, minor histocompatibility antigens are recognized by T lymphocytes only in the context of major histocompatibility complex molecules. The molecular nature and function of the minor histocompatibility antigens are not known; they are probably membrane bound and are usually present in a number of tissues. It is difficult to produce antibodies to minor histocompatibility antigens and they cannot usually be detected by serological assays. In contrast to the major histocompatibility complex-associated antigens, the minor antigens are not highly polymorphic.

***Minute.*** Dominant mutation of drosophila, lethal when homozygous, and thought to involve the coding sequences for transfer RNA. Affected heterozygotes develop slowly; the adults are small, sterile and possess an abnormal pattern of wing veins.

***Mismatch (in DNA).*** The presence of noncomplementary bases opposite each other in the double helix.

***Missense Mutant.*** Mutant in which a particular coding triplet changes to that specifying a different amino acid, the incorporation of which results in a defective protein.

***Mistranslation.*** Incorrect placement of an amino acid residue in a polypeptide chain during translation.

***Mitochondrial DNA (mDNA).*** DNA of mitochondria. It consists commonly of a closed circle of double-stranded DNA, of between 5 and 30 μm in length, comprising 15-20 kilobases in most animals (longer in high plants) and including about 50 gene sequences, of which about one-half code for transfer RNA. The DNA is not conjugated with histone and so is not in the form of nucleosomes. The mtDNA of a number of organisms such as Drosophilia melanogaster have been entirely sequenced.

***Mitochondrion (Chondriosome).*** Self replicating organelle found in the cytoplasm of all eukaryotic cells. The number of mitochondria per cell varies between one and 10000, and averages at about 200. Although of somewhat variable form, they tend to be sausage-shaped, bounded by two membranes, the inner one being elaborately infolded to form a series of cristae. The mitochondria of mammalian liver cells are approximately 1 x 3 μm in size, and these organelles have a tendency to move constantly, change shape, and fuse with an break away from one another. In some cells, such as those of insect flight muscle, they are aligned in long rows between the muscle myofibrils. They tend to concentrated in situations where large supplies of ATP are required, since they are sites of oxidative phosphorylation. Mitochondria have their own DNA and are distinct from the rest of the eukaryotic cell in possessing distinctive ribosomes, a single species of RNA elongation and termination factors. Most mitochondrial genes (except some in yeast cells) lack intron sequences. Only a minority of mitochondrial proteins are coded on the mitochondrial genome, most being coded by nuclear genes; they are thus self-replicating but only partially autonomous. They bear many resemblances to prokaryotic cells and are probably derived in the course of evolution from symbiotic bacteria within eukaryotic cells. See Figure M.10.

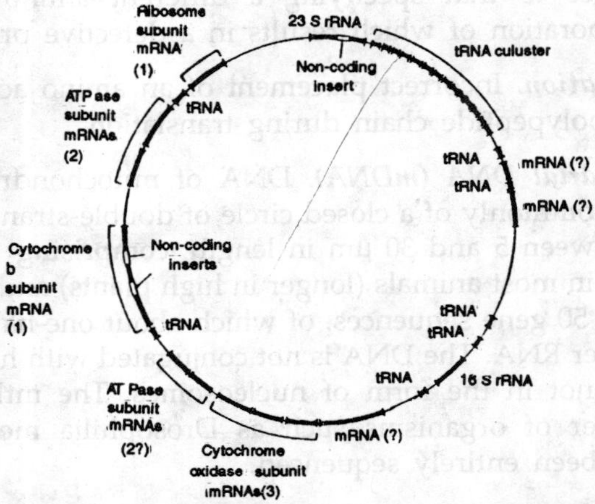


Figure M.10. Mitochondrial DNA. Approximate locations of mRNA and rRNA coding sequences in the yeast mitochondrrrial DNA circle.

***Mitogen.*** Substance that stimulates mitosis of cells. Mitogens, many derived from plants, particularly important in immunology where they may non-specifically stimulate polyclonal populations of lymphocytes to divide and transform. Both concanavalin A and phytohaemagglutinin stimulate mouse T lymphocytes, whereas pokeweed mitogen stimulates both mouse B and T lymphocytes. Some lymphokines called mitogenic factors, can act as mitogens for lymphocytes.

***Mitogen.*** Substance that induces mitosis of cells. As used by immunologists, the term refers to substances that induce transformation of diverse (polyclonal) lymphocytes. Some lectins (e.g. phytohem-agglutinin) transform T lymphocytes; other lectins (e.g. pokeweed) transform both T and B lymphocytes. Lipopolysaccharides transform mouse, but not human B lymphoytes.

***Mitomycin C.*** Antibiotic, derived from Streptomyces caespitosus, that inhibits DNA synthesis and mitosis by cross-linking DNA, being particularly potent against gram-positive, gram-negative and acid-fast bacilli. It is used in immunology to prevent immunologically reactive cells from dividing, and its use has also been suggested for cancer therapy.

***Mitosis (Karyokinesis).*** The process by which a cell nucleus divides into two daughter nuclei, each containing exactly the same chromosomes, and therefore genes, as the parent nucleus. The nuclear division is usually followed by cell division. Mitosis may be divided into four active stages; Prophase, metaphase, anaphase, and telophase, which are not distinct but grade into each other. When it is not undergoing mitosis, the cell is in interphase (the resting nucleus) and carries out activities such as duplication of chromosomes and protein synthesis. At the beginning of prophase the chromosomes appear as very long threads, which are tangled together and can be stained by basic dyes. They gradually become shorter and thicker by coiling into a spiral, a process known as spiralization. Each chromosome then appears as a double thread; each of the threads is called a chromatid. The chromatids are joined together at the centromere, a nonstaining region of the chromosome. Towards the end of prophase the nucleolus, which has been diminishing, disappears. The nuclear membrane begins to break down and by the end of prophase the chromosomes are dispersed in the cytoplasm. In metaphase (or, according to some authorities, at the end of prophase) a spindle is formed in the cytoplasm; in animals and lower plants it is associated with the centrioles. The chromosomes come to lie on the equatorial plate of the spindle, to which they are attached by their centromeres. In anaphase the centromeres divide into two, the chromatids separate, and the spindle elongates. This results in each chromatid being pulled to its respective pole, led by the centromere. Telophase is in many ways the reverse of prophase. The chromosomes become longer and less distinct as they uncoil, the nuclear membrane re-forms, and the nucleolus reappears. After telophase the cytoplasm usually also divides and two new cells are formed. Mitosis occurs whenever cells are formed. Mitosis occurs whenever cell division is necessary for growth or non-sexual reproduction; it is found in most animals and plants in either the haploid or diploid phase. See Figure M.11.

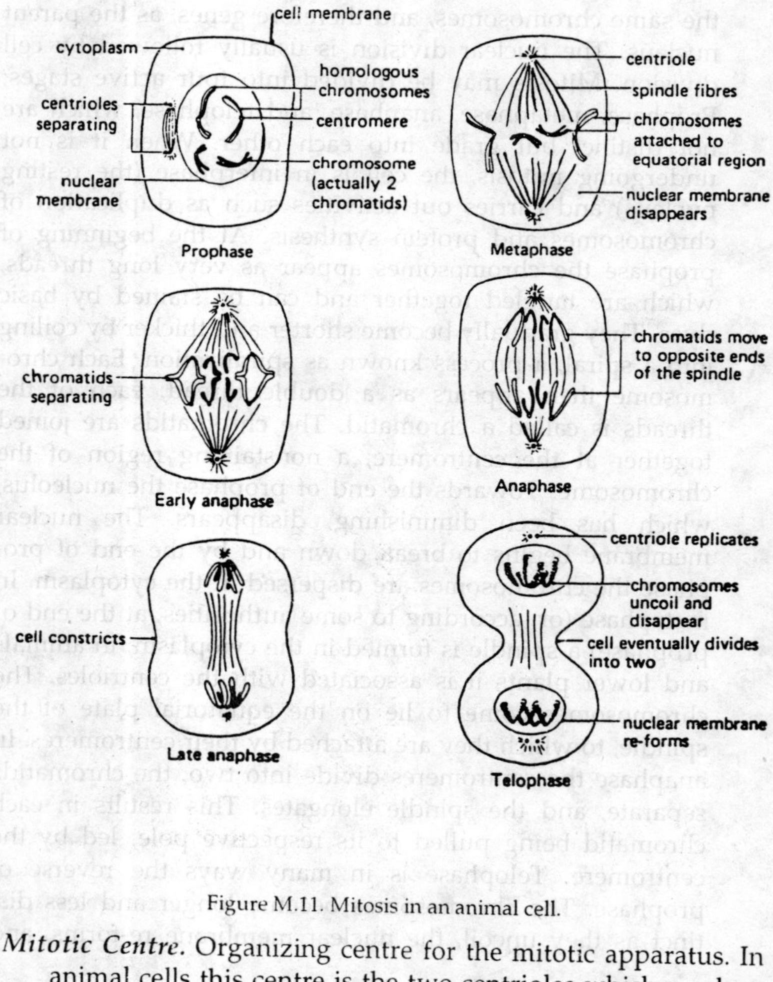


Figure M.11. Mitosis in an animal cell.

*Mitotic Centre.* Organizing centre for the mitotic apparatus. In animal cells this centre is the two centrioles which produce the asters, but no asters are found in plant cells and the nature of the mitotic centres is unclear.

***Mitotic Chromosome.*** Chromosome occurring at the mitotic stage of cell division.

***Mitotic Index.*** The proportion of cells in a population that are observed in mitosis. Mitotic indices vary from more than 10% for some cells in culture to less than 1% for tissues in vivo. A mitotic index of 0.1 means that 10% of the cell population are observed in mitosis.

***Mitotic Poison.*** Compound that specifically prevents mitosis, often by blocking spindle formation or operation, colchicine is a widely used mitotic poison in cytogenetic studies. Some mitotic poisons are used as cytotoxic drugs in cancer chemotherapy.

***Mitotic Recombination (Somatic Crossing Over).*** Recombination at mitosis between DNA of homologous chromosomes. Since such chromosomes do not normally associate at mitosis, this is a rare event and will have the effect of segregating heterozygous alleles, but will have little or any immediate genetic effect.

***Mixed Connective Tissue Disease.*** Disease in which patients have clinical features of systemic lupus erythematosus, systemic sclerosis and polymyositis. Patients have high serum titers of antinuclear antibody, with specificity for nuclear ribonucleo-proteins.

***Mixed Lymphocyte Reaction (MLR).*** Reaction that takes place upon culture of two sets of allogeneic leukocytes. The helper T lymphocytes (mouse or human CD4-bearing T cells) in either set recognize allogeneic class II histocompatibility molecules of the other set and undergo proliferation and differentiation, releasing a variety of lymphokines. In the 'one-way MLR', one set of cells is irradiated or treated with inhibitors of DNA synthesis and the cells therefore serve only as stimulators to the helper T lymphocytes in the other set. The mixed lymphocyte reaction is important in transplantation biology to study differences in histocompatibility antigens between donor and recipient. The degree of T cell proliferation, measured by the incorporation of [$^3$H]-thymidine into DNA gives an estimate of the degree of histoincompatibility.

***Mixed Lymphocyte Response.*** Situation that occurs when cells of one individual animal are mixed with lymphocytes of another in tissue culture. Helper T cells in both populations are stimulated to divide, and eventually cytotoxic T cells of each individual begin to kill the lymphocytes of the other.

***Mixoploid.*** Describing a population of individuals with differing chromosome numbers.

***M-N Blood Groups.*** Oligosaccharides present on human erythrocytes that form an antigenic system separate from the ABO blood group system and rhesus system. Individuals are typed as M, N or MN, since M and N are inherited without dominance. A further antigen, S, may be closely linked with M-N blood groups.

***MNSs Blood Group.*** Antigenic determinants of the glycophorins of human red blood cell membranes detected by alloantibodies. Red blood cell membranes have two types of glycophorins; glycophorin A ($M_r$ 31,000) and glycophorin B ($M_r$ 11,000). Glycophorin A bears the M (serine at position 1 and glycine at position 5) or the N (leucine at position 1 and glutamic acid at position 5) alloantigens. Glycophorin B bears the S (methionine at position 29) or the s (threonine at position 29) alloantigens. The MN alleles and Ss alleles are on chromosome 4 and are linked. Alloimmunization by MNSs alloantigens can cause hemolytic disease of the newborn.

***Moderately Repetitive DNA.*** Fraction of DNA obtained by renaturation of DNA fragments from a sample of eukaryotic DNA of reduced molecular weight. Such DNA hybridizes fairly fast because many copies of the same DNA sequence are present in the solution, but less speedily than does highly repetitive DNA or fold back DNA. Sequences that make up the moderately repetitious fraction include those coding for ribosomal and transfer RNA, widely represented promoter and other regulatory regions, and some families of genes where multiple copies are identical or near identical (e.g. histone genes).

***Modification.*** Any change to a nucleic acid or protein molecule made after its initial synthesis. DNA methylation, and the methylation, acetylation, and phosphorylation of histones are examples of such modification.

***Modification Enzymes.*** Methylases which attach methyl groups of DNA at special sites, especially adenine bases, in bacterial cells. Methylation prevents the genomic DNA from being digested by its own restriction endonucleases, most of which will not cut sequences containing methylated bases. The restriction enzymes thus protect the bacterium against invasion by DNA phages, the DNA of which is not methylated and is therefore subject to degradation.

***Modified Base.*** Base other than those bases from which DNA and RNA are normally synthesized (i.e. thymine, cytosine, adenine, guanine and uracil). Modified bases result from postsynthetic changes in nucleic acid and include 5-methylcytosine and 6-methyladenine.

***Modulating Codon.*** DNA coding triplets (codons) that code for rare transfer RNA (tRNA) molecules. Since the tRNA which carries the appropriate amino acid to the mRNA is in short supply in the cell, the presence of such codons tends to slow down translation of an m RNA containing them.

***Moiety.*** One of two subunits or parts of a molecule, each of approximately equal size.

***Molal Solution.*** Solution having a concentration of one mole per kilogram of solvent.

***Molar Solution.*** Solution having a concentration of one mole per litre.

***Mole (Mol).*** Amount of substance that contains as many elementary units as there are atoms in 0.012 Kg of carbon-12; one of the seven basic units of measurement of the International System of Units (SI Units). It is necessary to specify the elementary unit, which may be an atom, molecule, ion, radical, electron or a group of such entities.

***Molecular Evolution.*** Evolution viewed at a molecular level. It encompasses the evolution of molecules such as proteins and nucleic acids through the selective competition that occurs in the dynamic biochemistry of the cell, as well as the molecular aspects of the evolution of species and organisms resulting from the fact that although selection is at the level of the phenotype, this is itself partially determined by the genotype. Since mechanisms that translate genotype into phenotype are themselves molecular, it is clear that evolution has a very important molecular basis.

***Molecular Hybridization.*** Formation of duplexes of complementary RNA or DNA strands under controlled conditions in vitro, this single-stranded nucleic acids become double-stranded. The progress of the reactions is monitored using methods which can detect this change, such as spectrophotometry or SI nuclease sensitivity. The reaction normally contains one radioactively labelled strand as a probe to detect the presence and abundance of complementary sequences in unlabelled and uncharacterized nucleic acid from a different source. Molecular hybridization techniques are central to work in modern molecular biology.

***Molecular Hybridization Probe.*** Nucleic acid molecule that is made detectable by a labeling procedure (e.g. radiolabeling, fluorescent labeling) and that is used to detect nucleic acid molecules of complementary sequence by molecular hybridization.

***Molecular Mimicry.*** Sharing of an antigenic determinant by mammalian cells and microorganisms. For example, the M protein of streptococci shares antigenic determinants with membranes of human heart cells.

***Molecular Weight.*** Mass of a molecule on a scale where the mass of a carbon is 12. For macromolecules the molecular weight is sometimes given in units (Daltons); alternatively the relative nature of the term is acknowledged and the expression relative molecular mass ($M_r$) is used instead.

***Moltinism.*** Polymorphism in terms of the number of moults undergone by the larvae of a particular species. Thus the larvae of Bombyx mori can, in different strains, undergo three, four or five moults.

***Monera.*** One of the five kingdoms of living organisms, and including all prokaryotic species such as bacteria and cyanophytes.

***Monoamine Oxidases (MAO).*** Enzymes that inactivate monoamine neurotransmitters (e.g. dopamine, serotonin, noradrenaline). Inhibitors of monoamine oxidases are used clinically as antidepressant drugs.

***Monocentric.*** Describing a chromosome that, like most, has only a single centromere.

***Monoclonal.*** Related to or derived from a single clone.

***Monoclonal Antibody.*** Antibody derived from a clone of B lymphocytes. Usually a monoclonal antibody is obtained from a B lymphocyte hybridoma, which is a clone from a single B lymphocyte that was fused with a myeloma cell. Monoclonal antibodies are therefore homogeneous in structure. These antibodies are useful in structural studies and immunoassays (e.g. amino acid sequence analysis of antibodies, identification of single antigens in complex mixtures, identification of cell surface molecules, and measurement of drugs and hormones).

***Monoclonal Antibody.*** An antibody produced by a cell clone and therefore comprising only a single species of immunoglobulin molecule. Such cell clones are produced by the artificial fusion of antibody-forming cells from mouse spleen with mouse myeloma cells (which are cancerous). The hybrid cells multiply rapidly and are grown in vitro as clones of cells, each clone producing only a single type of antibody molecule.

***Monoclonal Gammopathy.*** Presence in serum of a monoclonal immunoglobulin (sometimes called 'M-component'), as in multiple myeloma, macroglobulinemia of Waldenstrom, benign monoclonal gammopathy and certain other diseases.

***Monoclonal Immunoglobulin.*** Immunoglobulin that is the product of a clone of B lymphocytes or plasma cells (e.g. myeloma protein, monoclonal antibody).

***Monocyte.*** Circulating immature cell of the mononuclear phagocyte lineage. Monocytes are considered to be more immature than macrophages because their cytoplasm contains fewer organelles and enzymes, their membranes have fewer receptors, and they are less active in pinocytosis.

***Monocyte.*** A large agranulocytic vertebrate white blood cell, 10-12 μm in diameter, that has an oval nucleus and stains with basic dyes, e.g. methylene blue. Monocytes comprise up to 7% of the white cells in human blood and have pronounced phagocytic properties, ingesting large particles and bacteria. In inflammatory conditions they migrate from the blood to the tissues and are thought to be identical with tissue macrophages.

***Monoecious.*** Designing a plant species in which separate male and female flowers are produced on the same plant.

***Monogamous Bivalency.*** Antigen-antibody complexes in which each bivalent antibody molecule combines with two determinant groups on a single antigen molecule or particle, rather than cross-linking two different antigen molecules or particles. Such monogamous binding requires that the antigens have repeating determinants that are suitably spaced to accommodate both Fab arms of a single antibody molecule. If this requirement is met, binding of the first Fab arm places the second Fab arm in a favorable position for forming the second bond. The functional affinity of such inter actions is very high; therefore, these binary complexes are extremely stable. A similar situation may occur if a single IgM antibody binds to several determinants on a multivalent antigen particle; this would be 'monogamous multivalency'.

***Monogenea.*** An order of the Trematoda (flukes), sometimes regarded as a separate class of Platyhelminthes.

***Monohybrid.*** An organism considered as heterozygous for one pair of alleles, such as Aa.

***Monokine.*** Polypeptide, secreted by monocytes and macrophages, that affects the functions of other cells (e.g. interleukin-1, tumor necrosis factor).

***Monolayer.*** Cells growing as a single layer, usually in culture. When such a cell culture is at maximum concentration the cells are all in contact with one another, and the culture is said to be confluent.

***Monomer.*** Molecule or molecular aggregate that exists as a distinct particle or is a subunit of a larger aggregate (e.g., 30S subunit of a 70S ribosomes, single histone molecules from nucleosomes).

***Monomorphic Locus.*** Locus at which a single allele or phenotypic morph is present in a population. More precisely it is a locus at which the commonest allele has a frequency of greater than 0.95 in the population.

***Mononuclear Phagocyte.*** Widely distributed cell characterized by its high rate of uptake of soluble and particulate materials. Mononuclear phagocytes derive from stem cells found in large numbers in the bone marrow and in other tissues. The young differentiated cells in this lineage are monocytes, which circulate in blood for 24-48 hours. The fully differentiated cells are macrophages, which in different tissues usually in a perivascular distribution. Monocytes and macrophages do not proliferate. Macrophages of liver are known as Kuppfer cells, those in the central nervous system as microglia, those in the lung alveoli as alveolar macrophages and those in the connective tissue as histiocytes. macrophages derive from stem cells found in the tissues and from the migration of blood monocytes. The contribution of one or the other source appears to vary among different tissues. The localization of macrophages to sites of inflammation results mostly from the emigration of blood monocytes. The multiplication of the stem cells is regulated by colony stimulating factor-1 (CSF-1) a specific mitogen that is abundantly secreted in cultured of fibroblasts.

Mononuclear phagocytes have receptors for carbohydrate (mannose and fucose), for the heavy chains of IgG and IgE (Fcγ and Fc∈ receptors), for C3 (complement receptor 1 and complement receptor3) and for denatured proteins. Through these receptors they are able to bind proteins, cells and micro-organisms. Monocytes and macrophages express class II histocompatibility molecules and can serve as antigen presenting cells. Expression of these molecules is in part stimulated by interferon-gamma, a lymphokine produced by activated T lymphocytes. Mononuclear phagocytes secrete a wide range of molecules such as eicosanoids (e.g. prostaglandins, thromboxane and leukotrienes), complement proteins (C2, C3, C4 and Factor B), enzymes (e.g. lysozyme, collagenase, elastase) and cytokines (e.g. interleukin-1, tumor necrosis factor interleukin-6). Many of these molecules are only released following stimulation by microbial products (e.g. lipopolysaccharide) or lymphokines.

Monocytes and macrophages participate in immunity by presenting antigen to T lymphocytes and in host defense after activation by lymphokines.

***Mononucleosis.*** Glandular fever, an infectious disease of the lymph nodes, usually of relatively mild character, caused by epstein-barr virus.

***Nononucleotide.*** Freely occurring single nucleotides including such molecules as coenzyme A and AMP.

***Monophyletic.*** Designating a group of species, genera, etc., that have descended from a common ancestor. All natural groups in classification are monophyletic.

***Monoploid.*** (1) Describing a somatic cell or an individual with one set of chromosomes. (2) The basic chromosome number in a series of polyploid variants.

***Monosaccharides.*** Group of carbohydrates with the general formula $C_nH_{2n}O_n$. The number of carbon atoms in the molecule is used as a basis for their classification, so that a triose has three carbon atoms, a tetrose four, a pentose five and a hexose six. The nature of the carbonyl group is also used in the nomenclature so that a ketose (e.g. fructose) has a keto group in that position, and an aldose (e.g. glucose) an aldehyde group. Most monosaccharides contain one or more asymmetric carbon atoms and therefore exist in different forms called stereoisomers. The simplest stereoisomers are referred to as dextro- or laevorotatory (D-or L+)thus giving D-glucose and L-glucose. Monosaccharides from the sub-units of disaccharides, oligosaccharides and polysaccharides, in which the monosaccharides are joined by glycosidic linkages. See Figure M.12.

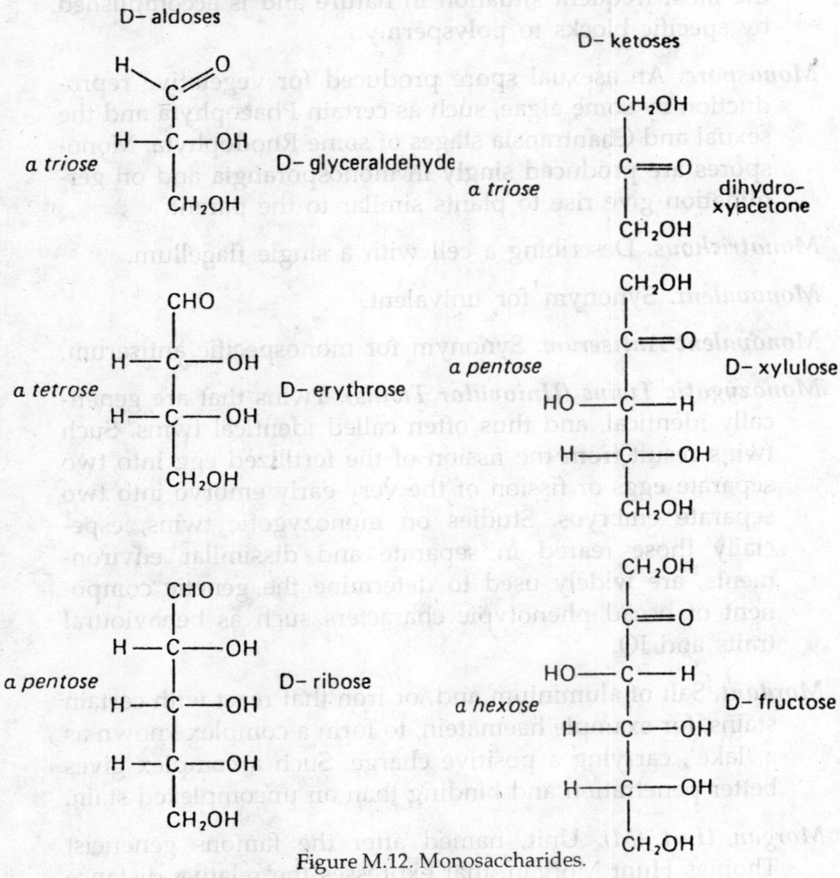


Figure M.12. Monosaccharides.

*Monosomy.* The condition in which one or more chromosomes are represented only once in a nucleus, cell, or organism, so that the diploid chromosome complement is 2n-1, where n is the haploid number. Monosomy is the normal condition for the males of some grasshoppers, which have only one sex chromosome and therefore a chromosome complement of 2n+X.

***Monospecific Antiserum.*** Antiserum containing antibodies against only one antigen or antigenic determinant.

***Monospermy.*** Fertilization of an egg by only one sperm. This is the most frequent situation in nature and is accomplished by specific blocks to polyspermy.

***Monospore.*** An asexual spore produced for vegetative reproduction by some algae, such as certain Phaeophyta and the sexual and Chantransia stages of some Rhodophyta. Monospores are produced singly in monosporangia and on germination give rise to plants similar to the parent.

***Monotrichous.*** Describing a cell with a single flagellum.

***Monovalent.*** Synonym for univalent.

***Monovalent Antiserum.*** Synonym for monospecific antiserum.

***Monozygotic Twins (Uniovular Twins).*** Twins that are genetically identical, and thus often called identical twins. Such twins result from the fission of the fertilized egg into two separate eggs or fission of the very early embryo into two separate embryos. Studies on monozygotic twins, especially those reared in separate and dissimilar environments, are widely used to determine the genetic component of broad phenotypic characters such as behavioural traits and IQ.

***Mordant.*** Salt of aluminium and/or iron that react with certain stains, for example haematein, to form a complex known as a 'lake', carrying a positive charge. Such a complex gives better penetration and binding than an uncomplexed stain.

***Morgan Unit (M).*** Unit, named after the famous geneticist Thomas Hunt Morgan, that expresses the relative distance between two genes located on the same chromosome. A cross-over value of 100 percent is equal to 1 morgan (M), a value of 10 percent is a decimorgan (dM) and 1 percent is a centimorgan (cM). Such usage depends upon the observation that the further apart two gene loci are on a chromosome, the more likely it is that crossing -over will occur between them.

*Morph.* Phenotypic variant in a population or organisms, most often applied to individuals within a conspicuously polymorphic population.

*Morphactins.* Plants growth regulators (morphologically active substances) that affect plant morphogenesis and growth. They consist of modified fluorene-9-carboxylic acids and inhibit shoot elongation and cell division in apical meristems. These and other effects are believed to result from antagonistic or synergistic interactions with other endogenous plant growth substances.

*Morphogen.* Substance that induces specific changes in morphogenesis. The word is most frequently applied to a substance that acts like a hormone, in that the target site or tissue is other than or distant from the site of synthesis. The term is probably synonymous with inductor.

*Morphogene.* Gene involved in the direct or indirect control of morphogenesis and growth, for example, genes coding for polypeptide hormones or cell cycle control factors.

*Morphogenesis.* Development of form and structure in a tissue or organism. Although morphogenesis often involves cell differentiation, certain aspects of the development of shape are clearly independent. A population of cells may be differentiated in a particular way, but due to a mutation affecting morphogenesis they do not collectively adopt the appropriate form of the tissue or organism containing them.

*Morphogenetic Movements.* Movements of cells that are responsible for or involved in the unfolding patterns of growth and form which characterize different stages of animal or plant development. Such movements may be in response to signals such as morphogens or other cell surfaces, or may be an intrinsic property of the cells concerned.

***Morphogenetic Stimulus.*** Stimulus exerted by one part of an embryo on another, such that the cells receiving the stimulus are induced to adopt a form or a movement characteristic of a pattern of morphogenesis.

***Morula.*** An animal embryo during cleavage, which comprises a solid group of cells that will later form the blastula.

***Mosaic.*** An organism consisting of two or more lines of genetically different cells. The term is almost synonymous with chimaera, but the latter should be reserved for organisms in which the multiple cell lines have arisen from different zygotes.

***Mosaic Development.*** Pattern of development in certain embryos such as those of molluscs, in which the fates of different cells in the embryo is fixed at or soon after fertilization. Such a pattern of development can be verified by the artificial removal of certain localized cells, which will result in an embryo and adult lacking the particular organ or tissue part normally developing from those cells. Mosaic development does not involve a change in fate, and the cells in such embryos are said to lack plasticity or to be non-regulative.

***Mosaic Egg.*** A fertilized ovum in which the direction of development of the cells of the embryo is determined in the early stages of cleavage (in some species, e.g. amphioxus, even before fertilization).

***Moth- Eater Mouse.*** Mouse of a mutant strain (me/me) derived from the inbred strain, C57BL/6J, characterized by patchy loss of hair, susceptibility to infection and autoimmune disease. Moth-eaten mice develop polyclonal hypergammaglobulinemia, impaired cell-mediated immunity and an autoimmune disease, characterized by deposition of immune complexes in the kidney.

***MRL/1pr Mouse.*** Mouse of a mutant strain, characterized by profound changes in lymphoid tissues. MRL/1pr mice have marked hyperplasia (excess tissue formation) of all lymphoid organs, produce multiple autoantibodies and deposit immune complexes in the kidney. The lymphoid hyperplasia is due to a proliferating cell derived from the thymus that bears little Thy-1 and no L3T4.

***Mouse Inbred Lines.*** Lines of mice that have resulted from repeated brother-sister matings within laboratory stocks. Such lines can be tested for genetic similarity by the fact that each should accept skin grafts from any other.

***M Phase.*** Phase of the cell cycle in which mitosis takes place.

***$M_r$.*** Relative molecular mass.

***MS2.*** Bacteriophage when an RNA genome and from which an RNA replicase has been isolated.

***MS222.*** Compound widely used as an anaesthetic for aquatic organisms such as fish and amphibians. The animal is immersed in a dilute solution of the anaesthetic.

***MU.*** (1) Map unit used in mapping distances between gene loci or chromosomes. (2) Virus particle that endows Paramecium cells containing it with mate-killing capacity.

***Mucilage.*** Complex of carbohydrate derivatives that forms a slimy compound and is produced by many plants and animals.

***Mucin.*** Chief constituent of mucus; a glycoprotein.

***Mucopeptide (Murein, Peptidoglycan).*** A macromolecule unique to be cell wall of prokaryotes, though often present in small amounts (less than 10% in Gram-negative bacteria). It is a complex heteropolymer of two amino sugars, N-acetylglucosamine and N-acetylmuramic acid, and the amino acids alanine, glutamic acid, and either diaminopimelic acid or lysine. Half the alanine and all the glutamic acid residues are of the D isomer. Mucopeptide is formed as a continuous molecular net around the cell membrane, conferring both shape and the strength to resist osmotic bursting in the usual hypotonic environment. See Figure M.13.

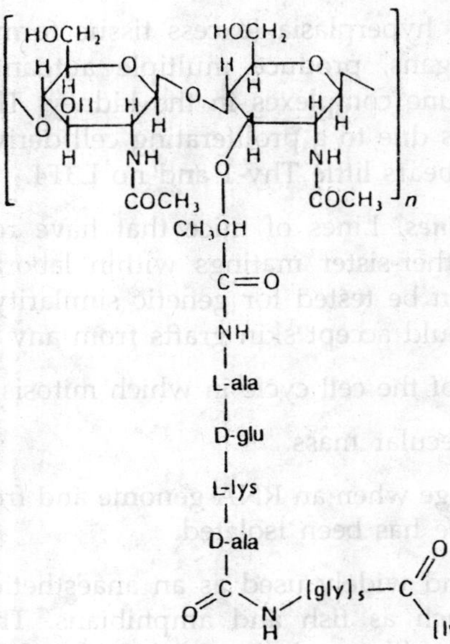


Figure M.13. Mucopeptide.

***Mucopolysaccharides.*** A group of polysaccharides that are present in animal connective tissue and consist of disaccharide repeating units, one monomer of which is always an amino sugar, such as glucosamine. The most abundant mucopolysaccharides are hyaluronic acid, chondroitin, and heparin.

***Mucoprotein.*** Protein containing a substantial carbohydrate group. Glycoproteins are very similar in structure, but have less carbohydrate (less than 4 percent).

***Mucosa (Mucous Membrane).*** Layer of moist surface epithelium that lines many vertebrate cavities in contact with the external environment. These include much of the respiratory, urinogenital and intestinal tracts. The mucus that covers the mucosa is rich in mucoproteins and glycoproteins, especially mucin, and is secreted by globlet cells found, for example, in intestinal villi. However, much of the mucosa or, for example, the urinogenital tract contains no globlet cells, and the mucus is secreted elsewhere.

***Mucus.*** Slimy, viscous substance composed of mucoproteins and glycoproteins, especially mucin, that is dispersable nut not truly soluble in water. It covers the mucosa of many vertebrate epithelial surfaces, as well as being a common protective layer on such invertebrates as marine and terrestrial worms.

***Mu Heavy Chain Disease.*** Form of myelomatosis, characterized by the presence in serum of abnormal monoclonal immunoglobulin mu chains and in urine of Bence-Jones protein. Mu chain disease is a rare complication of chronic lymphocytic leukemia or of reticulum cell sarcoma. Plasma cells, found in the bone marrow, produce immunoglobulin mu chains with extensive deletions and immunoglobulin light chains. The deletions in the mu chains are variable in location but usually start near the beginning of the variable region and extend through the $C_H1$ domain with resumption of the normal sequence in the $C_H2$ domain.

***Mule.*** Animal with a horse as mother and a donkey as father. Mules have 63 chromosomes, intermediate between the 64 of the horse and 62 of the donkey, and are sterile. The opposite cross is termed a hinny.

***Multicellular.*** Describing an organism or tissue that consist of many cells.

***Multicopy Plasmids.*** Plasmids that are present in cells in numbers exceeding one per cellular genome copy.

***Multienzyme Complex.*** Molecular aggregate containing molecules of more than one enzyme. Such complexes are an efficient way of increasing reaction rates since reaction intermediates of one enzyme are passed directly to the second. An example of such a complex is pyruvate dehydrogenase, which consists of eight trimers of dihydrolipoyl transacetylase, 12 molecules of dihydrolipoyl dehydrogenase and 24 molecules of pyruvate decarboxylase.

***Multigene Family.*** Sets of similar, but chiefly non-identical coding sequences in the same genome. Such gene families are a common feature of eukaryotic genomes, and most are presumed to have arisen during evolution by duplication of a single ancestral gene and the gradual adaptive increase in sequence divergence with time. Examples of such multigene families are those for ribosomal RNA, which number 450 in Xenopus, 250 in Drosophila and 140 in yeast, and those for transfer RNA which number 1150, 860 and 250, respectively, in these organisms. Other multigene families include those for histones, haemoglobins and keratins.

***Multilocus Theory.*** Genetical theory regarding the frequencies with which separate loci show correlated allelic tendencies.

***Multimer.*** Molecule, usually a protein, made up of two or more subunits.

***Multiparous.*** Describing female that has had more than one offspring.

***Multiple Alleles (Multiple Allelomorphs).*** Several (three or more) alleles, any two of which occupy the same relative position on homologous chromosomes in diploid cells. In some cases one of the alleles is dominant to the others; for example in Drosophila, the allele for red eye colour is dominant to that for cherry, eosin, apricot, etc. In other cases there is no dominance. In some plants, e.g. Nicotiana (tobacco), the presence of a series of multiple alleles, $S_1$, $S_2$, $S_3$ etc., produces incompatibility: if the same allele is present in the pollen grain and in the ovary the pollen grain cannot grow. The term multiple allelomorph is also used for the characteristic produced by a multiple allele.

***Multiple Myeloma.*** Neoplastic disease in humans involving excessive proliferation of plasma cells. The disease is normally clonal, so that all cells appear to have arisen from one original aberrant cell. Since such cells secrete proteins related to gammaglobulin, excessive amounts of such proteins are used as a diagnostic assay, and are termed bence-jones proteins.

***Multiple Myeloma.*** Malignant disease of plasma cells occurring most frequently in elderly men. Widespread tumors of plasma cells usually develop in bone marrow and cause destruction of bone. Myeloma cells usually secrete monoclonal immunoglobulin (myeloma protein) of the IgG, IgA, IgE or IgD class and/or bence-jones protein. The frequency distribution of immunoglobulin classes found in multiple myeloma is the same as the relative concentration of the immunoglobulin classes in normal serum. In very rare cases, a patient may have two myeloma proteins, derived from a single clone, and differing only in their heavy chain constant regions. Presumably this occurs because the cell that became transformed was in the process of switching from the production of one immunoglobulin class to production of another class. More frequently, two or more unrelated myeloma proteins are produced as a result of transformation of two or more distinct plasma cells. Patients with multiple myeloma frequently have impaired B lymphocyte function and susceptibility to infection with pyogenic organisms.

***Multipolar Spindle.*** Mitotic spindle with more than two poles, resulting from the activity of multiple centrioles. Although normally very rare, such aberrant spindles are common after irradiation of the cells concerned.

***Multituberculata.*** An extinct order of Jurassic to early Tertiary mammals containing the first herbivorous mammals, characterized by a gap (diastema) between the strong incisor teeth and molars with rows of cusps for grinding. The dentition and jaw musculature were similar to those of later placental herbivores but multituberculates were not ancestral to later groups.

***Multivalent.*** (1) Describing an association between three or more chromosomes at meiosis in polyploid individuals. (2) Describing an antiserum if it contains antibodies against several antigens.

***Multivalent.*** Having more than two binding sites.

***Multivalent Antiserum.*** Antiserum containing antibodies against more than two antigens.

***MU Phage.*** Type of bacteriophage whose genome acts as a natural transposon in bacterial host cells.

***Muramyl Antiserum.*** Antiserum containing antibodies against more than two antigens.

***Muramyl Dipeptide (MDP, N-acetylmuramyl-L-alanyl-D-isoglutamine).*** Synthetic peptide that can replace killed mycobacteria in complete Freund's adjuvant in the induction of antibodies and cell-mediated immunity. A number of derivatives of MDP have also been shown to have adjuvant activity. Some of these derivatives may be suitable for use in human vaccination.

***Muscular Dystrophy.*** Group of diseases of the human in which there is progressive degeneration of limb and girdle muscles. The diseases are inherited, some as autosomal recessive or autosomal dominant disorders, but one, Duchenne muscular dystrophy is inherited as a sex-linked recessive. The diseases are usually characterized by symmetrical muscle wasting without involvement of the nervous system, and by increased serum aldolase and creatine kinase levels, presumably due to muscle cell lysis. Single gene mutations in the mouse can result in a similar disorder.

***Mustard Gas.*** Chemical mutagen, used also as an antipersonal weapon in warfare.

***Mutable Gene.*** Gene with a significant rate of spontaneous mutation. Such genes can be detected in some multicellular organisms by somatic mutation leading to the development of a mosaic.

***Mutable Site.*** Location on a chromosome at which mutations are readily detected, especially spontaneous mutations.

***Mutagen.*** Any agent capable of causing a mutation or increasing the rate of mutation. Chemical mutagens cause chemical changes in DNA molecules leading to either changing of a base pair or addition or deletion of a base pair. Nitrous acid, for example, removes an amino group from cytosine, converting it to uracil. This ultimately leads to substitution of an adenine-thymine base pair for a guanine-cytosine base pair at DNA synthesis. Other chemical mutagens include alkylating agents, such as nitrogen mustard and ethyl methanesulphonate, which can produce base pair changes; and acridines, which cause deletions or additions of base pairs. Electromagnetic radiation can also induce mutation. X-rays, gamma rays, and beta particles all increase the frequency of mutation and ultraviolet light is known to produce pyrimidine dimers by covalent bonding between adjacent pyrimidine bases on the DNA chain.

***Mutagenesis.*** Induction of mutations.

***Mutagenic.*** Describing an agent that causes mutations.

***Mutant.*** Individual organism that carries a specific mutation at a gene locus and expresses it in the phenotype.

***Mutant.*** Descriptive of a mutation (adjective). Gene, protein, cell or individual bearing a mutation (noun).

***Mutation.*** Heritable change in the genome of an organism. Mutations are alterations in the sequence of DNA; they may occur either in germ cells or somatic cells. A mutation occurring in a germ cell can be inherited by subsequent generations; a mutation in a somatic cell is inherited in the descendents produced by mitotic division of that cell. Mutations range from changes in a single base pair (point mutation) to gross changes in a chromosome (e.g., duplication, translocation, inversion, deletion). Point mutations in the DNA encoding a protein may not be expressed (because of ambiguity in the genetic code) or they may result in an amino acid substitution (missense mutation) or in chain termination (nonsense mutation). The insertion or deletion of one of a few base pairs (not multiples of three) leads to a frame-shift. Mutations occur spontaneously at a low level; the mutation rate can be increased by mutagens (e.g. X-irradiation; chemicals such as nitrous acid, alkylating agents, acridines). Most mutations are deleterious or neutral, although some mutations may be advantageous and be selected during evolution.

***Mutation.*** A change in the amount or structure of DNA in the chromosomes or the resultant change in a characteristic of the organism. If this change occurs in the gametes the mutation is inherited by subsequent generations of offspring. If it occurs in any other cells (somatic cells) it is not inherited, except by the daughter cells produced by mitosis of the mutated cell, and is known as a somatic mutation. Inherited mutations produced by a change in the amount of DNA are known as chromosome mutations and are usually visible under the microscope. Inherited mutations produced by a change in the structure of DNA (by a change in one or more bases) are known as gene mutations and are not visible under the microscope. There are various types of chromosome mutations, including polyploidy, aneuploidy, deficiency, duplication, inversion, and translocation. Gene mutations are probably more common and result in the misreading of one or more codons in DNA leading to one or more wrong amino acids being substituted in the protein being made. This results in the formation of an ineffective protein or a protein that differs from the original.

The occurrence of mutations is one way of providing variations in a population on which natural selection can act, bringing about evolution of the species. When first produced, mutations are usually recessive and deleterious; if they are advantageous natural selection eventually causes them to become dominant. Gene mutations usually occur only in one chromosome of a homologous pair, and the mutated gene is allelomorphic to the unmutated one. Mutations are brought about by various means: some occur naturally, others can be induced by mutagens.

***Mutational Load.*** Accumulation of deletérious genes resulting from mutations: genetic disadvantages sustained by a population or organisms as a result of such mutations.

***Mutation Rate.*** Number of mutations occurring in a gene or an organism per unit time. In general terms the spontaneous mutation rate is one base-pair change per $10^9$ base-pair replications. This, in mammals, implies some three base-pair changes per haploid genome per cell generation, and for a gene 1000 bases long, one mutation per $10^6$ cell generations. This number agrees with estimates of mutation rates in evolution as being of the order of one mutation per gene every 200 000 years, assuming five cell generations per year in germ line cells.

***Mutator Gene.*** Mutant gene, the action of which induces spontaneous mutations in one or more other genes. Most mutator genes are mutant alleles of ger that code for DNA polymerase or DNA repair enzymes.

***Muton.*** Smallest unit of DNA that can be altered in the formation of a mutation. A muton is equivalent to a single nucleotide.

***Mutualism.*** State of symbiosis in which both species benefit from the relationship.

***Myasthenia Gravis.*** Autoimmune disease of young adults characterized by fluctuating muscle weakness due to faulty neuromuscular transmission. Patients with myasthenia gravis have IgG autoantibodies to acetyl choline receptors at the neuromuscular junction, resulting in a decrease in the number of functional receptors. The disease is often ameliorated by thymectomy. Infants of mothers with myasthenia gravis may also develop the disease due to passive transfer of maternal IgG antibodies to acetylcholine receptors.

***Mycelium.*** Mass of hyphae that constitutes the vegetative mass of a fungus.

***Mycetocyte.*** Specialized cell found in certain insects, containing symbiotic organisms such as yeasts or bacteria.

***MYC Oncogene.*** Oncogene from a retrovirus that causes carcinoma, sarcoma and leukaemia in chickens.

***Myc Oncogene.*** V-myc is a retroviral oncogene (from avian myelocytomatosis virus) that encodes a protein found in the nucleus of infected cells. c-myc is the related proto-oncogene found in normal eukaryotic cells; c-myc has been mapped to chromosome 8q24 in humans and to chromosome 15 in mice. In human Burkiti's lymphoma and in mouse myelomas, there are reciprocal rearrangements between one copy of the chromosome bearing c-myc and the chromosomes bearing immunoglobulin genes; these translocations deprive the myc gene of its normal transcriptional regulatory sequences (e.g. promoter, enhancer) and replace these with sequences from the immunoglobulin gene. This translocation deregulated the gene, its expression is enhanced and contributes to the neoplastic transformation of the cell. The c-myc gene may also become deregulated by the nearby integration of a retrovirus.

***Mycoplasmas.*** A group of minute non-motile bacteria with a flexible cell wall. The shape of the cell varies according to the stage of the life cycle. The group includes Mycoplasma, which causes various diseases in animals, and the nonpathogenic microorganisms formerly known as pleuropneumonia-like organisms (PPLO).

***Myelin Sheath.*** An insulating jacket surrounding the axon of most vertebrate and some invertebrate neurones. It is composed of closely packed double layers of plasma membrane that are derived from the continuous with the membranes of the Schwann cells and spiral tightly round the axon. The cytoplasm of the Schwann cells forms columns between the membrane lamellae. The regions of the axon ensheathed with myelin are termed the internodes; the unmyelinated spaces between the adjacent Schwann cells are the nodes of Ranvier.

***Myeloblast.*** Cell that give rise to leucocytes.

***Myelocyte.*** Cell in vertebrate bone marrow that is the immediate progenitor cell of polymorphs. Myelocytes are themselves produced by differentiation and cell division of multipotential stem cells in the marrow.

***Myelocyte.*** Immature cell of bone marrow that is the precursor of polymorphonuclear leukocytes. The most immature cells of this lineage are called myeloblasts. Myeloblasts are approximately 18 μm in diameter; the nucleus is large and has finely dispersed chromatin and two prominent nucleoli. The cytoplasm is sparse and stains intensely with basophilic dyes. As myeloblasts mature, large azurophilic (blue staining) primary granules appear in the cytoplasm (promyelocyte stage) and, subsequently, specific or secondary granules appear (myelocyte stage), the nuclear chromatin begins to form dense clumps and the nucleoli disappear.

As this process of nuclear condensation continues, the cells lose their capacity to divide (metamyelocyte stage); the nucleus elongates into a sausage shape (band stage) before turning into the characteristic trilobed structure of polymorphonuclear leukocytes.

***Myeloid Cell.*** Undifferentiated cell of the bone marrow from which are derived plate lets, monocytes, neutrophils, eosinophils, basophils and red blood cells.

***Myeloid Tissue.*** Vertebrate erythrocyte and leucocyte-producing tissue found in foetal liver and spleen, and the red marrow of certain adult bones.

***Myeloma.*** Neoplastic proliferation of a clone of plasma cells, particularly in bone marrow. Myelomas are found in the human disease multiple myeloma and can be induced experimentally in certain susceptible inbred strains of mice (e.g. BALB/c) by the injection of mineral oil into the peritoneal cavity. Myelomas can occur spontaneously in mice, rats, cats, dogs and other species.

***Myeloma Protein.*** Monoclonal immunoglobulin produced by a clone of neoplastic plasma cells (e.g. in multiple myeloma or in the experimentally induced disease myelomatosis in mice). Before hybridomas became available, myeloma proteins were the chief source of homogeneous immunoglobulins and were widely used in structural studies.

***Myelomatosis.*** Disease characterized by plasma cell proliferation (e.g. multiple myeloma, macroglobulinemia of Waldenstrom, alpha, gamma and mu heavy chain disease).

***Myeloperoxidase (MPO) Deficiency.*** Absence of myeloperoxidase from neutrophils and monocytes. MPO ($M_r$ 116,000) constitutes 7 percent of the weight of neutrophils and is found in primary granules. It is a deep green color due to a heme ring, which accounts for the color of pus. The deficiency is inherited as an autosomal recessive and causes a mild form of chronic granulomatous disease. Infections with Candida albicans are particularly common in MPO deficiency.

***Myoblast.*** Cell that, through fusion, forms the multinucleated cell of skeletal muscle.

***Myoepithelial Cell.*** Small, contractile epithelial cell found in such locations as the milk-secreting alveoli of the mammary ducts. Contraction of these cells leads to expulsion of milk from the alveolus during lactation.

***Myofibril.*** The structural unit of a striated muscle cell, consisting of the contractile apparatus, i.e. sarcomeres, surrounded by sarcoplasmic reticulum and mitochondria.

***Myofilament.*** Filaments of actin and myosin within muscle which form part of the structure of a myofibril.

***Myoglobin.*** Red respiratory pigment ($M_r$=17000) found in

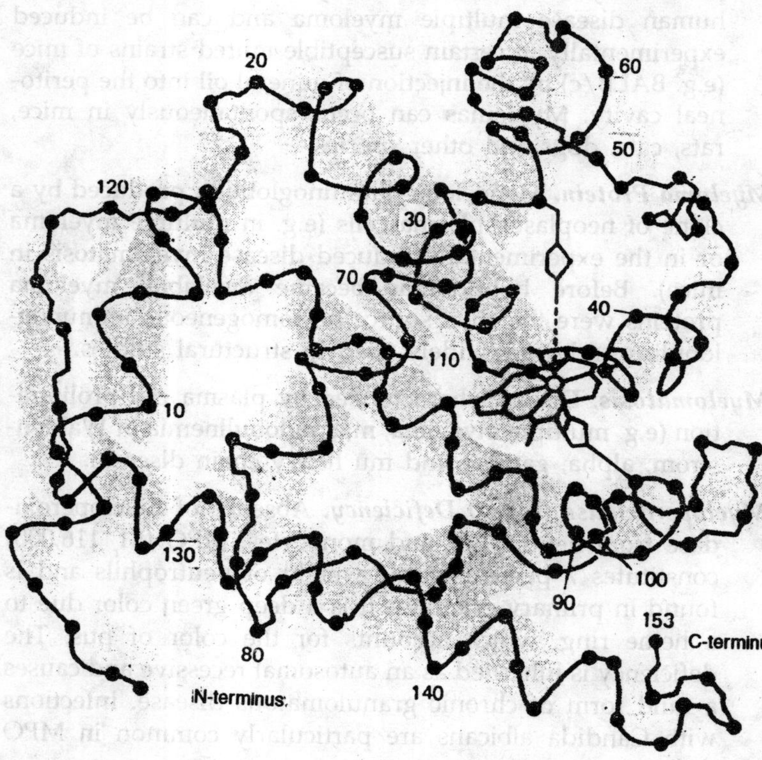


Figure M.14. Myoglobin. Outline of the myoglobin molecule, indicating the polypeptide backbone and regions of alpha-helical folding of the chain.

vertebrate muscles that binds oxygen reversibly. It consists of one polypeptide globin chain linked to an iron-containing haem moiety. By means of the haem, each molecule of myoglobin binds one atom of oxygen. See Figure M.14.

***Myoglobin Gene.*** Gene coding for the protein Myoglobin. Unlike the globin genes, which contain two introns each, the myoglobin gene contains three, and these are of such a length that the exons together make up less than 5 percent of the total gene coding sequence.

***Myoneme.*** Contractile fibril occurring in the outer cytoplasm of Protozoa.

***Myosin.*** A protein that, with actin, constitutes the principal element of the contractile apparatus of muscle. The myosin molecule consists of a tail, by which it aggregates with other myosin molecules to form filaments, and a globular head with sites for the attachment of actin and ATP. See Figure M.15.

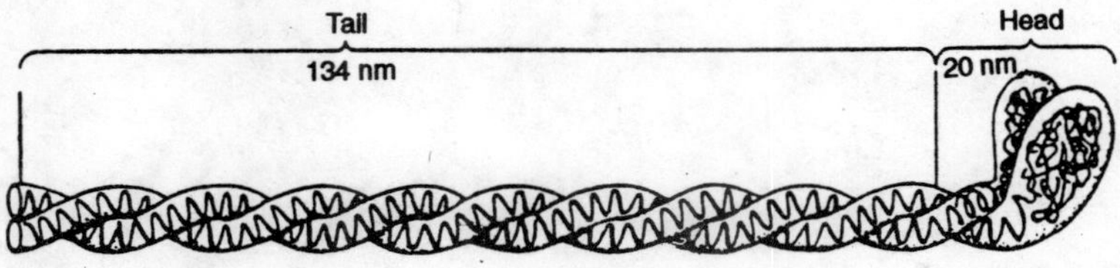


Figure M.15. Myosin.

***Myotonic Dystrophy.*** Single-gene congenital disorder in the human, caused by an autosomal dominant gene on chromosome 19. The disease is characterized by progressive muscle weakness in early adult life and frequent cataract formation.

***Myxamoeba.*** Cells resulting from germination of zoospores in Myxomycetes.

***Myxobacteria.*** A group of bacteria that lack a rigid cell wall and show a gliding movement in contact with a solid surface. They occur in soil, rotting wood, etc., and form loose colonies that, under certain conditions, produce stalked fruiting bodies.

***Myxomycetes.*** The true slime fungi (or moulds): a group of free- living fungi characterized by a plant body consisting of a plasmodium. Under certain conditions they will produce flagellate zoospores, which germinate to release one to four uninucleate amoeboid cells (myxamoebae). The Myxomycetes are usually placed with the mycelial fungi in the Eumycophyta but are sometimes classified as Myxomycophyta. The term Myxomycetes is sometimes used as a synonym for the Myxomycophyta.

***Myxoviruses.*** Group of enveloped viruses with single-stranded RNA genome and helical capsids including those viruses responsible for influenza, mumps, measles, rubella and rabies.

# N

*N.* (1) Normal solution, that is a solution containing one gram equivalent weight of solute in a total volume of one litre of solution. (2) Symbol for nitrogen.

*N.* Haploid chromosome number, the diploid number being given as 2N and tetraploid as 4N. When the number of copies of the genome is being indicated, as for example in different stages of the cell cycle, it is indicated as 2C or 4C rather than 2N or 4N.

*N.* Symbol for a neutron.

***NAA (α-Naphthaleneacetic Acid).*** Synthetic auxin.

***NAD (Nicotinamide Adenine Dinucleotide).*** A coenzyme functioning as a hydrogen carrier in oxidation-reduction reactions, for example in those of the electron transport chain in aerobic respiration. NAD and the closely related coenzyme NADP (nicotinamide adenine dinucleotide phosphate) are both derived from nicotinic acid. They are reduced to NADH and NADPH, respectively, when hydrogen atoms are transferred from the substrates to the coenzymes in reactions catalysed by substrate-specific dehydrogenases.

NAD was the first coenzyme to be recognized; its structure (and that of NADP) was elucidated in the 1930s. NAD was formerly termed DPN (diphosphopyridine nucleotide), and NADP TPN (triphosphopyridine nucleotide).

***NADP$^+$* *(Nicotinamide adenine dinucleotide phosphate, triphosphopyridine nucleotide, TPN).*** NADP$^+$ has the same chemical structure as NAD$^+$ except for an additional phosphate group on the ribose attached to the adenine. It functions in a way entirely analogous to that described fro NAD$^-$. Some dehydrogenases and monooxygenases that use NAD$^+$ or NADH are also able to use NADP$^+$ or NADPH. Some reactions are, however, specific for one or other of the coenzymes. NADPH is, for example, more often the coenzyme that is involved in biosynthetic reducing reactions such as those in fatty acid synthesis. See Figure N.1.

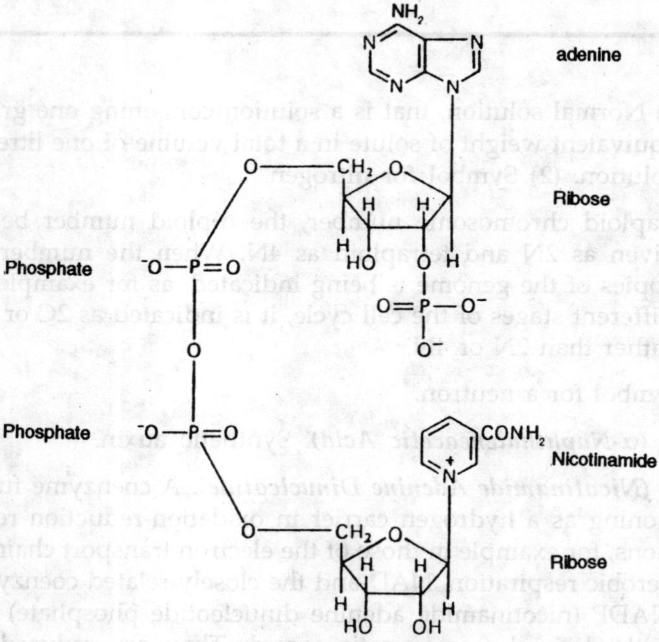


Figure N.1. NADP$^+$.

***Naegleria.*** Genus of amoebae found in the soil and best known for their transition from an amoeboid to a flagellated cell form in experimental conditions involving changes in ionic content of the solution in which the cells are suspended.

***Nail Patella Syndrome.*** Inherited disease in the human, due to a dominant gene on chromosome 9, and expressed in the phenotype as small or absent kneecaps and deformed fingernails.

***Nalidixic Acid.*** Drug used in molecular biology for its specific action in inhibiting DNA gyrase in E. coli.

***Nanometre (nm).*** Unit of distance, frequently used in microscopy, equal to one thousandth of a micrometer (μm) or 10 angstroms (A). (Angstrom units are now obsolete).

***Naproxen*** (2-naphthaleneacetic acid, 6 methoxy-α-methyl). Drug used in the treatment of rheumatoid arthritis, juvenile rheumatoid arthritis and ankylosing spondylitis because of its anti-inflammatory effects. See Figure N.2.

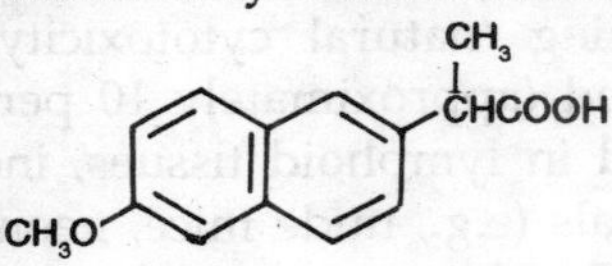


Figure N.2. Naproxen.

***Nascent.*** Describing a molecule that is in the process of synthesis and therefore still in complete. The term is applied chiefly to the growing chains to polypeptides or polynucleotides on ribosomes or on the DNA.

***Natural Acquired Immunity.*** Resistance to disease following exposure of the individual to the virus or organism causing the disease at some earlier time.

***Natural Antibodies.*** Antibodies that are not the result of known immunization. These antibodies may be the result of cryptic immunization (e.g., antibodies to the A and B blood grup in humans).

***Natural Immunity (Native immunity, non-specific immunity).*** Mechanisms for the neutralization and removal from animals of foreign organisms or non-self molecules that do not involve an immune response with its associated features of specific antigen recognition, activation of lymphocytes, synthesis of antibody or initiation of cell-mediated immune phenomena, and acquisition of memory for the evoking antigen. The production of interferon by virally infected cells, the action of lysozyme, ingestion of harmful agents by phagocytes, encapsulation of foreign bodies, cytotoxic activity towards virally infected or neoplastic cells by NK cells, and the action of various humoral lysins, agglutinins and precipitins are all characteristic of natural immunity. Some natural immunity results from the genetic constitution of the host (e.g., human immunity to canine distemper). Natural immunity is of vital importance in invertebrates for defence against harmful agents; in vertebrates it complements the specific immune system.

***Natural Killer (NK) Cell.*** Lymphoid cell capable of killing a variety of nucleated cells in the absence of antigenic stimulation. NK cells have been identified as distinct cells capable of expressing 'natural cytotoxicity'. NK cells are found in the blood (approximately 10 percent of the total lymphocytes) and in lymphoid tissues, including those of athymic individuals (e.g., nude mice, neonatally thymectomized mice, SCID mice and in infants with severe combined immunodeficiency). They are about 15 μm in diameter, bear a kidney-shaped nucleus, and two or three large granules in the cytoplasm (hence, the term large granular lymphocytes). NK cells can kill some, but not all tumor cells, some virus-infected cells and most nucleated cells coated with antibody. In the latter group, the killing takes place because of the adherence of the NK cells, which have an Fcγ receptor, to the opsonized target (a phenomenon termed antibody-dependent cell-mediated cytotoxicity (ADCC). Cells that mediate ADCC have been called killer (or K) cells but are thought to be the same as NK cells. NK cells may represent a first line of defense against spontaneously arising tumor cells and against spontaneously arising tumour cells and against viral infections. In experimental animals, there is a correlation between the number of NK cells and the degree of natural resistance to tumors. NK cells are distinct from monocytes, B lymphocytes and T lymphocytes and, hence, may represent a distinct lineage. It is noteworthy that some strongly activated cytotoxic T lymphocytes can show natural cytotoxicity (i.e., kill some tumor cells unrelated to the cellular antigens that induced them).

***Natural Selection.*** The main mechanism bringing about evolution according to Darwinian theory. Competition for food and space, the action of predators, etc., influence the composition of a population, resulting in the survival of organisms having variations advantageous to their environment and the elimination of those with unfavourable variations. When survivors of these selection pressures breed, their advantageous variations are passed on to the next generation, which eventually results in evolutionary change.

***Nature And Nuture.*** The genotype and environment, respectively, of an organism. The interaction between the two produces the phenotype (appearance of the organism).

***Nearest-Neighbour Analysis.*** Technique used in DNA sequencing, consisting of determining the relative frequencies with which pairs of each of the four bases occur in adjacent positions. DNA molecules from different sources, even if of identical base composition, may have strikingly divergent nearest-neighbour analyses.

***Nebenkern.*** Medial section of a spermatozoon, in which a helical arrangement of clumped mitochondria occurs at the proximal end of the tail filament.

***Necrosis.*** Death of tissue.

***Negative Complementation.*** Situation when complementation between alleles permits a mutant subunit to inactivate the wide-type subunit with which it associates in a multimetric protein.

***Negative Control.*** Control of gene expression by the binding of a specific controlling element to DNA and consequent prevention of transcription. Negative control of gene expression is probably the main mechanism operating in both eukaryotic and prokaryotic gene expression. The Lac operon of E. coli is controlled negatively, so that the transcription will occur provided the repressor protein is nor present to prevent operon activity. Induction of the operon is thus an act of derepression.

***Negative Interference (In genetic mapping).*** The effect that a cross-over event appears to have of reducing the probability of another cross-over in its vicinity. Thus double cross-overs within a short region of a chromosome are much less frequent than would be predicted from the frequencies of observed single cross-overs.

***Negative Staining.*** A method of staining for light or electron microscopy in which only the background is stained, so that the unstained specimen shows up clearly against it.

***Negative Supercoiling.*** Supercoiling of a duplex DNA molecule upon itself in a direction opposite to the turns of the double helix strands.

***Nematocyst.*** Stinging apparatus of a stinging cell or cnidoblast.

***Nembutal (Sodium pentobarbital).*** General anaesthetic commonly used by injection in mammals.

***Neoantigen.*** Newly expressed antigenic determinant. For example, a neoantigen may emerge: (1) upon conformational change in a protein; (2) as a newly expressed determinant on the surface of a transformed cell; (3) as the result of complex formation of two or more molecules or, (4) as a result of cleavage of a molecule with resulting expression of new determinants. Tumor-associated antigens are examples of neoantigens.

***Neolithic.*** The New Stone Age of human history, which succeeded the Palaeolithic about 10 000 years ago in Mesopotamia. It was characterized by advanced stone implements, following the invention of techniques of grinding and polishing to make very fine arrow-heads, axes, knives, etc. Farming replaced hunting and gathering as a method of obtaining food, with the cultivation of cereals and the development of animal husbandry.

***Neomorph.*** Mutant allele that produces a qualitatively new and different effect to that produced by the wild-type allele.

***Neomycin.*** An antibiotic, obtained from the bacterium Streptomyces fradiae and similar to Streptomycin, that acts by binding to bacterial ribosomes to cause misreading of the genetic code. It is used to treat intestinal bacterial infections and infectious dermatitis.

***Neoplasm (Tumour).*** Population of cells that have proliferated at an abnormal rate and are therefore not amenable to the factors normally governing growth and cell division in the organism. A neoplasm may be malignant and therefore cancerous if it displays properties of invasive growth and spreads by metastases, or benign if neither of these characteristics are apparent. A common wart, caused by the papillomavirus, is an example of a benign neoplasm, and a carcinoma an example of a malignant one.

***Neoplastic.*** Describing a cell with disordered cell growth, as in tumours. Neoplasms may be benign and non-invasive, as in the common wart, or malignant, as in cancer.

***Neoteny.*** The persistence in an animal of juvenile or larval features, or of the entire juvenile form, beyond the normal juvenile stage of development. It is thought that the evolution of some groups is due to neoteny; for example the Chordata are thought to be descended from neotenous echinoderm larvae, and man is thought to be a neotenous form of ape. Neoteny is also seen in certain ostriches bred for their plumes. Selected to retain their juvenile downy plumage, these birds also have juvenile characteristics of head and beak.

***Network Theory.*** Theory that views the immune system as a network of lymphocytes bearing idiotypes to which are directed corresponding lymphocytes bearing antiidiotypes. Antigen disrupts the balance of this network resulting in the increased production of certain idiotypes and the consequent increased production of the corresponding anti-idiotypes, which may then modulate the response. Anti-idiotypes have been found in the course of immunization with some antigens. When isolated and injected into experimental animals, such anti-idiotypes may inhibit the response to that antigen. The binding site of some anti-idiotypes resembles the immunizing antigenic determinant and is therefore called the internal image of the antigenic determinant. Not all anti-idiotypes are internal images. Immunization with anti-idiotypes bearing an internal image may result in the production of antibodies that bind the original antigen. Thus, anti-idiotypes have been used to protect mice against certain viruses. Anti-idiotypes may also bind to cellular receptors for the original antigen and have been used to isolate such receptors.

***Neural Crest.*** A band of ectodermal cells on each side of the neural tube in vertebrate embryos that gives rise to the dorsal root ganglia of the spinal nerves, chromaffin tissue, chromatophores, and many other ectodermal structures.

***Neural Fold.*** All vertebrates, with the exception of teleosts, form the major part of the CNS by a rolling up of the neurectoderm into a tube orientated longitudinally along the anterior/posterior axis of the embryo. This rolling morphogenesis is achieved by the formation of two, bilateral neural folds —elevations of the margin of the neural. Plate — which then proceed to move towards the midline. At the point of contact, fusion takes place resulting in a longitudinal orientated neural tube covered by ectoderm. This process is termed neurulation and the embryo at this stage a neurula.

***Neural Plate (Medullary Plate).*** A flat dorsal region of ectoderm in vertebrate embryos that develops after gastrulation and gives rise to the central nervous system.

***Neural Tube.*** A dorsal tube formed in vertebrate embryos after gastrulation by the joining together of the two edges of the neural plate (neural folds). The neural tube develops into the brain and spinal cord of adult vertebrates.

***Neuraminic Acid.*** Important constituent of many phospholipid membranes. It is a glycolipid and is particularly abundant in the plasma membranes of neurones. See Figure N.3 on next page.

***Neuraminidase.*** Enzyme capable of effecting removal of sialic acid (N-acetyl-neuraminic acid) residues from the outer surfaces of plasma membranes.

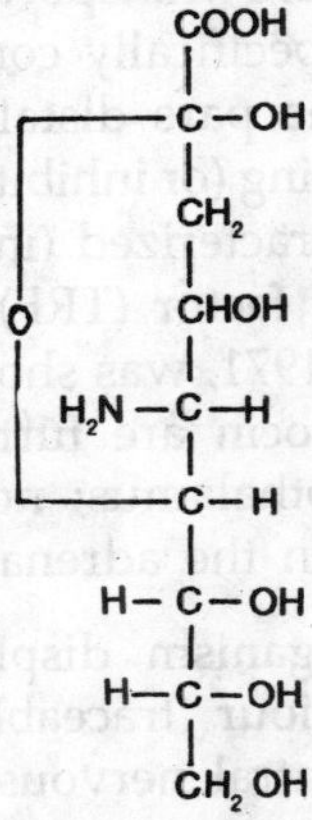

Figure N.3. Neuraminic acid.

***Neuroblast.*** Embryonic cell that, by division and differentiation, produces nerve cells.

***Neurofibromatosis.*** Single disorder in humans caused by an autosomal dominant gene with full penetrance. It is characterized by numerous skin neurofibromatoma tumours, coffee-coloured patches (cafe-aulait patches), and sometimes mental retardation and spinal cord compression.

***Neurofilament.*** Filament within a nerve cell, composed of three different intermediate filament polypeptides and thought to have a role in strengthening axons.

***Neurohormone.*** Any substance (often a peptide) that is released from specialized nerve cells (neurosecretory neurones) of animals and produces a specific effect at a distant site. Neurohormones are usually manufactured in the cell body and transported down the axon to the nerve ending, where they are released in response to impulses passing down the axon. They are usually transported to although some neurosecretory cells terminate in close proximity to the effector organ.

Following the pioneer work of G.W. Harris in the 1940s, it was established that the hypothalamus is the main region for producing and secreting neurohormones in mammals, birds, and possibly other vertebrates. Several small peptide neurohormones are transported in the blood to the pituitary gland and specifically control hormone synthesis and secretion from the pars distalis and pars intermedia. The first of these releasing (or inhibiting) factors or hormones to be isolated and characterized (in 1969) was a tripeptide, thyrotrophin-releasing factor (TRF). Gonadotrophin-releasing factor, isolated in 1971, was shown to be a decapeptide. Vasopressin and oxytocin are further neurohormones released from the hypothalamus; noradrenaline is secreted by chromaffin tissue in the adrenal medulla.

***Neurological Mutant.*** Organism displaying abnormalities of locomotion or behaviour traceable to malformation or malfunction of the central nervous system.

***Neuropathy.*** General term for behavioural or neuronal diseases, some of which are presumed to have a hereditary basis.

***Neurosecretion.*** Production of neurohormones by specialized secretory cells of the nervous system.

***Neurosecretory Spheres.*** Electron-dense particles of about 0.1 μm in diameter, visualized in electron micrographs of neuronal axons and known to be transported down the axon.

***Neurospora Crassa.*** Ascomycete fungus widely used in genetics. Together with Sordaria and yeast, Neurospora is an important organism in cell biology. As eukaryotic microbes they offer the possibilities of rapid growth and easy culture, while having a eukaryotic cellular structure. Neurospora grows as Mycelium of hyphae, and forms ascospores. Since the spores are arranged in a linear row of eight following meiotic division, it is possible to study the segregation of genes by growing each spore separately and studying the expression of a particular gene locus. This is termed tetrad analysis, since it analyses the products and cross-over events of meiosis.

***Neurotoxin.*** Toxin that affects the nervous system specifically. Neurotoxins are found in some snake venoms, as well as other sources, and include cobratoxin and α-bungarotoxin which act by binding to acetylcholine receptors on motor endplates.

***Neurula.*** The stage of a vertebrate embryo that succeeds the gastrula, when the neural tube develops from the neural plate and marks the first appearance of the nervous system.

***Neuter.*** An organism that does not have sex organs but is otherwise normal. For example, flowers that do not have stamens or pistils and have been produced as ornamentals in cultivation are called neuters.

***Neutralization Test.*** Test of capacity of an antibody to neutralize the biological activity of an antigen or of an organism (e.g., a virus) bearing an antigen.

***Neutral Mutation.*** Mutation that confers neither selective advantage or disadvantage on the organism concerned. According to a theory advanced by M. Kimura, most nucleotide substitutions result in neutral or near-neutral mutations. Such mutations may spread in a population by chance since there is no selective pressure against them. However, many geneticists disagee with Kimura's interpretation and hold that neutral mutations are rare or nonexistent, the argument turning on how fine an advantage or disadvantage must be to be significant or measurable.

***Neutral Red.*** Biological stain and acid/base indicator which gives a red colour in acid: and an orange-brown in basic conditions. It is normally employed as a solution in 70 percent ethanol.

***Neutral Substitution.*** Amino acid substitution in a protein that does not affect the activity of the molecule.

***Neutron Scattering.*** A technique employing the emission of neutrons from high-flux neutron generators to determine ordered structure of biological materials containing two or more components. Since scattering-length density is dependent on the elements present in a compound, patterns of neutron scatter can yield useful information about the biological molecules or materials causing the scatter.

***Neutropenia.*** Decrease in the number of neutrophils in the blood.

***Neutrophil.*** Type of polymorphonuclear leukocyte, characterized by secondary granules that stain pink with Wright or Giemsa stains. Neutrophils constitute approximately 60 percent of the white cells of blood; they are the most numerous phagocytes of blood.

***Neutrophil.*** A polymorph having fine cytoplasmic granules that stain faintly with acidic or basic dyes. Neutrophils comprise 55-60% of the white cells of human blood. They exhibit amoeboid movement and are highly phagocytic, appearing in large numbers in blood during pyogenic (pus-forming) infections and migrating freely into the tissues during inflammation.

***New Zealand Mice.*** Two inbred strains- the New Zealand black (NZB) and the New Zealand white (NZW)-used in the study of autoimmune disease. NZB develop autoimmune hemolytic anemia and low titers of anti-nuclear antibodies. NZB mice have spontaneously activated B lymphocytes and abnormalities of T lymphocytes, the nature of which is not clear. It is not known which abnormality is the primary defect. Several genes appear to be responsible for the manifestations of autoimmunity. NZW mice are asymptomatic, but the offsprig of NZW x NZB matings develop a severe immune complex disease, which resembles systemic lupus erythematosus, characterized by high titers of anti-nuclear antibodies and glomerulonephritis.

***Nexin.*** Protein that forms links between adjacent microtubule droplets in the outer ring of microtubules of eukaryotic cilia.

***NG (N-methyl-N'-nitro-N-nitrosoguanidine).*** Potent mutagen acting only in vivo. Its mode of action is primarily through alkylating the O-6 of guanine bases in DNA which leads to misparing or error-prone repair synthesis. NG has a tendency to produce clusters of mutations at the replicating fork of DNA, but is widely used to induce mutations in bacteria. See Figure N.4.

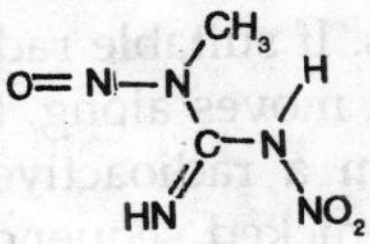

Figure N.4. NG.

***Niacin.*** Obsolete name for nicotinic acid.

***Niche.*** The sum of the abiotic and biotic components of the environment with which an organism reacts. For each resource, the biological activity of a species can be considered as a bell-shaped curve, whose height indicates the maximum level of activity or rate of resource utilization and whose breadth indicates the variety of resources used. Two such species curves show niche breadth, distance apart, and niche overlap: the closer the niches of two species, the more likely it is that inter-specific competition will occur between them. See Figure N.5.

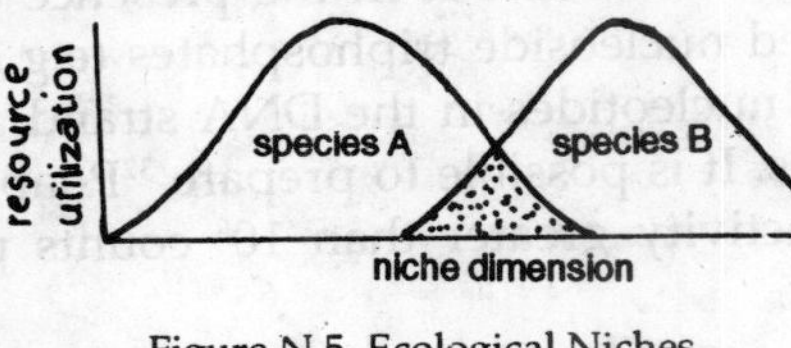


Figure N.5. Ecological Niches.

***Nicking.*** The production of single strand breaks in DNA. Some endonucleases nick DNA, and this has been widely exploited as a means of obtaining discrete DNA sequence lengths for sequencing or cloning.

***Nicking-Closing Enzyme.*** A DNA polymerase involved in DNA repair. It effects the introduction of a nick in the DNA chain next to an undesirable base, followed by excision of the unwanted base, insertion of an authentic base in its place, and closing of the nick by DNA ligase action.

***Nick Translation.*** A technique employed to produce radioactive prove DNA from double-stranded DNA. The controlled use of DNA polymerase I results in the progressive translation (movement) of a nick (break), one nucleotide at a time, along a length of DNA; the enzyme also has the ability to replace the extruded nucleotides with a new polymer as it moves. If suitable radioactive nucleotides are available as the nick moves along, they will be inserted nd polymerized to form a radioactive single-stranded molecule in place of the nicked sequence.

***Nick Translation.*** Term referring to the movement ('translation') of a nick along a duplex DNA molecule. A nick is a discontinuity in one strand of the duplex; at the nicked site there is a free 3'-hydroxyl and a free 5'-phosphoryl group, but no loss of nucleotides. Nicks are introduced at widely separated random sites in DNA by very limited treatment with deoxyribonuclease I. In the presence of DNA-directed DNA polymerase I (E.coli), nucleotides are progressively removed from the 5'-terminus of the nick (by virtue of the 5'—>3'exonuclease activity of this enzyme), and other nucleotides are added to the 3'-hydroxyl terminus; i.e., the nick translates along the duplex in the 5'—>3' direction. If the reaction is carried out in the presence of one or more radio-labeled nucleoside triphosphates (e.g., [$\alpha$-$^{32}$P]-dNTP), preexisting nucleotides in the DNA strand are replaced by labeled ones. It is possible to prepare $^{32}$P-labeled DNA with a specific activity greater than $10^8$ counts per minute per microgram.

***Nicotinic Acid (Niacin).*** A vitamin of the B complex that is essential to man nd other animals, who obtain it from such sources as milk, yeast, liver, etc. Deficiency of the vitamin in man results in the disease pellagra. Nicotinic acid is a constituent of the coenzymes NAD and NADP; it has the formula $C_5H_4NCOOH$ (pyridine-3-carboxylic acid).

***Nif Genes.*** Genes coding for proteins involved in nitrogen fixation. The genes occur in bacteria present in the root nodules of leguminous plants.

***Ninhydrin Reaction.*** A biochemical and chromatographic test for the presence of proteins or amino acids. Ninhydrin (triketohydrindene hydrate) is heated with the test substance and produces a blue colour for a positive result.

***Nissl Body (Nissl Granule).*** Ribonucleoprotein granules, probably associated with proteins synthesis, found in the cell bodies and dentrities of neurones, but not extending into the axon hillock.

***Nitrification.*** The process by which nitrifying bacteria in the soil convert complex organic compounds containing nitrogen into nitrates, which can be absorbed easily by plants. The process occurs in three stages: the decaying organic matter is converted to ammonia: this is oxidized to nitrites by Nitrosomonas bacteria, and the nitrites are converted to nitrates by Nitrobacter species.

***Nitroblue Tetrazolium*** (NBT) ***Dye Test.*** Quantitative blood test for the diagnosis of chronic granulomatous disease (CGD), NBT is a clear yellow dye that is taken up by neutrophils and monocytes during phagocytosis, NBT is reduced witthin tthe phagocytes to an insoluble deep purple dye. A negative test, the failure of NBT reduction, is diagnosttic of CGD.

***Nitrocellulose Filter.*** Widely used material in molecular biology, consisting of a paper-like mat of nitrocellulose fibres. Double-stranded nucleic acids adhere to it selectively, whereas single-stranded molecules pass through the filter. Filters are used in southern blotting of gels.

***Nitrogen Cycle.*** The circulation of nitrogen and its compounds in nature. The cycle involves the activities of nitrifying bacteria, which convert organic nitrogenous compounds to nitrates, and nitrogen-fixing microorganisms, which convert free nitrogen to nitrates. Some of the nitrates are reduced to nitrites and nitrogen by the action of denitrifying bacteria (denitrification); the rest are utilized by plants in protein synthesis. See Figure N.6 on next page.

***Nitrogen Fixation.*** The incorporation of gaseous nitrogen into compounds containing nitrogen. In nature this is brought about by some bacteria in the soil and some blue-green algae in the sea. The soil bacteria are either free-living or exist symbiotically in the root nodules of leguminous plants. Nitrifying bacteria bring about the conversion of the dead remains of these microorganisms and plants into nitrates, which can be utilized by plants. A small amount of nitrogen is fixed, as nitric oxide, by the action of thunderstorms in the atmosphere. Gaseous nitrogen is also fixed on a massive scale by industrial chemical processes for the production of nitrate fertilizers used in agriculture.

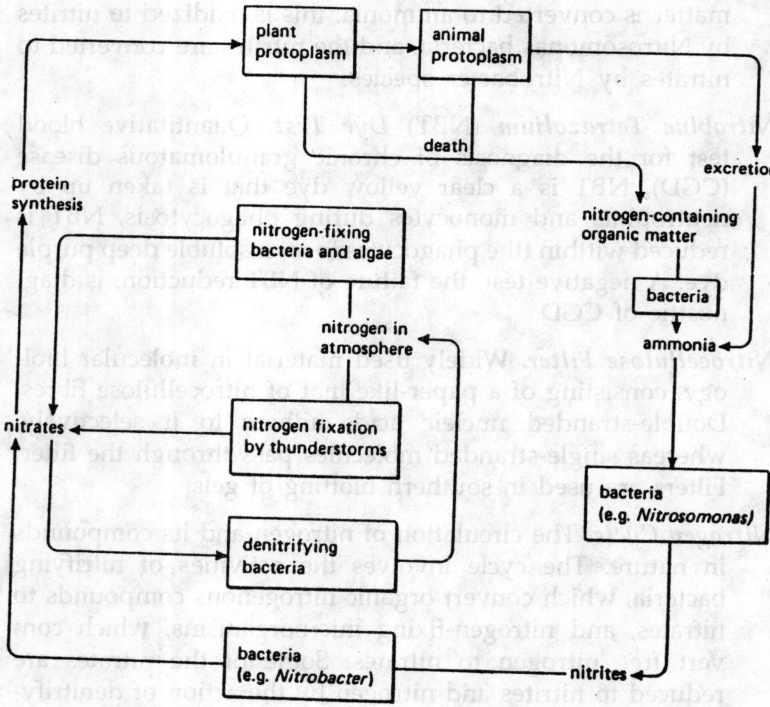


Figure N.6. Nitrogen cycle.

***Nitrogenous Base.*** Heterocyclic compound, containing both carbon and nitrogen in a ring structure; found as a component of nucleosides, nucleotides and nucleic acids. The term is usually applied to purine and pyrimidine bases, but in a broader sense is can refer to other nitrogen-containing heterocyclic groups such as flavin and nicotinamide occurring in nucleotide coenzymes.

***Nitrous Acid ($HNO_2$).*** Acid that acts on cells as a mutagen by converting the purine and pyrimidine base amino groups to hydroxyl groups.

***NK 1.1.*** Alloantigen found on natural killer cells (NK) of some inbred strains of mice (e.g., C57BL/6).

***NK Cell (Natural Killer Cell).*** Vertebrate cell that is spontaneously and non-specifically cytolytic for some cultured tumour cell lines and virus-infected cells. It is thought that the NK cell targets on a membrane glycoprotein with altered carbohydrate; the Ly5 differentiation antigen may be the NK cell receptor. Interferon and macrophage-stimulating agents enhance NK cell activity. NK cells play a role in natural immunity, and they may exist in invertebrates.

***N-linked oligosaccharide.*** Oligosaccharide attached covalently to asparagine residues of many proteins. All N-linked oligosaccharides have a brranched core structure consisting of two residues of N-acetylglucosamine and three residues of mannose. Three main types, differing in their outer branches, are distinguished: (1) high-mannose oligosaccharides, which typically have two to six additional mannose residues linked to the pentasaccharide core; (2) complex oligosaccharides, which contain two to five terminal branches composed of N-acetylglucosamine, galactose, usually N-acetylneuraminic acid (sialic acid), and sometimes other sugars such as fucose; (3) hybrid molecules, having features of both high-mannose and complex oligosaccharides.

The pentasaccharide core is derived from a branched precursor containing two residues of N-acetylglucosamine, nine of mannose, and three of glucose, linked by a pyrophosphoryl group to dolichol, a long-chain unsaturated lipid. This structure is transferred, by the enzyme oligosaccharide transferase on the luminal side of the rough endoplasmic reticulum, to a nascent polypeptide chain at a tripeptide acceptor sequence, asparagine-X-serine or asparagine-X-threonine (X is any amino acid residue except possibly proline or aspartic acid). Soon after transfer, while the polypeptide is still in the rough endoplasmic reticulum, the three glucose residues and at least one of the mannose residues are removed. The polypeptide is usually now transported to the golgi complex. Here, the high-mannose oligosaccharides may be trimmed further by removal of mannose. Extensive modification to form the complex and hybrid oligosaccharides takes place in the Golgi complex; additional mannose residues are removed and the branched arms are constructed by stepwise transfer from nucleotide sugar precursors, catalysed by individual glycosyl transferases. Fucose and N-acetylglucosamine may be added to the core.

Immunoglobulins of all classes contain N-linked oligosaccharides. These are usually attached to the constant region of the heavy chain, although some variable regions having a tripeptide acceptor sequence may also contain such oligosaccharides. Most of the oligosaccharides are of the complex type, but the mu, delta and epsilon constant regions also contain high-mannose oligosaccharides. The number of N-linked oligosaccharides varies from one in the constant region of human gamma chains to six in the constant region of human epsilon chains. Sialic acid is the only sugar residue of immunoglobulins that bears a charge (negative), and variations in content of sialic acid can lead to charge heterogeneity even of homogeneous immunoglobulins such as myeloma proteins and monoclonal anibodies.

The function of N-linked oligosaccharides differs for different glycoproteins. They may play a role in maintaining protein stability, and they may be important for movement within cells, for secretion, or for mediating clearance of glycoproteins from the blood. In some, but not all classes of immunoglobulins, glycosylation seems to be important in maintaining the conformation necessary for assembly and secretion. The presence of carbohydrate may protect immunoglobulins from proteolytic degradation. Removal of carbohydrate has variable impact on the effector functions of antibodies (e.g., complement activation, binding to Fc receptors).

***NMR Spectroscopy (Nuclear Magnetic Resonance Spectroscopy).*** A technique used in chemistry and biochemistry to obtain useful absorption spectra for different compounds by induction of small changes in the resonant frequency of the atomic nuclei.

***NOD Mouse.*** Mouse of a mutant strain, characterized by the early onset of autoimmune insulin-dependent diabetes mellitus. The NOD mutation is inherited as an autosomal recessive. Pancreatic islets of Langerhans in NOD mice are infiltrated with lymphocytes and β cells of the islets are destroyed. NOD is an abbreviation for non-obese diabetic.

***Nominal Allotype.*** Allotype that is expected according to the genetic constitution of the animal. The term nominal allotype is used in contrast to latent allotype.

***Non-adherent Cell.*** Cell that does not adhere to surfaces in vitro (e.g., lymphocyte).

***Non-Coding DNA.*** DNA that is the nonsense strand (Negative strand) of the DNA duplex, or is out with the coding sequence of any gene. It may or may not be taken to include intron sequences. Centromeric region DNA is non-coding.

***Non-Darwinian.*** Describing evolution in which changes in populations are produced by forces or factors other than natural selection.

***Nondisjunction.*** The process of misdivision during meiosis that brings about aneuploidy in a cell. During anaphase I of meiosis, when homologous chromosomes separate, both members of a bivalent migrate to the same pole instead of separating to opposite poles. Thus one of the daughter nuclei produced gains an extra chromosome and becomes a trisomic (2n + 1 ) while the other loses a chromosome and becomes a monosomic (2n — 1).

***Non-Histone Proteins.*** Proteins found in the nuclei of eukaryotic cells that are not histones. Such proteins are acidic, unlike the positively charged histones, and include HMG proteins, and the greaty variety of polymerases and gene regulatory proteins necessary for the control of transcription.

***Non-Mendelian.*** Describing ratios in the progeny of a cross which fail to follow mendel's laws, due to phenomena such as gene conversion.

***Non-Permissive Condition.*** Condition that prevents survivors of conditional lethal mutations.

***Non-Polar.*** Referring to chemical groups that are not water-soluble since they lack the polar group necessary for aqueous interaction.

***Non-precipitating Antibody.*** Antibody that does not precipitate with antigen. However, such antibodies may coprecipitate with insoluble complexes formed by antigen and other (precipitating) antibodies. Antibodies may be non-precipitating because of low affinity for antigen, or because they do not cross-link different molecules or particles of antigen.

***Non-Random Mating (Assortative Mating).*** Mating system in which the chances of a male gamete fertilizing female gametes in the population is non-random, because of some process of selection or specificity operating.

***Non-Repetitive DNA.*** DNA that shows reassociation kinetics indicative of unique DNA.

***Non-secretor.*** Person whose secretions (e.g., gastric juice, saliva, tears, ovarian cyst mucin) do not contain the ABO blood group substances. Non-secretors are homozygous for the gene se; they constitute approximately 20 percent of the population.

***Nonsense Codon (Stop Codon, termination codon).*** Any of three codons that do not code for an amino acid, but instead cause termination of protein synthesis. They are UAG, UAA and UGA, of which UAG is known as amber, UAA as ochre, and UGA as opal.

***Nonsense Mutation.*** Mutation which interconverts a nonsense codon to or from a sense-coding triplet, resulting in an abnormally foreshortened or elongated polypeptide chain.

***Nonsense Suppressor.*** Gene that codes for a molecule of tRNA which is able to respond to one or more nonsense codons.

***Non-Sibling Species.*** When two species that do not show close morphological identity and therefore would not be likely to be seen as sibling species.

***Non-specific.*** Not involving specific immune recognition.

***Non-Transcribed Spacer.*** DNA sequences that lies as a space between tandem copies of a transcribed gene sequence, but is not itself transcribed. Note that the so-called non-transcribed spacer between the copies of the large ribosomal genes in Xenopus is now known to be transcribed.

***Nopaline.*** One of the opine compounds that are synthesized by plant cells when present in a crown gall and stimulate the Agrobacteria causing the gall to grow rapidly.

***Noradrenaline (Norepinephrine).*** A neuro-transmitter in the sympathetic nervous system and a neurohormone released from the adrenal medulla. Noradrenaline was first extracted from adrenergic nerves (splenic nerves) and peripheral tissue (heart) by Von Euler, who concluded from its distribution and physiological activity that it was the transmitter of the sympathetic nervous system. Noradrenaline is present, together with adrenaline, in adrenal tissue and is partly responsible for the action of intravenously injected adrenal extracts in producing increased blood pressure. The excitatory effects of noradrenaline on the sympathetic nervous system include powerful vasoconstriction, in which vascular smooth muscle is the effector. Noradrenaline is widely distributed in sympathetically innervated effectors such as smooth muscle and glandular tissue. It is stored in synaptic vesicles in sympathetic nerve terminals and in chromaffin granules in the adrenal medulla. The release of noradrenaline from nervous tissue and its secretion from the adrenals are analogous, both processes being calcium-dependent and accompanied by the release of ATP and proteins. In the central nervous system, noradrenaline is localized in nerve terminals of the brain stem (as shown by fluorescent histochemistry), especially in the hypothalamus, where local application of noradrenaline inhibits the firing of certain neurones. This suggests that it is functioning here as an inhibitory transmitter.

***Normal Solution (N).*** Solution in which one litre of liquid contains one gram equivalent weight of solute.

***Northern Blotting.*** Procedure, analogous to southern blotting, except that the nucleic acids being transferred are RNAs and not DNAs. Nucleic acids, previously resolved into subfractions by agarose gel electrophoresis, are transferred to a nitrocellulose filter by capillary action. They are then bound to the sheet by heating and can be probed with radioactive labelled nucleic acids followed by auto-radiography. Note that although southern blotting was so called after its inventor. E. Southern, northern blotting was so called simply as a contrasting name.

***Northern Blotting.*** Technique for detecting sepecific RNA sequences within a population of RNA molecules that have been separated by gel electrophoresis. Either the RNA is denatured with glyoxal or dimethylsulfoxide before electrophoretic separation, or methylmercuric hydroxide or formaldehyde is added to the gel to achieve denaturation of the RNA. Following electrophoresis, the RNA is transferred, by 'blotting' (or electrophoresis), to diazobenzyloxymethyl (DBM) paper (no longer much used) or to nitrocellulose or nylon membranes, and is hybridized with a probe (e.g. radiolabeled DNA or RNA). The term Northern blotting or transfer was coined because the method is similar to the technique for transferring and detecting DNA fragments which had been descrribed by and named after E.M. Southern.

***Novobiocin.*** Antibiotic extracted from the fungus Streptomyces niveus. See Figure N.7.

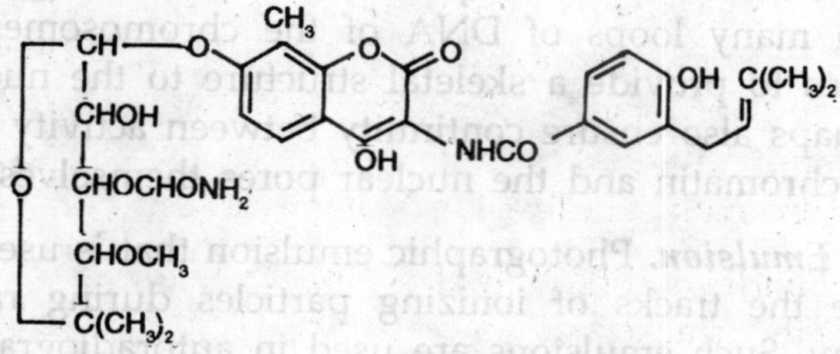

Figure N.7. Novobiocin.

***NP.*** Nucleotide pair.

***N region.*** Short portion of a variable region of an immunoglobulin or T cell receptor polypeptide chain that is not encoded by the germ line gene segments, but rather by short nucleotide (N) insertions at the recombinational juctions. Such 'N nucleotides' have been found both 3' and 5' to the D gene segment of rearranged immunoglobulin heavy chain genes and also at the V-J, V-D-J and D-D junctions of T cell receptor variable region genes. Before the insertion of N nucleotides, a few bases at these junctions may be removed by an exonuclease. It is thought that the N nucleotides are inserted at random by a nontemplate directed mechanism, perhaps catalysed by the enzyme DNA neucleotidylexotransferase (terminal transferase).

***nRNA.*** Nuclear RNA.

***NU Bodies.*** Nucleosomes which, when visualized, appear like breads on a string on interphase chromatin viewed using an electron microscope.

***Nucellus.*** The tissue within an ,ovule that is equivalent to the megasporangium (and is thus part of the sporophyte parent). A single cell of the nucellus becomes the megasporocyte while the rest acts as a nutritive tissue for the developing megaspore. In the seeds of some plants, e.g. Beta vulgaris (beetroot), the nucellus may be retained to form a food store, the perisperm, for the developing embryo.

***Nuclear Cage (Nuclear lamina, nuclear matrix).*** Fibrous layer that lies immediately inside the inner membrane of the nuclear envelope. This laminar structure is attached to all of the nuclear pore complexes, as well as being associated with many loops of DNA of the chromosomes. It thus serves to provide a skeletal structure to the nucleus and perhaps also ensure continuity between activity transcribing chromatin and the nuclear pores themselves.

***Nuclear Emulsion.*** Photographic emulsion that is used to visualize the tracks of ionizing particles during radioactive decay. Such emulsions are used in autoradiography.

***Nuclear Envelope.*** Envelope of two membranes surrounding the eukaryotic nucleus. The two membranes of the envelope are often some distance apart so that a distinct perinuclear cisterna is evident. The envelope is traversed by nuclear pores and is sometimes studded on its outer cytoplasmic surface by ribosomes.

***Nuclear Magnetic Resonance Spectroscopy (NMR Spectroscopy).*** Technique used in chemistry and biochemistry to identify different compounds in complex mixtures and to quantify the amounts present by analysing absorption specta following changes in the resonance frequencies of the atomic nuclei.

***Nuclear Pore.*** One of a series of hundred or thousands of differentiated structures is the nuclear envelopes of eukaryotic cells. Pores are often grouped in patches on the nuclear surface, and rather than being simple holes, each has an annulus within it to fill or partly fill the hole. Although some of the selectivity of transport into and out of the nucleus may be simply determined by the size of pore annuli, other effects involve active transport and are ATP-dependent. The entire structure is usually referred to as the nuclear pore complex, having an inner diameter of 80 nm and an outer one of 10 nm. Eight large protein granules arranged in an octagonal pattern make up the annulus. The hole through the pore is only about 9 nm in diameter as an open channel, and even this area is sometimes seen to be plugged by a central granule. There is also evidence that the granules of the pore complexes are part of a continuous protein latticework of protein underlying the nuclear envelope. This is known as the nuclear matrix, and probably helps in synthesis of new envelope and in attachment of chromatin fibres to the inner surface of the envelope. See Figure N.8.

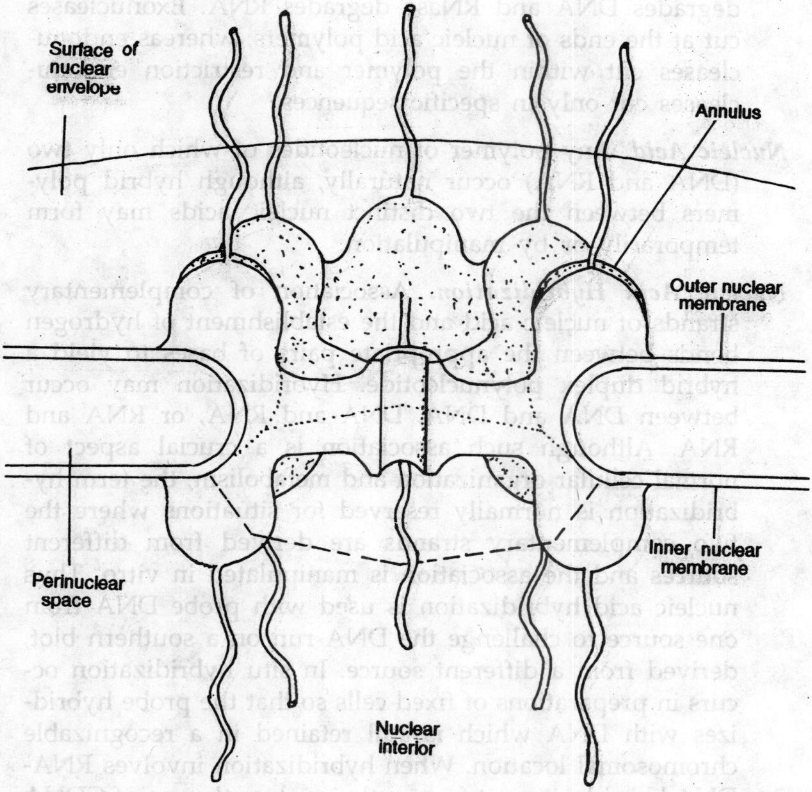


Figure N.8. Nuclear pore. Probable structure of a nuclear pore.

***Nuclear Transfer (Nuclear Transplantation).*** Exchange of nuclei between cells by micromanipulation using fine glass needles. Nuclei may be transferred between large cells of Protozoa (e.g. Amoeba proteus) so that one cell comes to have two nuclei. Alternatively a nucleus from a cell at one stage of the cell cycle is introduced into an enucleated cell at a different stage. In higher organisms, nuclear transfer usually involves insertion of somatic nuclei from differentiated tissues into enucleated egg cells. Many nuclei taken from one individual and injected into a series of egg cells can be used to obtain a population of cloned individuals.

***Nucleases.*** Enzymes that break down nucleic acids: DNase degrades DNA and RNase degrades RNA. Exonucleases cut at the ends of nucleic acid polymers, whereas endonucleases cut within the polymer and restriction endonucleases cut only in specific sequences.

***Nucleic Acid.*** Any polymer of nucleotides of which only two (DNA and RNA) occur naturally, although hybrid polymers between the two distinct nucleic acids may form temporarily or by manipulation.

***Nucleic Acid Hybridization.*** Association of complementary strands of nucleic acid and the establishment of hydrogen bonds between the appropriate pairs of bases to yield a hybrid duplex polynucleotide. Hybridization may occur between DNA and DNA, DNA and RNA, or RNA and RNA. Although such association is a crucial aspect of normal cellular organization and metabolism, the term hybridization is normally reserved for situations where the two complementary strands are derived from different sources and the association is manipulated in vitro. Thus nucleic acid hybridization is used with probe DNA from one source to challenge the DNA run on a southern blot, derived from a different source. In situ hybridization occurs in preparations of fixed cells so that the probe hybridizes with DNA which is still retained in a recognizable chromosomal location. When hybridization involves RNA-DNA hybrids, it most frequently involves the use of CDNA to probe a northern blot for specific mRNA.

***Nucleocapsid.*** Particle consisting of viral nucleic acid together with the surrounding capsid.

***Nucleocytoplasmic Ratio.*** Ratio of the nuclear volume to the cytoplasmic volume.

***Nucleoid.*** The DNA-containing area of a prokaryote cell, analogous to the eukaryote nucleus but not membrane bounded.

***Nucleolar-Organizing Centre.*** One or more areas located at specific chromosomal sites with which nucleoli are associated. They are in fact region in which multiple copies of the ribosomal RNA genes are to be found, the nucleoli being largely composed of the RNA transcripts from these genes.

***Nucleolonema:*** Central region of the nucleolus made up to dense, convoluted fibrillar material.

***Nucleolus (Plasmosome).*** Discrete part of the eukaryotic nucleus, visible by light or electron microscopy, in which ribosomes are synthesized. Most somatic cells have two to seven nucleoli in their nucleus, although amphibian oocytes may have more than 1000. The nucleolus consists of granular regions (newly synthesized ribosomes) and fibrillar regions (DNA, including the ribosomal cistrons), but is not bounded by any membrane.

***Nucleoplasm (Karyolymph, Karyoplasm).*** Protoplasmic phase of the nucleus (i.e. soluble phase, excluding chromatin and nucleolus).

***Nucleoprotein.*** A compound consisting of a nucleic acid (DNA or RNA) combined with a protein. In eukaryotic cells DNA in the nucleus is associated with histones and protamines; RNA in the cytoplasm is associated with protein in the form of the ribosomes. Viruses may be entirely nucleoprotein, consisting of DNA or RNA surrounded by a protein or lipoprotein coat.

***Nucleosidase.*** Enzyme that hydrolyses a nucleoside to a free nitrogenous base (a purine or a pyrimidine) and a pentose (Ribose or deoxyribose).

***Nucleoside.*** A molecule consisting of D-ribose or deoxyribose linked to a purine or pyrimidine base; it is formed by the partial hydrolysis of a nucleotide. Common nucleosides are adenosine guanosine, cytidine, thymidine, and uridine.

***Nucleosome.*** The basic unit of chromatin structure in eukaryotic cells. A nucleosome consists of eight histone molecules of four different types, together with about 140 base pairs of DNA coiled around it. Nucleosomes are arranged at intervals along a length of DNA, approximately one nucleosome per 200 base pairs, and evidence suggests that they are present both on active and inactive chromatin. A fifth type of histone, HI, links neighbouring nucleosomes together. Chromatin consists of stacks of nucleosomes, each stack resembling a solenoid.

***Nucleotide.*** A compound consisting of a pentose sugar, phosphoric acid, and a nitrogenous base. Nucleic acids consist of many nucleotides linked covalently to form a polynucleotide chain; the base is either a pyrimidine (cytosine, thymine, or uracil) or a purine (adenine or guanine) and the sugar is D-ribose (for RNA) or deoxyribose (for DNA). Two nucleotides can be linked through their phosphate groups to form a dinucleotide; two important dinucleotides are the coenzymes NAD and FAD. Nucleotides can also occur free in the cell; examples of mononucleotides are AMP and coenzyme A.

***Nucleus.*** 1. The organelle of the eukaryote cell that contains the chromosomes and hence ultimately controls cellular activity and inheritance through the activity of the genetic material, DNA. It is conspicuously large in most cells, commonly up to 20 μm long and usually spherical to ovoid in shape. It is surrounded by two membranes, forming the nuclear envelope; the outer membrane is continuous with the endoplasmic reticulum. The envelope is perforated by complex nuclear pores, 40-100 nm in diameter, which control exchange between nucleus and cytoplasm. The interphase nucleus contains chromatin (which condenses during nuclear division into chromosomes), and one or more nucleoli, in which ribosomes are manufactured, all within a ground substance called the nucleoplasm (or nuclear sap). True nuclei are absent from prokaryotes (bacteria and blue-green algae). Red blood corpuscles of mammals and sieve-tube elements of higher plants are virtually unique in losing their nuclei as they mature. In ciliates and some other Protozoa two types of nuclei, a micronucleus and a macronucleus (or meganucleus), exist. Cells with a macronucleus normally also possess one or more micronuclei. The macronucleus contains nucleoli and most of the DNA is polyploid. It controls normal cell metabolism, i.e. the vegetative functions of the cell, and divides amitotically. The micronucleus divides by mitosis and function in sexual reproduction.

2. An anatomically distinct mass of nerve cell bodies in the vertebrate brain. The nuclei resemble, and are often alternatively termed, ganglia.

***Nuclide.*** Atom designated according to the constitution of its nucleus in terms of proton and neutron numbers. Thus radioisotopes may be described as radionuclides.

***Nude Mouse.*** Mouse with a congenital absence of the thymus gland, and, as a consequence, severely depleted of T lymphocytes. Mice homozygous for the gene 'nude' are referred to as nu nu and also lack hair. Such mice will accept grafts of foreign skin and other organs.

***Nude Mouse.*** Mutant mouse, characterized by the complete absence of hair and thymus. These mice are homozygous for an autosomal recessive mutation (v) which maps to chromosome 11. The relationship between the absence of thymus and hair is not clear. Nude mice are used extensively to study the immunological effects of thymus deprivation. Nude mice cannot reject homografts, do not express cellmediated immunity, and do not make antibodies to most antigens. They lack T lymphocytes but have normal natural killerr cells and B lymphocytes.

***Null Allele.*** Allele that produces no functional product and therefore behaves as a recessive.

***Null Cell.*** Lymphocyte that cannot be identified as a T or B lymphocyte or a natural killer cell.

***Null Hypothesis.*** Statistical method bases on the proposition that, for example, there is no difference between the populations from which samples are drawn. The probability that one will find a difference equal to or greater than the one observed is then determined, and if this probability is low-less than 0.05—the null hypothesis can be rejected, and the differences in the populations scored as significant.

***Nulliparous.*** Describing a female that has had no offspring.

***Nullisomy.*** The condition in which both members of one pair of homologous chromosomes are absent, so that the chromosome complement is 2n - 2, where n is the haploid number.

***Numerical Response.*** The relationship between the numbers or fecundity of a population of predators or parasitoids and the density of their prey or hosts. Like functional response, it may reveal density dependence.

***Numerical Taxonomy.*** System of classification in which each taxonomic character in a population or individual is given equal weight and unitary value, permitting degrees of similarity between populations or individuals to be represented by numerical values.

***Nurse Cell.*** Cell in the ovary of insects that provides nutrition for the developing oocyte. The cytoplasm of the nurse cells streams into the occytes, which therefore grow at their expense. The cycles of DNA-replication in nurse cells are endomitotic (i.e. no nuclear division occurs).

***Nutrient Medium.*** Medium, for the cultivation of bacteria and other microorganisms, of undefined chemical composition. Nutrient media are based primarily on meat digests (tryptone, peptone), the soluble products of the enzymic digestion of meat or fish. Media are often supplemented with concentrated extracts of meat or yeast in provide vitamins and coenzymes. A typical nutrient medium has the following composition (in g/1): peptone (5.0), meat extract (1.5), yeast extract (1.5). NaCl (3.5), $K_2HPO_4$(3.7), $KH_2PO_4$(1.3), glucose (1.0). For fastidious bacteria, nutrient media can be further enriched with blood or serum.

***Nutritional Requirement.*** Although all living organisms have roughly similar chemical compositions, they vary in their nutritional requirements—their precursors for biosynthesis. Nutritional requirements of autotrophs are few; they include carbon dioxide as a carbon source, an inorganic source of nitrogen and trace elements (e.g. iron, copper, zinc, etc.). By contrast, heterotrophs require an organic source of carbon and energy. Many heterotrophs are unable to synthesize amino acids or coenzyme precursors (vitamins), and these must therefore be provided in the growth medium. In the study of microbial genetics many of the mutants used are auxotrophs. They differ from the parent strains (prototrophs) in their nutritional requirements. For example, a wild-type strain might require only an organic source plus nitrate for growth, whereas a nutritional mutant derived from. It might be unable to synthesize leucine. It would thus have acquired a 'new' nutritional requirement for leucine: it would be a leucine auxotroph.

***Nystatin.*** Fungicide used clinically to control oral, intestinal or urinogenital tract fungal infections. Nystatin is administered orally or locally. However, nystatin is not absorbed when taken orally and so cannot be used systemically. Nystatin can also be used to control fungal growth in cultures of eukaryotic cells; in bacterial cultures fungicides are not usually necessary as the bacterial cells outgrow any fungal contaminants.

# O

***O Antigen.*** Antigen of cell walls of entero-bacteria such as E. coli and Salmonella.

***O Antigen.*** Oligosaccharide antigen of the cell envelope of Gram-hegative bacteria. The designation O (German, 'ohne Hauch', 'without breath') was used becuase the non-motile bacteria, which contain O but not H antigens, do not form a film on agar plates. The O antigen is highly variable portion of the lipopolysaccharide (LPS) molecule, the major surface constituent of the cell envelope of these bacteria. It is composed of up to 40 repetitions of a unit consisting of a linear trisaccharide or a branched tetra- or pentasaccharide, often including unusual 3,6-dideoxyhexoses (abequose, tyvelose, paratose, colitose); the resulting chain is attached to a core polysaccharide which, in turn, is linked to lipid A. In each strain, the repeating oligosaccharide units are the same, although the length of the chains varies. The O antigens form the main basis for classification of strains of Salmonella in the Kauffmann-white scheme. The antigenic determinants consist of groups of sugar residues; dideoxyhexoses have an immunodominant role in many of these determinants. The O antigen is also known as the somatic (or cell-bound) antigen of these bacteria, in contradistinction to the H or flagellar antigen.

***Occam's Razor.*** Scientific principle that the simplest adequate hypothesis is preferred; named after the scholar William of Occam in 1347. Thus, when several possible explanations of a phenomenon are offered, the one favoured involves the fewest assumptions and is most consistent with the available data. It is also known as the parsimony principle.

***Ochre Mutation (Oc).*** Nonsense mutation that changes the nucleotide sequence of a gene to give the codon UAA. This results in premature termination of polypeptide biosynthesis.

***Octopine.*** Plant growth substance — an opine — produced by cells in crown galls on plants and active in promoting growth of the Agrobacterium in the crown gall cells.

***Octylglucoside.*** Chemically defined, neutral detergent.

***Odontoblast.*** One of a series of cells that lie along the periphery of the pulp cavity of a tooth, typified by their long cytoplasmic processes (fibres of Tomes), which extend into the canals of the surrounding dentine. They are thought to be involved in the formation and nutrition of dentine although the latter does not become necrotic when the odontoblasts are destroyed.

***Oenothera.*** Evening primrose; plant that has been intensively studied genetically. Because of the frequency of reciprocal translocation between chromosomes, the meiotic chromosomes are arranged in a ring rather than in pairs.

***Oestradiol-17β.*** The main natural oestrogen produced and secreted by mammals. It was first extracted from pig ovaries in 1935 and was later also isolated from cow placental extracts. See Figure O.1.

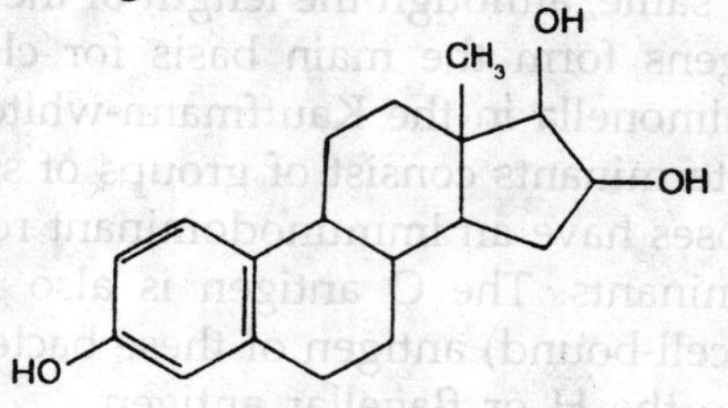


Figure O.1. Oestradiol-17β.

***Oestriol.*** An oestrogen isolated in 1930 from the urine of pregnant women. It is an excretion product of the ovary, but is probably also produced by the placenta. See Figure O.2.

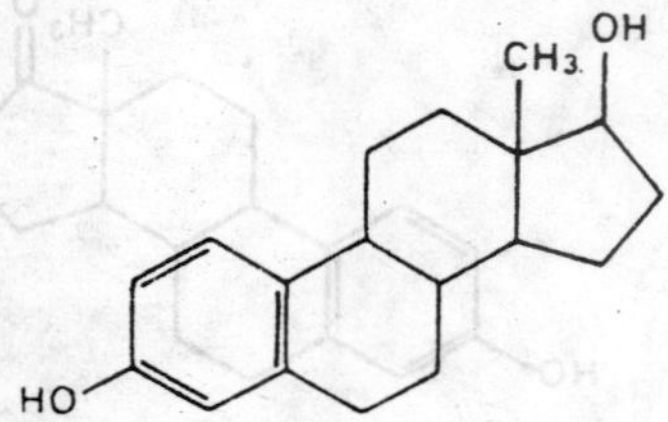


Figure O.2. Oestriol.

***Oestrogen.*** Any of a group of 18C (carbon) steroid hormones produced from acetate and cholesterol, chiefly by the ovaries and placenta but also by the testes and adrenal cortex in all vertebrates. They are also produced by many species of plants. Oestrogens have metabolic effects on many animal tissues but their best-known action is in female mammals, in which they stimulate the growth and maintenance of the reproductive organs (especially the uterus and vagina) and also of the female secondary sexual characteristics. Oestrogens also affect reproductive function and behaviour by actions on the hypothalamus and other regions of the central nervous system. The secretion of oestrogen from mature Graafian follicles is regulated by the pituitary gonadotrophins. Oestrogens have been shown to regulate the expression of genes in target tissues such as the uterus and brain by stimulating the synthesis of specific messenger RNA and protein in these organs; cytoplasmic and nuclear hormone receptors have been isolated. The predominant natural mammalian oestrogens are oestradiol-17β and oestrone. Many other oestrogenic substances found in the blood and urine are thought to be metabolites (e.g. oestriol) produced from the main hormones, although they may also have physiological significance. A number of potent synthetic oestrogens that are not steroids are used therapeutically.

***Oestrone.*** The first oestrogen to be identified. It was isolated in crystalline form from the urine of pregnant women in 1929 and was later shown to be produced by the ovaries. See Figure O.3.

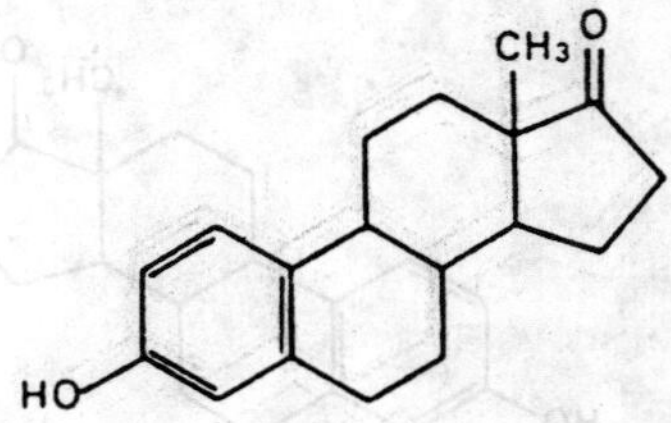


Figure O.3. Oestrone.

***Oestrone.*** Oestrogen synthesized by the ovaries.

***Oestrous Cycle.*** The reproductive cycle that occurs, either continuously or only during the breeding season, in sexually mature female mammals in the absence of pregnancy. Its length varies in different species from four to sixty days. The process is centrally regulated by the hypothalamus, which periodically release factors that stimulate the secretions of pituitary gonadotrophins. These, in turn, promote oestrogen and progesterone production, and the gonadal hormones themselves act as a feedback to modulate activity in the central nervous system. The following phases of the cycle generally occur :

(1) Oestrus (follicular phase) : the period of heat, during which copulation is permitted. In the ovary Graafian follicles mature and oestrogen secretion is at its highest; the endometrium (lining of the uterus) proliferates. Ovulation occurs forwards the end of this phase (it may be spontaneous, as in the rat, or activated by mating reflexes, as in the rabbit) and is probably triggered by a sharp rise in luteinizing hormone secretion.

(2) Metoestrus (luteal phase) : the period shortly after ovulation when mating is no longer permitted. The corpus luteum develops in the ovary and progesterone secretion increases, while the secretion of oestrogen decreases.

(3) Dioestrus : the beginning of the regression of the corpus luteum and uterine lining as well as the start of new follicular growth. Progesterone secretion diminishes. In some mammals this phase is lengthened if pregnancy does not follow mating and is termed pseudopregnancy.

(4) Pro-oestrus : the involution of the corpora lutea, coupled with the appearance of Graafian follicles, and a decrease in gonadal hormone secretion. It is followed by a slow increase in the secretion of follicle-stimulating hormone and oestrogen in preparation for the next oestrus.

If fertilization occurs following oestrus, the cycle becomes suspended in the luteal phase for the duration of pregnancy. Since the hormonal fluctuations during the cycle cause corresponding histological changes in the epithelium of the vagina, vaginal smears or scrapings of the vaginal wall can be examined under a microscope to determine the phase of the cycle.

***Ohno's Law.*** Genes present on the X chromosome in one species are likely to be X-linked in other species because of suggested unique regulatory features of the X chromosome; proposal advanced by S. Ohno.

***Okazaki Fragment.*** A short sequence of DNA that is the primary product of DNA polymerase during DNA replication. Okazaki fragments, of some 1000 to 2000 bases, are joined together by DNA ligase to yield a continuous new strand. Since synthesis can only proceed from a template strand going from the 3′ and towards the 5' end, synthesis of short fragments is inevitable using one of the parent strands as template. Although DNA replication could proceed continuously on the other strand, it also seems to be replicated initially as Okazaki fragments.

***Old Tuberculin (OT).*** Heat-concentrated filtrate from broth cultures in which Mycobacterium tuberculosis was grown. It was formed used in tuberculin skin tests.

***Oligoclonal.*** Related to or derived from a few clones.

***Oligo DA.*** Homopolymer of deoxyriboadenylate that can be made as an artificial polymer in vitro and used as a synthetic template for polyermases.

***Oligodendrocyte.*** Glial cell found in the vertebrate nervous system. These cells form insulating sheaths of myelin coiled around axons and other neuronal·processes in the nervous system.

***Oligo DT.*** Homoplymer of deoxyribothymidylate.

***Oligomer.*** Molecule made up of a few monomeric subunits.

***Oligomycin.*** Antibiotic active against fungi, but not against bacteria.

***Oligonucleotide.*** Nucleotide polymer containing somewhere between two and 10 nucleotides.

***Oligopeptide.*** Peptide polymer containing somewhere between two and 10 amino acids.

***Oligosaccharide.*** Carbohydrate made up of a small number of subunits. The carbohydrate moiety of glycoprotein is normally composed of such molecules.

***O-linked Saccharide.*** Sugar residues attached to the hydroxyl groups of serine, threonine or, sometimes, hydroxylsine residues of certain proteins. In most plasma proteins and in glycoproteins of mucinous secretions, the linking sugar residue is N-acetylgalactosamine and it is attached to serine or threonine. O-linked saccharides of plasma proteins usually consist of one to four residues. In addition to N-acetylgalactosamine, they frequently contain galactose and N-acetylneuraminic acid (sialic acid). The O-linked oligosaccharides in blood group substances are considerably larger and may contain more than a dozen saccharides. The sugar residues are added one at a time by different glycosyl transferases in the golgi complex. There is no known acceptor sequence for O-linked saccharides, but proline is often found adjacent to glycosylated serine or threonine residues and may promote beta turns in the polypeptide chain. In collagen and C1q, galactose (the linking residue) and glucose are attached to hydroxylysine residues.

Only two constant regions of human immunoglobulin chains contain O-linked saccharides. The hinge region of the alphal chain contains four disaccharides consisting of N-acetylgalactosamine and galactose and one monosaccharide, N-acetylgalactosamine, all linked to serine. The hinge region of the delta chain contains four to seven saccharides linked either to serine or threonine; these consist of N-acetylgalactosamine and galactose and, sometimes, one or two sialic acid residues.

***Onc Gene.*** Oncogene in a retrovirus. Such gene sequences are closely similar to proto-oncogenes which occur as normal coding sequences in vertebrate genomes.

***Oncofetal Antigens.*** Antigens normally expressed in fetal life that reappear in tumors.

***Oncogene.*** Gene that brings about or contributes to the neoplastic transformation of cells. The term may refer to:(1) genes, originally of cellular origin, that have been incorporated into retroviral genomes and, in the process, have acquired the ability to transform cells (e.g., v-src in Rous sacroma virus, v-abl in abelson murine leukemia virus, v-myc in avian myelocytomatosis virus); (2) genes from tumors that have arisen spontaneously or from cells that have been transformed by chemical carcinogens and that are responsible for maintenance of the neoplastic state; (3) genes from DNA viruses (e.g., polyoma, adenovirus) that can induce cellular transformation.

Retroviral and cellular oncogenes arise from cellular genes called proto-oncogenes (e.g., c-src, c-abl, c-myc), which play a role in normal growth and differentiation. An alteration in a growth regulatory signal (e.g., due to an increase in the amount of gene product or in its structure) may induce neoplatic transformation. This may occur by several different mechanisms: (1) as already noted, acquisition by a retrovirus, which places the cellular gene under the control of viral transcriptional promoters and enhancers; (2) nearby integration of a retrovirus; (3) gene amplification; (4) chromosomal translocation with resulting loss of normal regulation (e.g., translocation of the c-myc proto-oncogene from chromosome 8 to one of the chromosomes containing immunoglobulin genes); (5) mutation of protein-encoding sequences, which may occur as the only change responsible for mutagenesis or which may accompany the other mechanisms, contributing to the oncogenic transformation.

More than 20 cellular proto-oncogenes are known. Their products have been classified according to cellular location: secreted, cell surface, cytoplasmic, and nuclear. Some (e.g.,c-src and c-abl) encode protein kinases that phosphorylate tyrosine residues of specific cellular proteins; c-ras genes encode proteins that bind tightly to guanine nucleotides and possess GTPase activity. Some oncogenes have been identified as growth factors or growth factor receptors; c-sis encodes one chain of the platelet-derived growth factor; c-erbB encodes part of the epidermal growth factor receptor; c-fms encodes the receptor for the macrophage colony stimulation factor, CSF-1.

***Oncogenes***. Genes that have oncogenic or cancer-causing potential. They were initially discovered in retroviruses, although they are not native to these viruses. Oncogenes are found in both cancerous and non-cancerous cells, and are probably genes that are required for normal growth and development. Cellular oncogenes known more correctly as proto-oncogenes, have the split structural organization of normal cellular genes with exons and introns whereas viral oncogenes do not. The protein products of many of the oncogenes studied are protein kinases or protein phosphorylating enzymes. See Table.

**Oncogenes**

**List of viral oncogenes and the location and proposed function in the cell of the equivalent proto-oncogene. "Reproduced with permission from Biship. J.M. (1985) Cell. 42, 23-38**

| *Oncogene* | *Proto-oncogene Product; location in cell* | *Proto-oncogene product: function* |
|---|---|---|
| EIA (243)[b] | Nucleus; cytoplasm | Regulates transcription (?) |
| EIA(289)[b] | Nucleus; cytoplasm | Regulates transcription |
| EIB(21 kd) | Nuclear envelope endoplasmic | ? |

| | | |
|---|---|---|
| | reticulum;plasma membrane | ? |
| EIB(55 kd) | Nucleoplasm; perinuclear cytoplasm; cell-cell contacts | ? ? |
| Py-t | Cytoplasm | ? |
| Py-mT | Plasma membrane | Bind and stimulates pp60$^{c\text{-}src}$ |
| Py-T | Nucleus | Initiates DNA synthesis and regulates transcription |
| SV-t | Cytoplasm | ? |
| SV-T | Plasma membrane; nucleus | Initiates DNA synthesis; regulates transcription |
| v-abl | Plasma membrane (?) | Protein-tyrosine kinase |
| v-tesllps | Plasma membrane (?) | Protein-tyrosine kinase |
| v-tgr | ? | Protein-tyrosine kinase |
| v-src | Plasma membrane; juxtanuclear membranes | Protein-tyrosine kinase |
| v-erb-B | Plasma membrane; endoplasmic reti-culum; Golgi apparatus | Protein-tyrosine kinase |
| v-tms | Plasma membrane; endoplasmic reticulum; Golgi appa-ratus | Protein-tyrosine kinase |
| v-ros | ? | Protein-tyrosine kinase |
| v-yes | ? | Protein-tyrosine kinase |
| v-millral | Cytoplasm | Protein-serine/threonine kinase |
| v-mos | Cytoplasm | Protein-serine/threonine kinase |
| v-ras | Plasma membrane | Regulates adenylate cyclase |
| v-tos | Nucleus | ? |
| v-myb | Nucleus | ? |
| v-myc | Nucleus | Regulates transcription (?) |
| v-ski | Nucleus | ? |
| v-sis | Secreted; cytoplasm (?) | Analogue of PDGF-2/B |
| v-erb-A | Cytroplasm | ? |
| v-rel | Cytoplasm | ? |
| v-kit | ? | ? |
| v-ets | Nucleus (fused with product of v-myb) | ? |

"Symbols used are: A, adenovirus: Py, polyoma; SV, SV40; t, small T antigen; mT, middle T antigen; T, large T antigen;?, uncertain or unknown. PDGF, platelet-derived growth factor, pp60$^{c\text{-}src}$ is the 60 kilodalton protein product of the v-src oncogene. Numbers correspond to the number of amino acids in the gene product.

***Oncogenic.*** Having the capacity to induce cancer.

***Oncogenic Virus.*** A virus associated with cancer (because of the difficulty of establishing absolute causal relationships in biology, it is best not to regard these viruses as representing the cause of the disease). Both DNA and RNA viruses may be oncogenic, including some papovaviruses, adenoviruses, and leukoviruses. The Rous sarcoma of chickens and feline leukaemia are diseases in which viral causation is particularly likely. Many oncogenic viruses are capable of inducing cell transformation in vitro. And some other malignant diseases of the human are under suspicion of having a viral association, this remains speculative.

***Oncology.*** Study of cancer.

***Oncornaviruses.*** Acronym for oncogenic RNA viruses.

***One Gene-One Enzyme Hypothesis.*** The hypothesis that each gene is concerned with the synthesis of a single enzyme. However, since genes also determine the structure of all nonenzymic proteins, and many enzymes and other proteins are polymeric structures in which each monomer is coded by a separate gene, the concept is better expressed as the one gene-one polypeptide chain hypothesis.

***One Gene-One Polypeptide Chain Hypothesis.*** Modern restatement of an older proposition. Since many enzymes (e.g. eukaryotic RNA polymerases) are complex proteins made up of a number of differing polypeptide chains, it is clear that the relationship is 1 : 1 for the gene and the polypeptide chain. But, although each different polypeptide chain is the product of a different gene, many genes do not code for any polypeptide chains.

***ONPG (O-Nitrophenylgalactoside).*** Synthetic substrate for the enzyme β-galactosidase which is cleaved by the enzyme into two separate substances, one being the yellow-coloured o-nitrophenol. This compound is therefore used to assay for the presence of this enzyme, as for example in mutants of E. coli with lesions in the Lac operon genetic sequence.

*Ontogeny.* The development of an individual during its lifetime.

*Oocyte.* An egg cell of the animal ovary that undergoes meiosis to form an ovum. After a period of growth, the primary oocyte undergoes the first division to form a polar body (or polocyte), a cell with very little cytoplasm, and a secondary oocyte, a cell with a large amount of cytoplasm that undergoes the second division to form a further polar body and an ovum. In many species one of the two oocyte stages is released at ovulation and fertilization occurs without the formation of an ovum.

*Oogamy.* The sexual fusion of two dissimilar gametes. The male gamete is small, often motile, and has little food reserve; the female is larger, sedentary, and contains food reserves for the developing zygote.

*Oogenesis.* Production of the Ovum from the oocyte. The primary oocyte in the ovary undergoes its first meiotic division (during which prophase is arrested and growth and maturation occur before division is completed) to yield a secondary oocyte with much cytoplasm and a first polar body with little cytoplasm. The second meiotic division of the secondary oocyte yields the ovum and a secondary polar body. In some species, one or other of the oocyte stages is released at ovulation and fertilized without the ovum being formed.

*Oogonium.* 1. The simple female sexual organ of many algae and fungi, containing one to many oospheres.

2. A cell of the animal ovary that divides to produce oocytes.

*Oosphere (Ovum, egg cell).* A naked spherical sedentary haploid female gamete in plants, generally containing some food reserve. The term is sometimes restricted to a female gamete developed within an oogonium.

*Oospore.* A fertilized oosphere that develops into a thick-walled resting spore.

***Opal Mutation.*** Nonsense mutation that changes the nucleotide sequence within a gene to give the codon UGA, which codes for termination of polypeptide biosynthesis.

***Open Reading Frame (ORF).*** Region of a DNA sequence that has the potential to be read as codons specifying amino acids (i.e. it is not interrupted by nonsense codons as stop signals), ORF sequences are frequently encountered in the sequencing of gene banks and only occasionally can they be assigned to a particular known gene.

***Open Reading Frame (ORF).*** Stretch of DNA or RNA that may encode a protein or part of a protein. Open reading frames must not contain terminaion codons. A complete open reading frame would begin with the initiation codon ATG (AUG) and end at a termination codon (TAA (UAA), TAG (UAG), or TGA (UGA). The identification of an open reading frame may be the first indication for the existence of a previously unknown protein.

***Operator.*** Region of a DNA sequence capable of interacting with a specific repressor molecule, and in so doing, affecting the activity of other genes downstream from it.

***Operon.*** A group of closely linked genes that behave as a unit in determining the synthesis of the enzymes of a particular catabolic or biosynthetic pathway. It consists of an operator gene and one or more structural genes and its expression is controlled by a regulator gene, which is not part of the operon. The operator gene acts as an on/off switch controlling the transcription of the messenger RNA for the synthesis of all the proteins determined by the structural genes. The regulator gene produces a protein, the repressor, which can bind specifically to the DNA of the operator locus and prevent the synthesis of the messenger RNA.

Crown gall and used as a growth substance by the Agrobacteria within the gall. Nopaline and octopine are two examples of opines.

***Opine Synthetase (Opine synthase).*** Enzyme system responsible for the synthesis of opines of which there are a number of different types. The genetic information coding for opine synthetase resides in the T-DNA region of the TI plasmid. These plasmids confer virulence to strains of Agrobacterium, which are responsible for the crown gall disease. The T-DNA is transferred to the plant cells, where it is stably integrated into the nuclear genome and the opine synthetase gene is transcribed and translated.

***Opportunistic Infections.*** Infections that occur mainly in patients with defects in cell-mediated immunity (e.g., acquired immunodeficiency syndrome and severe combined immunodeficiency). Microorganisms causing opportunistic infections include Pneumocystis carinii, Candida albicans, Mycobacterium avium intracellulare, Toxoplasma, Cryptosporidia and herpes virus.

***Opsonin.*** Substance in serum that binds to particles (e.g. red blood cells or bacteria) and increases their suceptibility to phagocytosis. The term has been used to describe the following: (1) antibodies specific for antigenic determinants of the particles. The Fc fragment of the bound antibody attaches to Fc receptors of phagocytic cells, thereby facilitating phagocytosis of the particle. Antibodies are known as heat-stable opsonins. (2) Products of complement activation. C3b or C3bi, bound to particles by transacylation with the thiolester of C3, attach to complement receptor 1 or complement receptor 3, respectively, on phagocytic cells. C3b and C3bi are known as heat-labile opsonins. (3) Certain other substances that bind to particles (e.g., fibronectin).

***Opsonin.*** An antibody, present in blood serum, that reacts with the surface antigens of bacteria to promote phagocytosis. Opsonic adherence, which involves binding through complement components, is one of the most important defence mechanisms against infection.

***Opsonization.*** Deposition of opsonins onto particles, such as red blood cells or bacteria, thereby facilitating their phagocytosis.

***Optical Activity.*** Ability of a molecule to rotate the plane of polarized light when it is passed through a solution of the molecule. Sugars such as monosaccharides may exist in either of two isomeric forms, as a function of their asymmetric carbon atoms; they exist in two configurations known as D-form (dextrorotatory) and L-form (laevorotatory) bending light either to the right or to the left, respectively.

***Optical Density (OD).*** Degree of absorbence of light by a solution as a function of the concentration of the solute. For solutions that absorb light, the relative optical density provides information about concentration and the character of the solution. Spectrophotometers are machines designed to measure optical density, either of visible light, or with infrared or ultraviolet light. Scanning spectrophotometers provide an absorption spectrum over a range of wavelengths; this can be used to determine the precise composition and purity of a solution. Nucleic acids absorb light maximally at a wavelength of 260 nm, whereas proteins absorb maximally at 280 nm. Thus the protein content of an impure solution of DNA can be measured. Since the optical density of a DNA solution increases when the DNA is melted (the hyperchromic effect) changes in optical density can be used to provide detailed information about DNA complexity, especially in the use of reduction of optical density after melting, as is used to construct cot plots.

***Optical Isomers.*** Molecular isomers that induce rotation of a beam of plane-polarized light when it is passed through a solution of the molecule. The rotation, which results from the asymmetric form of the molecule may be to the right (dextro-) or to the left (laevo-) for different isomers of the same molecule. These isomers are referred to, as in the case of, for example, glucose, as d-glucose or l-glucose.

***Optimal Proportions.*** Synonym for equivalence.

***Orcein.*** Dye used in cytology, especially when dissolved in acetic acid as aceto-orcein for the staining of squash preparations of chromosomes.

***Ordered Tetrad.*** Linear sequence of the products of meiotic division as visualized in the row of eight ascospores of a fungal ascus, crossing-over events can be studied by growing each spore separately and scoring it for its expression of one allele at a particular locus.

***Ordovician.*** The second period of the Palaeozoic era, extending from 500 to 440 million years ago. It was named after a Celtic tribe that lived in the region of Wales where rocks of the period were first recognized. Ordovician fossils consist mainly of trilobites and brachiopods, but there are also gastropods, nautiloid cephalopods, and many echinoderms (including crinoids and some echinoids).

***Organ.*** A part of the body of an organism that forms a structural and functional unit and is composed of more than one tissue. An example of a plant organ is a leaf; animal organs include the heart and liver.

***Organ Culture.*** Growth of organs or pieces of organs in culture as compared to tissue culture, which involves the growth of cells without multicellular morphological structure. For whole organs, it is best illustrated by the culture of small embryonic gland primordia (e.g. salivary gland) or of skeletal primordia. Organ culture usually involves only short-term maintenance. The usefulness of the technique is limited by critical mass as continued growth leads to a point at which tissue necrosis occurs centrally due to the constraints of nutrient diffusion from the culture medium.

***Organic.*** (1) As applied to organisms, whether alive or dead, or to the chemicals derived from time. (2) Descriptive of chemical compounds based on carbon rings or chains, even if these have no direct connection with organisms. Thus oil and oil-based products are organic chemicals.

***Organizer.*** A region of cells in an animal embryo that, by the release of an evocator, can induce and direct cellular differentiation in another region. For example, if the dorsal lip of the amphibian blastopore (which itself develops into the notochord and somites) is transplanted into a region of prospective epidermis, it will induce prospective epidermal tissue to form a neural tube.

***Organizing Centres.*** Centres from which microtubules are organized or are grown. They include the cell centres and basal bodies.

***Organogenesis.*** Development of organs during embryonic life. It involves both the differentiation of individual cells and the structural form of the organ as it grows (morphogenesis).

***Original Anigenic Sin.*** Tendency to react to immunization by producing antibodies to a determinant on the stimulating antigen that resembles as a determinant on an antigen encountered previously. Antibodies that cross-react with the original antigen are produced preferentially. The term was first used to describe the response to reinfection with influenza when the host makes a secondary immune response to the strain of influenza of a previous infection. In the interval between infections, the influenza virus has undergone antigenic change.

***Origin of Life.*** Most modern organisms are dependent, directiy or indirectly, on two closely linked metabolic processes : photosynthesis and aerobic respiration. Although opinions differ as to what steps were involved in their evolution, it seems likely that photosynthesis evolved in the first third of the earth's history and aerobic respiration in the last half. Evidence from chemical fossils, morphological remains of microorganisms, and geochemistry regarding conditions present during rock formation suggests that six main stages of evolution are involved :

(1) abiogenic production of organic compounds. The earliest atmosphere probably consisted of ammonia, methane, hydrogen, and water vapour. Such a mixture has been shown to produce many of the organic compounds utilized by living organisms when energy in the form of an electric discharge, ultraviolet radiation, or sunlight is passed through it. These compounds include all the amino acids, some proteins, porphyrins and vitamins, and the precursors of nucleotides. The process of self-replication using DNA or RNA as a coding device for proteins is chemically extremely complex and a satisfactory theory of its evolution has

not yet been suggested. However, a compartmentalizing of such self-replicating systems within a membrane-bound unit would have resulted in the first primitive organisms.

(2) anaerobic heterotrophy. The first true organisms probably obtained energy by the partial oxidation of organic substances of nonbiotic origin. They evolved into organisms that used gaseous hydrogen for the reduction of carbon dioxide in the atmosphere to produce their carbohydrates, which they could then use as an energy source by partial oxidation.

(3) anaerobic photoheterotrophy. The first primitive type of photosynthetic system arose when anaerobic heterotrophs started using the light-absorbing porphyrins present in their cytoplasm for trapping light energy, as well as partially oxidizing hydrocarbons formed chemically.

(4) anaerobic phototrophy. Anaerobic photoheterotrophy was followed by the evolution of anaerobic organisms whose only method of organic molecule synthesis depended on light energy.

(5) lysis of water. The first oxygen in the atmosphere was produced by the photolysis of water. An important step in photosynthesis evolution occurred when organisms started dissociating water for themselves to yield hydrogen (the importance being that elemental oxygen was released into the atmosphere).

(6) oxygenation of carbon compounds. The final important stage occurred with the evolution of organisms capable to using oxygen to oxidize carbohydrates and yield much more energy than primitive fermentation processes.

An approximate time scale for these developments is indicate by the geological formations banded iron formations and red beds. The former were laid down 3.4-1.8 x $10^9$ years ago under reducing conditions (stages 1-3).The red beds have been laid down since 1.8 x $10^9$years ago in the presence of free oxygen, indicating that oxygen was present in the atmosphere and no longer toxic and that some organisms may have evolved the extra enzyme systems necessary for aerobic respiration (stages 4-5). Following oxygen evolution three levels of concentration in the atmosphere have been suggested as critical for the evolution of higher life forms:

(1) 1% PAL (present atmospheric level): allowed a completely modern type of metabolic system to function (probably around 6 x $10^8$ years ago, corresponding with the sudden blossoming of forms in the Cambrian).

(2) 10% PAL; provided enough oxygen in the atmosphere to shield the land against short-wave ultraviolet radiation (prior to this organisms needed the protection of water). This led to the invasion of the land by plants and thus to (a) the establishment of vegetation (providing possible habitats for the later invasion of the land by animals); and (b) increased oxygen production (probably) occurring about 4 x $10^8$ years ago - the Devonian expansion).

(3) 20% PAL; allowed land animal to emerge (about 3.4 x $10^8$ years ago, corresponding with the appearance of the amphibians at the end of the devonian.

***Origin of Species.*** Abbreviated form of the title of the book by Charles Darwin, first published in 1859.

***Ornithine.*** Basic amino acid that is an important intermediate in the urea cycle.

***Ornithine Cycle (Urea Cycle).*** Cyclic series of biochemical reactions responsible for conversion and detoxification of the nitrogenous products of protein metabolism. Ammonia and urea are derived from the metabolic pathway, the ammonia being used to convert ornithine to citrulline and the inocuous urea being largely excreted. Some genetic mutants in the human have blocks in the cycle, resulting in, for example, the citrullinuria and ornithine transcarbamylase deficiency.

***Orphan Viruses.*** Range of viruses that may be found in the respiratory and digestive tracts of healthy individuals; such viruses are not associated with any known pathology. Double-stranded RNA reoviruses are examples of orphan viruses.

***Orphon.*** Pseudogene that has become dispersed and isolated from the gene family in which it is presumed to have arisen. Orphons are probably important in the context of molecular evolution in that they may readily take on new functions following random changes in their sequence.

***Orthochromatin.*** Normal chromatin, as compared to unstable chromatin, deemed to be a reservoir of regulatory elements. The term is now little used.

***Orthogenesis.*** The theory that evolution can occur in a definite direction, which is predetermined by inherent factors in the genotype and does not rely on natural selection or genetic drift.

***Orthotopic.*** Descriptive of a tissue or organ graft to a site normally occupied by that tissue or organ.

***Osmium Tetroxide ($O_SO_4$).*** Compound used as a biological fixative for light and electron microscopy; sometimes wrongly termed osmic acid. It is highly toxic and readily vapourizes.

***Osmosis.*** Process whereby a solvent spontaneously moves from a region in a solution where its activity is high, to a region where its activity is lower. in practice, osmosis only occurs when a semipermeable membrane separate a solution, either from pure solvent or from a solution with the same solvent but having a different concentration of solute. In living systems the solvent is water, and its movement tends to equalize solute concentration on the two sides of a cell membrane. However, cell membrane are not truely semipermeable since they allow the passage of some solutes, consequently they are said to be selectively permeable.

***Osmotic Swelling.*** Increased in cell size (or in the size of other membrane-bound vesicles) due to osmosis.

***Ossification.*** Formation of bone. It is a process of replacement of pre-existing connective tissue, either in the form of cartilage (endochondral ossification) or simple connective tissue membrane (intramembranous ossification). The connective tissue is invaded by osteoblasts, which secrete an extracellular matrix of bone and finally become trapped in the matrix as osteocytes. When existing bone is being reformed in development or repair, some resorption of existing bone may occur, being accomplished by activity of osteoclasts.

***Osteoblast.*** Bone-forming cell typically found on the surface of bone matrix and which contributes to its appositional growth by depositing extracellular matrix and giving rise to osteocytes.

***Osteoclast.*** Multinucleate, giant cell responsible for resorption of bone matrix by extracellular enzymic action. Osteoclasts have a separate lineage from osteoblasts/osteocytes in that they are formed by the fusion of mononucleate precursor cells — monocytes.

***Osteoclast-activating Factor (OAF).*** Activity found in the cultures of antigen-stimulated lymphocytes that induces resorption of bone in vitro. Several molecules have been identified as having OAF activity including lymphotoxin elaborated by T lymphocytes and tumor necrosis factor, interleukin-1 and prostaglandins all elaborated by macrophages. OAF activity may be responsible for bone resorption found in patients with lymphoid cell malignacies such as multiple myeloma or T cell lymphomas.

***Osteocyte.*** Any of the principal cells of fully formed bone, found within the bone matrix and derived from osteoblasts. They are thought to participate in the release of calcium from the bone into the blood.

***Osteogenesis Imperfecta.*** Inherited disease of the human, but with varying genetic backgrounds (some diseases are autosomal dominant, and others are autosomal recessive). It is characterized by brittle bones, discoloured teeth and deafness, but is very variable in its severity from complete lack of symptoms to perinatal death.

***Otosclerosis.*** Progressive conductive hearing loss in middle age inherited as an autosomal recessive condition.

***Ouchterlony Tplate.*** Petri dish or slide used in the ouchterlony technique.

***Ouchterlony Technique (double diffusion technique).*** Precipitation test involving antibody-antigen interaction in gel diffusion systems. Two or more wells are cut in an agar slab, and a solution of antibody is placed in one central well. Other wells have various presumptive antigens in solution placed in them. By allowing simple diffusion, lines of precipitation are formed between the wells, each one representing a specific interaction.

***Oudin Technique.*** Test involving the formation of zones of precipitation resulting from antigen-antibody interaction; similar to the ouchterlony technique. A gel column is prepared with an even distribution of a selected antibody molecule. Following the deposition of an aqueous suspension of antigen molecules on the upper layer of the column, lines of precipitate form as the antigen molecules move into the column and interact specifically with the antibody.

***Outbreeding.*** The mating of individuals of the same species that are not closely related : also applied to cross-fertilization in plants. Many plants and animals have mechanisms (either physical or social) that encourage outbreeding, since this tends to be advantageous and to promote heterozygosity. However, extreme outbreeding - the crossing of two different species - is discouraged by various mechanisms because the products of the cross are infertile.

***Outbreeding.*** Mating of individuals less closely related than individuals chosen at random from a population. Outbreeding tends to promote genetic diversity in a populaton.

***Ovalbumin.*** One of the major proteins of egg white. It is the major nutritional protein of avian egg white and is a phosphoprotein of 386 amino acids.

***Ovalbumin Gene.*** Gene coding for ovalbumin; one of the first sequences in which the fragmented structure of introns and exons was demonstrated. It has been most thoroughly investigated in the chicken, where it is found to be some 7.8 kilobases in length and to consist of eight exons separated by six introns. Only a single copy of the gene exists in the chicken genome, but it is one of three genes in a small clustered multigene family. The other two genes in the family, code-named X and Y, are not as yet identified in terms of protein products. See Figure O.4.

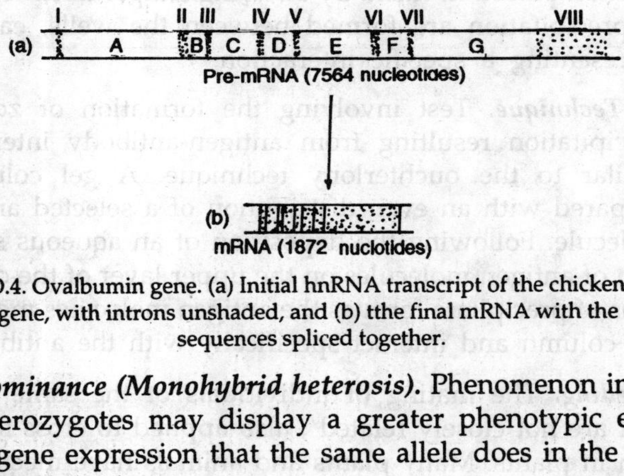


Figure O.4. Ovalbumin gene. (a) Initial hnRNA transcript of the chicken ovalbumin gene, with introns unshaded, and (b) tthe final mRNA with the exon sequences spliced together.

***Overdominance (Monohybrid heterosis).*** Phenomenon in which heterozygotes may display a greater phenotypic extreme of gene expression that the same allele does in the phenotype of the homozygote.

***Overlapping Code.*** The genetic code is in general non-overlapping, in that each triplet of bases codes for a distinct amino acid, and there is no sharing of common bases between adjacent triplets. Some overlapping genes do provide examples of uses of the same sequence with a change in reading frame, which involves triplet overlap.

***Overlapping Deletion.*** Compound deletion occurring as two separate events, in which one overlaps another.

***Overlapping Genes.*** Genes whose nucleotide coding sequences have some areas of overlap. Apart from some overlapping regulatory genes in bacteria, such as the operator and promoter sequences of the tryptophan operon of E. coli, the only clear example known is in the genes of certain phages. For example in the genome of the phage ϕx174, one gene lies entirely within the coding sequence of another, but is translated using a different reading frame.

***Overlapping Inversion.*** Situation in which a second inversion overlaps a previous existing inverted sequence.

***Overlap Syndrome.*** Synonym for mixed connective tissue disease.

***Overwinding.*** Situation in which the DNA double helix, already wound in a right-handed spiral, is placed under additional torsional stress in the same direction resulting in positive supercoiling of the double helix upon itself.

***Oviparity.*** A type of animal reproduction in which the fertilized eggs are laid or spawned by the mother. The eggs contain poorly developed embryos with a large supply of yolk. Oviparity occurs in many vertebrates, excluding marsupial and placental mammals, and in most invertebrates.

***Oviparous.*** Describing animals that lay eggs, in which the embryos develop and from which they hatch, all outside the body of the female.

***Ovotestis.*** Reproductive organ in certain hermaphrodite animals, either having both ovary and testis at the same time (a simultaneous hermaphrodite), or at consecutive times (a sequential hermaphrodite). Within the phylum Mollusca can be found species that display one or the other arrangement.

***Ovoviviparity.*** A type of animal reproduction in which the embryos develop within the maternal organism but make no apparent contact with maternal tissues for the purposes of nutrition. Ovoviviparity occurs sporadically in many invertebrate groups, fish, and reptiles.

***Ovulation.*** The discharge of an ovum or oocyte from a mature follicle of the vertebrate ovary. The process, although not fully understood, is initiated by hypothalamic factors that stimulate the secretion of luteinizing hormone from the pituitary. A rapid rise in the level of this hormone in the presence of follicle-stimulating hormone causes ovulation. See Figure O.5.

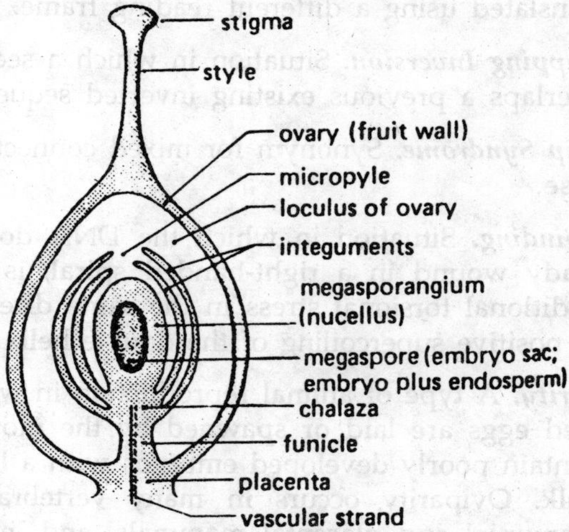


Figure O.5. Diagrammatic section through a monocarpellary angiosperm pistil containing a single ovule.

***Ovule.*** The structure in gymnosperm and angiosperm plants in which meiosis and megaspore formation occurs and which is borne on an ovuliferous scale in many gymnosperms and on the placenta within the ovary of angiosperms : an integumented megasporangium. It consists of a short stalk (termed the funicle in angiosperms) bearing a small mass of parent (sporophyte) tissue, the nucellus, which is surrounded by one or two integuments. These arise as folds at the funicular end of the nucellus (this region is known as the chalaza) and grow up round the nucellus; the small aperture usually left by their incomplete closure is termed the micropyle. A single cell at the micropylar end of the nucellus enlarges to become the megasporocyte and undergoes meiosis to produce sour cells, of which three abort and one becomes the functional megaspore. This cell undergoes either free nuclear division (division of the nucleus without division of the cytoplasm) or ordinary cell division to produce the embryo sac. This structure produces the archegonia (in gymnosperms) or contains the functional gametic nucleus (in angiosperms) and is usually regarded as a retained gametophyte prothallus. After fertilization of the archegonia or embryo sac, or by agamospermy, the ovule matures into the seed.

There are nine positions in which the ovule may be borne on the funicle. The simplest type (and probably the most primitive, from which the others evolved) is the orthotropous (or atropous) ovule, from which the hemitropous and anatropous ovules are derived. The orthocampylotropous (or campylotropus) ovule gives rise to the hemicampylotropous and anacampylotropous ovules, and the orthoamphitropous (or amphitropous) ovule gives rise to the hemiamphitropous and anamphitropous ovules.

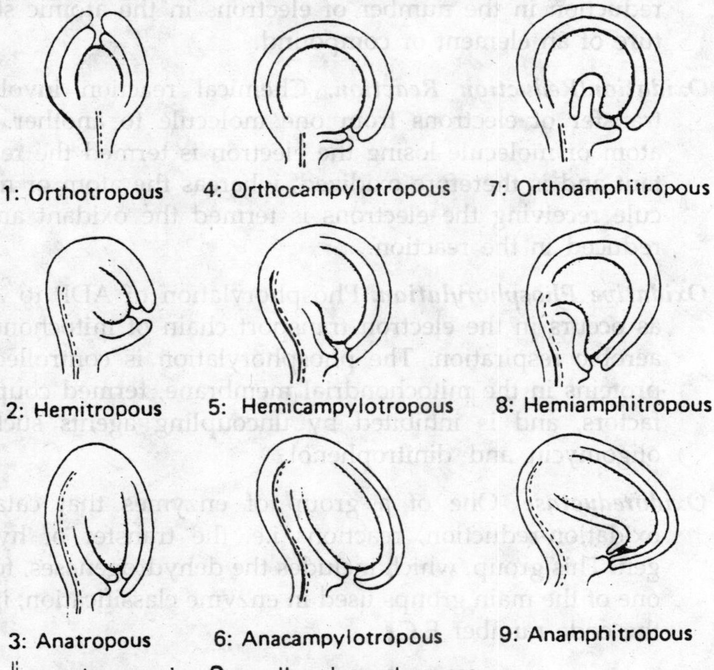


Figure O.6. Types of angiosperm ovules.

In gymnosperms such a wide variety is not shown; ovules are either erect or anatropous. See Figure O.6.

***Ovum (egg cell).*** Haploid non-motile, unfertilized female gamete of animals.

***Oxidases.*** Enzymes that catalyse oxidation reactions in which the electron acceptor (oxidant) is oxygen, the product is water or hydrogen peroxide ($H_2O_2$), and the oxygen atoms are not incorporated into the product of the reaction. For example, amino acid oxidases are flavoproteins that catalyse the oxygen-requiring oxidation of amino acids to keto acids with the concomitant formation of hydrogen peroxide. Perhaps the most important example of an oxidase is the cytochrome oxidase which uses electrons from an electron transport chain plus protons from the surrounding medium to reduce oxygen to water.

***Oxidation.*** Acquisition of oxygen, or loss of hydrogen, or reduction in the number of electrons in the atomic structure of an element or compound.

***Oxidation/Reduction Reaction.*** Chemical reaction involving transfer of electrons from one molecule to another. The atom or molecule losing the electron is termed the reductant and is therefore oxidized, whereas the atom or molecule receiving the electrons is termed the oxidant and is reduced in the reaction.

***Oxidative Phosphorylation.*** Phosphorylation of ADP to ATP, as occurs in the electron transport chain of mitochondrial aerobic respiration. The phosphorylation is controlled by proteins in the mitochondrial membrane, termed coupling factors, and is inhibited by uncoupling agents such as oligomycin and dinitrophenol.

***Oxidoreductase.*** One of a group of enzymes that catalyse oxidation-reduction, reactions i.e. the transfer of hydrogen. This group, which includes the dehydrogenases, forms one of the main groups used in enzyme classification; it has the code number E.C.I.

***Oxygenases.*** Enzymes that catalyse oxidation reactions (usually irreversible) in which oxygen is incorporated from molecular oxygen into the product. Oxygenase-catalysed reactions are often the first oxidative step in the metabolism of stable reduced compounds such as alkanes. Monooxygenases catalyse the incorporation of a single atom of oxygen, the second atom being reduced in the same reaction to water by an electron donor (reductant) which is usually NAD(P)H. Monooxygenase reactions often involve a number of electron transfer components between the electron donor and the substrate: these components may include Iron-sulphur proteins, flavoproteins or cytochromes. A typical example is the system occurring in mammalian liver for detoxification of foreign compounds; this contains a cytochrome called cytochrome $P_{450}$. Because reactions catalysed by monooxygenases often yield a molecule containing an extra hydroxyl group they are frequently called hydroxylation reactions. Dioxygenases differ from monooxygenases in that both atoms of oxygen from molecular oxygen are incorporated into the product, and a reductant is not involved in the reaction.

***Oxygen Quotient ($Q_{O2}$).*** Figure representing the rate of oxygen consumption of a tissue or organism, expressed as microlitres of oxygen per milligram dry weight per hour.

***Oz Isotypic Determinant.*** Antigenic determinant of human immunoglobulin lambda chains associated with lysine at position 190. This determinant is present on some of the lambda chains of every individual. It is, therefore, not the result of genetic polymorphism.

# ENCYCLOPAEDIC DICTIONARY OF GENETICS AND ORGANIC EVOLUTION

# Encyclopaedic Dictionary of Genetics and Organic Evolution

**Vol. 3**
[P — Z]

*Editor*
**Kiran Narang**

**ANMOL PUBLICATIONS PVT LTD**
**New Delhi-110 002**

**ANMOL PUBLICATIONS PVT LTD**
4374/4B, Ansari Road
Daryaganj, New Delhi-110 002

*Encyclopaedic Dictionary of Genetics and Organic Evolution*

First Edition 1995
**ISBN 81-7488-044-5 (Set)**

**PRINTED IN INDIA**

Published by J.L. Kumar for Anmol Publications Pvt. Ltd. and
Printed at Mehra Offset Press, Delhi.

# Preface

This encyclopaedic dictionary has been essentially a compilation and editing of the terms and concepts taken from genetics and organic evolution. Many words borrowed from more general usage have been endowed with very special meaning, sometimes not obvious to the uninitiated.

The entries have been represented in a clear and explanatory style to provide both straight forward definitions and invaluable background informations. This approach combined with an extensive cross referencing system enables the reader to place each entry into a broader scientific context. Many diagrams have been incorporated whenever the meaning of a term can be best conveyed by means of a diagram.

Every effort has been made to include certain entries which take into account of recent developments and trends in genetics and organic evolution.

The terms included in this encyclopaedic dictionary have been presented in brief analytical phrases thereby avoiding the more comprehensive type of treatment appropriate to large reference works. The extent of each entry has been determined by the need for definition of meaning, function and agricultural relevance. Also, certain entries have been added to take into account of recent developments and trends in agriculture.

This encyclopaedic dictionary will be of immense value to the students of genetics and organic evolution, botany, ecology, biology, microbiology, anthropology, biochemistry, archaeology, geography, geology, agriculture and environmental science.

**Editor**

**Vol. 3**

# P

***ϕX174***. Polyhedral, tail-less virulent phase about 25 nm in diameter containing a circular molecule of single-stranded DNA (5386 bases) coding for eleven proteins. On entering the host cell (E. coli) the DNA plus strand is converted into the double-stranded plus/minus replicative form (RF) by the host's DNA polymerase. Rolling circle replication then leads to the production of many plus strand genomes, while the minus strands of the RF are transcribed into mRNA by host RNA plymerase. Following the translation of capsid proteins,the phage genomes are packaged and released on cell lysis. Because the phage is dependent on many host functions for replication, it is believed that studies with ϕX174 will reveal how host proteins are involved in host chromosome replication.

***P150,95*** (CD11c,18). One form of complement receptor 4 composed of an alpha chain ($M_r$150,000) (CD11c) and a beta chain ($M_r$ 95,000) (CD18). The beta chain is identical to the beta chain of lymphocyte function associated antigen-1 (LFA-1) and of complement receptor 3 (CR3).

***$^{32}$P***. Phosphorus-32; radioactive isotope of phosphorus, widely used as a nucleic acid label. Its short half-life (14 days) limits its use, but its strong emission makes for ease of detection and high resolution.

$^{32}$***P Suicide.*** Death of cells or inactivation of viruses resulting from the decay of radiophosphorus molecules that they have incorporated.

***P.*** Referring (1) to phosphoric acid molecules as in CpG, or (2) to the short arm of a chromosome.

***$P_1$.*** Representing the immediate parents of the $F_1$ generation. Grandparents of $F_1$ are $P_3$,etc.

***P700 and P680.*** Modified forms of chlorophyll a with peaks of light absorption at wavelengths around 700nm and 680 nm respectively. P700 molecules comprise the energy traps of Pigment System I and P680 molecules are thought to be the traps of Pigment System II.

***Pachycaul.*** Designating angiosperms that have a large primary structure in which bud and leaf formation is slow and massive.

***Pachynema.*** Now little-used name for the pachytene stage of meiotic division.

***Pachytene*** (pachynema). Stage of meiosis in which following leptotene, the chromatid threads of the chromosomes separate, except at the centromere, so that each chromosome bivalent is now converted into a tetrad.

***Packing Ratio.*** Ratio expressing the degree of compaction of the DNA double helix into the fibres of chromatin that contain it. Each chromosome of the human complement of 23 in the haploid genome contains, on average, 5 cm of uncoiled DNA, this is reduced by packing to about 1 mm of 30-nm diameter chromatin fibre,and this fibre is further condensed by the higher-order structure of chromatin into a chromosome of average length of only 6 µm.

***Paedogenesis.*** A form of neoteny in which an organism becomes sexually mature while still in the larval or immature state. Paedogenesis is seen in the axolotl, which is the larval stage of the salamander but can breed in this form.

***Paedomorphosis.*** Phenomenon in evolution in which adult forms of a species may resemble the premature stages of ancestral species. In some cases it is believed to be at least partially explained by neoteny, and thus the human has been proposed to be a neotenous ape.

***Pairing (synapsis).*** The coming together in close association of the members of each pair of homologous chromosomes at prophase I of meiosis.

***Palaearctic.*** (Designating) a region of Arctogea consisting of Europe, north Africa, and Asia as far south as the Himalayas. This region has a basically similar fauna as the land masses are practically interconnected; differences are due mainly to climatic variations.

***Palaeocene.*** An epoch of the Tertiary period.

***Palaeoecology.*** The study of the interrelationships of living organisms and their environment that existed in the past. These relationships can be elucidated by the techniques of palynology and radioactive dating.

***Palaeogene.*** A collective name for the Palaeocene, Eocene, and Oligocene epochs of the geological time scale.

***Palaeolithic.*** The Old Stone Age of human prehistory, extending from the Pleistocene to about 7'-10000 years ago. Neanderthal and Cro-Magnon man and other species of Homo all contributed to Palaeolithic culture, which was characterized by the use of tools, mainly stones (especially flints) that came to hand. Food was obtained by hunting, fishing, and gathering (there was no agriculture).

***Palaeontology.*** The study of life in the past, including the structure of fossils, their evolution, and their environment.

***Palaeozoic.*** The first main era of the geological time scale, beginning with the Cambrian period and ending with the Permian and extending in time from 600 million to 225 million years ago.

***Palindrome.*** Group of letters (word or sentence) that read the same forward or backward, (e.g., 'able was I era I saw Elba'). In duplex DNA a palindrome is a sequence that is the same when each strand is read in the 5'—>3' direction, e.g.,

5' CATATG 3'
3' GTATAC 5'

***Palindromic Sequence.*** A nucleic acid sequence in which the code reads the same from either end. Such sequences are very common in DNA and their function is unknown. Most of these sequences are only true palindromes when both strands are considered. Thus

—AACTGCAGTT—
—TTGACGTCAA—

is palindromic. Such sequences are significant in two ways. Firstly, since they have a central axis of symmetry, they are capable of adopting special tertiary structures. For example, the sequence shown above can be alternatively folded as shown below and the specific hydrogen bonding requirements remain satisfied. See Figure P.1.

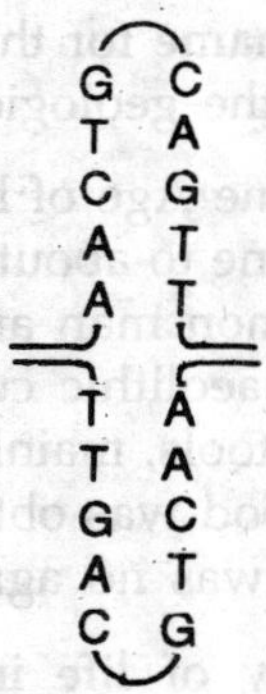


Figure P.1.

Secondly, palindromic sequences are the particular sites at which specific restriction endonucleases cut DNA, although not necessarily through the axis of symmetry. Palindromic sequences also reassociate very rapidly in Cot curve experiments; they are then known as foldback DNA.

***Pandemic.*** Descriptive of a disease that has reached epidemic proportions in different groups of the world human population more or less simultaneously.

***Pangenesis.*** Obsolete theory of development, which proposed that small particles from different parts of the body— known as pangenes — were collected together in the gametes and transmitted to offspring. A pattern of blending inheritance from the two parental lines would have resulted.

***Panmixis.*** Situation in which random mating occurs in a restricted population.

***Pantothenic acid.*** A water-soluble vitamin of the B complex, required in the diet of man and other vertebrates and occurring in yeast, liver, peas, etc. It functions as the precursor of coenzyme A.

***Pantotheria.*** An extinct order of Jurassic mammals, probably small carnivores or omnivores, e.g. Amphitherium. Pantotheres had long slender jaws with triangular premolars and molars. They are believed to have been ancestral to primitive marsupials and placental mammals.

***Papilloma.*** Benign neoplasm of the skin, many of which result from infection of the skin cells by papillomaviruses. The common wart is a papilloma, its non-invasive nature being betrayed by the fact that the cells of the wart do not grow down into the subcutaneous layers but simply pile up on the surface.

***Papillomaviruses.*** Group of the papovaviruses which cause papillomas in many mammalian species. These viruses have genomes of double-stranded DNA and are regular icosahedral units about 55 nm in diameter.

***Papovaviruses.*** Group of double-stranded DNA viruses which encompass two sub-groups; the papillomaviruses; and the slightly smaller polyomaviruses, which include SV40 virus.

***Parabiotic Intoxication.*** Disease that occurs when two outbred animals are surgically anastomosed or joined (parabiosis). The interchange of blood can result in graftversus-host disease in one or both animals.

***Parabiotic twins.*** Two animals joined together by functional connections as a result of surgery. Parabiotic twins are often used to study whether cells or substances depleted from one of the twins can be replaced by those of the other.

***Paracentric Inversion.*** Chromosomal inversion which does not include the centromere.

***Paracentrotus Lividus.*** Common sea urchin; widely used in studies on developmental biology and molecular genetics. It is very abundant around the North American coast, purplish in colour, and rarely more than 5cm in diameter. Sea urchin sperm, which is more than 50 percent pure DNA,is produced abundantly by sea urchins, and so they have become an important source of DNA in work on this molecule.

***Paracrystalline Aggregate.*** Regular array of molecules, such as occurs in some tissues with stored ribosomes, aggregates of virus or haemoglobin molecules within sickled cells from individuals with sickle cell anaemia.

***Paradigm.*** Hypothesis, model or situation that serves as an example of a general phenomenon.

***Parallel Evolution.*** The existence of similar adaptations in groups of animals and plants that are not closely related but have come to fill the same ecological niche. For example, marsupials in Australia and placentals elsewhere have undergone parallel evolution.

***Paramecin.*** Factor released by killer strain cells of Paramecium that has the capacity to kill non-killer, sensitive Paramecium cells. The factor is produced by the kappa particles, symbiotic bacteria of the species Caenobacter taenospiralis. There is some evidence that the paramecin factor is actually a DNA bacteriophage.

***Paramecium.*** Genus of ciliated Protozoa, abundant in freshwater, and much studied in terms of nuclear/cytoplasmic relations. P. aurelia is the species most studied, but P. caudatum and P. bursaria are also commonly kept. Paramecium species are noted for their possession of two nuclei per cell, a large polyploid vegetative nucleus— the macronucleus— and a small, diploid non-transcribed micronucleus, active only during conjugation. The pattern of cilia in rows of kineties on the surface cortex of these cells is also noteworthy, especially the fact that artificial changes in the kinety pattern, induced by microsurgery, are transmitted to progeny indeinitely, indicating that the pattern is not under precise control of nuclear genes.

***Paramutation.*** Situation in which an allele behaves as if it were mutant, but has no permanent change in its DNA sequence. Rather its phenotypic expression is modified and made to appear mutant by the activity of the other homologous allele in the heterozygous condition. The phenomenon is best known in the genetics of Zea mays.

***Paranemic Joint.*** Region in which complementary DNA sequences are associated like tram lines rather than intertwined in a helix.

***Paranemic Spiral.*** Spiral composed of twin parallel threads with opposite coiling directions.

***Parapatric.*** Describing a population or species that shares a common area of overlap in its geodgraphical distribution, within which area of overlap hybridizatioin regularly occurs.

***Paraprotein.*** Homogeneous immunoglobulin derived from an expanded clone of plasma cells and unrelated to known antigenic stimulation e.g., myeloma protein.

***Parasexual Cycle (mitotic recombination).*** A cycle of reproduction occurring in the Fungi Imperfecti that involves genetic recombination without meiosis or the fusion of gametes, processes associated with conventional sexual reproduction. It starts with a heterokaryotic mycelium with coexisting haploid nuclei, formed by hyphal fusion. Rare nuclear fusions yield stable heterozygous nuclei, dividing at the same rate as the more numerous haploid nuclei. During mitosis, recombination in the heterozygous diploid nuclei occurs at a low rate. Diploid daughter cells with different properties result; some of these cells undergo haploidization, in which the chromosomes are reassorted without crossing over taking place, giving rise to recombinants of the parents nuclei.

***Parasitism.*** State of relationship between two organisms in which one, the parasite, derives benefit from the other, the host; the latter organism frequently, but not invariably, suffers as a result of the relationship.

***Parathyroid Glands.*** One or two pairs of endocrine glands of tetrapod vertebrates lying near or within the thyroid glands and developing from the posterior gill pouches. They were first named and described in 1880, by Sandstrom, and their secretion of parathyroid hormone and calcitonin in the regulation of calcium and phosphate metabolism became evident during the 1920s and 1960s respectively. Parathyroid secretory activity is regulated not by the pituitary gland but directly by the concentration of calcium in the blood.

***Parathyroid Hormone*** (parathormone,PTH). Hormone secreted by the parathyroid glands, which are situated near the thyroid gland. It is a polypeptride hormone of about 75 amino acids (the inactive precursor has auextranine amino acids) and acts by raising blood calcium levels and modulating the calcium/phosphorus balance. Under its action, when blood calcium becomes low, calcium is reabsorbed from bone and calcium salts recovered by action of kidneys and gut absorption.

***Paratope.*** Synonym for antibody combine site.

***Parazoa.*** A subkingdom of invertebrates containing the phylum Porifera (sponges).

***Parenchyma.*** 1. A plant tissue composed of thin-walled living cells that is concerned with vegetative functions and forms the ground tissues of the plant. Parenchyma cells are the least modified of all plants cells and most closely resemble meristematic cells: they are regarded as the basic cell from which all other cell types have evolved. Collenchyma and sclerenchyma evolved by progressive thickening and lignification, respectively, of the cell wall.

Parenchyma cells occur in vascular tissue, in which they play an important role in the movement of water and food products in the xylem and phloem, respectively. In the secondary vascular tissue the parenchyma forms two major systems: the horizontal system of medullary rays, which provide radial transport, and the vertical system of axial parenchyma, which provides a link between the rays and also acts as a storage tissue for reserves such as oil and starch.

2. A loose spongy connective tissue of some invertebrates, e.g. the Platyhelminthes, consisting of cells lying in a matrix of fluid or gelatinous material.

3. The specific tissue of an organ, as distinct from the connective tissue, blood vessels, etc.

***Parental Type.*** Genetic constitution of parents in a genetic cross, particularly in terms of the genes being followed or studied in the cross.

***Parietal Endoderm.*** Outer layer of endoderm applied to the outer ectoderm layer at the neurula stage of embryonic development.

***Parity.*** Fact of having given birth to live young. A parous female has given birth to live young, and would be described as of parity 3 if she had given birth to three groups of young, whether the number per group was one or more.

***Paroxysmal Cod Hemoglobinuria.*** Form of hemolytic anemia in which patients have hemoglobin in their urine (hemoglobinuria) after they have been exposed to cold temperatures. A hemolysin, called the Donath-Landsteiner antibody, binds to red blood cells only in the cold, and the red cells subsequently lyse in the presence of complement when rewarmed to 37°C. Although classically associated with syphilis, Donath-Landsteiner antibodies can also appear following acute viral illnesses. Patients with these antibodies experience severe hemolytic eposides with fever and chills, in addition to hemoglobinuria.

***Paroxysmal Nocturnal Hemoglobinuria (PNH).*** Form of hemolytic anemia that resulsts from a clonal defect expressed in some erythorocytes, platelets and neutrophils. The affected cells are abnormally sensitive to lysis by complement. PNH cell membranes lack the decay accelerating factor, which downregulates the formation of the classical pathway C5 convertase on the cell membrane and the formation of the mebrane attack complex. The mebranes of PNH erythrocytes are deficient in all glycophospholipid anchored proteins (e.g., decay accelerating factor, LFA-3 and FcγRIII). Increased lysis of PNH red blood cells in acidified serum (Ham test) is used to diagnose the disease. For unknown reasons the hemolysis occurs predominantly at night.

***Parthenocarpy.*** The formation of fruits without the process of fertilization and therefore without the production of seeds.The ovary wall develops to form fruits that appear normal, e.g. seedless oranges and cultivated bananas. Parthenocarpy can be induced artificially by spraying the flowers with auxins; apples, tomatoes, and pears are often produced commercially in this way.

***Parthenogenesis.*** Reproduction in which eggs develop normally without being fertilized by a male gamete, producing an individual usually genetically identical to the parent.The main advantage of parthenogenesis is the acceleration of the reproductive rate and it occurs widely in plants. In animals, it is common in the Rotifera (males are unknown in one order) and in the Arthropoda. In some animals, e.g. aphids, several parthenogenetic generations alternate with a generation that reproduces normally (providing genetic recombination). In many cases artificial parthenogenesis can be initiated by chemical or physical stimuli, in plants and is quite frequent in certain groups of animals. Thus it is common in rotifers (in some species of which males are unknown), and is the explanation for the dramatic increase in the numbers of aphids in early summer.

***Partial dominance*** (semidominance). Development of a phenotype intermediate between the alleles in hetrozygous individuals.

***Partial Lipodystrophy.*** Loss of subcutaneous fat from the upper half of the body with concomitant obesity of the lower half of the body. C3 nephritic factor, an autoantibody to the alternative pathway C3 convertase (C3bBb), is present in the serum of patients with this syndrome. Most of the patients develop membranoproliferative glomerulonephritis. Partial lipodystrophy is presumed to be an immune complex disease, but its cause is unknown.

***Parturition.*** Expulsion of the foetus at the termination of pregnancy in mammals. The process is initiated by complex mechanisms not fully understood. Increased production of cortisol by the foetus has been suggested as the primary signal in sheep, but the premature removal of the foetus in other species does not prevent the placenta and empty membranes from being carried to term and delivered at the normal time.

***Passage.*** Subculturing of a cell line. Each repeated subculture is counted as one passaging event.

***Passage Cells.*** Cells in the endodermis, opposite to the protoxylem groups, that do not undergo secondary wall thickening but do possess Casparian strips and are thus assumed to allow the passage of solutes between the xylem and the cortex. Their occurrence may vary in a single axis; some parts possess passage cells, others have an endodermis composed entirely of thick-walled cells forming an impervious ring.

***Passenger Leukocyte.*** Leukocyte present within an allograft and contributing to the immunization of the host because it has class II histocompatibility molecules. Passenger leukocytes include monocytes, macrophages, B lymphocytes, langerhans cells.

***Passive Agglutination.*** Agglutination, by antibodies to a soluble antigen, of particles bearing the same antigen bound to their surfaces. Attachment of the antigen may be covalent or noncovalent (i.e., by adsorption). It is a very sensitive test for antibodies.

***Passive Cutaneous Anaphylaxis (PCA).*** Type of anaphylaxis induced in the skin after intradermal injection of antibodies (e.g., IgE) that bind to mast cells. The test animal is injected intravenously with antigen and a dye, such as Evans blue, hours or days after the intradermal injection of antibodies. A posotive reaction is indicated by the leakage of the dye at the site of the antigen-antibody interaction, resulting in a circumscribed area of blue skin.

***Passive Hemagglutination.*** Agglutination, by antibodies to a soluble antigen, of red blood cells bearing the same antigen bound to their membranes.

***Passive Hemolysis.*** Lysis of derivatized red blood cells by complement that has been activated by the combination of antibodies with antigens bound to the red blood cell membrane.

***Passive Immunity.*** Immunity acquired by the administration of antibodies from immune individuals (e.g., the immunity of newborns that results from the transfer of antibodies across the placenta or the ingestion of colostrum, the immunity that results from administration of antitoxins or antivenoms).

***Passive Immunity.*** Immunity that is not the product of an individual verterbrate's own immune system, but has been conferred by the acquisition of antibodies or sensitized lymphocytes from other, immune animals. The transfer of maternal IgG across the placenta confers passive immunity on the foetus in primates; in many mammalian species IgA and/or IgS are transferred from the mother to the newborn in colostrum and milk, and bird eggs contain maternal immunoglobulins. In clinical practice, artificial passive immunity is sometimes conferred, as when pooled human gamma-globulin preparations are given to immunodeficient patients who are suffering from measles or chickenpox, or to infectious hapatitis contacts. Horse globulins containing anti-tetanus and anti-diphtheria toxins have been used to confer passive immunity on patients exposed to these risks, although the use of such heterologous antibodies can elicit production of human anti-horse globulins which form immune complexes with the globulins, leading to serum sickness. Transfer of sennsitized lymphocytes to patients is sometimes known as adoptive immunity.

***Passive Transfer.*** Transfer of an immune reponse, or some component of it, from one individual to another by means of cells or serum. The transfer by means of cells is called adoptive transfer. Lymphocytes from an immunized mouse are transferred to a recipient mouse which, upon challenge with an appropriate antigen develops a secondary antibody response or delayed-type hypersensitivity. For successful passive transfer of cells, inbred animals should be used. Irradiation of the recipients may also be important perhaps because it reduces lymphoid mass that could interfere with the homing of lymphocytes. Antibodies are given to recipients for the passive transfer of humoral immunity. Passive transfer has been invaluable in identifying the functions of lymphocytes and of antibodies.

***Pasteurization.*** A process of heat treatment that kills pathogenic microorganisms in foods and drinks. For example,milk is maintained at a temperature of about 62°C for 30 minutes,which kills any pathogens but does not destroy harmless bacteria or affect taste. The process was orginally devised by Louis Pasteur (1822-95) to kill the spoilage microorganisms of wines and beers.

***Patau Syndrome*** ($D_1$ trisomy syndrome). Group of human congenital defects, resulting from the presence of an extra chromosome 13(i.e. trisomy 13).

***Patch Clamping.*** Technique for studying ion channel proteins in action in the plasma membrane. A fine glass needle is applied to the cell surface and a small area of membrane, containing only one or two ion channels, is allowed to bleb into the tube. Current can then enter the pipette only through the ion channels trapped inside,and using very sensitive electronic equipment transmission of low voltages with closed and open channels can be recorded.

***Patch Test.*** Method for establishing the cause of allergic contact dermatitis. The suspected provoking substance is applied to a small piece of linen, cotton, filter paper or aluminium foil, and placed on the skin for 24 to 48 hours. After removal of the patch, the skin is examined for erythema, vesiculation and edema, which indicate a positive result.

***Patching.*** Ligand-induced redistribution of membrane proteins into clusters as a result of cross-linking by bivalent or multivalent antibodies or lectins. Such redistribution can occur because the lipid bilayer is fluid and proteins can diffuse freely within the plane of the membrane. Redistribution into patches is a passive prrocess and does not require energy, but it can be prevented by chemically 'fixing' the cell membrane so that its proteins are immobilized. The distribution of membrane proteins can be visualized by reacting them with fluorescent-labeled or ferritin-labeled ligands followed by light or electron microscopy, respectively. Since a bivalent or multivalent ligand can itself induce redistribution, the organization of membrane proteins in the native state should be examined by attaching the label to a monovalent ligand (e.g., the Fab fragment of an antibody).

***Pathogen.*** Any microorganism that causes disease or a toxic response. Such organisms are described as pathogenic.

***Pathogenic.*** Causing disease or symptoms of toxicity.

***Patroclinous.*** Describing an offspring that resembles the father more closely than the mother.The male offspring of female Drosophila carrying an attached X chromosome are patroclinous for the sex-linked genes.

***Pattern Formation.*** Development in the embryo of recognizable patterns of tissue organization that may be serially repeated along the anterior/posterior axis (e.g. in a segmented animal), display bilateral symmetry (e.g., as in left and right appendages) or simply be faithfuly reproduced in successive generations of an organism (e.g., bristle patterns in insect cuticle, leaf veniation patterns); often used as a comnplement to morphogenesis. The molecular/cellular basis of pattern specification mechanisms is one of the central issues of developmental biology.

***Paul-Bunnell Test.*** Tes for heterophile antibodies in individuals suspected or having infectious mononucleosis. Test serum is absorbed with guinea-pig kidney to remove antibodies to forssman antigen. The titer of heterophile antibodies in test serum is then determined by the degree of agglutination of sheep red blood cells.

***pBR322.*** E.coli plasmid under relaxed control (can exist in high copy-number) that contains both ampicilin- and tetracycline-resistant genes and a number of convenient restriction sites and that is widely used as a cloning vector. pBR 322 consists of 4,363 base pairs. It was derived by methods of genetic engineering from naturally-occurring E.coli plasmids.

***pBR322.*** E. coli plasmid that is used very frequently as a

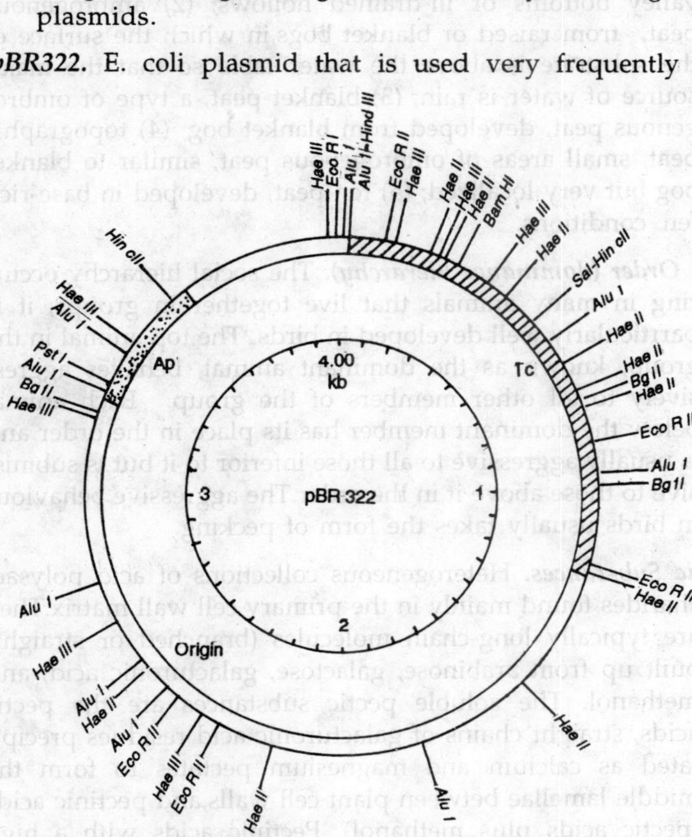


Figure P.2. pBR322. The physical map of pBR322, showing the restriction enzyme cleavage sites.

cloning vector for the propagation of other gene sequences. It grows in the cell under relaxed control and thus can be harvested in large numbers. It contains genes for tetracycline resistance and ampicillin resistance. See Figure P.2.

***PDGF.*** Platelet-derived growth factor.

***Peat.*** The plant remains of bog and fen vegetation. The wetness of the substrate leads to anaerobic acid conditions, which inhibits the microorganisms of decay and leads to an accumulation of vegetable remains in the substrate- the peat. Several types of peat are recognized:(1) basin peat (or topogenous peat), from bog vegetation, found in base-poor valley bottoms or ill-drained hollows; (2) ambrogenous peat, from raised or blanket bogs,in which the surface of the substrate is above the water table so that the major source of water is rain; (3) blanket peat, a type of ombrogenous peat, developed from blanket bog; (4) topographic peat, small areas of ombrogenous peat, similar to blanket bog but very localized; (5) fen peat, developed in base-rich fen conditions.

***Peck Order (dominance hierarchy).*** The social hierarchy occurring in many animals that live together in groups; it is parrticularly well developed in birds. The top animal in the group, known as the dominant animal, behaves aggressively to all other members of the group. Each animal below the dominant member has its place in the order and is usually aggressive to all those inferior to it but is submissive to those above it in the order.The aggressive behaviour in birds usually takes the form of pecking.

***Pectic Substances.*** Heterogeneous collections of acid polysaccharides found mainly in the primary cell wall matrix.They are typically long-chain molecules (branched or straight) built up from arabinose, galactose, galacturonic acid, and methanol. The soluble pectic substances are the pectic acids, straight chains of galacturonic acid residues precipitated as calcium and magnesium pectates to form the middle lamellae between plant cell walls,and pectinic acids (pectic acids plus methanol). Pectinic acids with a high degree of methylation and with the addition of sugars and acids form pectins. Polymers of pectin form the insoluble pectic substances, the large and complex protopectins that comprise the major pectic component of primary cell walls. In ripening fruits protopectin is converted to pectins. These form gels at low concentrations (when sugar is added) and are therefore used commercially as gelling agents.

***Pectin.*** Pectic acid with methylated carboxyl groups. It occurs in the cell walls or middle lamella of plant tissue.

***Pediatric AIDS.*** Form of acquired immunodeficiency syndrome (AIDS) in infants due to intrauterine or intrapartum infection with human immunodeficiency virus (HIV). Infected infants usually develop symptoms between three weeks and 24 months of age. Like adults with AIDS, affected infants have enlarged lymph nodes, fever, thrombocytopenia and elevated numbers of circulating B lymphocytes and a marked increase in the serum concentration of IgG, IgM and IgD. Unlike adults with AIDS, they are prone to infections with Epstein-Barr virus resulting in interstitial pneumonia and inflammation of the salivary glands, have normal numbers of T lymphocytes in the blood, and frequent blood stream infections with pyogenic bacteria (e.g., pneumococci or Hemophilus influenzae b). Affected infants only rarely have Kaposi's sarcoma and opportunistic infections that are typical of adult AIDS. Growth and development of these infants are retarded. Pediatric AIDS is almost always fatal.

***Pedigree.*** Ancestral history, with particular genetic traits often emphasized. It is customary in pedigree diagrams to symbolize females by circles and males by squares, and,in a diagram for a particular trait, those individuals expressing the trait are symbolized in solid figures.

***Pelagic.*** Living in the open waters of a sea or lake, as distinct from on the bottom. Pelagic plants and animals included the plankton and the nekton.

***P Elements.*** Group of transposable elements (transposons) occurring in Drosophila melanogaster. P elements have been widely cloned in E. coli and are responsible for one form of hybrid dysgenesis. P elements may be integrated and transmitted in the germ line and have been used successfully as vectors in the artificial integration of novel genes into the Drosophila germ line.

***Pellagra.*** Disease resulting from a deficiency of dietary nicotinic acid. It is characterized by extreme reddening of the skin when exposed to sunlight, digestive disturbance and eventual dementia.

***Pemphigoid.*** Blistering disease of the skin, differentiated from pemphigus by the absence of acantholysis (intraepidermal bullae). The bullous formation in pemphigoid is subepidermal, and linear deposition of IgG can be detected by immunofluorescence in the basement membrane zone. IgG antibodies to basement membrane of skin are present in the serum. Pemphigoid is seen most frequently in the elderly.

***Pemphigus.*** Blistering autoimmune disease of the skin, characterized by intraepidermal bullae, so-called acantholysis. Deposition of IgG, C1q, C4 and C3 is deteced by immunofluorescence in the skin lesions. The disease is caused by autoantibodies to antigens in the intercellular spaces of the skin. The cause of autoantibody formation is not known. Pemphigus is improved by treatment with corticosteroids. Pemiphigus occurs at all ages.

***Penetrance (expressivity).*** The extent to which the effects of a gene are shown in the organism possessing it. It is expressed as the percentage of organisms showing the effect of a gene out of the total number known to possess it. Penetrance can vary considerably with different genes and with different organisms possessing the same gene. In mendelian genetics, penetrance is assumed to be 100%. Variations in penetrance are thought to be due to the modifying action of other genes present and to the effects of the environment.

***Penicillins.*** A class of antibiotics that act by disrupting cell-wall synthesis in Gram-negative bacteria. They have the general formula shown, in which R is a variable side chain. Penicillin itself (i.e. penicillin G, in which R= $C_6H_5CH_2$) is produced by the mould Penicillium notatum; various chemical substitutions of the side chain R produce penicillins with different properties. See Figure P.3.

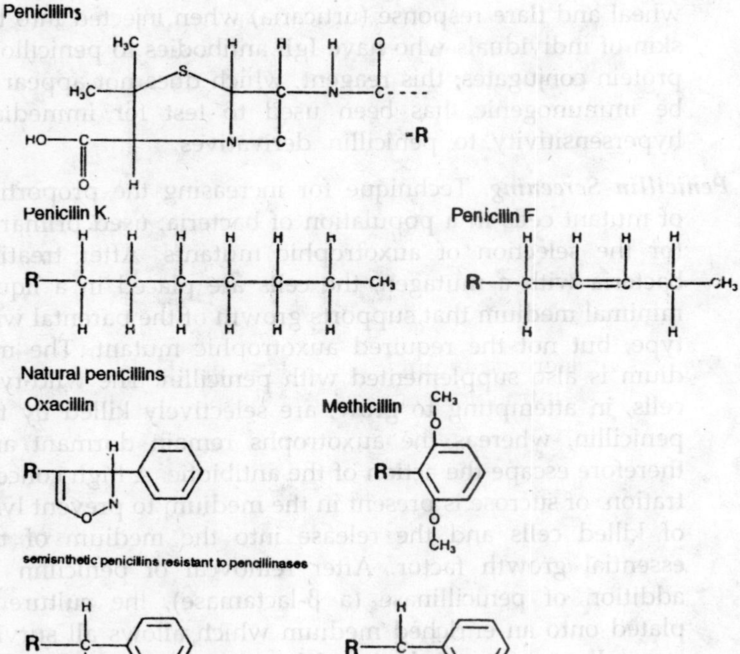


Figure P.3. Penicillins.

*Penicillin Allergy*. Allergy (hypersensitivity) to penicillin or to its breakdown products or to contaminants in penicillin preparations. Some derivatives (e.g., penicilenic acid) become conjugated to proteins, forming penicillloyl derivatives, and act as haptens in inducing an allergic response, which may be antibody-mediated or cell-mediated. Antibody-mediated reactions include anaphylaxis (due to IgE antibodies), serum sickness (rash, fever, joint pains) and hemolytic anemia. Cell-mediated reactions may be manifest as allergic contact dermatitis; this is quite common in individuals (e.g., nurses, pharmacists) who handle penicillin. Patch tests with penicillin are used to detect cell-mediated reactions to the drug. Penicilloyl-polylysine may induce a wheal and flare response (urticaria) when injected into the skin of individuals who have IgE antibodies to penicilloyl-protein conjugates; this reagent, which does not appear to be immunogenic, has been used to test for immediate hypersensitivity to penicillin derivatives.

***Penicillin Screening.*** Technique for increasing the proportion of mutant cells in a population of bacteria; used primarily for the selection of auxotrophic mutants. After treating bacteria with a mutagen, the cells are placed in a liquid minimal medium that supports growth of the parental wild type, but not the required auxotrophic mutant. The medium is also supplemented with penicillin. The wild-type cells, in attempting to grow, are selectively killed by the penicillin, whereas the auxotrophs remain dormant and therefore escape the action of the antibiotic. A high concentration of sucrose is present in the medium to prevent lysis of killed cells and the release into the medium of the essential growth factor. After removcal of penicillin by addition of penicillinase (a β-lactamase), the culture is plated onto an enriched medium which allows all surviving cells to form colonies. Mutant colonies are distinguished from wild type (now present with much decreased frequency) by replica plating.

***Penis.*** The unpaired erectile intromitent organ of all male mammals, some reptiles (chelonians and crocodilians), and a few birds. In mammals the terminal part of the urethra lies within the penis.

***Pentose.*** A monosaccharide with five carbon atoms, e.g. ribose.

***Pentose phosphate pathway (hexose monophosphate shunt).*** A pathway of glucose oxidation occurring in the cytoplasm of cells. The pathway requires NADP as an electron acceptor and the NADPH generated provided the reducing power for many biosynthetic reactions, e.g. the synthesis of fats.

In animals the pathway occurs mainly in the liver, adipose tissue, mammary glands, and adrenal cortex, where fatty acids and steroids are synthesized (as much as a third of the glucose oxidized in these tissues may be via the pentose phosphate pathway). Other important products include glyceraldehyde-3-phosphate (which can participate in glycolysis), ribose-5-phosphate (which is used for the synthesis of nucleotides and nucleic acids), and ribulose-5-phosphate (which, in photosynthetic organisms, combines with carbon dioxide to form sugars).

***Pentoses.*** Group of monosaccharide sugars with five carbon atoms. Ribose, which occurs in RNA , is a pentose.

***Pepsin.*** A proteolytic enzyme, secreted by glands of the vertebrate stomach, that acts as an endopeptidase in the presence of hydrochloric acid in the gastric juice.

***Peptidase.*** One of a group of enzymes that hydrolyse peptides into their constituent amino acids.

***Peptide.*** One of a group of compounds consisting of two or more amino acids linked by covalent bonds between the amino group of one and the carboxyl group of the next. This type of bond is known as a peptide bond and peptides of three or more amino acids are called polypeptides. Polypeptides made up of only a few amino acids are called oligopeptides.

***Peptide Bond*** (amide bond). Joining of α-carboxyl group of one amino acid to the α-amino group of another. Formation of the bond involves loss of a water molecule from the two amino acids, and the bond can be broken by hydrolysis. The equilibrium is in favour of hydrolysis; the reverse reaction, as in protein synthesis, requires an input of energy and information with respect to the sequence of amino acids. The orientation of the carbonyl group in the peptide is usually trans to the amino group, and because the bond has a partial double bond character (due to resonance) the bond is rigid and planar. This rigidity limits the number of configurations of a polypeptide chain and is a major determinant of the shape of proteins.

***Peptidoglycan.*** Mucopeptide unique to bacterial cell walls.

***Peptidyl Transferase.*** Enzyme that catalyses the movement of amino acid-charged tRNA molecules (aminoacyl-trna) on the ribosome during the translation stage of protein synthesis. The charged tRNA molecules engage consecutively with the A site and the P site on the ribosome prior to discharge, and the transferase facilitates the movements of the tRNAs from one site to another.

***Peptone.*** Large protein fragment produced from a protein molecule following partial hydrolysis by a degradative enzyme.

***Perforin.*** Protein ($M_r$75,000) isolated from the cytoplasmic granules of natrural killer cells (NK) and cytotoxic T lymphocytes that is thought to mediate the lysis of target cells. Following intimation contact of the NK cells or cytalytic T lymphocytes with target cells, intracellular granules are released with subsequent polymerization of perforin in the presence of $Ca^{2+}$. Polymerized perforin inserts into the membranes of target cells causing depolarization, abnormal ion flux and cell lysis. The mebranes of target cells have characteristic round lesions, resembling those seen in complement-dependent lysis. Antibodies to complement component C9 cross-react with perforin.

***Periarteritis Nodosa.*** Synonym for polyarteritis nodosa.

***Pericentric Inversion.*** Inversion in a chromosome that involves the centromere in the piece which is inverted.

***Perichondrion.*** Compact layer of collagenous connective tissue that surrunds most masses of cartilage.

***Periclinal.*** Describing any layer of cells that is located so that it is parallel to the surface of the part of the plant concerned. Meristematic cells in plants often divide periclinally, and the pericycle is located periclinally.

***Periclinal Chimaera.*** Plant made up of two or more tissues of distinct genetic constitution, arranged so that the tissues are circumferentially distinct from one another (i.e. one is inside another).

***Pericycle*** (pericambium). Normally a single layer of parenchyma cells lying just within the endodermis and peripheral to the vascular tissues. The cells retain an ability to divide and give rise to lateral root primordia and parts of the vascular cambium. The phellogen, the meristem which produces cork, also arises from the pericycle.

***Periderm.*** The outer protective secondary tissue of the roots and stems of woody gymnosperms and angiosperms, which replaces the axial epidermis when it is destroyed by secondary growth.

It comprises three layers. The outermost layer is the phellem (cork), which is produced to ther outside of the phellogen and forms the true protective layer of the periderm. It consists of tightly packed prismatic cells, which in the mature state have suberized walls and have lost their living contents. The surface of the phellem is interrupted at intervals by lenticels, which provide aeration passages in this otherwise impervious layer. The innermost layer is the phelloderm, which is produced to the inside of the phellogen and consists of living cells that resemble cortical cells in wall structure and contents. Between these layers lies the phellogen (or cork cambium). This is the lateral secondary meristem that produces the other two layers by periclinal divisions on both its inner and outer surfaces. It usually arises in the subepidermal layer, but it may arise (according to species) anywhere between the epidermis and the phloem (and occasionally in the xylem, forming anomalous secondary thickening).

***Perikaryon.*** Part of the cell in a neurone that surrounds the nucleus and forms the central cell body as distinct from the extending axon and dendrites.

***Perinuclear Space.*** Space between the inner and outer membranes of the nuclear envelope.

***Periodic acid Schiffls reagent (PAS).*** Staining procedure used to detect polysaccharide.

***Periodicity.*** As applied to DNA, number of base pairs per double-helical turn.

***Periosteum.*** Layer of connective tissue that surrounds bone and provides attachment for muscle and tendons. The inner layers of the periosteum are loose and highly vascular, and osteoblasts are formed in it before their migration into the bone proper. The outer layer is largely composed of which elastic fibres.

***Periplasmic Space*** (Periplasm). Space between the lipoprotein periplasmic membrane, which provided the osmotic barrier of the bacterial cell, and the rigid cell wall. It may consist of up to 20 percent of the volume of the bacteria. The periplasm contains a number of soluble proteins. These include the solute-binding proteins that are invcolved in transport of solutes such as amino acids and sugars into the bacteria, and which are also involved in chemotaxis. It also contains a number of components of the electron transport chain such as cytochrome c, blue copper proteins (e.g., azurin and amicyanin) and some dehydrogenases are usually inorganic (e.g., hydrogen or $Fe^{2+}$), but methanol dehydrogenase and methylamine dehydrogenase are also periplasmic.

***Perisperm.*** A storage tissue in the seeds of certain angiosperms that develops from the nucellus.

***Peripolesis.*** Clustering of cells around a different type of cell (e.g.,lymphocytes around a macrophage).

***Peristome.*** A single or double row of teeth (usually hygroscopic) at the apex of most moss capsules, through which the spores are shed.

***Perithecium (Pyrenocarp).*** A flask-shaped ascocarp whose inner surface is lined with a hymenium that produces the asci. At maturity the ascospores are ejected through the apical ostiole by the bursting of the asci.

***Peritrichous.*** Descriptive of bacteria that are entirely covered with cilia.

***Permeability.*** Ease with which a membrane or porous surface can be penetrated by molecules. Biological membranes are semipermeable, allowing some small molecules through, but excluding or partially excluding many larger ones. The movement of many molecules through permeable membranes results from simple diffusion.

***Permeases.*** Bacterial enzymes present in the plasma membrane that facilitate the movement of specific substances into or out of the cell. In the lac operon of E.coli, the lac Y gene codes for a permease that transports lactose into the cell.

***Permian.*** The sixth and last period of the Palaeozoic era, extending from 270 million years ago. It is named from Perm, on the River Volga in Russia, where rocks of the period were first recognized. In some places the Permina system grades into the Triassic and the two can be considered as a single system, the Permo-Triassic (or Permo-Trias). In many regions Permian fossils are scarce; they consist of land-living animals such as lungfish and labyrinthodont amphibians and xerophytic plants, indicating an increasingly dry climate. Marine fossils of the Permian include foraminiferans, ammonites, brachiopods, corals, and sponges. At the end of the Permian many marine groups died out, including the trilobites, many Palaeozoic crinoids, and some corals.

***Permissive Host.*** Host cell in which a particular strain of virus can reproduce and yield progeny virus. Cells that do not support such growth are defined as non-permissive. With certain viruses such as polyomavirus, a productive infection may occur in cells of one type, and no productive infection in non-permissive cells of another type, but transofmration may occur instead of the latter.

***Permissive Strain.*** Strain of cell capable of acting as a permissive host.

***Permissive Temperature.*** Temperature, or temperature range, at which a particular conditional lethal mutation will survive and reproduce.

***Pernicious Anemia (PA).*** Autoimmune disease characterized by autoantibodies to intrinsic factor and to gastric parietal cells. Parietal cells normally secrete a heat-labile substance, called intrinsic factor ($M_r$ 60,000), which binds dietary vitamin B12 and facilitates its absorption in the distal small intestine. Pernicious anemia results from a deficiency of vitamin B12. For unknown reasons pernicious anemia is a frequent complication of common variable immunodeficiency.

***Peroxisome.*** Ovoid, membrane-bound organelle (0.6-0.7μm in diameter) found in the cells of liver, kidney and other tissues. In animal cells, peroxisomes appear to be formed at the endoplasmic reticulum and contain catalase and other oxidases. Peroxisome enzymes are involved in the metabolism of hydrogen peroxide ($H_2O_2$), which is toxic to the cell. Plant peroxisomes, in combination with chloroplasts, are involved in photorespiration.

***Petite Mutants.*** Yeast mutants characterized by slow growth, so that the colonies they form are much smaller than those of wild-type cells. Such mutants are best known in the budding yeast Saccharomyces cerevisiae, but are not confined to that species. The slow-growing phenotype results from defective mitochondria and affected cells carry mutations in their mitochondrial DNA. The mutation can be induced at high frequency by drugs such as acriflavine and also result from growth at temperatures above 40ºC or exposure to ultraviolet light. Different types of petite mutants are known; vegetative petites in which all progeny cells are affected and result from one or more mutations in the mitochondrial genome (many yeast cells have a single, branched mitochondrion); segregational petites in which a nuclear gene coding for a mitochondrial protein is involved. The aberrant mitochondria, which can be visualized by electron microscopy of petite cells, are known as promitochondria, and are deficient in cristae.

***Petri Dish.*** A shallow flat lidded container made of glass or clear plastic in which bacteria, moulds, or tissue cultures can be grown in a nutrient medium or on a nutrient agar.

***pFc' Fragment.*** Fragment produced by digestin of IgG (or Fc fragment) with the enzyme pepsin. It consists of the twc $C_H3$ domains (probably the carbooxy-terminal 116 residues of both chains), which form a non-covalently bonded dimer.

***Pfeiffer Phenomenon.*** Rapid lysis of cholera bacteria by complement after these bacteria have been injected into the peritoneal cavity of an animal immune to cholera.

***pH.*** A measure of the concentration of hydrogen ions in a solution. It is defined as $-\log[H^+]$, where $[H^+]$ is the concentration of hydrogen ions. Pure water at normal temepratures dissociates only very slightly into hydrogen ions and hydroxyl ions, the concentration of each type of ion being $10^{-7}$ mole per cubic decimetre. The pH of pure water is therefore $-\log 10^{-7} = 7$ and this figure represents neutrality on the pH scale. A pH below 7 indicates acidity and a pH in excess of 7 indicates alkalinity.

***Phage Induction.*** Transition from the prophage state to lytic growth of a temperate phage in response to an external stimulus. Induction results in the initiation of transcription of phage genes, excision of the prophage from the host chromosome, and the synthesis of phage genomes and capsid proteins. Ultraviolet light (in doses too small to inactivate the phage), alkylating agents (e.g., mitomycin c), disruption of DNA replication (e.g., by nalidixic acid or by thymine deprivation) all act as inducers. Where a phage carries a temperature-sensitive mutation in the repressor gene, induction can be achieved by transferring the lysogen to the non-permissive temperature when the repressor is destroyed.

***Phagocyte.*** A cell that has the ability to ingest extracellular particles by engulfing them with its own cytoplasm, a process known as phagocytasis. Although many protozoans are phagocytic the word is more commonly applied to those cells that occur throughout vertebrate tissues and are responsible for the ingestion of bacteria and foreign particles, i.e. polymorphs and macrophages.

***Phage Neutralization.*** Abolition of the activity of bacteriophage by antibodies, thereby preventing the infection of a bacretial host. The neutralizing activity can be quantitated by determining the reduction in number of plaques when phage are incubated with antibodies before plating on bacteria. It is a very sensitive assay for antibody activity.

***Phagocyte.*** Cell that ingests particulate material. Neutrophils and mononuclear phagocytes are the principal phagocytes of the body.

***Phagocytosis.*** Ingestion of relatively large particles (e.g., bacteria or parts of a cell) by phagocytes (e.g., neutrophils, macrophages). The first event in phagocytosis is the binding of the particle to the plasma membrane of the phagocyte. Some particulate materials bind only when coated with specific antibody or complement. Following binding, the plasma membrane expands along the surface of the particle by means of actin-containing microfilaments that lie just under the cell surface. The particle is enveloped by the interaction of receptors on the surface of the phagocyte with ligands distributed on the particle's surface (called 'zipper interaction'). The invaginated membrane-enveloped particle is a large (1-2 µm) vesicle called a phagosome; this may fuse with a primary lysosome to form a phagolysosome (secondary lysosome), wherein the particle may be digested by hydrolytic enzymes. The fate of the intracellular particle varies depending of its nature and on the type of phagocytic cell. Some pyogenic bacteria are rapidly killed as a result of the oxidative processes that accompany phagocytosis. Some intracellular pathogens (e.g., Mycobacterium leprae, Leishmania, Toxoplasma, Legionella pneumophilla) remain viable inside the phagolysosome unless the macrophage is activated by interferongamma.

***Phagocytosis.*** Form of endocytosis involving the entrapment of extracellular particles within membrane-bound vesicles by the extension of pseudopodia or filopodia; it literally means cell eating. The particle more or less fills the vesicle which is of large size (1-2µm) and is referred to as a phagosome. Breakdown of the particle takes place following fusion of the phagosome with a primary lysosome to form a phagolysosome. Phagocytosis occurs in all classes of animals, but may be restricted to specialized cells generally referred to as phagocytes. It is the means whereby Protozoa ingest bacteria and other food particles and whereby macrophages in higher vertebrates remove antigen-antibody complexes.

***Phagolysosome.*** Membrane-bound vesicle formed within a cell as a result of fusion of a phagosome, or other endocytic vesicle, with a lysosome, and in which digestion of entrapped material takes place.

***Phagosome.*** Cytoplasmic particle that results from budding off of part of the plasma membrane and enclosing material recently phagocytosed. They are therefore found only in phagocytic cells and will fuse with lysosomes to produce phagolysosomes or digestive vacuoles.

***Phalloidin.*** Drug that stabilizes actin filaments, and by binding to them can prevent such processes as cytoplasmic streaming. It is derived from the poisonous mushroom Amanita phalloides.

***Phase Contrast Microscope.*** Variant of the compound light microscope, in which differences in refractive index of the different parts of an unstained specimen are optically converted into variations of light intensity and contrast. The phase contrast microscope thus greatly facilitates observations on living cells viewed in suitable media.

***Phaseolin.*** Glycoprotein storage molecule from the bean Phaseolus vulgarus, making up some 50 percent of the cotyledon storage protein. These proteins are coded by a small gene family of about 10 genes.

***Phaseolus.*** Genus of the family Leguminosae that includes kidney beans and mung beans, and is widely used in commerce and genetical research.

***Phasing.*** Arrangement of nucleosomes along a DNA strand in some sequence-specific manner. Since nucleosomes are not so arranged in most chromatin, this represents an unusual situation. Phasing of nucleosome has been detected by the controlled digestion of chromatin with micrococcal nuclease or DNase I, but its significance for the cell and gene regulation are not clear. If phasing is frequent, it could imply that nucleosomes on the same gene were arranged in different phases in different cells, so determining whether or not the genes were expressed.

***Phasmid.*** Plasmid gene cloning vector carrying the att site from lambda phage. It is thus able to insert into a phage genome (just as lambda phage does into the bacterial genome).

***Phellem*** (cork). Cellular tissue that replaces the epidermis in plants which undergo pronounced secondary growth; it acts as a compact protective layer. It is derived from the phellogen and consists of more or less isodiametric cells arranged in radial rows. At maturity the cells are devoid of cellular contents and have thick cell walls impregnated with suberin.

***Phelloderm*** (secondary cortex). Secondary plant tissue derived from the phellogen and situated internally to it. The cells retain their living contents and are only distinguishable from the cortical cells by their radial alignment with the phellogen and phellem. The phelloderm, together with the phellogen and phellem, makes up the periderm.

***Phellogen*** (cork cambium). Lateral meristem giving rise to the periderm, a protective layer replacing the epidermis in stems which undergo pronounced secondary thickening. Cells of the phellogen divide periclinally to give radially seriate files of cells. Those produced internal to the phellogen form the phelloderm or secondary cortex and those towards the outside differentiate as phellem or cork.

***Phene.*** Phenotypic character controlled by genes. Note however, that in fact all genetically determined characteristics are more accurately understood as resulting from an interaction of gene expression and environmental influence.

***Phenetic.*** Designating a classification based on observed similarities and differences in appearance, as opposed to one based on evolutionary descent.

***Phenocopy.*** An environmentally produced change in an organism, induced early in development, that is very similar to a gene mutation but is not inherited. For example, irradiation of mammalian embryos at sensitive stages of their development in the uterus produces abnormalities that are phenocopies of mutations.

***Phenocopy.*** Production of a characteristic phenotype by enviornmental factors such as stress or nutrition, in a form closely similarr to or indistinguishable from that normally resulting from the expression of a specific gene or gene mutation.

***Phenogenetics.*** Genetics of phenotypic expression and therefore covered by the more frequently recognized discipline of developmental genetics.

***Phenon.*** Group of organisms as recognized by the methods of numerical taxonomy.

***Phenotype.*** The physical characteristics, collectively, of an organism, determined by the genotype and the environment. Organisms with the same genotype may have different phenotypes in different environments. For example, two plants may be genotypically short, but if one is grown under conditions of poor light, it will become etiolated and hence taller than the other. Organisms with the same genotype may also show different phenotypes if the penetrance of the gene differs. On the other hand, organisms with different genotypes may have the same phenotype if each contains a dominant gene: in the same environment the homozygous organism AA is phenotypically identical to the heterozygous Aa in respect of gene A.

***Phenotypic Lag.*** Delay in the expression of a newly acquired character, the latter phrase usually meaning a recent mutation. Such a lag may result from a mitochondrial mutation where the presence of numerous mitochondria at first dilutes out any evidence of phenotypic expression, or the lag may be simple because the cytoplasm carries a large or long-lived store of the immediate gene product, and only when the store is exhausted is the effect of the mutant gene evident.There is a phenotypic lag of some weeks following the transplantation of nuclei between species in the unicellular alga Acetabularia.

***Phenotype.*** Detectable characteristics of a cell or organism. The characteristics considered to be the phenotype may vary according to the methods used for detection. The phenotype results from the interactions of the genotype with the environment.

***Phenotypic Mixing.*** Phenomenon resulting from a cell being infected by viruses of more than one strain. This may result in new genetic material of one viral strain being packaged within a protein capsid characteristic of the other strain, resulting in the production of intact virions of mixed phenotype.

***Phenotypic Mutant.*** Mutant that displays a characteristic phenotype and may be categorized by that phenotype. Most phenotypic mutants result from analysis of characters determined by additive factors, such as the Drosophila apricot-coloured eye, instead of the red eye, a situation that results from changes in the pigment gene dosage. Other phenotypic mutants may be detected only by allozyme analysis in electrophoresis.

***Phenotypic Variance.*** Total variance observed in a character: it is usually greater that the genotypic variance, which takes no account of the additional effect of the environment.

***Phenylalanine (phe).*** An amino acid, $C_6H_5CH_2CH(NH_2)COOH$, one of the 20 common amino acids occurring in proteins and an essential amino acid for man.

***Phenylbutazone*** (4-butyl-1,2-diphenyl-3,5-pyrazolidinedione). Drug used for the treatment of ankylosing spondylitis and rheumatoid arthritis. It inhibits prostaglandin synthesis and is a potent anti-inflammatory agent. See Figure P.4.

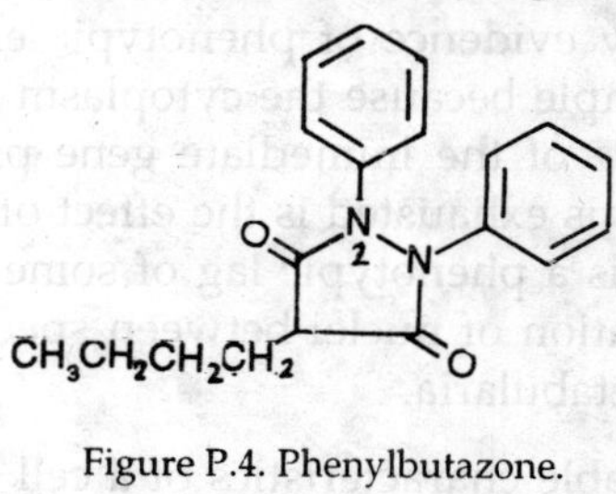


Figure P.4. Phenylbutazone.

***Phenylketonuria.*** A hereditary disorder, carried as a single recessive gene, in which the amino acid phenylalanine fails to be metabolized to tyrosine. The disorder results in excretion of phenylpyruvic acid (a precursor of phenylalanine) in the urine and, usually, severe mental retardation. Phenylketonuria can be detected soon after birth and a diet low in phenylalanine minimizes the symptoms.

***Pheromone.*** A substance excreted by an animal in small amounts that causes specific reproductive, developmental, or behavioural responses in neighbouring members of the same species. The earliest and best studied pheromones are the sex attractants produced by Lepidoptera and the queen-bee substance excreted by the queen of a hive. Characterized as 9-ketodecanoic acid, queen-bee substance is eaten by the workers, in which it inhibits the development of the ovaries (thus making them sterile) and prevents their manufacture of queen-bee cells in the hive.

***pH Gradient.*** Gradient employed in techniques such as isoelectric focusing, in which proteins migrate to positions equivalent to their own isoelectric point.

***Philadelphia Chromosome.*** Aberrant chromosome evident in bone marrow metaphase spreads from patients suffering from chronic myelogenous leukaemia. It results from a translocation in which half of the long arm of chromosome 22 is moved to the long arm of another chromosome, most often chromosome 9. The site of the break on chromosome 22 is adjacent to the locus of an oncogene, and so the resulting cancer may be in some way associated with the altered regulation of expression of this gene.

***Phloem.*** Chief food-conducting tissue of vascular plants. The phloem is composed substantially of living cells. The cell types of phloem include the conducting sieve elements—phloem parenchyma cells— and companion cells, which are all thin-walled and, in the case of the phloem sieve elements, no longer nucleated. Fibres are often also present, usually thick-walled, and often lignified. The nutrient fluid conducted in the phloem moves in different directions in different elements and is therefore quite distinct from the water transport in xylem, which is almost always root to stem to leaf.

***Phloroglucin.*** Staining material used in conjunction with concentrated hydrochloric acid to stain lignin in plant cells red.

***Phocomelia.*** Syndrome in which hands or feet are attached directly to the trunk by a single bone. It is a rare autosomal recessive in the human, but is best known in children born to mothers taking the tranquillizer thalidomide.

***Phorbol Ester.*** Ester of myristic acid and phorbol alcohols. The most commonly used phorbol ester is 12-O-tetradecanoylphorbol-13-acetate (TPA), also called phorbol myristate acetate (PMA). TPA is a tumor promoter (substance that facilitates induction of tumors by carcinogens). TPA exerts pleiotropic effects on a number of cell types, including lymphocytes. TPA binds to and activates protein kinase C, resulting in the phosphorylation of serine and threonine residues in the cytoplasmic domains of transmembrane proteins (e.g., CD2, CD3). These biochemical reactions increase the expression of interleukin-2 receptors on T lymphocytes and stimulate their growth when interleukin-1 is present in addition to TPA. TPA induces degranulation of polymorphonuclear leukocytes mast cells and platelets.

***Phosphatses.*** Enzymes that catalyse the removal of phosphate groups. Acid phosphatase is particuarly abundant in lysosomes.

***Phosphate Group.*** Phosphorus atom, with three oxygen atoms attached. Phosphate groups form important part of molecules such as AMP, ADP and ATP.

***Phosphatidic Acid.*** A simple phosphoglyceride with two fatty-acid residues esterified to carbons 1 and 2 of glycerol phosphate. It is formed in the biosynthesis of the more abundant phosphoglycerides.

***Phosphodiester Bond.*** Linkage bond between nucleotides forming a nucleic acid polymer. It involves attachment of the phospohate group of the 5'-position of one sugar to link with the hydroxyl group of the 3'-position of the sugar of an adjacent nucleotide.

***Phosphoenol Pyruvate (PEP).*** Compound, with a high phosphate group transfer potential, involved in glycolysis.

***Phospholipases.*** Enzymes capable of hydrolysing phospholipids and therefore important in studies of the cell plasma membrane.

***Phospholipids (Phosphatides).*** Polar lipids that are important components of cell membranes. Phospholipids can be divided into two groups: the phosphoglycerides and the sphingomyelins.

Phosphoglycerides are fatty-acid esters of glycerol phosphate with an alcohol group (e.g. ethanolamine, choline, serine, inositol) esterified to the phosphate. The most important phosphoglycerides are phosphatidyl ethanolamine (cephalin) and phosphatidyl choline (lecithin), the former being particularly abundant in the brain. Also belonging to this group are the plasmalogens, in which an α,β-unsaturated fatty aldehyde and a carboxylic acid are esterified to the glycerol and a base (e.g. ethanolamine) is often esterified to the phosphoric acid. Plasmalogens are concentrated in the brain and heart.

Sphingomyelins are derivaties of sphingosine with a fatty acid in amide linkage to the amino group of sphingosine phosphate and a base, usually choline, esterified to the phosphate. They are abundant in the brain.

Phospholipid molecules are amphipathic, containing a polar head of the negative phosphate group and the positive alcohol group and a hydrophobic tail of the fatty-acid chains.

***Phosphoprotein.*** One of a group of conjugated proteins in which phosphoric acid is bound to the protein portion of the molecule. The group includes casein.

***Phosphoprotein.*** Conjugated protein in which a phosphoric acid residue is coupled to the polypeptide chain (e.g., casein).

***Phosphorylases.*** Enzymes that catalyse the attachment of a phosphoric acid group to another molecule.

***Phosphorylation.*** Addition of a phosphate group to another molecule such as a protein. Enzymes that catalyse such a reaction are termed phosphorylases or if the phosphate is transferred from ATP kinases.

***Phosphoserine.*** Phosphorylated serine formed during protein phosphorylation, as, for example, in the phosphorylation of histones.

***Phosphovitin.*** Phosphoprotein that is abundantly present in yolk. Along with lipovitellin, it is a product of the large precursor molecule vitellogenin, which is synthesized in the liver.

***Photoautotroph*** (photolithotroph). Organism that uses light as its energy source and carbon dioxide as its main carbon source. Photoautotrophs include higher plants, algae and many photosynthetic bacteria.

***Photoauxotroph.*** Organism that requires only light plus inorganic compounds to provide all of its energy and nutritional requirements.

***Photoheterotroph*** (photoorganotroph). Organism that uses light as its energy source, and an organic compound as the principal carbon source. This group includes some of the purple and green bacteria.

***Photon.*** Quantum of electromagnetic energy. Light is measured in photons.

***Photoperiodism.*** The response by an organism to length of day (photoperiod). Flowering of most plants and certain other plant responses (such as tuber and bulb formation, leaf fall, bud dormancy) can be controlled by photoperiod. Plants may flower in response to short or long days and are called short-day and long-day plants respectively. Examples of the former include chrysanthemum and cocklebur, and of the latter spinach and certain cereals. The critical factor is, in fact, the length of the dark period. For instance, a brief flash of white or red light during a long night will inhibit flowering of a short-day plant but stimulate flowering of a long-day plant. The red flash effect can be reversed by a far-red flash, indicating that phytochrome is the photoreceptive pigment. The leaves are the sensitive organs and the stimulus is transmitted from them to the terminal bud. Some plants, e.g. tomato, flower independently of day length: they are known as day-neutral plants. The breeding season of many animals and many other seasonal activities, such as migration (in birds) are determined by photoperiod.

***Photophosphorylation (photosynthetic phosphorylation).*** The synthesis of ATP from phosphate and ADP during photosynthesis, using light energy.There are two types: cyclic photophosphorylation, coupled to cyclic electron flow, in which ATP is the only product; and noncyclic photophosphorylation, which is coupled to noncyclic electron flow, the electrons being used to reduce $NADP^+$ as well as to make ATP.

***Photophobic Response.*** Response in which an organism shuns or turns away from light.

***Photoreactivating Enzyme.*** Enzyme that is operative in a light-sensitive reaction to repair DNA. It is a nuclease that removes thymine dimers from DNA, such linked nucleotides resulting from prior ultraviolet damage.

***Photoreactivation.*** DNA repair that requires the presence of light. One type of mutation incurred by DNA, especially by irradiation with ultraviolet light, is the formation of thymine dimers between two adjacent thymine bases in the same DNA strand. Such dimers are cleaved by enzymes in the presence of visible light of wavelength 300-400 nm.

***Photoreceptor.*** Any biological light receptor. These include eyes, pineal bodies in some lower vertebrates, and other specialized groups of cells among invertebrates.

***Photorespiration.*** A light-dependent type of respiration that occurs in most photosynthetic plants and differs from normal (or dark) respiration. Glycollate, produced in chloroplasts by oxidation (using oxygen) of a Calvin cycle carbohydrate, is the substrate. It is oxidized to glyoxylate in peroxisomes and recycled to form a Calvin cycle carbohydrate via intermediates including the amino acids glycine and serine.The wasteful loss of carbon dioxide and energy in the form of ATP and $NADPH_2$ that this entails reduces the efficiency of photosynthesis. Some plants, characterized by very low carbon dioxide compensation points, have very low rates of photorespiration. These are mostly $C_4$ plants, whose special type of carbon dioxide fixation apparently reduced glycollate production and hence increases photosynthetic efficiency.

***Photosynthesis.*** The synthesis of organic compound by reduction of carbon dioxide using light energy absorbed by chlorophyll. In green plants, in which water is the hydrogen donor and source of released oxygen, it can be represented by an empirical equation:

$$CO_2 + 2H_2O \xrightarrow[\text{light}]{\text{chlorophyll}} [CH_2O] + H_2O + O_2$$

The evolution of photosynthesis was responsible for the switch from an anaerobic to the present aerobic atmosphere of the earth. Photosynthesis serves directly or indirectly as the source of carbon and energy for all forms of life except chemosynthetic organisms. In eukaryotes it takes place in chloroplasts.

Photosynthesis comprises light and dark reactions. The light-dependent reactions take place on thylakoid membranes and produce the ATP and $NADPH_2$ used in the subsequent dark reactions. The light-absorbing pigments are distributed in two systems, Photosystems or Pigment System I and II (PSI and PSII), probably in photosynthetic units. Each system contains chlorophyll a and accessory pigments, the latter mainly in PSII. Each also has photoreactive centres, or traps, containing one molecule of P700 (PSI) or P680 (PSII). These are probably modified chlorophyll a molecules; they collect energy absorbed by the other pigments, become excited, and emit high-energy electrons that are accepted by electron carriers. Electrons from PSII flow down an electron transport chain between the two systems; their energy is used to generate ATP (noncyclic photophosphorylation) and finally they replace electrons lost from PSI. Electrons from PSI flow down a second chain, either reducing $NADP^+$ or recycling to PSI causing cyclic photophosphorylation. The electrons (and hydrogen) used to reduce $NADP^+$ are derived ultimately from water (since water supplies electrons to replenish PSII), with the evolution of oxygen . Photosynthetic bacteria, which may lack PSII, use other electron donors to PSI and therefore do not evolve oxygen. For example, green and purple sulphur bacteria use hydrogen sulphide and release sulphur; purple nonsulphur bacteria use an organic molecule.

The dark (light-independent) reactions of photosynthesis use the energy (ATP) and reducing power ($NADPH_2$) produced in the light reactions to reduce carbon dioxide ($CO_2$). In eukaryotes it takes place in the chloroplast stroma. There are two possible routes. In some plants, the $C_3$ plants, the first product is a 3-carbon ($C_3$) compound, phosphoglyceric acid (PGA), two molecules of which are formed when $CO_2$ combines with a $C_5$ sugar, ribulose diphosphate. PGA may be used for fatty acid or amino acid synthesis, but is usually reduced (using $NADPH_2$ and ATP) to phosphoglyceraldehyde, a troise phosphate. This feeds a complex cycle, the Calvin cycle (or Benson-Calvin-Bassham cycle), that produces hexoses (e.g. glucose and fructose) and regenerates ribulose diphosphate. Similar cycles probably operate in photosynthetic bacteria and in chemosynthetic organisms, in which oxidative metabolism supplies ATP and $NADPH_2$. $C_3$ plants also produce glycollate in varying amounts, as well as PGA, as a result of photorespiration.

The second route is typical of tropical grasses and certain other plants. These are called $C_4$ plants becuase the first products are $C_4$-dicarboxylic acids. Oxaloacetate, the first, is made by combination of $CO_2$ with the $C_3$ compound phosphoenolpyruvate (PEP) in mesophyll chloroplasts. The enzyme involved has a very high affinity for $CO_2$, resulting in low $CO_2$ compensation points in $C_4$ plants, and a greater efficiency of $CO_2$ fixation. Oxaloacetate is rapidly converted to the $C_4$ acids malate and aspartate, which are transported to specialized chloroplasts (longer and with reduced grana) of the large cells surrounding the vascular bundles (bundle-sheath cells) typical of $C_4$ plants. Here they release $CO_2$, which is refixed as in $C_3$ plants. Thus a carbon dioxide pump operates between mesophyll and bundle sheath chloroplasts. This modified pathway is known as the $C_4$-dicarboxylic acid pathway (or Hatch-Slack pathway). The concentrations of $CO_2$ built up in the bundle sheaths are high enough to inhibit photorespiration; $C_4$ plants are therefore photosynthetically more efficient than $C_3$ plants (in which photorespiration largely wastes $CO_2$ and energy) and are capable of more rapid growth. Optimum growth in these plants occurs at higher light intensities and temperatures than in $C_3$ plants and they use only half the water per unit increase in dry weight. $C_4$ plants are therefore well adapted to tropical climates.

***Photosynthetic Pigments.*** The light-absorbing pigments of photosynthesis, located on thylakoid membranes. Several classes exist; some are accessory pigments, whose function is to collect light energy and pass it to a principal pigment. The pigments are distributed in two systems, Pigment Systems I and II. See Figure P.5.

All photosynthetic organisms contain chlorophylls and carotenoids. Chlorophylls absorb mainly red and blue-biolet light, reflecting green light, and therefore (unless masked by other pigments) to part a green colour to the organism. Actually, the chlorophyll molecule has a roughly square head (porphin (or tetrapyrrole) ring) with magnesium at its centre and a long tail (a long chain alcohol, phytol). Different chlorophylls have different side-chains. Chlorophyll a (and its bacterial equivalents), the most important pigment, has various forms with different absorption peaks, e.g. Chl a 670, 695, 700, 680. The latter two form the energy traps of Pigment System I and II respectively.

Carotenoids are yellow, orange, red, or brown pigments that absorb strongly in the blue-violet range. They are usually masked by chlorophylls, which they may protect

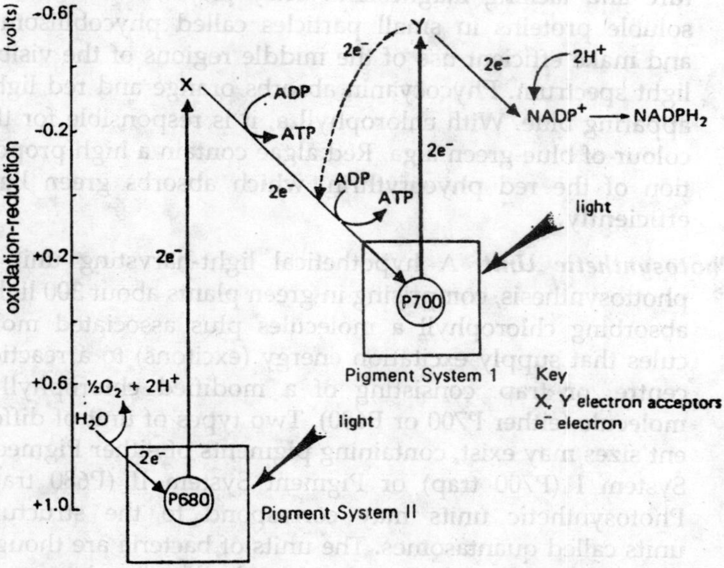


Figure P.5. The main photosynthetic pigment.

from oxidation by molecular oxygen. With anthocyanins they contribute to autumn foliage shades when chlorophyll is lost. They are also widely distributed in nonphotosynthetic tissues, usually in plastids.Thus they form the bright yellows and oranges of many flowers and some fruits, e.g. tomato. There are two types: the carotenes, which are hydrocarbons (tetraterpenes), and the xanthophylls, which are similar but contain oxygen. β-carotene is the most widely distributed carotene (well known as the orange pigment of carrots); it is converted to vitamin A by vertebrates. The major xanthophylls of higher plant leaves are lutein, violaxanthin, and neoxanthin. Another xanthophyll, fucoxanthin, which has an especially broad absorption spectrum, is responsible for the brown colour of diatoms and brown algae.

Phycobilins are related to bile pigmntts. They are trapyrroles, like the chlorophylls, but with an opn-chain structure and lacking magnesium. They are bound to water-soluble proteins in small particles called phycobilisomes and make efficient use of the middle regions of the visible light spectrum. Phycocyanin absorbs orange and red light, apparing blue. With chlorophyll a, it is responsible for the colour of blue-green alga. Red algae contain a high proportion of the red phycorythrin, which absorbs green light efficiently.

***Photosynthetic Unit.*** A hypothetical light-harvsting unit of phottosynthesis, comprising in green plants about 300 light-absorbing chlorophyll a molecules plus associated molecules that supply excitation energy (excitons) to a reaction centre, or trap. consisting of a modified chlorophyll a molecule (either P700 or P680). Two types of unit of different sizes may exist, containing pigments of either Pigmeent System I (P700 trap) or Pigment System II (P680 trap). Photosynthetic units may correspond to the structural units called quantasomes. The units of bacteria are thought to contain about 50 bacteriochlorophyll molecules.

***Phototrophic (photosynthetic).*** Designating organisms (phototrophs) that use light energy to synthesize their organic requirements, either from inorganic precursors (photoautotrophic organisms) or from organic precursors obtained from the environment (photoheterotrophic organisms). Most phototrophs are photoautotrophic and include all green plants.

***Phototropism (heliotropism).*** Tropic movement in response to light.Coleoptiles and most stems are positively phototropic, i.e. they grow towards light; since leaves are usually plagiotropic to light, the combined effect is to ensure the optimum arrrangement of leaves to trap light energy for photosynthesis. The tip of the stem or coleoptile is photosensitive; auxin accumulates on its shaded side and moves down the organ causing faster growth on that side, and hence bending towards the light. Most roots are insensitive to light; others are negatively phototropic, e.g. sunflower.

***Phragmoplast.*** The region between the daughter nuclei of a dividing plant cell. It consists initially of spindle fibres (microtubules) only, which proliferate rapidly to form a barrel-shaped birefringent structure containing ribosomes, Golgi apparatus, microtubules, and endoplasmic reticulum. It contains the cell plate and functions in cytokinesis; the microtubules may serve to guide Golgi vesicles to the plate during its formation.

***Phycobilin.*** Acessory pigment in photosynthesis, consisting of phycoerythrin and phycocyanin, and occurring chiefly in red algae and the prokaryotic blue-green algae.

***Phycobilisome.*** One of many particles, about 35 nm in diameter, that contain phycobilins and coveer the photosynthetic lamellae of red and blue-green algae.

***Phycocyanin.*** Blue phycobilin photosynthetic pigment that is abundant in the prokaryotic blue-green algae, but also occurs in red algae.

***Phycoerythrin.*** Red phycobilin photosynthetic pigment, constituting the main phycobilin of red algae, but also present in the prokaryotic blue-green algae.

***Phyletic Evolution*** (anagenesis, vertical evolution). Transformation of one species into a distinct species in the course of evolution without any side-branching, which would indicate some involvement of other species.

***Phylogenetic.*** Indicating that a classification is based on evolutionary descent.

***Phylogenetic-associated Residues.*** Amino acid residues found preferentially at certain positions in a protein of one or more species. The term has been used to describe such residues in immunoglobulin variable regions.

***Phylogenetic Tree.*** Diagram indicating the supposed sequence of historical relationship linking together species or high taxa. Lineages are commonly presented in relation to geological time, the taxonomic groups often being represented as line segments, the line brranches being the presumed times of separation of the species or other taxa.

***Phylogeny.*** Relationshiop between individuals, species, populations or other taxa as a reflection of their evolutionary history.

***Phylum*** (pl.Phyla). A unit used in the classification of animals. A phylum consists of a number of classes, or occasionally of only one class, with certain important characteristics in common, implying that all members are descended from a common ancestor. For example the phylum Protozoa consists of unicellular organisms; the phylum Arthropoda contains invertebrates with exoskeletons and joined appendages. Large phyla are divided into subphyla; for example the phylum Chordata is divided into the subphyla Urochordata, Cephalochordata, and Vertebrata. Subphyla are then divided into classes.The corresponding unit in plant classification is the division (although the phylum is used in some plant classification schemes).

***Physarum.*** Non-cellular slime moulds belonging to the phylum Myxomycota, and not closely related to the cellular slime moulds, the Acrasiomycota. P.polycephalum is the best known species and the most commonly grown in laboratories. It exists for much of its life history as a multinucleate plasmodium without plasma membranes between the nuclei, and has been widely used for studies on the cell cycle because of the natural synchrony of the nuclear division and DNA synthesis.

***Physical Map.*** Map, produced by nucleotide sequencing and electron microscopic heteroduplex assays, that indicates the linear order of DNA sequences on a chromosome or chromosome segment.

***Physiological Saline.*** Balanced salt solution of specified molarity and pH, crudely approximating to in vivo tissue fluids, and in which organs/tissues can be perfused or bathed during short-term experimentation.

***Phytoalexin.*** A nonspecific antibiotic produced by a plant in response either to infection by a microorganism (usually a fungus) or occasionally to chemical or environmental factors or injury. Phytoalexins are produced in appreciable amounts and contribute to disease resistance. Many phytoalexins are phenolic compounds; more than twenty have been chemically identified.

***Phytochrome.*** A blue-green proteinaceous pigment found in low concentrations in nearly all parts of higher plants. There are two forms, one ($P_R$ or $P_{660}$) absorbing red and the other ($P_{FR}$ or $P_{730}$) far-red light; these forms interchange rapidly and reversibly as shown in the Figure P.6.

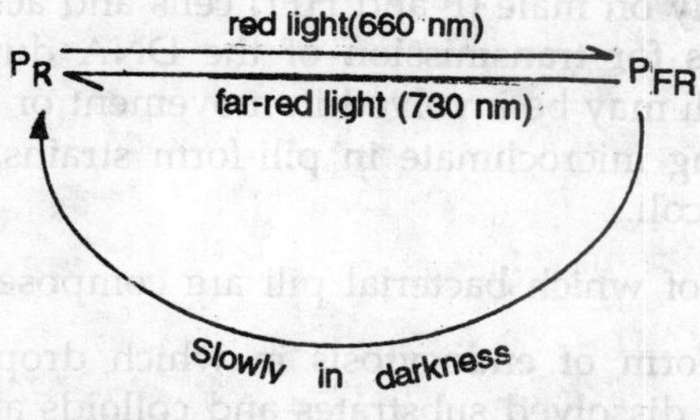


Figure P.6. Interchangeable forms of phytochrome.

The physiologically active $P_{FR}$ form mediates a range of important morphogenetic responses to light, being formed in red (and hence white) light, even of very low intensity and short duration. Processes controlled include photoperiodism (and hence floral initiation); greening and expansion of young or etiolated leaves and cotyledons; inhibition of etiolation; breaking of dormancy of certain seeds; and anthocyanin formation.

***Phytohaemagglutinin (PHA).*** A lectin that is bound by the glycoproteins at the cell surface and thereby stimulates some cells to divide. PHA is commonly used to stimulate in vitro division of circulating lymphocytes.

***Phytohormone.*** Any of the plant growth substances or plant hormones (e.g., auxins).

***Pico-carmine.*** Water-soluble cytological due that stains the cytoplasm yellow.

***Picogram.*** Unit of mass equal to $10^{-12}$ gram.

***Picornaviruses*** (enteroviruses). Small viruses with single-stranded RNA genomes, capsids of non-enveloped icosahedral form, and including a range of enteric viruses common in the human and other mammals. Examples include foot and mouth disease virus, polio virus, and cold viruses (rhinoviruses). The name is derived from an aggregate of pico (meaning small), RNA and virus.

***Pili.*** Filamentous·appendages attached to some bacterial cells, consisting of hollow tubes of pilin. Differing types of pili can be recognized, varying in size and number. Sex pili are present only on male (F and HFr) cells and act as conjugationb tubes for transmission of the DNA during mating. Normal pili may be involved in movement or in creating a surrounding microclimate in pili-form strains and species such as E.coli.

***Pilin.*** Protein of which bacterial pili are composed.

***Pinocytosis.*** Form of endocytosis in which droplets of fluid containing dissolved substrates and colloids are taken into cel!s usually by an intucking of the plasma membrane to form a vesicle; it litherally means cell drinking. Micropinocytosis involves the formation of vesicles (about 0.1 μm in diameter) visible only in the electron microscope; formation of vesicles visible under the light microscope is called macropinocytosis. Smooth-walled pinocytic vesicles (i.e. those lacking a clathrin coat during their formation) are thought to be non-selective with respect to materials pinocytosed (fluid pinocytosis). Pinocytosis is characteristic of amoeboid protozoans, leucocytes, certain endothelial and epithelial cells lining ducts and body cavities, and cells in tissue culture.

***Pinosome.*** Cytoplasmic vesicle, surrounded by a plasma membrane and containing liquid taken up by the cell during pinocytosis. Pinosomes form by budding off from the internal surface of the plasma mebrane during pinocytosis.

***Pisum Sativum.*** Graden pea. It was used by Gregor Mendel for his pioneering work on genetics.

***Pit.*** Cavity in the secondary wall of certain plant cells which extends down to the primary cell wall. The primary wall and the attendant middle lamella act as the pit membrane or pit-closing membrane. A pit usually occurs opposite a complementary pit in the wall of an adjacent cell to form a pit pair. These pit pairs allow the exchange of substances between adjacent cells. Pits may occur as either simple pits or as bordered pits.

***Piltdown Man.*** A fraudulent fossil man that was found at Piltdown, Sussex, and given the name Eoanthropus. Skull fragments were first found by Charles Dawson (1864-1916), in 1911 and subsequent discoveries led to the reconstruction of part of a skull. Chemical tests on the skull from 1949 to 1953 showed that the jaw bone was that of a modern ape and that the braincase was Pleistocene, but its origin unknown. The skull had been artificially coloured and the teeth artificially ground down, indicating that the skull fragments had been deliberately planted. Despite much speculation and circumstantial evidence, the perpetrator of the hoax has never been positively identified.

***Pitressin.*** Name for a commercially available form of vasopressin.

***pK.*** pH at which the concentrations of dissociated and undissociated forms are equal in a solution of a weak acid or base. It is numerically equal to the negative of the $\log_{10}$ of the dissociation constant (or $\log_{10}$ of the reciprocal of the dissociation constant).

***Placenta.*** 1. A temporary flat organ within the uterus of mammals and other viviparous animals that establishes a close association between the foetal and maternal blood circulations. It consists of both embryonic and maternal tissues and enables the foetus to depend entirely on maternal systems for obtaining oxygen and nutrients as well as for the removal of metabolic waste products. The degree of union of the tissues (placentation) varies between mammalian types; in ungulates the outer chorionic tissues of the embryo are merely closely applied to the maternal endometrium. In many groups, however, maternal tissue is eroded in such a way that direct contact is made with the maternal blood vessels. In primates (including humans) foetal tissue is directly bathed in maternal blood. The placenta also produces hormones (gonadotrophins, oestrogens, and progesterone) and in some species takes over the reproductive endocrine roles of the pituitary and ovaries during pregnancy. Soon after parturition the placenta is delivered as the afterbirth.

2. The part of a plant ovary to which the ovules are attached, which often corresponds to the line of fusion of the carpel edges. There are typically two placentae per carpel (one on each lateral margin) but the various types of infolding and fusion of the carpels in ovary formation have led to a variety of placentations.

3. The tissue to which sporangia or spores are attached.

***Placodermi.*** A class of extinct fishes common in the Devonian. They had a heavy bony armour over the head and front part of the body, an endoskeleton of bone, autostylic jaw suspension, paired fins, and a heterocercal tail. The first gill slit was not modified as a spiracle, as in other fishes. Placoderms were probably more closely related to the Chondrichthyes than to the Osteichthyes. There are several orders, including the Antiarchi and Arthrodira.

***Placodontia.*** A suborder of the Sauropterygia containing large exinct Triassic reptiles, e.g. Placodus, specialized for life in shallow coastal waters. Placodonts had long limbs with flattened paddle-like feet with which they rowed themselves through the water.

***Plankton.*** Minute plants (phytoplankton) and animals (zooplankton) that float in the surface waters of a sea or lake, they are of great economic and ecological importance. The chief constituents of phytoplankton are unicellular algae, which carry out photosynthesis and form the basis of the food chains that support all aquatic life. The zooplankton, typically consisting of animals with weak locomotory powers, includes protozoans, small crustaceans, and various invertebrate larvae.

***Plant Geography (Phytogeography).*** The study of the distribution of plant species over the surface of the earth.

***Plantigrade.*** Designating a gait of mammals in which the entire foot, i.e. digits and metacarpals (or metatarsals), remains flat on the ground. This is the most primitive gait and is characteristic of primates, insectivores, bears, etc.

***Plaque.*** Small area within a bacterial lawn where cells are being lysed or their growth is being inhibited, by the multiplication of a bacteriophage. Virulent phages produce clear plaques; temperate phages produce turbid plaques.

***Plaque Assay.*** Assay based on counting bacteriophage plaques on bacterial lawns, each lawn having a different dilution of phage to ensure that a correct estimate of the number of infective phage in a solution is achieved.

***Plaque-forming Cells.*** Cells that cause a clear plaque in a monolayer of erythrocytes due to haemolysis. These are normally antibody-secreting cells, which act as haemolytic agents in the presencre of complement.

***Plasma.*** Uncoagulated blood from which cells have been removed.

***Plasma Cell.*** Terminally differentiated B lymphocyte that synthesizes and secretes immunoglobulin. Plasma cells are round or ovoid and have a mean diameter of 14 μm. The nucleus is eccentric and its chromatin is distributed in a pattern resembling the spokes of a wheel ('cartwheel nucleus'). Plasma cells have abundant cytoplasm with prominent rough endoplasmic reticulum and golgi complex. The cytoplasm stains red with pyronin ('pyroninophilic') due to its high content of RNA. Plasma cells do not divide and have a half-life of about two to four days. They are identified by reactions with fluorescein-labeled antibodies to immunoglobulin in the cytoplasm. Plasma cells are usually found in secondary lymphoid organs (e.g., lymph nodes and spleen). In contrast to B lymphocytes, plasma cells have no surface immunoglobulin or complement receptors.

***Plasma Cell Antigen*** (PC-1, PC-2). Alloantigen in the membranes of mouse plasma cells.

***Plasma Cells.*** Connective tissue cells usually found in large numbers in areas of inflammation associated with chronic infection. They are thought to be derived from lymphocytes or lymphocyte precursor cells (lymphoblasts) and are responsible for the production of antibodies.

***Plasmagel.*** The gel-like state of protoplasm, which may be reversible transformed to plasmasol. Ectoplasm is typically a plasmagel.

***Plasmagene.*** A self-duplicating cytoplasmic entity containing its own set of genes independent of the nucleus. Its inheritance is therefore non-Mendelian since it does not involve fusion of nuclei (gametes).

***Plasma Membrane*** (cell membrane, plasmalemma). Essential membrane that surrounds all prokaryotic and eukaryotic cells and defines the interface between the cell's interior and exterior. Althought its basic structure is like all biological membranes its protein composition and asymmetry reflect its functions at the cell surface (e.g., membrane receptors to bind signalling molecules, such as hormones, in the cells environment; ion pumps to maintain the normal ioninc equilibrium with the environment). All oligosaccharide residues (of membrane glycolipids and glycoproteins) are found on the non-cytoplasmic aspect of the membrane as a glycocalyx, which is thought to have important but undefined influences on plasma membrane function. See Figure P.7.

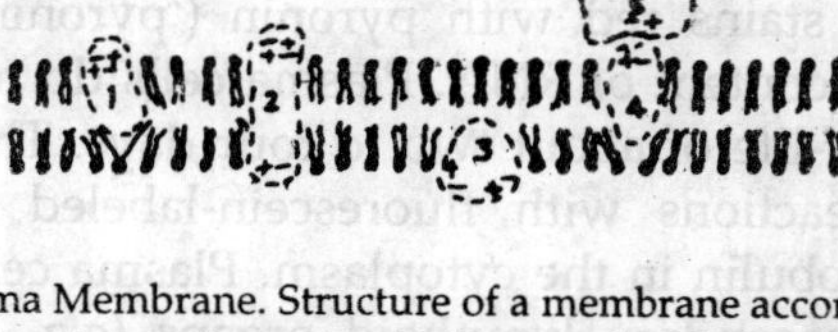

Figure P.7. Plasma Membrane. Structure of a membrane according to the fluid mosaic model. Four integral proteins (1-4) are embedded into a lipid bilayer so that the hydrophobic surface of each protein (dashed lines) is in the membrane and the polar regions (indicated by + and —) are external. Peripheral proteins (e.g., 5) are on the surface and bound to a polar region of an integral protein. Integral proteins can drift laterally, but cannot flip-flop.

***Plasmapheresis.*** Procedure in which blood is removed from an individual, centrifuged, and the cells are then re-infused into the patient. Plasmapheresis is used in the treatment of autoimmune disease (e.g., goodpasture's syndrome) to remove the antibodies that cause the disease. It is also used in the treatment of macroglobulinemia of waldenstrom to remove the macroglobulin that, in excessive amounts, increases blood viscosity and causes symptoms.

***Plasma Proteins.*** Proteins dissolved in blood plasma. In vertebrates such proteins include albumins, alpha-, beta-, and gamma-globulins (including immunoglobulins which constitute the majority of anti-bodies), transferrins, and proteins involved in blood clotting. The plasma proteins confer on the plasma a colloidal osmotic pressure which is important in osmoregulatory control.

***Plasmasol.*** The sol-like (fluid) state of protoplasm, which may be reversibly transformed to plasmagel. Endoplasm is usually in a plasmasol condition.

***Plasmid.*** A genetic element, often found in bacterial cells, that is separate from the genomic DNA and replicates independently of it. At one time plasmids capable of integration into the genome were called episomes, but the term plasmid is now generally used for all independent DNA factors. Plasmids include some bacteriophages and the factors bearing genes for bacteriocins (Col factors), drug redsistance (R factors), and bacterial sex (F factors). All consist of circles of double-stranded DNA. Chimaeric factors contain sequences of eukaryotic genes; they are produced by modern techniques of gene manipulation and are widely used as a means of cloning genes in bacterial hosts.

Plasmids are widely used as carriers of cloned genes, as for example the E.coli pasmid pBR322, and numbers of such plasmids may be amplified by treating the donor cells with chloramphenicol, which stops host cell DNA synthesis but not that of the plasmid. At one time plasmids were referred to as episomes if they were capable of integration into the genome of the host cell, but the term is now less commonly used. Some bacteriophages may exist either as integrated or free copies in the cell, and in either case can be termed plasmids. Yeast cells have been found to harbour some plasmids, and the Ti plasmid of Agrobacterium can survive in either bacterial or plant cells (although in a partial form in the later). When plasmids are used as cloning vectors and carry a novél DNA sequence they are referred to as chimaeric plasmids.

***Plasmid.*** Extrachromosomal double-stranded circular DNA molecules found in most bacterial species and in some eukaryotes. Ordinarily, a plasmid is not essential to its host cell. However, many plasmids contain genes (e.g., for antibiotic resistance) that may be essential in certain environments. Plasmids range in size from 1 to 200 kilobases. Although plasmids are dependent on the replication machinery of the host cell, they contain their own genes for regulating the time of synthesis and the number of plasmid copies per cell. The replication of plasmids under stringentt control is coupled to that of the host, and only one or a few copies of such plasmids are found per cell. Plasmids under relaxed control have copy numbers of 10-200; in such plasmids tthe copy number can be increased to several thousand per cell if host protein synthesis is shut off (e.g., by treatment with chloramphenicol).

Plasmids are frequently used as cloning vectors. To be useful for cloning, a plasmid should have the following properties: (1) small size and relaxed mode of replication; (2) presence of one o moe selectable markers (e.g.,antibiotic resistance) to allow identification of transforrmants and to prevent loss of the plasmid from the bacteria; (3) a single recognition site for one or more restriction enzymes in rregions of the plasmid that are not essential forr replication and into which foreign DNA can be inserted. If there are two o more genes for antibiotic resistance on the plasmid, it is useful if the site for DNA insertion is located within one of them, so that insertion inactivates the gene, allowing identification of bacteria containing the recombinant. Another useful marker is the E. coli lac gene, which may be inactivated as the result of insertion of exogenous DNA into the coding region. In this case, recombinants that do not produce β-galactosidase can be recognized by their failure to produce a colored product when the bacterial colonies grow on medium containing an appropriate chromogenic substrate.

***Plasmid Cloning Vector.*** Plasmid used as a cloning vector by the incorporation of novel DNA sequences into the plasmid DNA and transfection of bacterial cells with the chimaeric plasmids. Plasmids chosen for this role are usually small and under relaxed control within the bacterial cell. As carriers of recognition sites for specific restriction endonucleases and antibiotic genes, they may be readily manipulated, and bacteria carrying such plasmids are selected by treatment with the appropriate antibiotic. pBR322 is a commonly used cloning vector in E.coli.

***Plasmid Rescue..*** Procedure whereby plasmid genes, and other genes integrated into plasmid, can be transformed into the genome of a bacterium (e.g., Bacillus subtilis). Plasmids are linearized by cutting with a restriction enzyme and transfected into a bacterium which already carries a homologous plasmid. If part of the linearized plasmid is cut in the homologous sequence, then recombination between the newly acquired and existing plasmid copies occurs, leading to integration of some of the novel plasmid and its stable integration into the plasmid population of the bacterial cell.

***Plasmin.*** A nonspecific enzyme that is responsible for the dissolution of blood clots (fibrinolysis). It exists in normal blood as the inactive precursor plasminogen, which is converted into active ·plasmin by several proteolytic factors, e.g.trypsin.

***Plasminogen.*** Precursor molecule that is cleaved to yield plasmin, under the influcence of several proteolytic factors (e.g., trypsin).

***Plasmodesma*** (pl.Plasmodesmata). A narrow tube traversing the plant cell wall through which the protoplasm of adjacent cells is continuous. The tube is lined by the plasma membrane and contains a central, possibly tubular, core normally associated at either end with endoplasmic reticulum. The number per cell varies; they are sometimes cioncentrated in primary pit fields. Sieve plate pores are derived from plasmodesmata.

***Plasmodium.*** An acellular multinucleate amoeboid protoplasmic mass bounded by a plasma membrane, such as forms the vegetative phase of the Myxomycetes (slime fungi). Growth by plasmogamy may occur between plasmodia of the same species. In the Acrasiales (cellular slime fungi) the constituent amoebae retain their individuality within the protoplasmic mass, which is then termed a pseudoplasmodium.

***Plasmodium.*** Malarial parasite; parasitic protozoan of the class Sporozoa.

***Plasmogamy.*** The union of two or more protoplasts, which occurs in the formation of a heterokaryon or precedes karyogamy in sexual reproduction.

***Plasmolysis.*** Shrinkage of eventual lysis of a plant cell protoplast within the rigid cell wall. This phenomenon occurs by the osmotic loss of water if plant tissue is placed in a hypertonic solution.

***Plasmon.*** Collective name for all of the extrachromosomal hereditary factors of a cell (i.e. the mitochondria, plus protoplasts, plus any plasmids or other genetic factors present).

***Plasmosome.*** Little used name for the nucleolus.

***Plastid.*** An organelle present in all plants except bacteria, blue-gren algae, and fungi; it is enclosed by two membranes (the envelope) and has various functions. Plastids are classified according to their pigmentation. Chloroplasts contain photosynthetic pigments, including chlorophyll, and carry out photosynthesis. In chromoplasts, the pigments are predominantly or exclusively carotenoids, whose red or yellow colour masks any chlorophyll that may be present. Chromoplasts are usually derived from chloroplasts or leucoplasts and are found particularly in fruits and flowers of higher plants, in which their bright colours may serve to attract animals for pollination and seed dispersal. Leucoplasts are colourless plastids, lacking pigments, and are often modified for the storage of food, particularly starch. They occur in a variety of tissues, including the epidermis, root parenchyma, and young leaves. Interconversion between all three plastid types can occur. Plastids may be modified for storage of food reserves and can alternatively be classified according to the storage product: amyloplasts store.

***Platelet.*** Small (2-4 μm in diameter), spherical, colorless, refractile, non-nucleated particle of the blood that is derived from megakaryocytes of bone marrow. Platelets are required for the clotting of blood. Platelets contain serotonin and histamine; their release from plateles conributes to immediate hypersensitivity reactions. Mammalian platelets (except those of primates) bear complement receptor 1 on their surfaces and are important in immune adherence in these species.

***Platelet-activating Factorr (PAF).*** Phosphorylcholine derivative released from mast cells, polymorphonuclear leukocytes and macrophages when antibodies bound to Fc receptors on these cells encounter antigen. PAF aggregates platelets and releases intracellular platelet constituents (e.g., serotonin, histamine). Administration of PAF causes transient thrombocytopenia, hypotension, and increased vascular perrmeability. PAF is thought to play a role in immediate hypersensitivity reactions. See Figure P.8.

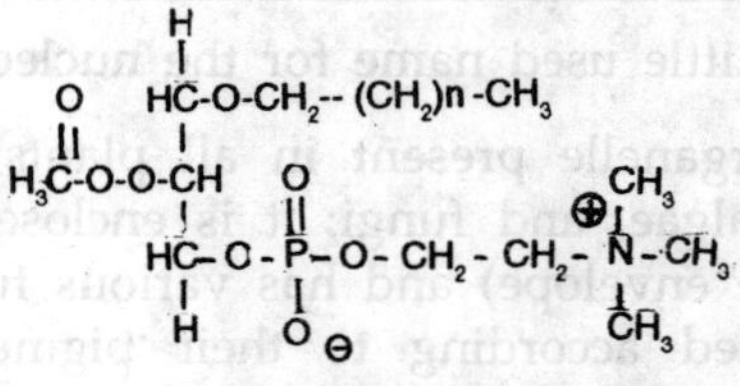

Figure P.8. Platelett activating factor.

***Polyadenlyic Acid.*** Polynucleotide chain composed only of adenine resudues. Messenger RNA molecules carry a tail of such residues at their 3'-ends.

***Polyacrylamide Gel.*** Medium used for electrophoretic separation of proteins and nucleic acids. Acrylamide in solution is polymerized and cross-linked, and allowed to set into a gel in tubes or between glass plates. The porosity of the gel can be varied, allowing the separation of molecules in different size ranges. Separations are influenced by both size and charge.

***Polyacrylamide Gel Electrophoresis in Sodium Dodecyl Sulfate*** (SDS-PAGE). Technique for separating proteins according to their molecularr weights. The proteins or mixture of proteins is incubated in excess SDS, usually at an elevated temperature and in the presence of a rreducing agent to ensure complete denaturation. Under these conditions, the amount of sodium dodecyl sulfate (SDS) bound to most proteins, per unit weight, is approximately constant. Therefore, different protein-SDS complexes have essentially identical charge-to-mass ratios and migrate in poly acrylamide gels of the correct porosity according to polypeptide size. Unlabeled proteins can be detected by staining with dye (e.g., Coomassie blue) and radiolabeled proteins by autoradiography. A plot of log molecular weight against mobility is approximately linear, and the molecular weight of an unknown potein can be estimated by comparison with standard proteins. However, some proteins (e.g., glycoproteins) bind relatively less SDS and others (e.g., membrane proteins) bind relatively more SDS than the proteins used as standards. Consequently, such proteins migrate anomalously in SDS gels, the apparent molecularr weight of a glycoprotein being higher and that of a membrane protein lower than the true molecular weight.

***Polyamines.*** Compounds that contain two or more amino groups. Examples are putrescine, $NH_2(CH_2)_4NH_2$, cadaverine, $NH_2(CH_2)_5NH_2$, and spermine, $NH_2(CH_2)_3NH(CH_2)_4NH(CH_2)_3NH_2$. At phsiological pH these compounds are multivalent cations and are found associated with the anionic sites (i.e. phosphate groups) of DNA helices in some viruses and bacteria. This neutralizing effect is analogous to the action of histones in eukaryotic cells and gives the DNA molecules greater flexibility.

***Polyandry.*** Pairing of one female with more than one male.

***Polyarteritis Nodosa.*** Segmental vasculitis of small and medium-sized muscular arteries of all organs. In 30 percent of cases, hepatitis B antigen is found in the blood, and this suggests that the disease is cuased by immune complexes. Affected blood vessel walls are infiltrated with neutrophils; ultimately necrosis of the arteries occurs. The male-to-female ratio among patients is 3:1. The disease may respond favorably to treatment with cyclophosphamide.

***Polycistronic Message.*** Molecule of messenger RNA that is the product of transcription of a series of tandemly located genes on the DNA. Although some polycistronic messages are later processed by cleavage into separate messages, some are translated intact. The messages of bacterial operons such as the lac operon of E.coli are polycistronic.

***Polyclona.*** Describing cells or molecules that are derived from more than one clone. An antibody would be described as polyclonal if it had been raised against several antigens, or several groups of one antigen. Similarly the cells of some tissues, especially neoplasms, may be monoclonal in that they are all derived from one original cell, whereas most tissues such as liver or spleen are polyclonal in that it can be shown that they are derived from more than one committed cell in early development.

***Polyclonal Activator.*** Substance that stimulates T or B lymphocytes, regardless of their antigen specificity. Polyclonal activators include plant lectins that activate T lymphocytes and/or B lymphocytes and bacterial products (e.g., lipopolysaccharides) that activate B lymphocytes.

***Polyclonal Antibodies.*** Antibodies, derived from many different clones of antibody forming cells, all of which react with a particular antigen. This term is used to contrast to the term, monoclonal antibodies. Immunization usually results in a polyclonal antibody response.

***Polycomplex.*** Fused synaptonemal complex, detached from diplotene chromosomes, found in the oocyte nuclei of some insects.

***Polycystic Disease.*** Autosomal dominant traint in the human affecting about one in 500 of the population, in which renal cysts occur and may lead to renal failure and hypertension. Infantile polycystic disease, which involves cysts in liver, pancreas and kidneys, is a rare condition. It is autosomal recessive and results in death in early childhood.

***Polycythaemia.*** Increase in the number of circulating erythrocytes per unit volume of blood. Polycythaemia may be the result of dehydration, or a compensatory phenomenon to increase the oxygen-carrying capacity of the blood (e.g., at high altitude, or in certain cardiac diseases). Polycythaemia vera is an extreme condition of unknown aetiology. Polycythaemia can be induced emperimentally by administering erythropoietin.

***Polydeoxyribonucleotide Synthase (ATP-requiring)*** (DNA ligase; EC 6.5.1.1). Enzyme that catalyses the formation of phosphodiester bonds between 5'-phosphoryl and 3'-hydroxyl groups in DNA and that requires ATP as a cofactor. Such enzymes have been isolated from a variety of sources including bacteriophage T4 and rat liver. DNA ligases seal single-stranded breaks in duplex DNA. In vivo they function in DNA replication and recombination and may play a role in DNA repair. It has been shown that the DNA ligase isolated from bacteriophage T4 can also catalyse blunt-end ligation of DNA (i.e., ligation between molecules lacking complementary single-stranded termini). This property makes the T4 DNA ligase useful in various manipulations of DNA in vitro (e.g. addition lof synthetic linkers to duplex DNA). In the presence of high concentrations of any of several types of macromolecules (e.g., polyenthylene glycol and bovine serum albumin), DNA ligase from rat liver has also been shown to catalyse blunt-end ligation. The T4 enzyme is a single chain of 487 amino acid residues and can be isolated frrom T4-infected E.coli. During catalysis, the cofactor is split to form an enzyme-AMP complex.

***Polydeoxyribonucleotide Synthase (NAD⁺-requiring)*** (DNA ligase; EC 6.5.1.2). Enzyme that catalyses the formation of phosphodiester bonds between 5'-phosphoryl and 3'-hydrroxyl groups and that requires $NAD^+$ as a cofactor. Such an enzyme has been isolated from E.coli. Although under ordinary assay conditions, the E.coli DNA ligase does not catalyse blunt-end ligation, this activity can be demonstrated when the assay is carried out in the presence of high concentrations of macromolecules and may, therefore, occurr in living cells. During catalysis, the cofactor is split to form an enzyme-AMP complex.

***Polyembryony.*** The formation of more than one embryo from a single zygote. It occurs in seed plants, in which several embryos are found in one ovule, and in many group of animals, e.g. the Platyhelminthes. Identical twins are produced by polymbryony.

***Polyimmunoglobulin Receptor.*** Receptor for polymeric immunoglobulins, which mediates the transcytosis of polymeric IgA and IgM into external secretions. These receptors are found on the surfaces of epithelial cells and hepatocytes; in the gut, they are located on the basolateral surface of epithelial cells. After the polymeric immunoglobulin is bound, the receptor-ligand complex undergoes endocytosis and is transported across the cell in vesicles; exoċytos of ths complex occurs at the apical cell surface, releasing the immunoglobulin into the lumen of the gut. Similar processes occur in hepatocytes iin some species, resulting iin transport of IgA into the bile. Before release into the secretions the receptor is proteolytically cleaved close to the membrane and discharged while still bound to the polymeric immunoglobulin. Thus, the receptor is used for only one round of transport. The portion of the receptor bound to immunoglobulin and released wiith it into the secretions is called the secretory component.

The primary translation product of one form of rabbit polyimmunoglobulin receptor, deduced from the cDNA sequence, was found to consists of 773 amino acid residues; a single sequence (18 residues), an extracellular portion (629 residues), most of which becomes the secretory component, a transmembrane segment (23 residues), and a long cytoplasmiic segment (103 residues). There are two sites for N-linked oligosaccharides. Analysis of the primary structure indicates that the protein is composed of seven domaiins, each containing approxmately 110 residues. The amino-terminal five domains have a high degree of homology with each other. As in immunoglobulin domains, each has a pair of cysteiine residues that could form an intradomain disulfide bridge spanning 60-70 amino acid residues. The five amino-terminal domains have significant similarity in amino acid sequence to immunoglobulin variable regions, especially to those of kappa chains, as well as to Thy-1. Thus, the polyimmunoglobulin receptor is a member of the immunoglobulin superfamily. The sixth domain, which contains the membrane-spanning segment, also has some resemblance in sequence to immunoglobulin kappa variable regions, but it does not have a pair of cysteine residue positioned to form a loop of the size characteristic of immunoglobulin domains. The seventh (cytoplasmic) domain has no similarity in sequence to immunoglobulins.

Human secretory component is similar in amino acid sequence to the first five domains of the rabbit polyimmunoglobulin receptor; after appropriate alignment there is about 55 percent identity.

***Polymorphism.*** Occurrence, with appreciable frequency in a population, of two or more variants at a particular genetic locus. The variants may or may not code for a protein. In human populations, appreciable frequency is usually taken to be at least 1 percent. The existence of polymorphisms can be established by direct analysis of DNA (e.g., determination of restriction fragment length polymorphisms) or by analysis of gene products (e.g., by electrophoretic and/or immunological techniques). Examples of polymorphisms in human populations are the ABO and Rh blood groups, molecules of the HLA complex (class I, II, and III), the Gm allotypes of immunoglobulin gamma chains, and the Km allotypes of immunoglobulin kappa chains.

***Polygamy.*** Pairing of one male with more than one female or one female with more than one male.

***Polygenes.*** Group of genes that combine to affect a quantitative charactger such as weight or growth rate.

***Polygyny.*** Pairing of one male with more than one female.

***Polylinker.*** Oligonucleotide DNA sequence that effectively joins DNA sequences colinearly.

***Polymer.*** Macromolecule composed of an aggregation of covalently bonded repeating subunits (monomers). Thus a linear polypeptide is an amino acid polymer, and a single-strand of nucleic acid is a polymer of nucleotide monomers.

***Polymerase.*** An enzyme responsible for synthesizing a polymer. Two classes of such enzymes are the DNA polymerases and the RNA polymerases (or transcriptases). In eukaryotic cells there are a number of DNA polymerases, only one of which is responsible for general DNA replication; the others are DNA repair enzymes. There are four main types of RNA polymerase in eukaryotic cells: Types I to IV. Type I is responsible for transcription of ribosomal RNA genes (except 5S RNA genes), Type II for messenger RNA transcription, Type III for transfer RNA and 5S ribosomal RNA transcription, and Type IV for transcription from the mitochondrial DNA. Bacteria possess a single type of RNA polymerase; they also have repair polymerases in addition to the general DNA polymerase involved in DNA replication. Some special polymerases are associated with viral replication, notably reverse transcriptase (RNA-dependent DNA polymerase), which synthesizes DNA from an RNA template. It occurs in the replication cycle of some oncogenic viruses.

***Polymorph (Polymorphonuclear Leucocyte).*** One of a group of white blood cells, about 10-12 μm in diameter, having lobulated nuclei and distinct cyctoplasmic granules. This name is commonly applied to the three principal granulocytic white cells in blood: neutrophils, basophils, and eosinophils, which usually represent about 60-65% of the white cells of human blood. All polymorphs are phagocytic and migrate freely from the blood vessels into tissues during inflammation.

***Polymorphism.*** The existence of two or more different forms (morphs) of individuals in the same species. There are two basic types of polymorphism. Balanced polymorphism is characterized by the coexistence of the different morphs all the time in the same population. It is seen in animal populations in which the two sexes differ in appearance or where a caste system exists and in plant populations of pin- and thrumeyed forms of primorses. In transient polymorphism, the two morphs exist in the population together for only a short time, while one form is replacing the other. This occurs in months undergoing the process of industrial melanism.

***Polymorphonuclear Leukocyte*** (PMN). White blood cell of myeloid lineage (13 μm in diameter), characterized by a nucleus composed of three distinct lobes that are connected by thin strands of chromatin. PMNs are classified by the staining properties of the specific or secondary granules in the cytoplasm: eosinophils (5 percent), basophils (2 percent) and neutrophils (approximately 90 percent). All PMNs contain primary granules. The term 'poly' (an abbreviation for polymorphonuclear leukocyte) is frequently used to mean neutrophil.

***Polymyositis.*** Inflammatory disease of muscle that is presumed to have an imunological cause. Patients experience muscle weakness and pain. Microscopically, the muscle is infiltrated with lymphocytes. Extracts of normal muscle are mitogenes for T lymphocytes from patients with polymyositis. Serum of patients contains autoantibodies to some tRNA synthetases.

***Polyneme Hypothesis.*** Proposition that a chromatid contains more than one duplex of DNA running in parallel. This has been largely superceded by the present understanding that a single duplex of DNA is present in a chromatid, but that it is elaborately packaged by supercoiling and looping out from a central axis, and so only at a superficial level can seprate gene loci be regarded as being in purely linear order along a chromosome length. Genes adjacent to one another on a DNA molecule might be regarded correctly as being at the same locus of a chromosome considered in linear terms.

***Polynucleotide 5'-hydroxyl-kinase*** (polynucleotide kinase; EC 2.7.1.78). Enzyme, usually obtained from E.coli infected with bacteriophage T4, that catalyses the tansfer of the $\gamma$-phosphate group from ATP to the 5'-hydroxyl terminus of DNA, RNA, oligonucleotides or even nucleoside-3'-phosphate. Since naturally occuring nucleic acids have 5'-phosphoryl, not 5'-hydroxyl groups, the 5'-phosphoryl group must first be removed, e.g., with alkaline phosphatase. When [$\gamma^{32}$P]-ATP is used, the label is incorporated at the 5' end of the DNA or RNA strand. The enzyme is used for labeling 5'ends of DNA, e.g., for sequencing by the Maxam-Gilbert technique and for S1 nuclease mapping. The function of polynucleotide kinase in vivo is not known.

***Polynucleotide Ligase.*** Enzyme that catalyses phosphodiester bond formation between adjacent 3'-hydroxyl and 5'-phosphorus termini in nucleic acids.

***Polynucleotide Phosphorylase.*** Enzyme that catalyses the production of polymers of RNA from random ribonucleotides without reference to a template strand. It is used in the synthesis of synthetic polynucleotides such as polyuridic acid.

***Polyomaviruses.*** Members of the papova-viruses; small, double-stranded DNA viruses about 45 nm in diameter and capable of in vitro cell transformation and tumour induction. SV 40 is a polyoma-type virus.

***Polyphensim.*** Existence of several phenotypic types in a population not resulting from genetic difference in the individuals, but from different genetic expression due to dissimilar environmental experience by the individuals, or simply due to differences in developmental stage of the organism.

***Polyphyletic.*** Group of individuals which are classified together but include some members that are known to have a quite distinct ancestral origin from others.

***Polyploid.*** Descriptive of an individual organism that has more than two sets of chromosomes (i.e. it is more than diploid). Low-number polyploidy may be designated as triploidy, tetraploidy or even, say 23-ploidy.

***Polypide.*** The polyp-like individual of a colony of Ectoprocta or Entoprocta.

***Polyploidy.*** The condition in which the basic (haploid) number of chromosomes in an organism is multiplied by three, four, five, or more. If the haploid number is n, and the diploid 2n, a polyploid may be 3n (triploid), 4n (tetraploid), 5n (kpentaploid), and so on. Polyploidy occurs in both animals and plants but is more common in the later; it may arise naturally but can be induced by treating cells with colchicine or similar chemicals.

There are two types of polyploidy. Autopolyploidy occurs when the chromosome number of an otherwise normal organism becomes multiplied. It has been used commercially in breeding crop plants (including sugar beet, tomatoes, and tobacco plants) to produce a more vigorous or sturdy growth. The main disadvantage of these autopolyploids is that they are usually less fertile than diploids. Although animals are probably never entirely autopolyploid, many have some polyploid cells, produced by endomitosis.

Allolpolyploidy occurs when the chromosome number in a sterile hybrid becomes doubled. It results in the new organism increasing its fertility and becoming a new species that is fertile with polyploids like itself but infertile with its diploid parental species. Many species of flowering plants are thought to have originated by allopolyploidy and can be recognized by the fact that their chromosome number is the sum of those of the parents. For example the cross between Triticum (wheat) (2n = 42) and Secale (rye) (2n = 14) gave a sterile hybrid with 2n = 28. This then doubled its chromosome number to give a fertile allotetraploid, Triticale, with 2n = 56. Bread wheat itself is a hexaploid (6n) that has been produced in cultivation during the last 3000 years. Animals rarely, if ever, form new species by allopolyploidy.

***Polyprotein.*** Situation in which more than one distinct protein results from cleavage of a long polypeptide chain (e.g, vitellogenin).

***Polysaccharides.*** Carbohydrates formed by the polymerization of simpler monosaccharide subunits. Important polysaccharides include starch, glycogen and cellulose.

***Polysomy.*** The condition in which one or more chromosomes are represented more than twice in a nucleus, cell, or organism so that the diploid chromosome complement is 2n + x, where n is the haploid number.

***Polyspermy.*** Entry of two or more male gametes/spermatozoa into a single egg/ovum at fertilization. Normally only one male pronucleus will fuse with the female pronucleus, and those derived from further spermatozoa will simply be resorbed (as in very yolky meroblastic eggs), but in some forms, to prevent any risk of disturbance to development, blocks to polyspermy have evolved.

***Polytene Chromosome.*** Chromosome that has an increased number of chromatids, having arisen by many rounds of DNA replication without nuclear division or separation of the chromatids. Polytene chromosomes are found in some protozoan ciliates, in certain ovule cells of some angiosperms, and in various tissues of some dipteran flies. They are best known as experimental material in cytogenetics from the giant salivary gland cells of third instar larvae of Drosophila, and also from analogous tissues in Chironomus, Sciara, Rhyncosciara and Smittia, all dipteran flies. The novel feature of these giant chromosomes is that, since they have replicated many times but remain adjacent, the polytene structure consists of a flat, ribbon-like chromosome, the DNA of which is no longer than in non-polytene chromosomes, but in which the chromosome is giant in terms of width. The structure prevents the disappearance of the chromosome structure during interphase, so these are essentially interphase chromosomes and are transciprionally active. Polytene chromosomes have a characteristic banded appearance due to the condensed bands and un-

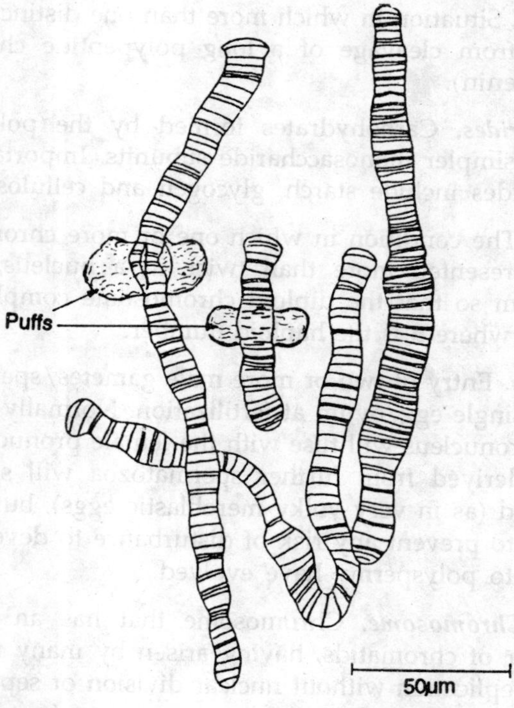


Figure P.9. Polytene chromosome. Chromosomes from the salivary gland of the fly Chironomus.

condensed interbands remaining in register across the breadth of the chromosome. The interbands are believed to represent housekeeping genes which are constantly transcribed into products required in all cells. The condensed bands are thought to represent tissue-specific genes, and, when transcriptionally active, they are evident as a conspicuous puff. Some very large puffs which can be discerned in Chironomus and other species are termed balbiani rings. Polytene chromosomes are also of considerable importance in genetics because inversions, deletions and translocations in the heterozygous condition are readily seen in the microscope as discontinuities of the flat chromosome ribbon. This is because both homologous chromosomes of the diploid set are lying together in register in the single chromosome ribbon. See Figure P.9.

***Polythetic.*** Designating a method of classification in which organisms belonging to any taxon must possess a large number of characteristics in common.

***Polytopic.*** Designating organisms of a taxonomic group that occur in more than one region.

***Polytopy.*** Phenomenon in which subspecies are distributed in two or more distinct and discontinuous geographical areas. The distribution of the hooded and carrion crows in the UK is an example of polytopic subspecies.

***Polytypic.*** Describing a species with a number of specialized races, such as the negroid and caucasian races in the human.

***Polyvalent.*** Synonym for multivalent.

***Polyvalent Antiserum.*** Synonym for multivalent antiserum.

***Polyvalent Vaccine.*** Vaccine composed of several antigens, such as various strains of poliovirus, or pneumococcal polysaccharides, or DPT (diphtheria, pertussis, tetanus).

***Population*** (in ecology). A group of individuals of the same type, particularly of the same species, within a community. Populations have certain characteristics not shown by individual organisms or the community as a whole, and the study of these can elucidate the ecology of the species and of the community. Characteristics of a population include density (size in relation to unit space), birth and death rates (natality and mortality, respectively), age distribution, sex ratio, dispersion (distribution of the individuals within the area), and growth rate.

***Pore Complex.*** The structure that makes up a nuclear pore in the eukaryotic nuclear envelope. There may be hundreds or thousands of nuclear pores per nucleus and they tend to be concentrated in patches on the envelope. The pores are not simply holes: each is largely filled by an annulus, fitting like a grommet in a pipe. Although some of the sieving effect of the pores may operate simply on particle or molecule size, other effects are similar to active transport and involve the expenditure of ATP.

***Progomy.*** Situation in some angiosperm plants in which the pollen tube enters the ovule through the micropyle.

***Porphyria.*** Disease characterized by abnormal porphyrin metabolism. The most frequent are the haematoporphyrias in which porphyrins occur widely in the tissues, are secreted in the urine and lead to marked facial pigmentation and sensitivity of the skin to sunlight.

***Porlphyrin.*** One of a group of pigments, widely distributed in living organisms, that are derived from porphin, a ring structure of four pyrrole nuclei linked by carbon atoms. The most comon porphyrin is protoporphyrin IX. The nitrogen atoms of porphyrins are often coordinated to metal ions (e.g. iron, magnesium) to form chelates, of which haem (protoporphyrin combined with FeII) is the most important. See Figure P.10 on next page.

***Portable Genetic Element.*** DNA element that has no vegetative form of existence and can only replicate in covalent association with its host chromosome.

***Positional Information.*** Hypotheses relating to mechanisms of pattern formation; synonomous with the name of Lewis Wolpert, a British developmental biologist. Derived, in part, from earlier gradient theories, which attempted to

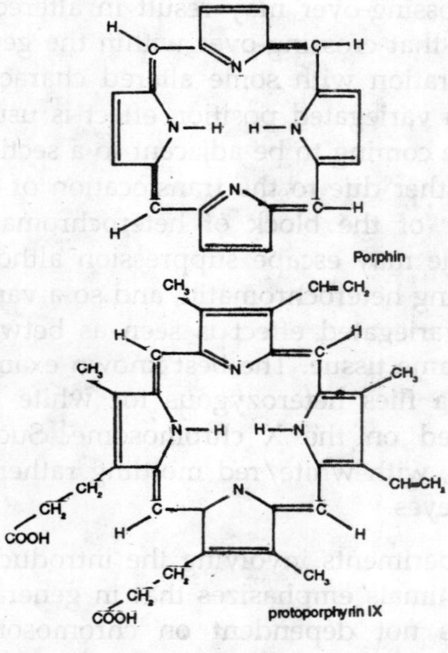


Figure P.10. Porphyrin.

explain how a cell's fate could be specified according to its position in the embryo. It is proposed that within a morphogenetic field, there is positional information generated across that field. Also cells can, and do, detect local positional information in their microenvironment, and respond by assuming a positional value which, because of their individually unique lineage position/developmental history will determine their subsequent differentiative and morphogenetic activity. Positional information can apparently be spatial (e.g., a diffusible morphogen) or temporal (e.g., putative mitotic clocks'). Corroboration at the cellular and molecular level of such theoretical hypotheses is still awaited.

***Position Effect.*** Any change in the phenotypic expression of a gene that follows from a change in its chromosomal position or of other adjacent gene sequences that normally lie beside it. Two distinct kinds of position effects are known — stable and variegated — the former also known as cis/transposition effects. In the former stable position effect, intragenic crossing-over may result in altered expression, so indicating that crossing-over within the gene leads to a trans-configuration with some altered characteristics. The better known variegated position effect is usually a result of a sequence coming to be adjacent to a section of heterochromatin, either due to the translocation of the sequence concerned or of the block of heterochromatin. In some cells, the gene may escape suppression although close to the suppressing heterochromatin, and so a variable or phenotypically variegated effect is seen as between different cells in the same tissue. The best known example is found in Drosophila flies heterozygous for white gene for eye colour, carried on the X chromosome. Such flies have mottled eyes, with white/red mottling rather than all red or all white eyes.

Recent experiments involving the introduction of novel genes into animals emphasizes that in general phenotypic expression is not dependent on chromosomal position, since such sequences integrate randomly and yet are most frequently correctly expressed.

***Positive Control.*** Mechanism of gene regulation in which a gene sequence must interact with a regulatory protein before transcription can occur.

***Positive Interference.*** Phenomenon observed when the occurrence of one chromosomal crossing-over between homologous chromosomes at meiosis reduced the likelihood of another crossing-over occuring in the vicinity on either side of the chromosomal position of the first crossing-over.

***Positive Supercoiling.*** Supercoiling of a DNA duplex in the same direction as the double helix itself is wound. Thus the normal B form of DNA is a right-handed double helix, and its further positive supercoiling will be right-handed.

***Postcardiotomy Syndrome.*** Fever, chest pain and pericardial effusion occurring days to weeks after cardiac surgery or any traumatic injury to the heart. Patients have autoantibodies to antigens of the heart, detectable by immunofluorescence. The symptoms respond rapidly to corticosteroid therapy. A similar syndrome has been observed in patients who have had myocardial infarctions.

***Postmeiotic Fusion.*** Fusion of two identical haploid nuclei in eggs produced by parthenogenesis. Mitotic division of the egg nucleus provides twin haploid nuclei, and if these are induced to fuse, diploidy is restored and the egg may develop normally.

***Postmeiotic Segregation.*** Segregation of genes after meiosis due to the presence of a mismatched heteroduplex of DNA in a postmeiotic chromosme. This segregation can be detected in organism such as Neurospora as an unexpected pattern of segregation of spores in the ascus.

***Post-transcriptional.*** Describing any cellular event that occurs after transcription of RNA from a DNA template. Most frequently the term is applied to nuclear events such as the modification of RNA by tailing and capping which occur prior to translation.

***Post-Translational.*** Describing any cellular event that occurs in the process of protein synthesis after translation of the messenger RNA into a polypeptide chain. These events are usually cytoplasmic and include protein modifications (e.g., cleavage of vitellogenin into its constituent subunits) or differential rates of protein degradation.

***Poxviruses.*** Group of double-stranded DNA viruses with enveloped capsids. They include those viruses causing smallpox, cowpox and myxomatosis.

***PP60 v-src.*** Protein encoded by the Rous sacroma virus oncogene v-src. The prefix pp indicates that it is a phosphoprotein. Its activity is that of a protein kinase, phosphorylating the tyrosine subunits of some cellular proteins.

***PPM.*** Parts per million.

***PPT.*** Precipitate.

***Prader-Willis Syndrome.*** Chromosomally based congenital disorder of humans resulting from a small deletion in the long arm of chromosome 15 (in order 50 percent of affected individuals only). Sufferers are mentally retarded, with small hands and feet, some narrowing of the head and a tendency for obesity to develop.

***Prausnitz-Kustner Reaction.*** Skin test in humans for immediate hypersensitivity to a particular allergen. Test serum is injected intracutaneously into a normal recipient who is challenged 24-48 hours later with a putative allergen. A positive reaction is indicated by a wheal and flare reaction at the injection site within 20 minutes. The positive reaction results from the transfer of antibody. This reaction, which is named after the two physicians who were donor and recipient in the original test, is now only of historic interest.

***Pre-B Cell.*** Earliest cell in the B lymphocyte lineage. Pre-B cells are identified by the presence of immunoglobulin mu chains in the cytoplasm and by the absence of surface immunoglobulin. Pre-B cells are present in the bone marrow of adults and in the liver of the fetus at 10 weeks of gestation. Pre-B cells are found in normal numbers in the bone marrow of males with X-linked agammaglobulinemia, but B lymphocytes do not develop. Studies of immunoglobulin genes show that the heavy chain, V, D and J gene segments have become contiguous in pre-B cells. However the light chain genes segments are not rearranged.

***Preadaptation.*** Acquisition of a function or character by an organism as a result of random mutation that proves beneficial to the organism following a subsequent environemental changes.

***Pre-Cambrian.*** The unit of geological time that preceded the Cambrian period, i.e. the time before 600 million years ago. Pre-Cambrian rocks contain no definite (i.e. structural) fossils, but some structures found in these rocks may be the remains of the precursors or products of organisms. In some Pre-Cambrian limestone rocks of Australia, Siberia, and parts of the USA there are structures known as stromatolittes, which may have been formed by blue-green algae. Frond- and disclike impressions of a supposed plant (Charnia) have also been found. Amino acids have been idenfied from Pre-Cambrian rocks dated at 1700 million years old.

***Precipitin.*** An antibody that combines specifically with and precipitates soluble antigen. This activity is utilized in the precipitin reaction, which detects and identifies antigens.

***Precipitin.*** Antibody that forms precipitates with the appropriate antigen. At one time, it was though that the ability to form precipitates was the property of a particular type of antibody, but it is now known that most antibodies are capable of precipitating with antigen.

***Performation.*** The theory that a whole miniature adult organism (homunculus) exists inside an egg or sperm and that development consists merely of thee expansion of this miniature. Some 17th-centuary theorists considered that the homunculus existed inside the egg (ovist theory) and that the sperm merely triggered development; others that it was found inside the sperm (spermatist (spermist) theory) and that the egg was merely an aid to development. The theories of preformation culminated in the box theory, which stated that the egg or sperm of the homunculus must contain the homunculus for the next generatioln, and so on for all succeeding generations.

***Precipitin.*** Antibody that combines with a soluble antigen and in so doing, forms a precipitate. The precipitin reaction is frequently used to identify a specific antibody or antigen.

***Precipitin Curve.*** Plot of results of a set of recepitin reactions in which increasing amounts of antigen are added to a constant amount of a mixture of antibodies (antiserum). The total amount of precipitate or the amount of antibody precipitated is plotted against the amount of antigen added. The curve is divided into three zones; antibody excess, equivalence and antigen excess, according to the presence or absence of detectable antibody or antigen in the supernatant. See Figure P.11 on next page.

***Precipitin Reaction.*** Reaction in which antibodies combine with soluble antigen to form a precipitate.

***Preformation.*** Theory that an entire miniatture adult organism -homunculus- exists inside an egg or sperm add that development consists of an increase in the size of this miniature adult, rather than a progressive and radical change in its form. The theory was widely held in the 17th century, but has now been replaced by the concept of epigenesis.

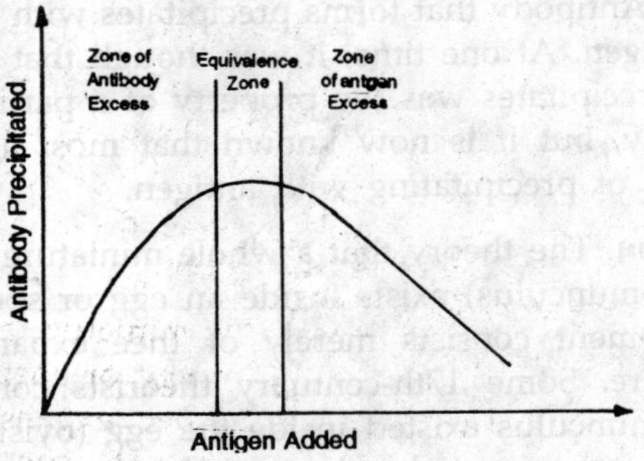


Figure P.11. Precipitin curve.

***Premature Chromatin Condensation.*** Condensation of some or all chromosomes in an interphase nbucleus following its introduction by artificial cell fusion into another cell in which the nucleus is entering mitosis. Signals are exchanged between nucleus and cytoplasm in such heterokaryons so that chromosome condensation is initiated earlier than usual in the interphase nucleus.

***Prenatal Diagnosis.*** Assessment of disease or normality in the human foetus. This is often accomplished by analysis of the amniotic fluid surrounding the foetus, but can involve use of ultrasound and analysis of the mother's blood.

***Prepupal Period.*** Beginning of pupation when an insect larva is proceeding through metamorphosis, but prior to the emergence of appendages with imaginal disc primordia.

***Preribosomal RNA.*** Primary product of the genes coding for ribosomal RNA is most organisms, prior to its cleavage to yield the 18S, 28S and 5.8S rRNAs utilized in the ribosomnes. The precursor varies between 38S and 45S in different organisms and has some parts of its sequence cleaved out and discarded during processing. These are the spacer sequences.

***Presumptive.*** Indicating the normal fate of a defined tissue or localized group of cells in an embryo. For example, 'presumptive mesoderm' indicates that, in the course of normal development, those cells will become mesoderm. Applied later in development, it is possible to descripe groups of cells as 'presumptive optic cup' or 'presumptive forebrain'.

***Presynaptic Membrane.*** Specialized region of the membrane of a nerve cell at the synapse. A nerve impulse in conducted along the axon as an action potential and is relayed between nerve cells at a synapse by a neurotransmitter (e.g., acetylcholine) released by the presynaptic nerve. The transmitter diffuses across the small synaptic cleft between the two cells before binding to receptors on the postsynaptic membrane, initiating an action potential in the postsynaptic nerve. The presynaptic membrane is adapted for the secretion of the neurotransmitter, which is stored in small intracellular vesicles, with a proportion of these synaptic vesicles being attached to the inside of the presynaptic membrane.

***Pribnow Box.*** Semiconserved sequence of nucleotides rich in A-T base pairs found in the promoter regions of prokaryotic genes. The concensus sequence of the Pribnow box (i.e. the average of many different genes), which is one of two main parts of the promoter responsible for RNA polymerase binding, is TATAAT. The Pribnow box is centred about 10 base pairs upstream of the point at which RNA synthesis begins and is important in directing the specificity of this process.

***Prickle Cells.*** Flattened cells that form a layer between the outer keratinized cells and the innermost basal layer of the mammalian epidermis. The name derives from the thick tufts of keratin filaments inserted in the numerous spot desmosomes of each cell.

***Primary Billiary Cirrhosis.*** Chronic disease of the liver, characterized by progressive destruction of intrahepatic bile ducts. The disease is seen predominantly in middle-aged women. Almost all patients (more than 90 percent) have antibodies to mitochondrial membrane antigens, as well as circulating IgM-containing immune complexes. The relationship of the immunological abnormalities to the pathogenesis of the disease is unclear.

***Primary Culture.*** Culture of cells that are directly derived from cells or tissues taken from an organism without intermediate culture. The cells or tissue from which a primary culture is derived is termed an explant. Non-primary cultures are either described as an established cell line or as passaged cells.

***Primary Granule.*** Cytoplasmic organelle (0.8 μm in diameter) of polymorphonuclear leukocytes that stains blue (azurophilic) with Wright or Giemsa stains. Primary granules contain myeloperoxidase, collagenase and elastase. They constitute 10-20 percent of the cytoplasmic granules of polymorphonuclear leukocytes.

***Primary Immune Response.*** Immune response that takes place following the first encounter with antigen. The rate of development and magnitude of this response depends upon the immunogenicity of the antigen; it is usually slower and of smaller magnitude than the secondary immune response to the same antigen. In the primary response there is usually a lag period of several days between introduction of the antigen and the appearance of antibody or specific T lymphocytes in blood; the serum antibody is of low titer and usually of low affinity with a relative predominance of IgM. In contrast, the secondary antibody response has a short latent period and consists mostly of IgG antibodies. The distinction between primary and secondary immune response may be less apparent when highly immunogenic antigens, such as bacteria, viruses and particulate antigens, are used or after immunization with adjuvant.

***Primary Immunodeficiency.*** Any failure or compromise of specific immunity caused by an intrinsic defect in B and/or T lymphocytes.

Primary immunodeficiency diseases

A. *Predominantly antibody defects*

1. X-linked agammaglobulinemia
2. X-linked hypogammaglobulinemia with growth hormone deficiency
3. Austosomal recessive agammaglobulinemia
4. Immunoglobulin deficiency with increased IgM (and IgD)
5. IgA deficiency
6. Selective deficiency of other immunoglobulin isotypes.
7. Kappa chain deficiency
8. Immunodeficiency with thymoma
9. Transient hypogammaglobulinemia of infancy

B. *Combined immunodeficiency*

10. Common variable immunodeficiency
    a. Predominant antibody deficiency
    b. Predominant cell-mediated immunity defect
11. Severe combined immunodeficiency
12. Reticular dysgenesis
13. Adenosine deaminase deficiency
14. Purine nucleoside phosphorylase deficiency
15. MHC class I deficiency ('bare lymphocyte syndrome')
16. MHC class II deficiency

C. *Immunodeficiency associated with other major defects*

17. Wiskott-Aldrich syndrome
18. Ataxia-telangiectasia
19. Third and fourth pouch syndrome (DIGeorge's syndrome)
20. Transcobalamin 2 deficiency

21. Immunodeficiency with partial albinism
22. Immunodeficiency following hereditary defective response to Epstein-Barr virus

This classification is modified from the WHO Committee on Immunodeficiency Diseases.

***Primary Interaction.*** Binding of antigen and antibody. Primary interaction does not refer to subsequent events such as precipitation or complement fixation. It can be measurred by tests such as equilibrium dialysis, fluorescence quenching and various radioimmunoassays.

***Primary Lymphoid Organ.*** Lamphoid organ where T or B lymphocytes mature. In primary lymphoid organs, stem cells mature in the absence of antigenic stimulation. The thymus is the primary lymphoid organ for T lymphocytes in all vertebrate species. The bursa of fabricius is the primary lymphoid organ for B lymphocytes in birds. In adult mammals, the primary lymphoid organ for B lymphocytes is the bone marrow.

***Primary non-disjunction.*** Non-disjunction in diploid organisms involving the sex chromosomes. For example, in the homogametic sex, the gametes would carry two X chromosomes or none, with progeny being XXY or YO.

***Primary Oocyte.*** Stage in vertebrate egg production in which oogonial cells in the ovary differentiate to yield primary oocytes. During the first meiotic division the primary oocyte divides to yield two secondary oocytes, one of which is the first polar body.

***Primary Pit Field.*** Area of the primary wall of plant cells where the wall thickness is substantially reduced and often where numbers of plasmodesmata penetrate the wall. In those cells that develop a secondary wall with pits these are often, but not always, positioned over the primary pit fields.

***Primary Ray*** (medullary ray). Parenchymatous tissue extending radially out from the pith between the vascular bundles of the primary tissues of the stem.

***Primary Sexual Characters.*** Reproductive organs, ovaries and testes.

***Primary Structure.*** That aspect of the structure of a protein or polynucleotide that depends on covalent bonding, i.e. the linear sequence of amino acids in a polypeptide chain and any covalent bridging within it or of nucleotides in a single strand of DNA or RNA.

***Primary Structure.*** Linear amino acid sequence of a polypeptide or protein.

***Primary Transcript.*** Initial form of RNA as it is transcribed from DNA, commonly containing both introns and exons, but lacking such modifications as cap and tail which may be added after initial synthesis.

***Primary Wall.*** Initial cell wall laid down by plant cells, and, in some cells such as those of the leaf mesophyll, it is the only wall.

***Primase.*** Bacterial polymerase probably also found in eukaryotes that makes the precursor primer RNA molecule on the lagging strand during DNA replication. In E.coli. it is a protein ($M_r$=60,000) and, unlike RNA polymerase, is not inhibited by rifampicin.

***Primates.*** An order of the Eutheria containing basically arboreal mammals characterized by a very highly developed brain, quick reactions, and binocular vision (the eyes face forward and are separated from the temporal fossa by a bony plate or ring). The skeleton is unspecialized; the thumb and usually the big toe are opposable for grasping and the digits have sensory pads and nails replacing claws. Only a few young are produced at one birth, and these undergo a long period of growth and development, allowing learning. The most primitive group is the Prosimii (Lemuroidea), e.g. Galago (bushbaby) and Lemur (lemurs). The Anthropoidea contains the New World monkeys, e.g. Alouatta (howler), which have prehensile tails, and the Old World Monkeys, e.g. Macaca (rhesus monkey, Barbary ape), which never have a prehensile tail. The Hominoidea includes the great apes, e.g. Pongo (orang-utan), and man and his precursors; tailless primates with brachiating arms.

***Primed.*** Preconditioned or presensitized, as of lymphocytes primed by antigen to produce antibody.

***Primed Lymphocyte.*** Lymphocyte from an immunized individual or lymphocyte that has been exposed to antigen in vitro.

***Primer DNA.*** Single-stranded molecule of DNA, usually of short sequence, required by DNA polymerase III for the further replication of DNA.

***Primer RNA.*** Short RNA sequence of about 10 nucleotides that is synthesized by a primase on the lagging strand during DNA replication. These short lengths of RNA are then extended by DNA polymerase to yield the okazaki fragments, from which the primer RNA molecules are then erased and the pieces 'sitched' together by DNA ligase to yield a continuous new DNA strand.

***Primitive Streak.*** In birds and mammals, a relatively broad, longitudinal band of mesodermal cells in the embryo that develops in a dorsal trough along the length of the gastrula. Cells build up in the primitve streak before migrating downward through the streak and spreading in an anterolateral direction to form a seprate sheet of mesoderm betwen the hypoblast and the surface layer.

***Primordial Germ Cells.*** Cells that are singled out in early development as progenitors of gametes. These cells migrate to the developing gonads, and, after a period of mitotic proliferation, undergo meiosis and differentiate into mature eggs or sperm.

***Primordium.*** Group of cells that functions as the mitotic progenitor of an organ or tissue in later development.

***Primosome.*** Protein complex that is involved in the primary action to produce the okazaki fragments of DNA on the lagging strand during DNA replication. The complex includes a primase that synthesizes that primer RNA.

***Prion.*** Protein believed to be the infectious agent for scrapie, a transmissable disease of the nervous system of sheep and goats. There is no evidence that the scrapie agent possesses nucleic acid, and therefore it cannot be a virus or a viroid.

***Private Idiotypic Determinant*** (IDI). Idiotypic determinant that is unique to an antibody produced by a single individual. Typically, private idiotypic determinants reflect unique amino acid sequences in the hyper-variable regions of antibody heavy and/or light chains.

***Private Specificity.*** Antigenic determinant that is unique to one member of a family of proteins (e.g., a group of alloantigens). The term is often used to refer to determinants on molecules in the major histo-compatibility complex (e.g., a determinant associated with a single H-2 allele (H-2K or H-2D).

***Privileged Site.*** Tissue where allografts are protected from rejection (e.g., the anterior chamber of the eye or the brain) perhaps because of poor lymphatic drainage. The slow diffusion of antigen from privileged sites to lymphoid organs appear to retard graft rejection.

***Proband Method.*** Technique in human genetics in which the propositus of the genetic trait is used as a basis for determinating gene frequency rather than an affected child. Such a method avoids bias towards affecting siblings in such computation.

***Probe DNA.*** A DNA molecule radioactively labelled (most frequently with $^{32}P$) and used to detect nucleic acid molecules of complementary sequence by molecular hybridization. Autoradiography is often used to reveal the presence of the probe DNA and thus to localize the complementary hybridizing sequences.

***Pro-C3.*** Single-chain polypeptide that is cleaved into the alpha and beta chains of C3. The beta chain is amino-terminal.

***Pro-C4.*** Single-chain polypeptide that is cleaved into the alpha, beta and gamma chains of C4. The beta chain is amino terminal, the gamma chain is carboxy-terminal.

***Pro-C5.*** Single-chain polypeptide that is cleaved into the alpha and beta chains of C5. The beta chain is amino-terminal.

***Procambium*** (provascular tissue). Plant tissue from which the primary vascular tissues differentiate. It develops from derivatives of the apical meristem and consists of highly meristematic and densely cytoplasmic cells elongated· in the longitudinal plane of the axis.

***Processed Gene.*** Pseudogene in the eukaryotic genome that lacks introns, but contains a poly A sequence at its 3'-end. These characteristics suggest that such genes are derived from reversed copying of a processed mRNA molecule, perhaps involving a reverse transcriptase. Commonly such genes also contain numerous stop condons which prevent their effective transcription.

***Processing.*** (1) Modication of RNA following initial transcription, including capping, tailing, intron excision and exon splicing. (2) modification of antigen by macrophages to a form such that the antigen appears in the macrophage surface membrane and is then stimulatory to the appropriate lymphocytes.

***Processive Enzyme.*** Enzyme that continues to act on a substrate even during repetitious catalytic events and release of poroduct.

***Prochloron.*** Member of the group of Prochlorophyta, a group of prokaryotic organisms, found living commensally with ascidians (squirts), which possess chlorophylls a and b and thus have some affinity with eukaryotic algae and may represent an ancestral relative of these organisms.

***Procollagen.*** Large precursor of collagen, found associated with endoplasmic reticulum in collagen-making cells. These molecules later have terminal extension peptides trimmed away to provide collagen.

***Productive Infection.*** Infection of cells by virus such that progeny virus are produced via vegetative growth and/or a lytic cycle.

***Proembryo.*** Developmental step that follows from fertilkization prior to the formation of a discrete embryo. In animals, it includes the blastula and gastrula stage. In some eggs, such as those of mammals, there is a discrete group of cells within the developing eggs that will form the embryo proper, namely the inner cell mass. Similarly discrete proembryo cells can be found in early development of many plants.

***Proenzyme.*** Molecule that is the inactive precursor molecule for an enzyme.

***Profilin.*** Protein ($M_r$=16,000) that binds to unpolymerized actin, thereby retarding polymerization. It is though to modulate the availability of free actin in cells and is particularly abundant in sperm and blood platelets.

***Proflavine.*** Acridine dye that is a powerful mutagen by dint of initiating the insertion of reading frame shifts. It is particularly effective as a mutagen for mitochondrial DNA and thus freely induces the petite mutation in yeast cells. Sometimes proflavine is used as a topical antibiotic.

***Progeny.*** Siblings; offspring of a given mating or members of the same biological family and having the same father and mother.

***Progeny Testing.*** Study of progeny under controlled conditions, both in terms of phenotype and genotype, as a means of evaluating the genotype of an individual parent.

***Progeria*** (Hutchinson-Gilform syndrome). Hereditary disease in humans characterized by signs of premature ageing and often resulting in the death before the age of 20. There is evidence from studies on cells from affected individuals established in tissue culture that DNA repair is less efficient, and there is a reduced number of expected mitoses in the replicative life span of the cell.

***Progesterone.*** A steroid hormone produced chiefly by the corpus luteum of the mammalian ovary but also by the testis, adrenal cortex, and placenta. Its most important role in the female is to prepare the reproductive organs for pregnancy and to maintain the uterus throughout gestation, but progesterone is also an intermediate in the biosynthesis of all steriod hormones. It was first isolated from pig ovaries in 1934. See Figure P.12.

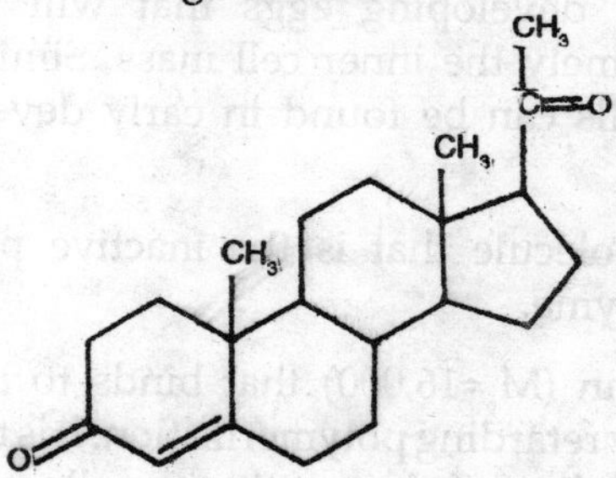


Figure P.12. Progesterone.

***Progestogen.*** Any of a group of substances that show progesterone-like effects on the female mammalian reproductive organs.

***Programmed Cell Death.*** Theory that proposes that as cells differentiate they become programmed to die after a fixed number of divisions. For example, mammalian fibroblasts, grown in culture, will divide between 20 and 50 times (depending on the age of the source of animal). Later division cycles take longer until the divisions cease and the cell population dies. Neoplastic cells (e.g., HeLa cells) will go on dividing indefinitely.

***Progressive Systemic Sclerosis.*** Synonym for systemic sclerosis.

***Progressive Vaccinia.*** Relentless progression of a smallpox vaccination lesion, spreading from the intial site of vaccination, and resulting in death. This complication of smallpox vaccination occurs in children who have primary immunodeficiency of cell-mediated immunity (e.g., severe combined immunodeficiency).

***Prohormone.*** A large precursor protein from which polypeptide hormones are produced by enzymic cleavage. The first to be established was proinsulin in 1967.

***Proinsulin.*** Prohormone of the hormone insulin. It is synthesized in the beta-cells of the islets of Langerhans and consists of a polypeptide chain of about 80 amino acids. The central section of 30 amino acids is cleaved out by specific proteolytic action, leaving the two terminal peptides which, by association, form the active insulin molecule.

***Prokaryote (Procaryote).*** An organism whose genetic material is not contained within a true nucleus but lies free in a special region of the cytoplasm called the nucleoid. Prokaryotic organisms comprise mainly the bacteria and blue-green algae.

***Prolactin (Lactogenic Hormone, luteotrop(h)ic hormone,LTH).*** A protein hormone secreted by the pars distalis of the pituitary gland in mammals and by corresponding tissue in all other vertebrates. In mammals it stimulates and maintains lactation and (in some) the secretion of progesterone from the corpus luteum. In birds it promotes secretion of 'milk' from the crop glands - an ability utilized in bioassays of the hormone before the more sensitive radioimmunoassays were available. The association of the pituitary with lactation was first demonstrated in 1928; prolactin was isolated in 1937 and its structure determined in 1969. It consists of a single chain of 198 amino acid residues with three disulphide linkages and is structurally similar to growth hormone. In lower vertebrates prolactin shows a wide range of effects on activities such as osmoregulation, reproduction, growth, catabolism, and associated behaviour responses and its functional adaptability may have contributed to the diversification of the vertebrates.

***Prolamine.*** One of a group of simple plant proteins that are soluble only in aqueous alcohol. The group includes gliadin, a constituent of gluten.

***Proline*** (pro). One of the 20 common amino acids and one with a non-polar side-chain. It is a cyclic molecule and gives rise to a bend in a polypeptide chain where it occurs. See Figure P.13.

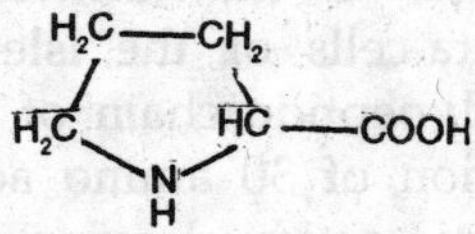

Figure P.13. Proline.

*Prometaphase.* Early part of the metaphase during which alignment of the chromosomes on the metaphase plate occurs.

*Promiscuous DNA.* Segment of DNA integrated in the nuclear genome for which there is clear evidence of an earlier mitochondrial or chloroplast location.

*Promitochondrion* (protomitochondrion). Mitochondrion with incomplete cristae found in petite mutants of yeast.

*Promoter.* Region on a DNA molecule upstream from the coding sequence: area to which the RNA polymerase initially binds prior to the initiation of transcription. The nucleotide sequence of the promoter, or at least part of it, determines the nature of the polymerase that associates with it. This is significant since a range of different RNA polymerases occur in eukaryotic cells. Some genes have internal promoter sequence for example the small ribosomal RNA gene coding for 5S RNA. Certain consensus sequences within the promoter region seem to be particularly important in the binding of RNA polymerase, and these are known as CAT and TATA boxes. The promoter region extends from some 40 nucleotides to about five nucleotides upstream from the start of the gene-coding region, the CAT and TATA boxes being located within the promoter region as short six or seven nucleotide sequence.

*Promoter.* Region of DNA that plays an essential role in the initiation of transcription of a gene. In bacteria, it is the DNA segment(s) to which RNA polymerase binds when transcription is initiated. Two hexamer sequences, centered at about 10 and 35 nucleotides upstream (5') from the origin of transcription, appear to be particularly important. The sequence at -10 is called the 'Pribnowl box' and its consensus sequence is TATAAT; the sequence at -35 has the consensus sequence TTGACA. Strong promoters (high levels of transcription) generally match the consensus sequence more closely than do weak promoters. Sequences further upstream may also influence promoter efficiency.

Initiation of transcription by the RNA polymerase of eukaryotes is considerably more complex than it is in the case of prokaryotes. For transcription by RNA polymerase II, there are important sequences in the region just 5' to the transcriptional start site. The most conserved of these is the 'TATA' box, a conserved AT-rich segment centered about 25 base pairs upstream from the start site and usually flanked by G/C-rich sequences. Additional promoter elements may lie further upstream, e.g., a consensus sequence containing the nucleotides CAAT about 70 bases from the start site; there may also be more distant upstream sites. Genes transcribed by RNA polymerase III contain internal promoters downstream (~50-100 nucleotides 3') from the transcriptional start site. For transcription by RNA polymerase I, a number of sequences surrounding the start site appear to be important. In addition to the RNA polymerases, a variety of 'transcription factors' (proteins that regulate transcription by interacting with specific promoter elements or that bind directly to polymerases) are required. Such factors may confer species, stage and tissue specificity on the promoter.

Transcription of immunoglobulin genes depends on a 'TATA' box and also requires a promoter element, the octamer ATTTGCAT, which is 70 $\pm$ 10 nucleotides upstream from the start site of K and $\lambda$ transcription; the complement (ATG-CAAAT) is found at the same location with respect to heavy chain genes. This octamer element is also found in other promoters. There are at least two proteins that bind to the octamer sequence, one of which is found only in lymphoid cells and probably confers tissue specificity. This octamer is also found in the heavy chain enhancer.

*Pronase.* Protease extracted from Streptomyces, that is relatively specific for mucoproteins.

***Pronephros.*** The first (anterior) part of the kidney to appear in the embryonic development of vertebrates. It is functional in larval fishes and amphibians but in amniotes it is transient and never functional. It is drained by the Wolffian duct.

***Pronucleus.*** Nucleus of an egg, sperm or pollen tube. Such nuclei are haploid and are derived by meiotic divisions from the original diploid nuclei of the pregametic cells. Fertilization results from fusion of the male and female pronuclei. The pollen tube contains two pronuclei, both being involved in the double fertilization event characteristic of many plants.

***Proof-reading.*** Mechanisms involved in correcting errors during nucleic acid replication, transcription or translation. Proof-reading during DNA replication is a function of the activity of a DNA polymerase, often termed a proof-reading of editing enzyme.

***Properdin (P).*** Protein of the alternative pathway of complement. Properdin binds to the alternative pathway C3 convertase (C3bBb) and stabilizes it. C3 nephritic factor has similar activity.

Properdin is composed of a single polypeptide chain of 441 amino acid residues. There are two sites for attachment of N-linked oligosaccharides (asparagines at positions 370 and 400). By electron microscopy, properdin is seen to form cyclic oligomers. (mainly dimers, trimers and tetramers) by interaction between the 30-40 amino acid residues at the amino- and carboxy-termini. Properdin contains six repeating motifs of approximately 60 amino acid residues (between positions 53 and 413). In these motifs, 11 of the positions are always occupied by the same amino acid residues: cysteine at positions 10, 14, 17, 48 and 54, tryptophan at 7, serine at 8 and 11, valine at 12, threonine at 13 and arginine at 23. The repeating motif is homologous to 60 amino acids at the amino- and carboxy terminal ends of C7, C8α and C8β and the amino terminal end of C9. This 60 residue motif is also found in three repeats in each chain of the homotrimer, thrombospondin, which binds fibrinogen, plasminogen, fibronectin and other matrix molecules. It is also found in a circumsporozoite protein of several species of malaria and is thought to facilitate entry of circumsporozoites into hepatocytes.

Properdin was the first protein described in the alternative pathway of complement, which was formerly called the properdin system.

***Properdin Deficiency.*** Rare genetic deficiency inherited as an X-linked recessive. Affected males have less than 2 percent of the normal amount of properdin in serum and they are susceptible to neisserial infections. In one kindred, a mutant form of properdin has been found in serum of affected males. Heterozygous females have half-normal to normal amounts of properdin in serum and may also be susceptible to neisserial infections.

***Prophage.*** Integrated form of a bacteriophage in a lysogenic bacterium, carrying all the genetic information necessary for phage production, but unless specifically induced (e.g., by ultraviolet irradiation) remains quiescent within the bacterial genome. It is constantly replicated as part of it.

***Prophage-mediated Conversion.*** Acquisition by a bacterium of new genetic properties following its infection by a lysogenic bacteriophage.

***Prophase.*** First stage of mitosis and meiosis. The chromosomes become evident but are not aligned on the spindle. Indeed the spindle has not yet fully formed, but is evident as an extra nuclear series of microtubules joining the two centrioles. Meiotic prophase is subdivided into different stages; leptotene, zygotene, pachytene, diplotene and diakinesis.

***Proplastid.*** Small body found in meristematic plant cells that constitute a form of plastid in an early stage of development.

***Prophylactic Immunization.*** Protection against infections usually by active immunization and sometimes by passive immunization.

***Propositus.*** Family member who is clinically affected with an inherited trait and through whom the pedigree of interest is first traced.

***Prosenchyma.*** Plant tissue composed of more or less elongatged cells with tapering ends. The term is also used for a form of plectenchyma in which the loosely packed tissue is composed of long fused hyphae.

***Prostaglandin.*** One of a group of chemically related hormone-like substances that are formed from essential fatty acids and occur in most mammalian tissues, particularly in human seminal fluid. They were first discovered in human semen in the early 1930s and many varieties, including prostaglandin $E_1$ ($PGE_1$), have now been isolated. Prostaglandins have a wide spectrum of pharmacological activity but are best known for their potent effects on smooth muscle, particularly in stimulating contraction and relaxation of the human uterus. Their main therapeutic use has been to induce abortion and labour in women. By their vasodilatation (or vasoconstriction) of blood vessels, they can regulate blood flow and have been shown to assist hormone secretion by increasing the blood flow through endocrine glands. Prostaglandins have also been implicated in various hormone effects because of their ability to modify cyclic AMP levels. They are known to be released during the inflammatory response of damaged tissue, and the analgesic effects of aspirin are thought to be due to an inhibition of prostaglandin synthesis.

***Prostaglandin (PG).*** Molecule derived from arachidonic acid by the action of an enzyme called cyclooxygenase. $PGD_2$ is released from mast cells following IgE-meditated reactions; it causes dialation of small blood vessels and constriction of bronchi and blood vessels in the lung. $PGE_2$ is released from mononuclear phagocytes following binding of antigen-antibody complexed to Fcγ receptors. $PGE_2$ inhibits expression of class II histocompatibility molecules in macrophages and T lymphocytes and also inhibits the growth of T lymphocytes.

$PGD_2$ and $PGE_2$ (as well as $PGI_2$ or prostacylin released from endothelial cells) inhibit platelet aggregation and thus antagonize the action of thromboxane $A_2$, the principal PG metabolite released from platelets.

Aspirin and indomethacin, two potent anti-inflammatory drugs, inhibit PG synthesis. Prostaglandins were so named becuase they were first found as a substance(s) in seminal fluid that contracts uterus and were thought to come from the prostate gland.

***Prosthetic Group.*** Part of an enzyme that does not form part of the polypeptide chain. The prosthetic group is at the active site of the enzyme and is changed during the course of the reaction. Prosthetic groups are tightly bound to the enzyme (sometimes covalently to form the holoenzyme). They differ from coenzymes in that regeneration of the prosethetic group occurs in situ; it does not need to dissociate from the enzyme for regeneration. Examples of posthetic groups include FAD (in flavoproteins), thiamine pyrophosphate (in decarboxylases), biotin (in carboxylases) and pyridoxal phosphate (in amino acid aminotransferases). The part of the enzyme without the prosthetic group is the apoenzyme.

***Protamines.*** Small basic proteins found associated with the chromatin of sperm. Although they replace histones in sperm, they are not known to adopt a nucleosome-like configuration. Some such as salmine, found in salmon sperm, are named invidually.

***Proteases.*** Enzymes that degrade protein.

***Protein A (SpA).*** Constituent of the cell wall of many strains of Staphylococcus aureus that binds to some immunoglobulins. Protein A has been used extensively as a reagent for identifying and isolating immunoglobulins and antigen-antibody complexes (e.g., immunoblotting). Protein A has also been used to remove antibodies and immune complexes from serum of patients by extracoporeal filtration. The usual source for protein A is the Cowan I strain of S.aureus.

Protein A binds to the Fc region of human IgG subclasses (except IgG3), to mouse IgG subclasses, and to IgG of many other mammalian species; the strength of the interaction varies according to the immunoglobulin. Other classes of immunoglobulin (e.g., IgM, IgA) may also bind protein A, but these so-called alternative interactions appear to be mediated by the Fab region, and are weaker. Protein A can be used in soluble form or it can be coupled to insoluble matrices (e.g., agarose); whole staphylococci (usually heat-killed and formalin-fixed) with protein A on their surfaces can also conveniently be used for immunoprecipitation.

Protein A is covalently linked to peptidoglycans in the bacterial cell wall. The gene encoding a precursor protein has been sequenced from strain 8325-4. The corresponding protein consists of 524 amino acid residues. There is a putative signal sequence of 36 amino acid residues, five repeats of a 58-residue unit, which display considerable (about 65-80 percent) identity in amino acid sequence and are responsible for IgG binding, 12 repeats of an eight amino acid unit and a carboxy-terminal region containing a hydrophobic stretch that may serve as a membrrane anchor. Due to processing at the amino-and carboxy-terminal ends, the $M_r$ of the protein isolated from the Cowan I strain is about 42,000 and it amino-terminus is blocked. Cleavage of the protein by trypsin releases four IgG-binding domains. The fifth domain encoded by the cloned gene may be specific to strain 8325-4 or may not bind IgG due to sequence differences. X-ray diffraction studies indicate that the main contacts between human IgG1 and protein A are formed by nine residues in $C_H2$ and $C_H3$ of Fc and eleven residues in each of the repeat-units of protein A. The inability of human IgG3 to bind protein A may by the result of a single amino acid substitution in $C_H3$.

The physiological function of protein A is not clear. It has been suggested that it may help the bacterium evade the immune response by covering its antigenic determinants with immunoglobulins, which are autologous or self-antigens (i.e., not foreign), and therefore not immunogenic.

***Protein G.*** Constituent of the cell wall of group G streptococci that binds to the Fc region of most IgG molecules. Protein G binds to all four sub-classes of human IgG (including IgG3 to which protein A does not bind). Compared to protein A, protein G reacts more strongly and with a wider range of IgGs from different mammalian species. (The only IgG to which protein A is reported to bind more strongly is that from the cat). Protein G does not appear to bind to other immunoglobulin classes (e.g., IgM and IgA) and is therefore a more versatile and specific reagent for complex formation with IgGs.

Like protein A, protein G is covalently attached to the bacterial cell wall. It has been solubilized by treatment with papain to yield a product of $M_r$ 30,000. The gene encoding protein G has been cloned from several strains of streptococci. That from strain GX7809 encodes a protein of 448 amino acid residues including a putative signal sequence of 33 residues, two sets of repeated sequences, each occurring twice (A1 and A2, each of 37 residues; B1 and B2, each of 55 residues), a proline-rich section, five repeats of a highly-charged pentapeptide, and a carboxy-terminal segment that may function as a membrane anchor. The IgG binding activity has been localized to the B repeats. A protein G gene isolated from another streptococcal strain specifies three A and three B repeats, but is otherwise similar. Group C streptococci produce IgG-binding proteins that resemble those from group G in structure and function. Except for the putative signal seqnece and membrane anchor, there is little if any significant similarity in sequence between protein G and protein A. However, in general organization, these proteins share some structural features (e.g., repeated immunoglobulin binding segments).

***Protein S.*** Vitamin K-dependent plasma protein that acts as a cofactor for protein C in the clotting system. It is a single polypepdtide chain ($M_r$ 69,000) that, like other vitamin K-dependent clotting factors, contains approximately 10 gamma-carboxyglutamic acid residues. About half of plasma protein S is bound to the C4 binding protein; the bound form of protein S is inactive.

***Proteins.*** Biological molecules composed of one or more polypeptide chains, each chain comprising a series of amino acids covalently linked by peptide bonds.

***Proteinases*** (endopeptidases). Group of enzymes whose action is to split proteins into smaller peptides. Such enzymes are abundant in lysosomes, especially in liver. Proteinases are used widely to digest protein in the purification of nucleic acid from chromatin, but these enzymes are also a source of considerable difficulty in the isolation of purified proteins from cell homogenates.

***Protein Kinase.*** Enzyme responsible for the phosphorylation of protein by the attachment of phosphate groups to serine, threonine or tyrosine.

***Proteinoid.*** Polymer of amino acids produced by heating together amino acids and phosphoric acid in a dry state. Such aggregates are not antigenic, but are presumed to be possible primeval molecules in theories of the origin of life.

***Protein.*** One of a group of macromolecules that are fundamental to the structure and function of all living organisms. Proteins are made up of one or more chains of amino acids; consecutive amino acids are linked covalently between the $\alpha$-amino group of one and the $\alpha$-carboxyl group of the next with the elimination of a molecule of water.

This linkage is called a peptide bond. Protein molecules containing three or more amino acids (some may contain several hundred) are known as polypeptides. About 20 amino acids are found in naturally occurring proteins and the specific sequence of amino acids in a polypeptide chain is genetically controlled by the cell in which it is made. Proteins such as albumins, globulins, and protamines, consisting solely of amino acids, are known as simple proteins; those consiting of an amino-acid sequence with nonprotein prosthetic groups attached are conjugated proteins.

There is a great variety in the size and structure of proteins. Molecular weights range from a few thousand (for protein hormones, e.g. insulin) to several million (e.g.

for enzyme complexes). The three-dimensional structure of a protein, i.e. its conformation, determines its specific biological properties. The variation in protein conformation enables a wide range of functions; for example, some proteins (e.g. collagen, keratin) are structural, others are enzymes, antibodies, or hormones. There are four levels of protein conformation. The primary structure is the specific amino-acid sequence in the polypeptide chain. The secondary structure is maintained by hydrogen bonds at regular intervals. Intramolecular hydrogen bonding produces a regular coiling, commonly in the form of an alpha-helix, which is characteristic of fibrous proteins and also present in globular proteins. Intermolecular hydrogen bonding gives rise to the beta-pleated sheet, found in silk. The tertiary structure is formed by the folding of the chain upon itself and is maintained by disulphide (S-S) bridges and noncovalent bonds such as hydrophobic interactions. It results, for example, in the formation of active sites in enzymes. Quaternary structure is the arrangement of polypeptide chains in proteins, such as haemoglobin, that have more than one polypeptide per molecule.

***Protein Structure.*** Composition of protein molecules and the ways in which the molecules are arranged. It is customary to divide protein structure into four separate levels of hierarchy.

Primary structure. Refers to the order of amino acids in the polypeptide chain.

Secondary structure. Refers to the helical configuration adopted by the chain and is most frequently a form known as the alpha-helix, but many proteins adopt a conformation known as a beta-pleated sheet.

.Tertiary structure. Refers to the way in which such helices or sheets are folded upon themselves by means of hydrogen bonds and disulphide bridges to yield the unique three-dimensional structure of the particular protein. Active sites of enzymic proteins involve unique configurations of tertiary structure involving many amino acids. Such amino acids, adjacent in the active site, may be relatively distant in the primary amino acid sequence of the protein. Thus mutations in the protein distant from one another may yet have commcn phenotypic effects since they relate to a common active site.

Quaternary structure. Displayed by some proteins; refers to the way in which two or more polypeptide chains, each the product of a gene sequence, are associated to yield a more complex protein structure. The protein may thus comprise an aggregate of identical or non-identical subunits, or a mixture of the two. For example, adult haemoglobin is a tetramer, consisting of two identical alphaglobins and two identical beta-globins.

***Protein Synthesis.*** The synthesis of protein molecules from their constituent amino acids takes place on the ribosomes of cells. The information for determining the sequence of amino acids in a particular protein in encoded in the base sequence of messenger RNA (mRNA), which is transcribed from DNA in the nucleus; the sequence of nucleotides in the mRNA determines the sequence of amino acids in the protein, each nucleotide triplet (codon) specifying a single amono acid. The mRNA migrates into the cytoplasm and becomes associated with the ribosomes, usually forming polysomes. It acts as a template for the synthesis of a particular protein, the sequence of base triplets in the mRNA determining the sequence of amino acids in the protein.

***Proteoglycan.*** Extracellular matrix macromolecule produced by the covalent linking of unbranched glycosaminoglycan side-chains to the serine residues of a core protein. Size range is potentially enormous and, given the possible tissue specificity of the core protein (and therefore diversity of glycosaminoglycan side-chain number, type and length), the potential for structural complexity becomes equally enormous.

***Proteolysis.*** Degradation of proteins into peptides or amino acids by enzymic or other means.

***Proteoplast.*** Plastid in plant cells that stores proteins.

***Prothrombin.*** Thrombin precursor; glycoprotein of two polypeptide chains. It is present in normal blood plasma in an enzymically inactive form, and is converted to thrombin by a complex process requiring cofactors such as calcium ions and thromboplastin.

***Protista.*** Kingdom of original classification that comprised all microorganisms including bacteria, thus distinguishing them from plants and animals. Since this classification system is now obsolete, the grouping of the Protista can now be seen to be misleading. The term remains in use, however, being used to designate any one-celled organism. Single-celled eukaryotic organisms are now classed as Protoctista.

***Protoctista.*** One of the five kingdoms of the classification of living organisms. It includes eukaryotic microorganisms and their relatives, such as Protozoa, slime moulds and many algae.

***Protodaeum.*** Posterior invagination into the embryonic ectoderm that is the progenitor of the terminal part of the alimentary canal. In the embryo it joins up the exterior with the archenteron and during development goes to form rectum, cloaca or anus, depending on the animal group.

***Protoderm.*** Meristematic tissue located in an apical meristem, giving rise to the epidermal structures associated with the new shoot.

***Protofilament.*** Filament extending along the axonieme of a cilium and flagellum. Each axoneme is composed of a nine-plus-two arrangement of microtubule doublets, and each microtubule is composed of 13 protofilaments of tubulin, one microtubule in the doublet being composed of α-tubulin, the other of β-tubulin.

***Protogyny.*** Situation in some hermaphrodite animals in which the ova are poroduced from the ovary before sperm is produced from the testis.

***Protomer.*** Single chain of a polymeric protein.

***Proton Channel.*** Protein channel located in the inner membrane of a mitochondrion, allowing the pumping of protons out of the matrix during oxidative phosphorylation.

***Protonema.*** Structure produced by a germinating spore. It is most often applied to the filamentous structure that develops from bryophyte spores and which produces buds that sprout into gametophyte plants.

***Proton Gradient.*** Electrochemical gradient across the inner membrane of a mitochondrion, due to both membrane potential and a proton concentration gradient. This energy is harnessed to produce ATP for mitochondrial energy conversion.

***Proton Motive Force*** (pmf, $\Delta U_{H+}$, $\Delta p$). Electrochemical potential across a closed membrane system made up of a proton gradient ($\Delta pH$) plus a transmembraneous electrical potential ($\Delta\psi$). These components are related by a formula in which R is the gas constant, T is the temperature (K) and F the Faraday constant. The proton motive force is expressed as :

$$\Delta p = \Delta\psi - 2.3\ RT\ pH/F$$

***Proton Pump.*** Protein system that is active in producing a gradient of protons across a closed membrane system. Some proton pumps are single proteins, such as bacteriophodopsin which pumps protons on activation by light. The membrane-bound ATP synthetase of mitochondria or bacteria pumps protons when it is acting as an ATPase, hydrolysing ATP to ADP and inorganic phosphate. The combined vectorial reactions in the electron transport chain which lead to a proton gradient across, for example, the mitochondrial or bacterial membrane are also sometimes referred to as a proton pump.

***Proton Symport.*** Proton channel in bacterial surface membranes that admits not only protons but also, along with them, many desired metabolites.

***Proto-oncogene.*** Cellular gene, found in the genome of a eukaryote such as a mammal, that is closely similar or identical to an oncogene. Proto-oncogenes are presumed to provide the evolutionary ancestral origins of retroviral oncogens. The oncogenic effects of retroviruses are presumed to result from alterations in the regulated expression of a proto-oncogene, or to some qualitative difference between oncogene and proto-oncogene. Proto-oncogenes specify a variety of cellular products, but many are protein kinases or cellular growth factors, and this may in some way be linked to the altered growth properties of neoplastic cells.

***Protophloem.*** The part of the primary phloem formed before the axis or structure in which it occurs has finished elongating. Protophloem elements are short-lived and soon crushed since they lose their nucleus during formation and so cannot keep pace with the growth and extension of the surrounding tissues.

***Protoplasm.*** Living substances of cells, including both nucleoplasm and cytoplasm, as well as various organelles found in these media.

***Protoplast.*** The total protoplasm of a cell, excluding material outside the plasma membrane. Protoplasts of plant cells and some prokaryotes can be prepared by enzymic digestion of the cell walls, using cellulase or lysozyme respectively.

***Protoplast.*** Protoplasm of a cell, including the cytoplasmic membrane (cell membrane, plasma membrane), but excluding the cell wall that surrounds the cytoplasmic membrane. In Gram-positive bacteria, this cell wall consists of a thick (20-80 nm) layer of peptidoglycan. In Gram-negative bacteria, the cell wall is bipartite, consisting of a thin (~1nm) peptidoglycan layer surrounded by the lipopolysaccharide-containing outer membrane. Protoplasts are osmotically fragile, but can be protected from lysis by placing them in hypertonic solutins (e.g.,20 percent sucrose). Protoplasts can be prepared from Gram-positive cells either by inhibiting cell wall synthesis (with antibiotics such as penicillin) or by enzymatic digestion of the peptidoglycan layer (with lysozyme). Protoplasts of Gram-negative bacteria can be prepared by similar treatment although in this case the outer membrane limits access to the peptidoglycan layer and may require disruption (e.g.,with EDTA) to allow protoplast preparation; such protoplasts usually contain remnants of the outer membrane and are often called spheroplasts.

***Protoplast Fusion.*** Method for transfer (transfection) of DNA from bacteria into other bacteria or into cultured animal cells such as myeloma cells. Protoplasts, which may be prepared by lysozyme-EDTA treatment of E.coli carrying an appropriate plasmid, are fused with myeloma cells by methods similar to those used in production of B cell hybridomas (e.g., treatment with polyehylene glycol).

***Prototroph.*** (1) Bacterium capable of growing on a defined minimal medium. (2) Any organism requiring only inorganic compounds plus a single carbon source for food. Thus green plants use only carbon dioxide in photosynthesis, and for most bacteria the carbon source can be sugar or starch.

***Protoxylem.*** The part of the primary xylem formed before the axis or structure in which it occurs has finished elongating. Protoxylem elements are short-lived and soon crushed since they lose their living contents during formation and so cannot keep up with the growth and extension of the surrounding tissues.

***Protozoa.*** Subkingdom of the Protoctists, which includes most unicellular eukaryotes that are not plants, such as amoebae, ciliates and flagellates.

***Provirus.*** Viral genome integrated into the genome of a eukaryotic cell. Provirus are thus transmitted from cell to cell since they are treated as a normal part of the cellular genome and are replicated with it, but no vegetative virla production or cell lysis occurs. Viruses such as retroviruses and polyomavirus may be integrated in this way, and the integration is often a step that leads to cell transformation. In some situations,, provirus may be induced to enter a replicative and potentially lytic cycle. There is also evidence to suggest that vertical transmission of provirus through the germ line from parent to progeny may occu r, and this might explain some familial patterns of tumour development.

***Prozone.*** Zone in a titration at which high concentrations of antibodies apparently fail to react even though less concentrated solutions of the same antibodies do react. In agglutination reactions, cells in the prozone do not agglutinate but may have antibodies on their surface; the failure to agglutinate may be the result of saturation of each particle with antibodies so that no cross-linking occurs. In some precipitin reactions, the antigen-antibody complexes formed in antibody excess may be relatively small and remain soluble.

***Pseudoalleles.*** Distinct genes that are functionally related and so closely linked that they behave as if they are allelic.

***Pseudogamy.*** Development of an egg by parthenogenesis, but involving activiation or stimulation (but not fertilization) by a male gamete.

***Pseudogene.*** A DNA sequence that is largely homologous to a structural gene sequence but is apparently never transcribed. Pseudogenes have been discovered by genetic engineering techniques and some (e.g. globin pseudogenes) are situated close to the locus of the active structural gene. The function of pseudogenes is unknown by they are commonly believed to represent redundant DNA and may be a by-product of the evolution of the genome.

***Pseudogene.*** DNA sequence that resembles a gene but that is not expressed because of one or more defects that impair some stage of gene expression (e.g.,faulty promoter, deficient splice signal, in-frame stop signal). Once the normal gene product is no longer produced, there is no selective barrier to the further accumulation of mutations, so pseudogenes typically have a number of defects. Some pseudogenes, which resemble mRNA in that they have 3'-poly-A tracts and correctly excisd introns, are thought to originate from the insertion of reverse transcripts (possibly carried by a retrovirus) into the genome.

***Pseudoglobulin.*** Globulin that is sparingly soluble in water, as distinct from a euglobulin, which is insoluble in water.

***Pseudomonas.*** A genus of strictly aerobic bacteria widely distributed in soil and water. The cells are rod-shaped and usually motile. A few species are pathogenic to man, including P.aeruginosa, which can cause septicaemia, abscesses, and urinary-tract infections.

***Pseudoparenchyma.*** A plectenchyma in which the filaments or hyphae have lost their individuality, their cells separating and becoming isodiametric. It becomes indistinguishable from parenchyma in its mature state while differing from it in ontogeny.

***Pseudopodium.*** A temporary projection from the cell of some Protozoa, especially the Sarcodina (e.g. Amoeba), used for locomotion and food capture. Pseudopodia, which are thought to be formed by changes in the consistency of the cytoplasm, may be in the form of fine threads (flopodia), blunt projections (lobopodia), or a branching network (rhizopodia); some (axopodia) have an internal supporting rod. Pseudopodia are also formed by macrophages.

***Pseudopregnancy.*** A state resembling pregnancy in certain mammals, including rodents, without the formation of embryos.

***Psoralens.*** Cross-linking reagents that are light-sensitive mutagens through their effects on nucleic acids.

***Psoriasis.*** Disease affecting between 1 and 2 percent of the population in which skin cells are overproduced, resulting in considerable problems with itching and sloughing off of dead skin. Inheritance patterns are complex, and there is evidence of immunological involvement with the HLA system.

***Psychrophilic.*** Designating microorganisms that can grow at temperatures below 20°C. Obligate psychrophiles require an optimum temperature of 15-18°C (they are killed at 20°C); facultative psychrophiles have an optimum similar to that of mesophiles (i.e. 30-45°C) but can grow, although more slowly, at 20°C or lower.

***Ptyalin.*** Amylase that occurs in the salive of some mammals.

***Public Idiotypic Determinant*** (IdX or CRI). Idiotypic determinant that is found in many members of the same species, usually on antibodies specific for a particular antigen. However, such shared determinants can also occur on apparently unrelated antibodies. These determinants are also known as cross-reacting idiotypic determinants, hence the abbreviations IdX or CRI. Public idiotypic determinants reflect similarities in amino acid sequence of antibody heavy and/or light chains; they have been used as markers for the gene segments encoding variable regions.

***Public Specificty.*** Antignic determinant that is shared by more than one member of a family of proteins (e.g., a group of alloantigens). The term is often used to refer to determinants on molecules in the major histocompatibility complex. Public determinants may be shared by many proteins or by as few as two.

***Puff.*** Highly decondensed area of a polytene chromosome, visible using light microscopy. A puff is an area of transcriptional activity believed to represent the activation of cell-specific genes. Puffing, which can be specifically induced in isolated preparations of Drosophila salivary glands by edysone, or by heat shock, has been extensively studied since it represents a unique example of transcriptional activity of interphase chromatin visible in the light micrscope. See Figure P.14 on next page.

***Pulsed field gradient gel electrophoresis (PFGE).*** Technique for separating large pieces of DNA by application of alternating electric fields to an agarose gel matrix. The field may be alternated in one dimension by reversing the anode and cathode (field inversion gel electrophoresis or FIGE) or it may be alternated in two directions (orthogonal field alternation gel electrophoresis or OFAGE). With present technology, molecules of several thousand kilobases (e.g., yeast chromosomes) can be resolved. PFGE is being used for studies of chromosomal organization in a variety of orgtanisms including humans.

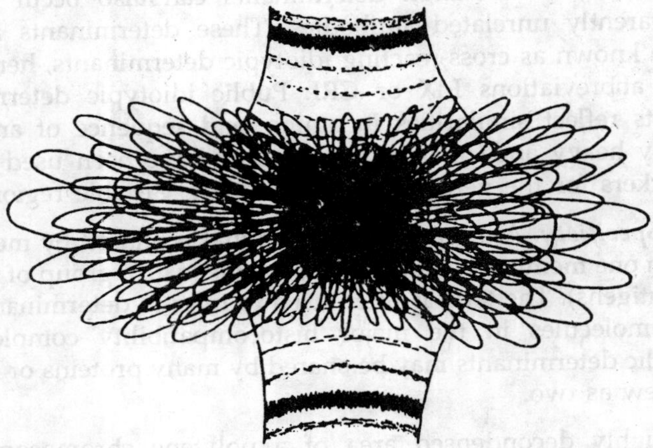

Figure P.14. Puff. Presumed structure of a large puff on a giant-polytene chromosome. The long loops of material in the puff are individual strands of decondensed chromatin, peerhaps in the form of single, extended DNA duplexes.

***Punctuated Equilibrium.*** The theory that speices usually arise relatively quickly in geological time rather than through a long process of gradual change. This is opposed to the traditional neo-Darwinian theory of evolution.

***Punnett Square.*** Square chequerboard pattern, invented by R.C.Punnett, that is used to plot and assign the genotypes resulting from fusion of gametes of a particular cross. Phenotypic assignment can also be made on the basis of the genotypic one.

***Pupa.*** The nonfeeding immobile form of an endopterygote insect, in which the transformation from larva to adult (metamorphosis) occurs. Pupae are usually exarate, with movable wings and limbs, but the chrysalids of the Lepidoptera (butterflies and moths) are obtect, with wings and limbs fused to the body, and the pupae of some Diptera (flies) are coarctate, with a hard barrel-shaped puparium protecting the exarate pupa.

***Purebred.*** Describing progeny from an inbred line of animals or plants. The term is used fairly loosely to designate progeny with a stranded phenotype within a particular breed of cattle, dogs, etc. Such animals may, however, be relatively heterozygous at many loci and may show considerable individual variation. Intense inbreeding may be used to produce an inbred line of stock that is highly homozygous and that, in the case of animals, will accept tissue grafts from one another. Laboratory strains of small mammals are an example of such highly inbred lines.

***Pure Culture.*** Culture that contains only one cell type, or one strain of cells, or is made up of individuals of only one species.

***Pure Line.*** A continuous series of generations of an organism that are consistently homozygous for one or more characters or genes. A pure line is produced by crossing two organisms homozygous for the genes. In practice this is best achieved by self-fertilization in plants and by inbreeding animals. Organisms of a pure line are said to breed true for the character(s) under consideration.

***Purified Protein Derivative (PPD).*** Soluble protein fraction precipitated by trichloroacetic acid from medium in which Mycobacterium tuberculosis has been grown. It is widely used in tuberculin tests.

***Purine Nucleoside Phosphorylase Deficiency.*** Form of severe combined immunodeficiency that results from the inheritance of mutant forms of purine nucleoside phosphorylase (EC 2.4.2.1) (PNP). The immunodeficiency is caused by accumulation of metabolites that are toxic for T lymphocytes; B lymphocytes are usually present in normal numbers. PNP, which is present in all mammalian cells, catalyses phosphorolysis of guanosine, deoxyguanosine and inosine. PNP deficiency results in increased intracellular concentrations of guanosine, deoxyguanosine, guanosine triphosphate (GTP) and deoxyguanosine triphosphate (dGTP). dGTP inhibits ribonucleoside-diphosphate reductase, an enzyme involved in DNA synthesis. Precursors of T lymphocytes are more vulnerable to destruction by the accumulation of these metabolites than are other cells. Unlike adenosine deaminase, PNP is not more abundant in lymphoid tissue compared with other tissue.

PNP is a trimer of $M_r$ 32,000 subunits. The gene encoding PNP has been mapped to chromosome 14q13.1; it encodes a polypeptide chain of 289 amino acid residues. PNP deficiency is inherited as an autosomal recessive. Levels of PNP (usually measured in red blood cells) are half-normal in heterozygotes. PNP deficiency has been treated successfully with transplants of bone marrow cells.

***Purines.*** One of two classes of organic bases found in nucleic acids, but are also present in coenzymes: the other class are the pyrimidines. The two most abundant purines are adenine and guanine, uric acid is the chief end-product of purine breakdown.

***Purkinje Cell.*** Type of neurone found in the vertebrate brain, especially in the cerebellum, and characterized by a dense basket work of dendritic extensions.

***Purkinje Fibres.*** Large muscle fibres found in the ventricular walls of some mammals and responsible for the conduction of contractile waves through the ventricular muscle.

***Puromycin.*** Antibiotic that inhibits protein synthesis in eukaryotic cells. It acts by complexing to the growing end of a nascent polypeptide chain, thus blocking its further growth and resulting in dissociation of the peptide-puromycin complex from the ribosome.

***Purpura.*** Hemorrhage into the skin causing the appearance of a purple or purple-blue rash.

***Purpura Hyperglobulinemia.*** Skin hemorrhages of the lower extremities, particularly about the ankles. The phonomenon is observed in patients with markedly elevated serum immunoglobulins as in Sjogren's syndrome, macroglobulinemia of waldenstrom, multiple myeloma, etc.

***Putrescine.*** Polyamine found associated with DNA in certain species of bacteria.

***Pycnosis.*** Condensation of chromatin in chromosomes, especially involving the staining characteristics and phase contrast appearance of the chromatin. Chromatin in the Y chromosome, for example, is described as heteropyknotic since it is more described as heteropycnotic since it is more highly condensed than most other chromatin and can be stained more readily.

***Pyloric Stenosis.*** Syndrome in the human in which affected infants have an abnormal pyloric sphincter, with frequent vomiting apparent. It responds well to surgery. It is a polygenic disorder with a complex pattern of inheritance, and there is a three to one male excess of the disease.

***Pyogenic Infection.*** Bacterial infection that induces the formation of pus. Bacteria causing pyogenic infections include Staphylococcus aureus, Streptococcus pyogenes, Streptococcus pneumoniae and Hemophilus influenzae. Susceptibility to pyogenic infections is found in patients with antibody deficiency syndromes and in patients having defects in phagocytic cells or complement components (e.g., C3 deficiency, Factor H deficiency, Factor I deficiency).

***Pyramid of Biomass.*** A diagrammatic representation of the total biomass at all trophic levels in a food chain. The biomass decreases slightly at each successive level up the food chain.

***Pyramid of Numbers.*** A diagrammatic representation of the numbers of animals at all trophic levels in a food chain. A decrease occurs at each successive level, which is more noticeable than the decrease in biomass because animals at the end of a food chain tend to be fewer, although larger, than those at the lower levels. See Figure P.15 on next page.

***Pyranose.*** A monosaccharide that exists in the form of a six-membered ring of five carbon atoms and one oxygen atom. An example is α-D-glucopyranose, one form of glucose.

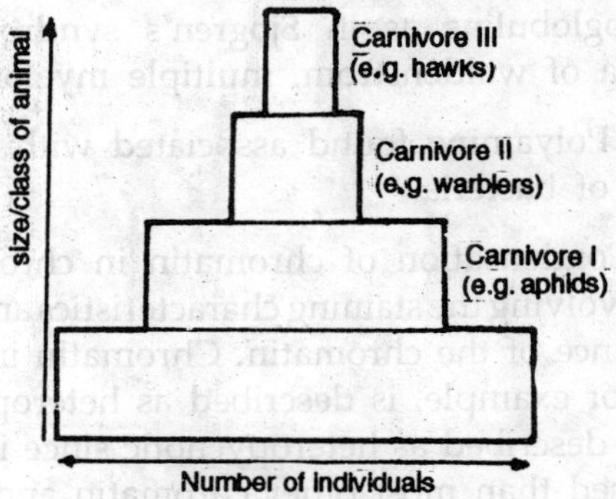


Figure P.15. Pyramid of numbers.

***Pyridoxal Phosphate.*** Coenzyme of transaminating enzymes and of amino acid decarboxylation. See Figure P.16.

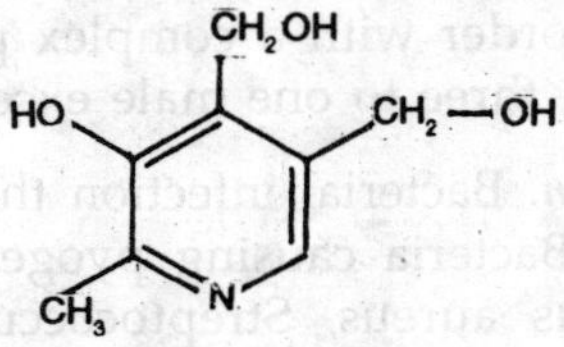

Figure P.16. Pyridoxine.

***Pyridoxine*** (Vitamin $B_6$). Water-soluble vitamin of the B complex, required by many animals and microorganisms, and acting as a precursor of pyridoxal phosphate. Its deficiency causes dermatitis and anaemia in mammals.

***Pyrimidine Dimers.*** Compounds formed following irradiation of DNA by ultraviolet light. The dimer involves the covalent joining of two adjacent thymines or cytosines, or an adjacent thymines and cytosines, but thymine dimer formation is much the most significant. Dimer formation blocks DNA replication, but may be repaired by photoreactivation.

***Pyrimidine.*** One of a group of nitrogenous bases whose parent compound has the formula shown. The three most abundant pyrimidines are cytosine, thymine, and uracil, which are constituents of nucleic acids.

***Pyrogen.*** Substance that causes fever.

***Pyroglobulin.*** Monoclonal immunoglobulin (e.g., myeloma protein) that precipitates irreversibly at 56°C, in contrast to Bence-Jones protein, which precipitates at 56°C but redissolves upon boiling.

***Pyrrole.*** Organic compound containing one nitrogen and four carbon atoms; four pyrroles join to form the porphyrin ring, which occurs in haem, cytochromes and chlorophyll.

***Pyrroloquinoline Quinone (PQQ).*** Novel prosthetic group of a number of bacterial dehydrogenases including those responsible for oxidation of methanol, methylamine and glucose. The dehydrogenase react with the electron transport chains at the level of cytochrome c, amicyanic (a blue copper protein) and ubiquinone, respectively.

***Pyrophosphate.*** Product of ATP hydrolysis. It is also an intermediate in providing energy for DNA replication.

# Q

***$Q_{10}$.*** Temperature coefficient; increase in the rate of a reaction for a rise of 10ºC, the rate being expressed as a multiple of the initial rate.

***Qb.*** RNA bacteriophage, best known as the source of an RNA replicase.

***Q banding.*** Chromosome banding technique so called because it involves the use of quinacrine dyes (quinacrine mustard or quinacrine dihydrochloride). The technique is most useful in demonstrating areas of heterochromatin, especially the Y chromosomes.

***Quadrivalent.*** Describing an association of four homologous chromosomes at meiosis.

***Quantasome.*** One of many small regularly arranged particles, about 18 x 16 x 10 nm, located on or in chloroplast thylakoid membranes, visible with the aid of electgron microscopy and isolated by suitable fragmentation techniques. They are thought to be either artefacts or structural units of photosynthesis, containing pigments and other molecules. They are just large enough to be the postulated photosynthetic units.

***Quantitative Preciptin Reaction.*** Immunochemical reaction in which the amount of precipitate, formed as a result of mixing antigen and antibodies in various proportions, is determined quantitatively, usually by washing the precipitates and then measuring the amount of protein in each. The determination of protein content can be make by several procedures, e.g. micro-Kjeldahl analysis (to determine nitrogen content), measurement of the optical density (at approximately 280 nm) of the dissolved precipitin.

***Quantum Speciation.*** Evolution of new species within small peripheral populations by genetic drift and founder effect, on a much smaller time scale than normally involved in the evolution of new species.

***Quantum Yield (Quantum Efficiency).*** The number of molecules of carbon dioxide fixed, or oxygen evolved, per light quantum absorbed in photosynthesis. It is the reciprocal of the quantum requirement (or quantum number), the number of light quanta required for the reduction of one carbon dioxide molecule. The theoretical minimum quantum requirement for photosynthesis is three, but in practice it is usually postulated to be eight (a quantum yield of 1/2). The higher the quantum yield of a photochemical reaction, the higher it^ efficiency.

***Quaternary.*** The second period of the Cenozoic era, extending from one million years ago to the present day. It consists of two epochs, the Pleistocene and Holocene.

***Quaternary Structure.*** The arrangement of polypeptide chains in a protein molecule that is made up of more than one polypeptide.

***Quaternary Structure.*** Packing of two or more filded polypeptide chains into a higher-order structure.

***Quick Stop.*** Type of bacterial mutant in which DNA and cellular replication cease abruptly at 42°C.

***Quiescent Centre.*** A group of cells at the very tip of an apical meristem that differ physiologically from the surrounding cells of the apex. It appears to be common to most root apices but has also been demonstrated in some shoot apices. Its principal feature is a much lower rate of mitosis than the surrounding tissue. However, its size appears to fluctuate and occasionally it may become indistinguishable from the rest of the apex, suggesting that it may be intermitently quiescent. The quiescent centre may be a site of auxin formation and seems to be the source of the active initials in the meristem by its (infrequent) mitoses. It also provides a reservoir of cells whose inactivity makes them less prone to damage such as chromosomal aberrations.

***Quiescent Culture.*** Culture of cells in which active cell growth and replication are minimal, but in which cells continue to survive adequately. Confluent cell cultures may behave in this way.

***Quin-2.*** Quinoline derivative that increases in fluorescence intensity when it binds to free $Ca^{2+}$. Quin-2 is administered as an ester so that it can enter cells; subsequently it is de-esterified. The fluorescence intensity of B and T lymphocytes loaded with Quin-2 increases upon activation, an indication of an increase of free $Ca^{2+}$ in the cytosol. See Figure Q.1.

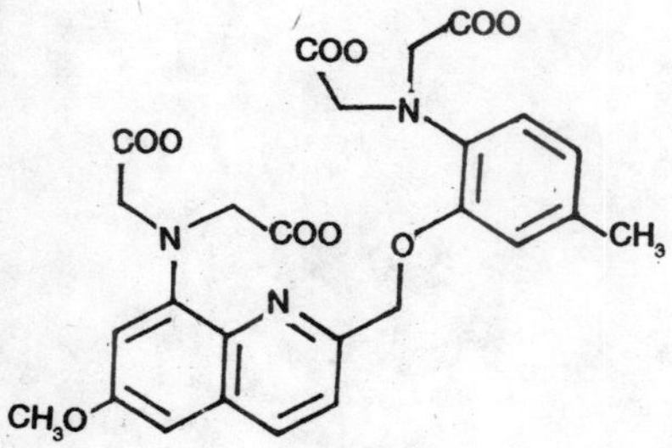


Figure Q.1. Quin 2.

***Quinacrine.*** Derivative of acridine used as an antimalarial drug and also in cancer chemotherapy. Quinacrine dyes (quinacrine mustard or quinacrine hydrochloride) are also used as chromosome stains and will fluoresce under ultraviolet light.

***Quinacrine Mustard.*** Cytotoxic drug; alkylating agent used as an anticancer drug.

***Quinone.*** One of a class of molecules active in biological oxidation/reduction systems.

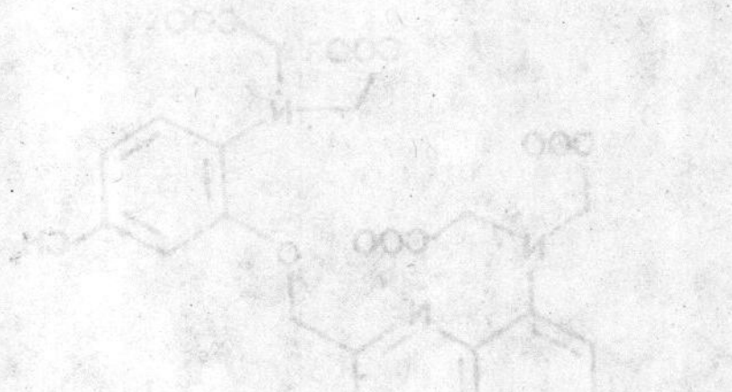

# R

***R.*** Roentgen; measure of level of ionizing radiation.

***RII Locus.*** Part of the genome of the bacteriophage T4, made famous because it was subjected to detailed study by Seymour Benzer and was the first DNA segment to be subjected to fine structure mapping analysis.

***Race.*** Subspecific group of population that can be distinghished by phenotypic character and/or geographical isolation from other groups or populations within the species. The degree of differences between races is variable, and the word is used according to convenience. Races may or may not be recognized as subspecies, and are only so recognized when the racial differences are considerable and deemed to be of taxonomic importance.

***Rad.*** Term derived as a contraction for radiation absorbed dose; defined as 100 ergs of radiation per gram of tissue.

***Radial Cell.*** Glial cell that extends from the lumen to the outer surface of the spinal cord and occurs throughout the central nervous system. Radial cells are thought to guide the migrations of other nerve cells to their correct destinations.

***Radiation.*** Wave energy emitted and propagated through medium or space. It includes ionizing particles and electromagnetic radiation, such as gamma rays, X-rays, and the light rays in ultraviolet, visible and infrared wavelengths.

***Radiation Chimaera.*** Chimaera that is the result of damage to the genome of a constituent cell of the organism by ionizing radiation. Radiation chimaeras have been of use in clonal analysis in developmental biology to distinguish between lineage-dependent and position-dependent differentiation in the ommatidia of insect eyes: clones of cells can be marked by X-irradiation and their fates followed.

***Radiation Sickness.*** Syndrome that characterizes exposure to high and potentially lethal doses of radiation, usually above 400 r for the human. Symptoms include nausea, diarrhoea and mental depression; death usually follows within a few days. The immediate cause of the disease is not mutation alone, but a generalized loss of capacity for mitotic division of the body's cells. Thus tissue with high mitotic rates is likely to be the first to show dramatic change.

***Radioactive Contamination.*** Discharge of radioactive materials, resulting in increased levels of radiation in previously low background radiation areas. Contamination may result from fall-out from the atmosphere following an atomic explosion, or from accidental discharge of radioactive gases or liquids. The seriousness of such contamination depends greatly on the isotope concerned. Thus isotopes with long half-lives, intense radioactive discharges and involving elements incorporated into vital biological structures are the most serious. These include: radiolabelled thymidine, which is incorporated into DNA; radioactive strontium and caesium which are incorporated into bone; labelled iodine which is concentrated in the thyroid gland; powerful emitters such as plutonium.

***Radioactive Dating.*** Any of various dating techniques that give the absolute age of a sediment or fossil. All methods depend on the fact that naturally occurring radioactive isotopes (radioactive forms of an element) decay at a known rate. By calculating the amount of isotope left in a sediment or fossil, and by knowing the amount present when it was first laid down and the rate of decay, it is possible to work out the age of the specimen. This method depends on several assumptions, the most important being the known proportion of radioactive to nonradioactive isotopes at the time the fossil or sediment was laid down. The radioactive isotopes most often used are carbon (carbon-14), potassium-argon, and uranium.

The carbon-14 method (radiocarbon dating) can be used to date organic material directly, up to an age of 7000 years, since carbon-14 has a half life of 5730 years, i.e. the radioactivity decreases to half in this time. Carbon-14 is produced in the upper atmosphere by the action of cosmic radiation on nitrogen and becomes incorporated into atmospheric carbon dioxide in a known proportion to nonradioactive carbon. The carbon dioxide is absorbed by plants during photosynthesis and becomes incorporated into the animals that eat them. When a plant or animal dies, the carbon-14 present begins to decay. The amount of residual radioactivity can be measured, enabling the absolute age to be calculated.

Potassium-argon dating utilizes the fact that naturally occurring potassium contains the radioisotope potassium-40, which decays to the gas argon-40; this becomes trapped in minerals containing potassium. The decay is much slower than that of carbon-14 (potassium-40 has a half life of 1300 million years), which considerably extends the range of absolute dating.

***Radioactive Decay.*** Disintegration of the nucleus of an unstable atom, resulting in emission of photons or charged particles such as alpha- or beta-particles. Since decay is a random process it is usually expressed as a half-life, being the time taken for 50 percent of a radionuclide to decay.

***Radioactive Isotope*** (Radioisotope). Isotope of an element that is intrinsically unstable and is likely to emit ionizing radiation as a result of radioactive decay to a more stable form.

***Radioactive Labelling.*** The incorporation of radioactive isotopes (e.g. $^{14}C$, $^{3}H$, $^{32}P$), or tracers, into chemical compounds. The technique is widely used to study biological processes, in which labelled molecules can be traced during such experimental procedures as chromatography and electrophoresis. Using labelled precursors, the fate of radioactive molecules within cells can also be studied and metabolic pathways worked out. Radioactively labelled compounds can be detected and quantified by such means as autoradiography and liquid scintillation counting.

***Radioactivity.*** Random disintegration of unstable radioactive isotopes to produce different atoms with concomitant emission of energetic particles (e.g., electrons) or radiation (e.g., gamma-rays). Radioactivity can be detected in various ways. Electrons (beta-particles) can be detected and quantitated in a geiger counter or in a liquid scintillation counter. Radioactivity can also be located by its action on a photographic emulsion.

***Radioallergosorbent Test (RAST).*** Test to measure IgE antibody specific for an alltergen. The allergen is bound to an insoluble carrier, such as dextran beads. The serum to be tested is reacted with the insolubilized allergen, the particles are washed and then reacted with a radiolabeled antibody to human IgE. The labeled antibody binds only to the IgE antibody in the test serum that has been taken up by the particle-bound allergen. The allergen must be in excess relative to the total antibodies (all classes) in the test serum to assure complete uptake of the antibodies. The anti-IgE antibody must be in excess relative to the bound IgE antibodies. The amount of radioactivity bound to the beads is then proportional to the amount of specific IgE anitbody to the allergen in the test serum.

***Radioautographic Efficiency.*** Efficiency of an autoradiographic process.

***Radiobiology.*** Branch of biology that involves the study of the effects of radiation on biological materials and organisms.

***Radioimmunoassay.*** The most widely used technique for measuring polypeptide hormones in biological tissues and fluids. It is based on the ability of an unlabelled hormone to inhibit competitively the binding of labelled hormone by specific antibodies. The hormone concentration of the unkown sample is determined by comparing the degree of inhibition with that produced by a series of standards cokntaining known amounts of the hormone. This technique has outstanding advantages in sensitivity, specificity, practicability, and precision over other procedures and can measure normal circulating levels of hormones (in the range $10^{-8}$ to $10^{-4}$ kg/m$^3$) with reasonable reliability. The method was first described by Berson and Yalow in 1960 for the measurement of plasma insulin in man. It has also been used to assay nonpeptide substances, such as steroids, prostaglandins, and nucleotides.

***Radioimmunoassay (RIA).*** Any method for detecting or quantitating antigens or antibodies utilizing radiolabeled reactants. RIA can be used to detect very small quantities of antigens or antibodies, even in complex mixtures. In one frequently used version of RIA for antigen detection, the antigen is radiolabeled and reacted with a limiting amount of specific antibody (Ab1). The complex containing bound antigen is then separated from free antigen (e.g., by reaction with a second antibody (Ab2) specific for Ab 1). Unlabeled antigen in a test sample is used to complete with the binding of labeled antigen. The amount of test antigen is determined from the extent of inhibition obtained with standards containing defined amounts of the same antigen.

***Radioimmunoelectrophoresis.*** Variant of immunoelectrophoresis in which radio-labeled antibody or antigen is used to react specifically with particular precipitin .arcs, followed by autoradiography to localize the radiolabel.

***Radioimmunosorbent Test*** (RIST). Test to measure total IgE concentration in serum. Anti-IgE is bound to an insoluble carrier such as dextran beads. The serum to be tested is reacted with a standard amount of radiolabeled IgE and the mixture is then reacted with the insolubilized anti-IgE. After appropriate incubation and washing, the amount of radiolabeled IgE adhering to the beads is determined. The IgE in the test serum competes with the radiolabeled standard IgE for binding to the beads. The decrease in amount of labeled IgE relative to a control (no unlabeled IgE) is a measure of the IgE concentration in the test serum. The assay can be made quantitative by determining the degree of inhibition obtained with known IgE standards.

***Radiomimetic.*** Descriptive of chemicals (e.g., nitrogen mustards) that mimic ionizing radiation in the way in which they cause lesions in the nucleic acids.

***Ragweed.*** Weed of the Ambrosiae family whose pollen contains the most common respiratory allergens in North America. The two common species are the short and giant ragweed: Ambrosia artemisiifkolia (eliator) and Ambrosia trifida. Their characterized allergens are listed in the table. The amino acid sequences of Ra3 (101 amino acid residues), Ra5S (45 residues) and Ra5G (40 residues) have been determined.

***Raji Cell Assay.*** Test for immune complexes in human serum. Raji cells are a line of transformed human B lymphocytes that lack surface immunoglobulin, but have Fcγ receptors, complement receptor 1, complement receptor 2 and receptors for C1q. Test serum is mixed with Raji cells, and the amount of immune complex bound is quantitated with radiolabeled $F(ab')_2$ antibodies to IgG.

***Ramapithecus.*** A genus of manlike fossil apes of the Miocene or early Pliocene, dated 12 to 14 million years ago. They show hominid dental features and may be the ancestors of true hominids.

***Rana.*** Genus of frogs; widely used in biological research.

***R and K Selection.*** Two distinct types of theoretical selection which operate in population ecology. r denotes the inherent rate of natural population increase, and k the selection imposed on a population by limited food reserves. r selection occurs when food reserves are not limiting, thus a population expands purely as a result of natural increase. When k selection is in operation the population will always be close to the environmental carrying capacity, and species are favoured that reproduce slowly and are well adapted to a relatively stable environment. Such organisms are described as k strategists. Where r selection is the main force in determining population size the food reserves may fluctuate considerably, but are not the ultimate determinants of population size. High reproduction rate and large progeny sizes are favoured; such organisms are described as r strategists. Thus predatory mammals such as lions and tigers are k strategists, whereas insects such as aphids are r strategists.

***Random Assortment.*** Referring to the fact that different combinations of chromosomes are distributed among the separate gametes at meiotic division. It follows from the fact that each pair of homologous chromosomes in an individual consists of one derived from a paternal chromosomes and one from a maternal. Since assortment is random, a single sperm or egg will acquire a paternal chromosome from one homologous pair but a maternal one from some other pair, the origin of the chromosomes being randomly determined.

***Random Breeding.*** Random mating of individuals in a population. If the random-bred population is sufficiently large, it will remain genetically diverse. However, small closed populations, even if randomly bred, tend to become genetically uniform.

***Random Genetic Drift.*** Referring to the fact that genetic drift is based on random processes.

***Random Mating.*** Mating system in a population in which every female gamete has an equal opportunity of being fertilized by every male gamete.

***Random X-inactivation.*** Referring to the fact that in the homogametic sex for example the human female, the X chromosome which is inactivated in each cell is more or less randomly determined, being in some cells the X of paternal origin, in others the X of maternal origin. The process is not completely random, however, in that groups of adjacent tissue cells often tend to have the same X inactivated, as examplified by the tortoiseshell cat whose coat colour betrays the phenotypic expression of two distinct X-linked alleles determining pigment colour. Since the coat colour is patchy, the X chromosomes are randomly inactivated at a whole animal level, but not at a tissue level. The inactivated copy of the X chromosome is called the barr body, and the inactivation process is also discussed under the lyon hypothesis.

***Rapidly Reassociating DNA.*** Fraction of DNA that anneals or renatures rapidly after denaturation. The annealing involves the recovery of double-strandedness by specific hydrogen bonding, and its rate in solution is a function partly of the frequency of a particular sequence in the mixture and partly of the nature of the sequence involved. The DNA that reassociates most rapidly is the palindromic sequences material, which can hybridize with itslf by doubling over of a single-stranded molecule. It is thus called snap back or fold back DNA. A fraction that reassociates somewhat more slowly than fold back DNA, but still much faster than bulk eukaryotic DNA, is highly repetitive, largely composed of centromeric DNA. DNA of intermediate speed of reassociation is termed moderately repetitive DNA and comprises material such as ribosomal and transfer RNA genes, as well as genes coding for histone which are present in multiple copies.

***Rapid Lysis Mutant.*** Type of E.coli mutant in which infection by T even phage leads to particularly fast cell lysis.

***Rare Bases.*** Purine and pyrimidine nucleoside phosphates that occur infrequently in nucleic acids. They include such compounds as 1-methylguanosine, ribothymidine and 5-ribosyluracil which are found in the molecules of transfer RNA. See Figure R.1 on next page.

***Rare Genotype Advantage.*** Hypothesis in connection with frequency-dependent selection which suggests that some genotypes would be advantageous only when rare. If it is increased in frequency due to selection the fitness of such individuals would decrease, thus stabilizing the correlation between rarity and fitness.

***Rare Phenotype Advantage.*** Situation in a polymorphic population in which commoner phenotype or phenotypes are disadvantage, in some or all circumstances; for example, predation may be selective for commoner phenotypes. In this way a rare phenotype may be at an advantage, at least in some circumstances, and thus persist in the population.

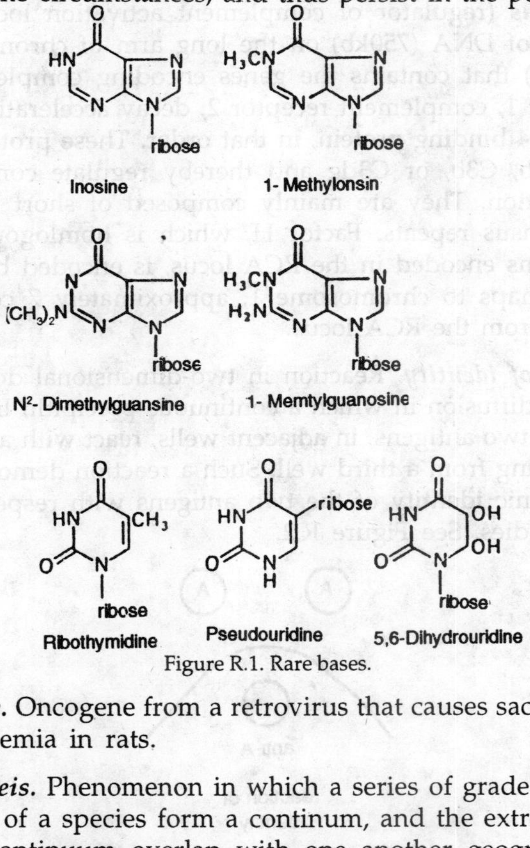

Figure R.1. Rare bases.

***Ras Gene.*** Oncogene from a retrovirus that causes sacroma and leukaemia in rats.

***Rassenkreis.*** Phenomenon in which a series of graded populations of a species form a continum, and the extremities of the continuum overlap with one another geographically, but are then found to be reproductively isolated from one another. The herring gull and lesser black-backed gull in the UK form the overlapping ends of such a continuum stretching around the world in subpolar regions.

***Ratt Syndrome.*** Rare X-linked dominant trait, which is lethal in hemizygous males.

***Raynaud's Phenomenon.*** Sudden, painful vasospasm of the fingers usually upon exposure to cold that may occur alone or in many connective tissue diseases (e.g., systemic lupus erythematosus, systemic sclerosis) and in cryoglobulinemia.

***RCA Locus*** (regulator of complement activation locus). Segment of DNA (750kb) on the long arm of chromosome 1 (1q3.2) that contains the genes encoding complement receptor 1, complement receptor 2, decay accelerating factor and C4 binding protein, in that order. These proteins bind to C4b, C3b, or C3dg and thereby regulate complement activation. They are mainly composed of short and long consensus repeats. Factor H, which is homlogous to the proteins encoded in the RCA locus, is encoded by a gene that maps to chromosome 1, approximately 7 centi-Morgans from the RCA locus.

***Reaction of identity.*** Reaction in two-dimensional double immunodiffusion in which a continuous precipitin line forms when two antigens, in adjacent wells, react with antibodies diffusing from a third well. Such a reaction demonnstrates antigenic identity of the two antigens with respect to the antibodies. See Figure R.2.

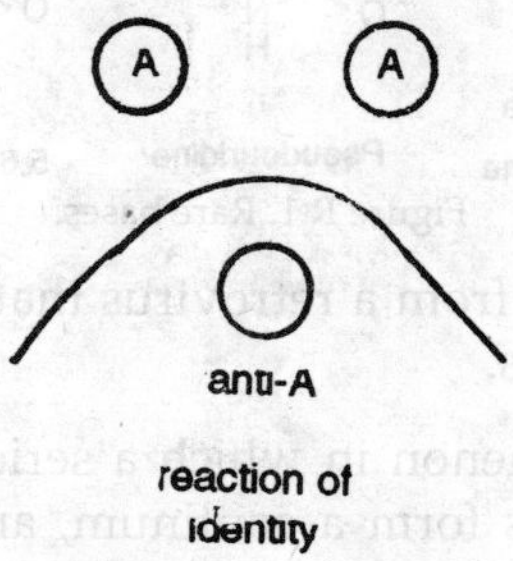


Figure R.2. Reaction of identity.

***Reaction of non-identity.*** Reaction in two-dimensional double immunodiffusion in which two distinct precipitin lines form when two antigens, in adjacent wells, react with a mixture of antibodies to each of them diffusing from a third well. The precipitin line formed by each of the two antigen-antibody systems is not affected by the presence of the other; typically the two precipitin lines cross. Such a reaction demonstrates that the two antigens do not share any determinants that can be detected by these antibodies. See Figure R.3.

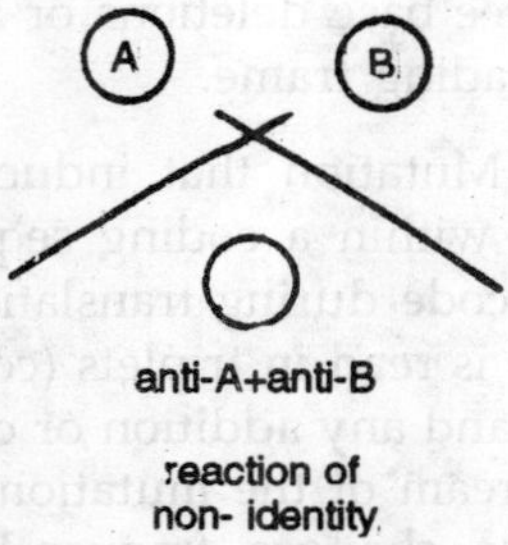


Figure R.3. Reaction of non-identity.

***Reaction of Partial Identity.*** Reaction in two-dimensional double immunodiffusion in which a continuous precipitin line plus a spur form when two antigens, in adjacent wells, react with antibodies diffusing from a third well. Such a reaction demonstrates that the two antigens are related but not identical. (Some of the antibodies react with both antigens, but other antibodies—those that form the spur—react with only one of the antigens). See Figure R.4.

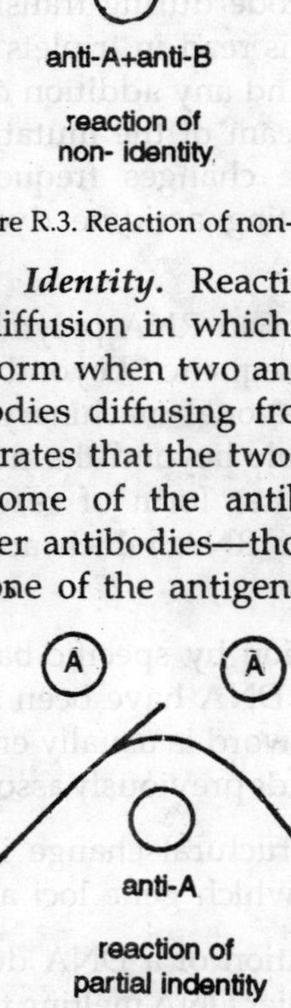


Figure R.4. Reaction of partial identity.

***Reactive Lysis.*** Lysis of unsensitized red blood cells (not coated with antibody) initiated by complexes of C5b and C6 in the presence of C7, C8 and C9. Reactive lysis occurs as a bystander phenomenon when complement is activated.

***Reading Frame.*** Particular sequence of nucleotide triplets (codons) employed in translation. The reading frame depends on the location of the initiation codon; addition or deletion of one base (or two bases) will alter the reading frame, whereas three base deletions or additions will have no effect on the reading frame.

***Reading Frame Shift.*** Mutation that induces the addition or deletion of a base within a coding sequence, resulting in misreading of the code during translation. This is because the DNA sequence is read in triplets (codons) from a fixed point of initiation, and any addition or deletion will lead to all triplets downstream of the mutation differing from the original. Such base changes frequently result from the actions of intercalating acridine dyes such as acriflavine and acridine orange.

***Read Through.*** Action of an RNA polymerase in continuing to transcribe a DNA sequence beyond a stop codon, or the action of the translational machinery in translating a messenger RNA molecule beyond the normal codon for chain termination. The latter form of read through results, for example, in transfer RNA which acts as a nonsense suppressor.

***Reannealing.*** Renaturation by specific base pairing of complementary strands of DNA have been seperated by denaturing or melting. The word is usually employed to refer to the renaturation of strands previously associated prior to melting.

***Rearrangement.*** Any structural change in a chromosome that alters the order in which gene loci are arranged.

***Reassociation.*** Reformation of a DNA double helix by renaturation following earlier DNA melting to form single-stranded molecules.

***Reassociation Kinetics.*** Study of rates of DNA reassociation in controlled conditions as in the determination of cot curves. Following the melting of a sample of DNA, the rates of reassociation, measured by reduction in absorption at 260 nm, can be used to deduce the proportions of DNA having different Cot values and therefore of differing repetition frequencies in the DNA sample.

***Recapitulation.*** A theory put forward by Ernst Haeckel (1834-1919) in the 19th century that ontogeny repeats phylogeny, i.e. that each organism in its development from zygote to adult climbs its own family tree. For example, a mammal strats life as a single cell, resembling its protozoan ancestors, then becomes a two-layered embryo, resembling a coelenterate ancestors, and later goes through a stage of having gill slits, similar to its fish ancestors. This theory has been largely discredited; the evidence indicates only that there is a closer resemblance between embryos of related animals than between the adults themselves.

***Rec A Protein.*** Protein produced in some bacteria, including E.coli; product of the rec A locus. It has important functions in DNA repair, especially in sos repair. The rec A protein is a protease that cleaves the hex A repressor. Such cleavage activates a number of genes involved in repair. Since SOS repair is error-prone, its efficiency modulates mutation rate in important ways.

***Receptor.*** Molecule or molecular complex that specifically recognizes and associates with another specific molecule (ligand). Often the receptor, when so complexed, will initiate new molecular processes within the cell. Bacteriophages have specific receptors on the surfaces of sensitive strains of bacteria, many hormones bind with receptor sites on cell surfaces, and, at a nucleic acid level, different DNA sequences act as receptors for polymerase molecules, transcription factors and regulatory molecules that operate in the activation or repression of operons.

***Receptor-mediated Endocytosis.*** Form of endocytosis highly specific for certain vital macromolecules present in the extracellular fluid. Uptake is effected through the presence of high-affinity, highly specific protein receptors which become localized in coated pits of the plasma membrane and which concentrate the ligand at this site. With the formation of a coated vesicle the ligand is then internalized. The fate of the ligand and receptor varies. Both may be recycled to the cell surface as in the case of transferrin which brings iron into the cell. Alternatively, the ligand may be broken down in secondary lysosomes, and the receptor recycled as in the case of low-density lipoprotein which is a source of cholesterol. Both receptor and ligand may be degraded in secondary lysosomes as in the case of epidermal growth factor and insulin where the action of certain hormones needs to be regulated.

***Recessive.*** (Designating) the member of a pair of alleles that does not show its effect in the presence of any other allelic partner. Therefore a recessive shows up in the phenotype only when it is homozygous in the genotype; it is then known as a double recessive. If a dominant gene A has a recessive allele a, the phenotype of the recessive shows only in the homozygous double recessive aa. Recessives arise from dominant genes by mutation and are frequently deleterious. There is sometimes more than one recessive corresponding to a dominant.

***Recessive Gene.*** Gene that is recessive when present in a diploid cell which contains a dominant allele on the other homologous chromosome.

***Recessive Lethal.*** Descriptive of an allele that is lethal only when in the homozygous state.

***Recipient.*** A person or animal that receives organs, tissues, or blood derived from another individual of the same or of a different species.

***Reciprocal Cross.*** A pair of matings in which the genotypes of the male and female gametes are reversed in the second cross. For example, if a male AA is crossed with a female aa in the first cross, a male aa is mated with a female AA in the second. It is used to determine whether the sex has any influence on the result of the cross.

***Reciprocal Translocation*** (balanced translocation). Chromosome aberration following chromosome breakage in which a precise exchange of chromosomal segments occurs between two non-homologous chromosomes. If such a translocation occured between homologous chromosomes it might easily be undetectable. Reciprocal translocation does not normally alter the length or appearance of the chromosomes concerned.

***Rec Mutant.*** Family of mutants that are characterized by defective recombination. It results from lesions in the enzymes involved in ligation of recombination DNA fragments and also results in impaired repair following irradiation.

***Recombinant.*** Cell or organism that reveals the results of a recombination event.

***Recombinant DNA.*** DNA formed when single strands combine by complementary base pairing to yield double helices. Such reactions occur in nature during crossing over in meiosis and between sister chromatids during normal cell division. Recombination also occurs in bacterial conjugation and transformation and it is widely used in vitro in genetic engineering (recombinant DNA technology).

***Recombinant DNA.*** DNA strand resulting from the physical joining of two or more pre-existing DNA strands. Traditionally, in eukaryotes, the term refers to the result of DNA exchange during meiosis or mitosis or by gene conversion. Recently, the term has come to be used to describe DNA constructs created in vitro.

***Recombinant DNA technology.*** Methodology associated with the isolation, purification and replication of genes from one organism in another. It usually involves ligation of genomic or cDNA into a plasmid or viral vector in which the DNA can be replicated.

***Recombinant Inbred (RI) Strain.*** Strain derived by inbreeding two members of the $F_2$ generation of a cross between two inbred strains. A distinct line can be produced from each randomly chosen pair. This results in the genetic fixation of alleles present in the original $F_2$ pair. Recombinant inbred strains are useful in establishing genetic linkages. For this purpose, the distribution of genes among a group of different recombinant inbred lines is compared. To date, recombinant inbred strains are available only in the mouse.

***Recombination.*** The formation of a zygote containing combinations of genes that are different from the combinations in either parent. For example, if a parent AAbb is crossed with aaBB, it is possible to produce an individual containing AaBb, which is both phenotypically and genotypically different from the parents. Recombination results from the process of crossing over during meiosis in eukaryotes or from simple DNA exchange in prokaryotes. Some recombination events, however, appear to involve the addition of a new sequence to an existing DNA molecule, without exchange. Recombination is an important means of producing variation, upon which natural selection can act to bring about evolutionary change.

***Recon.*** The unit of genetic recombination, now known to be an individual base pair in a DNA molecule. Although recombination of only one nucleotide lengths is unlikely to occur, there is no larger sequence that cannot be broken and in which recombination cannot occur.

***Red Blood Cell (Red Blood Corpuscle, Erythrocyte).*** The principal type of cell of vertebrate blood, responsible for the transport of oxygen from the lungs to the tissues and of carbon dioxide from the tissues to the lungs. In mammals red cells are flattened non-nucleate biconlcave discs; in all other vertebrates the nucleus is retained and the cells tend to be oval and larger. Their size varies considerably in different mammals; in man they are 7-8 μm in diameter. There are about 5000000 red blood cells in one cubic millimetre of human blood, each having a lifespan of about 120 days. Each red cell has a colloidal matrix containing a solution of the respiratory pigment haemoglobin, which is responsible for binding oxygen and carbon dioxide.

***Redifferentiation.*** Change in cellular specialization from one state of differentiation to another. It is arguable whether all cells must undergo a process of dedifferentiation before the further specialization or redifferentiation ensues. A classic case of redifferentiation is that undergone by cells of the iris following removal of the lens from amphibian eyes. Previously pigmented iris cells lose their pigment and become lens cells, changing shape and synthesizing substantial quantities of the lens-specific protein crystallin.

***Redox Potential.*** Atoms or molecules that can take part in oxidizing and reducing reactions exist in two forms: the reduced form, which can act as an electron donor, and the oxidized form, which can act as an electron acceptor. The two forms together constitute a redox couple (e.g., $Fe^{3+}$/$Fe^{2+}$; $NAD^+$/NADH; ethanal/ethanol). The redox potential of such a couple is a measuree of its tendency to donate or accept electrons from any other couple. Electrons flow from a couple having a lower (more negative) redox potential to one with a higher (more positive) potential. The redox potential is measured in volts compared with a standard hydrogen electrode whose midpoint potential is zero by definition. The redox potential of a couple when it is half oxidized and half reduced is the midpoint redox potential. If an overall redox reaction shows an imbalancee of protons then the redox potential will be affected by the pH. For convenience the midpoint redox potential measured at pH 7.0 ($E_m$) is the standard midpoint potential used for biological systems.

***Reductases.*** Enzymes that carry out a reduction.

***Refractive Index(n).*** Ratio of the velocity of light in a vacuum to that in the substance.

***Regeneration.*** Regrowth of lost tissue or organs by an organism, most frequently following injury. Such growth is very common in plants, largely because of the retention of meristematic tissue in stems, roots and leaves. Thus vegettative propagation of plants from cuttings of all three tissues is frequently possible, its ease varying with species, age, etc. Regeneration is common in lower animals, and becomes progressively less evident as complexity increases. Complete new organisms can be grown from tissue explants in many planarians, coelenterates, and other invertebrates. Crustaceans will readily regenerate legs or antennae, and amphibians and reptiles will regenerate complete limbs or tails. In mammals, however, regeneration is limited to skin wounds, repair of broken bones and regrowth of partially severed nerves. A special phenomenon—compensatory hypertrophy—takes place in some mammals when pieces or lobes of liver or pancreas are removed, involving increase by cell division of the remaining tissue to make up for the mass lost, but the actual lobe severed is not replaced. In mmany animals, regeneration is accomplished by the aggregation of undifferentiated or dedifferentiated cells into a blastema prior to the organized reassembly of the tissues or organs being replaced. A somewhat similar situation occurs in plants where the mass of undifferentiated cells is referred to as a callus.

***Regression Line.*** Line superimposed on a graph that indicates to what extent an increase or decrease in one variable will affect the increase or decrease in a second variable.

***Regressive Curve.*** Curve that expresses the change in rate of a dependent variable, with respect to an independent variable.

***Regulation.*** Ability of an organism, usually an embryo, to develop normally despite manipulative interference (e.g., transplantation or removal of cells). Regulation is therefore a compensatory mechanism which tends to permit the continuation of normal development in spite of some abnormal insult or injury.

***Regulation Egg.*** A fertilized ovum in which the direction of development of the cells of the embryo is not determined until cleavage is well adavanced. Regulation eggs can recover from early damage or disturbance to complete normal development.

***Regulative Development.*** Type of development seen in echinoderms and vertebrates in which removal of cells during cleavage, or altering cleavage planes, does not affect development.

***Regulative Egg.*** One in which the cells of the fertilized ovum retain equipotentiality during cleavage stages. Thus removal of a blastomere can be compensated for by others in regulative eggs and a blastomere isolated experimentally may in certain cirucmstances give rise to a normal individual.

***Regulator Gene.*** Gene whose function is to control the transcriptional activity of other genes, either adjacent or distant in the genome. In the case of the lac operon of E.coli the regulator gene laci produces a protein product that represses the operator gene of the operon. In bacterial regulons, the same regulator gene may affect a series of non-adjacent operons. Probably most proteins synthesized by regulator genes act by allostery. The presence of regulator genes is eukaryotes is in may situation hypothetical, although the products of genes with homeo boxes seem likely to have regulatory functions in regard to other sequences.

***Regulon.*** Complex of non-adjacent bacterial operons under the control of a common regulatory gene. The enzymes involved in arginine metabolism in E.coli arre coded by a family of genes forming a regulon, and many other bacterial pathways are similarly organized at a genetic level.

***Reichert's Membrane.*** Thin, non-cellular, freely premeable extraembryonic membrance peculiar to rodents. It is in addition to the amnion and the yolk sac found in most mammals.

***Reiter's Syndrome.*** Rare disease of humans strongly, but not absolutely, associated with the HLA antigen B27.

***Relapsing Polychondritis.*** Episodic, progressive inflammatory disease of cartilage, most frequently involving the external ears and presumed to have an immunological cause. Patients have antibodies to collagen in serum.

***Relative Fitness.*** Indication of fitness comparatively between individuals, usually by dividing the fitness of the individual being assessed by that of the most fit individual in the population.

***Relaxation Complex.*** Aggregate of three proteins responsible for converting some plasmids of E.coli from a tightly supercoiled form to a nicked open circle of DNA. Such nicking requires a stimulus (e.g.,alkali, heat treatment) and occurs at only one specific site in the plasmid DNA. On nicking, two of the proteins in the complex fall off, but the third remains covalently bound to the 5'-end of the nicked DNA. Plasmid nicking is essential for transfer during conjugation.,

***Relaxed Control.*** Situation in which the numbers of a particular plasmid present in a bacterial cell are not closely regulated by coupling of plasmid DNA synthesis to host cell DNA synthesis. In relaxed control up to 100 copies of plasmid per cell may be found; this may be further increased using chloramphenicol.

***Relaxed Mutant.*** Bacterial mutant that does not shut down RNA synthesis abruptly in a depleted growth medium.

***Relaxin.*** Mammalian polypeptide hormones synthesized in the late stages of pregnancy by ovary, uterus, or placenta. The hormone facilities temporary softening of collagen and cartilage in the pelvic ligaments, thus facilitating parturition.

***Release Factors*** (termination factors). Factors that facilitatte the release of completed polypeptide chains from the messenger RNA in the presence of a nonsense codon.

***Relict*** (Relic). Group of organisms that commonly from a small, discrete population, being the descendants of a previously much larger population. The existence of relict populations frequently follows from geographical isolation in favoured localities or refugios during ice ages.

***Rem*** (Roentgen Equivalent Man). Dose of ionizing radiations that has the same effect as one rad of X-rays.

***Renin.*** Enzyme that stimulates angiotensis formation from liver globulin and is synthesized in the kidney. It is released in increased amounts in humans suffering from high blood pressure.

***Rennin.*** Enzyme that coagulates casein in milk. It is secreted in the stomachs of young mammals.

***Reoviruses.*** Group of double-stranded RNA viruses that have been isolated from human respiratory and enteric tissues, but have not been clearly associated with any known pathology. The are therefore orphan viruses. The prefix reo- is derived from the words 'respiratory and enteric orphan'.

***Rep*** (Roentgen Equivalent Physical). Amount of ionizing radiation that results in a tissue absorption of 93 ergs per gram.

***Repair Nuclease.*** Nuclease that recognizes a DNA stand with a missing base and cleaves out the damaged nucleotide, plus some neighbouring nucleotides, allowing later repair by insertion of an undamaged sequence by DNA polymerase plus DNA ligase.

***Repair Synthesis.*** Recognition of damage in DNA, followed by its enzymic removal and replacement with the correct structure. Several different repair systems are present in both prokaryotic and eukaryotic cells to deal with damage caused by a variety of agents (e.g., ionizing radiation, ultraviolet light, chemical mutagens). Excision repair of thymine dimers involves the UvrABC endonuclease. The enzyme cuts the strand both sides of the dimer to release a 12-base pair oligonuleotide containing the lesion leaving a gap that is filled by DNA polymerase and sealed by DNA ligase. Unnatural (e.g., methylated) bases and uracil (present as a result of misincorporation, or through deamination of cytosine in situ) are removed by specific DNA glycohydrolases. The 'apurinic'or 'apyrimidinic' DNA is recognized by an AP endonuclease which cuts the strand lacking the base leaving a primer end from which DNA polymerase can initiate nick translation to replace the missing nucleotide together with a few adjacent nucleotides. Mismatch correction enzymes recognize mismatched base pairs in duplex DNA and remove a single-stranded segment containing the wrong nucleotide. The gap can then be filled in with the correctly matched sequence by DNA polymerase.

***Repetitious DNA.*** A fraction of DNA comprising nucleotide sequences that are repeated many times in the genome of any one cell. It can be subdivided into highly repetitious

DNA and moderately repetitious DNA (intermediate repetitive DNA). Highly repetitious DNA consists of sequences represented more than 1000 times per genome; many of these sequences are very short, consisting of less than 100 base pairs. Such material is concentrated in heterochromatin and, in chromosomes, is largely located at and around the centromere. Moderately repetitious DNA consists of sequences that are repeated between 10 and 1000 times per genome. This fraction of DNA reassociates at intermediate Cot values and can be isolated by DNA reassociation experiments. In consists mainly of relatively long sequence (between 1000 and 3000 bases) and there is evidence to indicate that many of these are interspersed with the so-called single-copy (or unique) sequences. Moderately repetitious DNA accounts for between 10% and 20% of the geneome of an average eukaryotic organism; it includes the genes for ribosomal and transfer RNA, structural genes for histone, and a large remaining fraction, often assumed to have a regulatory function.

***Replacement Site.*** Site within a gene sequence at which a mutation causes a change in the amino acid determined.

***Replica Plating.*** Technique by which identical patterns of bacterial colonies are transferred from one petri dish to others. It is achieved by pressing a pad of valvet on to the master plate with growing colonies and then on to a series of sterile agar-coated plates. By using media of varying compositions in the secondary replica plates, the nutritional requirements of the various colonies can be analysed simultaneously, and nutritional mutants identified and isolated.

***Replicase.*** RNA-dependent RNA polymerase, extracted from the bacteriophage Qb.

***Replicating Form*** (Y fork). Open Y formation adopted by the double helix of DNA to allow replication to occur.

***Replication.*** The process by which two molecules of DNA are formed from a parent molecule in such a way that each of the daughter molecules is identical to the parent. It involves the splitting of the double-stranded parent molecule into two single strands, each of which controls the synthesis of a new strand complementary to itself. The enzyme responsible for the synthesis of the complementary strand (a DNA polymerase) uses deoxyribonucleoside triphosphates as substrates. Because of the specificity of base pairing, the new double-stranded molecules are exact duplicates of the old. One half of the parental DNA goes to make up half of each of the daughter strands, i.e. the replication is semiconservative.

Since each newly synthezied strand of DNA has an orientated sequence of nucleotides running from a 5' end to a 3'end, and since the DNA polymerase can only utilize the template strand running from 3' to 5', it follows that one of the parent strands cannot be copied in a straightforward fashion. For this template, the polymerase molecule synthesizes short pieces of DNA termed Okazaki fragments, which are later spliced to form a continuous strand. Each new DNA sequence, including each Okazaki fragment, is primed by a very short sequence of newly synthesized RNA. This RNA is later cleaved out and the space filled in with DNA. See Figure R.5.

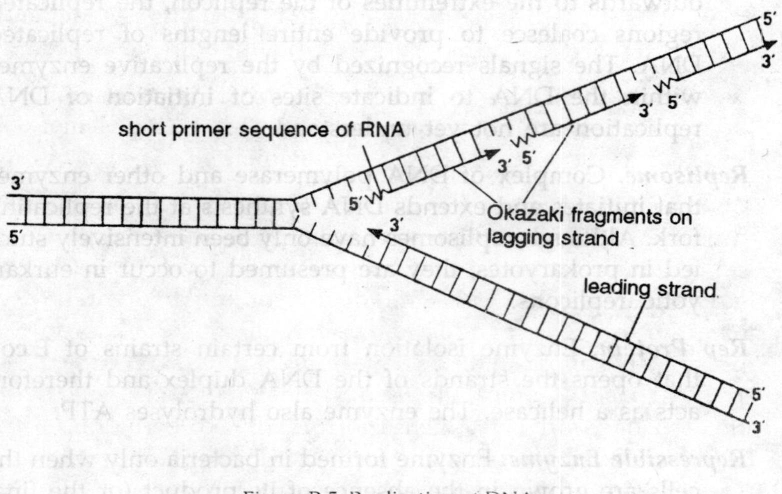


Figure R.5. Replication of DNA.

***Replication Bubble*** (Replication Eye). Open eye-like formation seen in the electron microscope when replicating DNA is visualized. The bubble results from replicating forks extending outward, flanked by regions of unreplicated DNA.

***Replication Origin.*** Site in the DNA at which a replicating fork originates. The site tends to be activated in groups of 20-80 such origins in a cluster, a so-called replication unit. The precise manner of activation and the recognition site for the rreplication origin remain unclear. Origins are usually spaced about 30,000-30,0000 bases apart.

***Replicative Forms.*** Forms of single-sranded DNA and RNA viruses at a time of replication, when they adopt a temporary double-stranded form.

***Replicon.*** Length of DNA that acts as a unit of replication during DNA synthesis. In prokaryotes the entire circular genome is a single replicon, but in eukaryotes many hundreds of replicons exist within a single chromosome length of DNA. DNA replication commences at an initiation site in the centre of the replicon, and two replicating forks extended outwards in either direction to form a temporary replication bubble. When all the bubbles have extended outwards to the extremities of the replicon, the replicated regions coalesce to provide entire lengths of replicated DNA. The signals recognized by the replicative enzymes within the DNA to indicate sites of initiation of DNA replication are not yet understood.

***Replisome.*** Complex of DNA polymerase and other enzymes that initiates and extends DNA synthesis at the replicating fork. Although replisomes have only been intensively studied in prokaryotes, they are presumed to occur in eurkaryotic replicons.

***Rep Protein.*** Enzyme isolation from certain strains of E.coli that opens the strands of the DNA duplex and therefore acts as a helicase. The enzyme also hydrolyses ATP.

***Repressible Enzyme.*** Enzyme formed in bacteria only when the cells are grown in the absence of its product (or the final product of the metabolic pathway of which the repressible enzyme is a component).

***Repression.*** Cessation of synthesis or biochemical activity due to the action of a specific factor, termed the repressor. Thus catabolite repression involves cessation of enzyme synthesis by inhibition by the product of the synthetic pathway. Transcription or translation may be repressed by specific repressor proteins interacting with the DNA or messenger RNA at specific sites.

***Repressor Molecule.*** A protein molecule that binds to a specific DNA sequence (e.g. the operator of an operon) and prevents transcription of adjoining genes.

***Repulsion.*** Situation that compares with the coupling configuration. In the repulsion situation two homologous chromosomes carry two non-allelic mutants in a configuration of (a+/+b); in other words in the trans-configuration. This cis/trans terminology is usually only applied when genes are pseudogenes.

***Rescue.*** Phenomenon in which multiple infection of cell permits recombination of phage plasmids resulting in the retention of viability, either of the cell, the virus, or some genetic or biochemical property of either.

***Residual Body.*** Secondary lysosome containing indigestible substances within cells.

***Resistance Factor*** (R plasmid). Type of plasmid that carries genes for antibiotic resistance and confers the resistant property on bacteria which carry such a factor.

***Resistance Transfer Factor (RTF).*** Plasmid carrying genes conferring antibiotic resistance. The resistance genes themselves are normally part of transposable elements, and the plasmid also carries DNA coding for its own transfer between bacterial cells.

***Resolution.*** Phenomenon whereby a lens resolves into separate images two closely adjacent structural components of a specimen. The term can be applied equally well to electron optics and to light optics.

***Resolvase.*** Enzyme that facilitates site-specific recombination between two transposons which represent direct copy repeats in a cointegrate structure.

***Resolving Power.*** Ability of a lens, in a light or electron microscope, to resolve. The resolving power of a lens is determined not simply by its magnifying power, but the wavelength of the illumination source. Thus, the shorter the wavelength, the greater the resolving power of the lens and of the microscope.

***Respiration.*** Release of energy by oxidative breakdown of energy-rich molecules, usually following the acquisition of oxygen from air (aerobic respiration).

***Respiratory Pigment.*** Coloured compound that combines reversibly with oxygen, thus increasing the oxygen transport capacity of the circulatory system. Such pigments include haemoglobin, haemerythrin, chlorocruorin and haemocyanin, some of which occur in erythrocytes in some organisms, others are free in the plasma of different organisms.

***Resting Cell.*** Cell whose nucleus is in interphase, the stages during the cell cycle when the nucleus is not undergoing mitosis or meiosis. Resting cells carry out chromosome duplication, and protein and other synthetic activity.

***Resting Potential.*** Potential difference existing across the membrane of a cell when it is not in a state of stimulation.

***Restitope.*** In antigen presentation, the part of a T cell receptor that interacts with a class II histocompatibility molecules.

***Restitution Nucleus.*** Nucleus that remains diploid at meiotic division or becomes tetraploid at mitosis due to failure of the nuclear spindle to function.

***Restriction Endonuclease (Restriction Enzyme).*** An enzyme that cuts a DNA sequence internally at a particular site with a characteristic sequence of bases. Most restriction endonucleases cut DNA at palindromic sequences, although not necessarily through the axis of symmetry. They are produced by many bacteria as protection against the foreign DNA of invading viruses. Bacteria modify their genomic

DNA by methylation to protect it from attack by the restriction enzymes. Viral DNA appearing in a bacterial cell is not methylated and is therefore degraded by the restriction endonuclease present. These enzymes are now important tools in genetic engineering.

***Restriction Endonuclease.*** Bacterial endonuclease that recognizes and binds to a short sequence of DNA; binding is followed by cleavage, either within the recognition site of elsewhere, depending on the enzyme. In addition, for each restriction activity, a bacterial strain possesses a DNA methylase that recognizes the same sequence and 'modifies' it by adding methyl groups to either adenine or cytosine residues. As a rule, the methylation blocks binding of the restriction enzyme, rendering the DNA resistant to cleavage. However, certain restriction enzymes specifically cleave only methylated sequences. In either case, the effect of the restriction-methylase activities in a bacterial strain is to provide a mechanism for degrading foreign DNA molecules, while protecting the bacterium's own DNA.

The restriction-modification systems were originally discovered by their effects on bacteriophage DNA. Phage DNA can pass from one bacterium to another within the same strain because it has the same methylation pattern as that of the host DNA. When the phage DNA enters a new bacterial strain, it is subject to attach by the host endonuclease activity. Hence, the phage tends to be 'restricted' to one strain of bacteria. However, a small fraction of the phage DNA may escape cleavage in the new host. If such DNA survives one cycle of replication, it acquires the methylation pattern of the host since it has been replicated in the presence of host methylase. These phage can now continue to replicate efficiently in the new host. The non-heritable change ( a specific methylation pattern) that confers on the phage the ability to grow on a new host is called modification.

The name of a restriction or methylation activity is derived from the first letter of the genus name and the first two letters of the species name of the bacterium (Escherichia coli = Eco; Hemophilus aegyptius = Hae); strain or type identification follows as an additional letter, which may be either lower or upper case (e.g., Bam HI). If a particular host has several different restriction-modification systems, these are identified by romal numerals (e.g., Hae I, Hae II, Hae III).

Restriction enzymes, all of which require $Mg^{2+}$, have been classified into three types. Type I restriction enzymes (EC3.1.21.3) are large and complex proteins, consisting of three types of subunit, which carry both the restriction and methylation activities. These enzymes have an absolute requirement for ATP (or dATP) and S-adenosyl-L-methikonine. They recognize bipartite asymmetrical DNA sequences (e.g., Eco B: $TGAN_8TGCT$) and cleave the DNA at sites that are probably random and at least 1,000 base pairs from the recognition site. Methylation occurs at the recognition site. Type II restriction endonucleases (EC 3.1.21.4) are relatively simple enzymes; the methylation activity is associated with a separate protein. For example, the Eco RI enzyme is a single polypeptide of 276 amino acid residues, which interacts with the recognition sequence as a dimer; the methylase is a somewhat larger polypeptide. The recognition sequences for type II enzymes are four to six (rarely eight) nucleotides long and usually, but not always, have a twofold axis of symmetry (i.e., a palindrome). The cleavage may be at the axis of symmetry, but is frequently 'straggered', yielding DNA fragments with proturding cohesive ends. For example, Eco RI makes single-stranded breaks four nucleotides apart in opposite strands, generating a 5' 'overhand', thus:

$$5'\ G^{\downarrow}AATT\ C\ 3'$$

$$3'\ C\ TTAA_{\uparrow}G\ 5'$$

The overlapping segments can associate by hydrogen bonding with other fragments having similar cohesive ends. Other type II restriction endonucleases generate protruding 3' termini; still others generate blunt-ended fragments with no cohesive ends. A few recently discovered type II restriction endonucleases (e.g., Hga I) cleave DNA at a measured short distance to one side of the asymmetric target sequence. Type III restriction enzymes (EC 3.1.21.5) consist of two different types of subunit. These enzymes require but do not hydrolyse ATP; S-adenosyl-L-methionine stimulates the reaction but is not absolutely required. Type III enzymes cleave the DNA 24-26 base pairs 3' to the recognition sequence. Type II, but not types I or III, restriction endonuclease are extensively used in recombinant DNA technology.

***Restriction Fragments.*** Products of the complete digestion of a chosen target DNA with a restriction endonuclease. Fragments are flanked by the specific reognition sites for that restriction endonuclease.

***Restriction Fragment Length Polymorphism (RFLP).*** Polymorphism in the genome that is detected by comparing restriction maps of DNAs from different individuals. Variations in positions of restriction sites (ie., sites where restriction endonucleases cleave the DNA) may be detected as differences in lengths of restriction fragments, as revealed by southern blotting with suitable molecular hybridization probes. It is possible to find such polymorphisms in any type of DNA sequence (e.g., exons, introns, flanking sequences). The DNA sequence variations detected by this procedure display Mendelian inheritance and can be used as genetic markers in linkage studies. RFLPs are used in family studies to provide markers linked to defective genes that cause inherited diseases.

***Restriction Map.*** Map of a DNA sequence indicating the sites of cutting of one or more restriction endonucleases. Since enzymes are very specific in their cutting characteristics, such a map can be predicted from a known DNA base sequence.

***Restriction Mapping.*** Technique of ordering type II restriction endonuclease cleavage sites on a DNA fragment. Restriction maps are usually constructed by complete digestion of a target molecule with a number of different restriction endonucleases. Sequential complete digests allow the relative position of different restriction sites to be determined. Restriction fragments produced in such analyses are then sized by electrophoresis using agarose gel. In this system the mobility of DNA fragments within defined size ranges is proportioned to the $\log_{10} M_r$. The use of DNA standards of known molecular weight allows the construction of calibration curves from which the size of unknown restriction fragments can be determined. The diagram shows how a simple restriction map may be constructed. See Figure R.6.

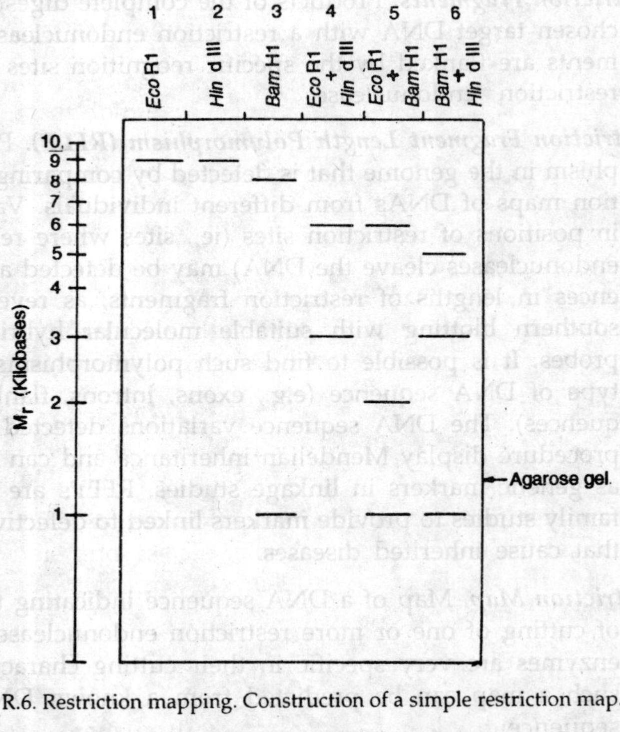


Figure R.6. Restriction mapping. Construction of a simple restriction map.

***Restriction Mapping.*** Localization of the positions of restriction endonuclease cleavage sites on a DNA molecule. The DNA is digested with one or a combination of restriction endonucleases, the fragments are separated by gel electrophoresis, and their sizes are determined by comparing their mobilities with those of DNA fragments of known size. The fragments in the gel can be visualized either by staining with ethidium bromide or, for end-labeled fragments, by autoradiography. It is often useful to start with an end-labeled fragment and carry out partial digestion so that, on average, only one cleavage occurs per molecule. From the sizes of the various fragments, the positions of the restriction sites can be deduced; e.g., the difference in size between a pair of adjacent fragments on the gel corresponds to the distance between neighbouring sites.

***Reticular Dysgenesis.*** Very rare form of severe combined immunodeficiency in newborns characterized by profound T lymphocyte and B lymphocyte deficiencies and an absnece of neutrophils. The syndrome results in rapid death of affected infants, unless they are salvaged with a transplant of bone marow. Reticular dysgenesis is inherited as an autosomal recessive.

***Reticulocyte.*** Immature red blood cell that is an intermediate between an erythroblast and an erythrocyte. Reticulocytes are so-called because they retain a faintly staining cytoplasmic reticulum, the remains of the earlier endoplasmic reticulum of the erythroblast. In the human the reticulocyte has already lost its nucleus, but in some animals (e.g., fish, amphibians, reptiles, birds) it is nucleated cell.

***Reticuloendothelial Blockade.*** Reduction in the rate of clearance of particles injected into the circulation as a result of previous administration of particles (e.g., colloidal gold) that have an affinity for, or are taken up my, macrophages of the liver and spleen.

***Reticuloendothelial System (RES).*** Cells capable of taking up vital dyes and particles. The term was originally used to include a variety of cells that are highly active in endocytosis and/or phagocytosis (e.g., macrophages) or less active (e.g., fibroblasts and endothelial cells). The major function of the RES- the clearance of particles from the blood- is carried out by macrophages in the liver and, to a lesser extent, in the spleen. The activity of the RES can be measured by the rate of elimination of radiolabeled albumin or of [$^{51}$Cr]-labeled red blood cells, sensitized with antibodies.

***Reticuloendothelial System (RES).*** Macrophage cells of vertebrate spleen, liver and bone marrow. The cells capture particulate material such as dead cells, bacteria and viruses from blod and plasma.

*Retinal* (Retinene). Carotenoid pigment derived from vitamin A, of which it is an aldehyde; it is light-absorbing, and combines with opsin to form rhodopsin, the light-sensitive compound in the rods of the optic retina.

***Retinitis Pigmentosa.*** Single gene disorder in humans in which clumps of retinal pigment cause progressive visual loss. There are both X-linked and autosomal genes involved in different forms, with an overall prevalence of about one in 5000.

***Retinoblastoma.*** Malignant tumour of retinoblast—epithelial neurological cells from the retina of the eye—occurring exclusively in children. It is a celebrated example of autosomal dominant inheritance of a tumour. Retinoblastomas are amenable to treatment by surgery and irradiation.

***Retroregulation.*** Ability of a sequence downstream from a coding sequence to affect the translation of parts of a messenger RNA molecule upstream from it.

***Retroviruses*** (Leucoviruses). Group of single-stranded RNA viruses that are characterized by their possessing reverse transcriptase, which transcribes the RNA genome into DNA during the replicative cycle. The transcribed viral DNA is then integrated into the host cell DNA and is replicated with it. The genomes of most retroviruses consist of a set of four genes: gag, which codes for the capsid protein of the virus; pol, which codes for the reverse transcriptase; env, which codes for a protein forming spikes on the outer envelope; onc, which is an oncogene. Many retroviruses are oncogenic, owing this property to the possession of oncogenes. Closely related sequences that are present in cellular genomes and code for normal proteins are termed proto-oncogenes. The termini of the retroviral genome consists of repeat sequences, which facilitate the integration of the retroviral DNA into the genome of the host cell. Retroviruses include rous sarcoma virus, mouse leukaemia viruses such as malony leukaemia virus, mouse mammary tumour viruses such as bittner mouse milk factor virus, feline leukaemia viruses, and the human HTLV viruses including the AIDS virus. Retroviruses have, in the past, been known as leucoviruses or oncornaviruses. See Figure R.7.

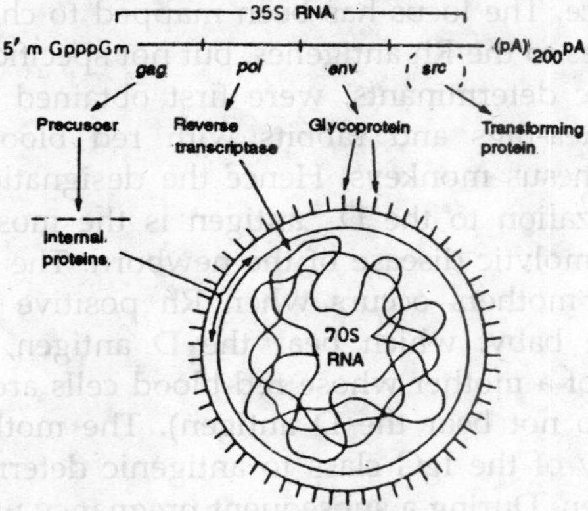


Figure R.7. Retroviruses.

*Reverse Mutation* (Reversion). Second mutation in a mutant gene which restores the sequence to that of the wild-type allele and thus permits the production of a functional product.

*Reverse Selection.* Artificial selection that reverses the trend of a previous selection pressure.

*Reverse Transcriptase (RNA-dependent DNA polymerase).* An enzyme that directs the synthesis of DNA from an RNA template (reverse transcription). It is found in certain RNA viruses, such as the Rous sarcoma virus, that replicate by means of a DNA intermediate called the provirus. This enzyme is widely used in genetic engineering technology to produce complementary DNA (cDNA) from a purified preparation of a specific messenger RNA.

*Revertant.* Allele that is the result of a reverse mutation or the organism carrying such a gene.

***Rh Blood Group.*** Antigenic determinants of human red blood cells detected by alloantibodies, usually obtained from women who have had a child with hemolytic disease of the newborn. The Rh alloantigens are proteins, which have not yet been biochemically characterized. The Rh locus is thought to consist of three closely linked pairs of alleles: Dd, Cc and Ee. In Caucasians the most common linkage groups are DCe and dce. The locus has been mapped to chromosome 1. Antibodies to the Rh antigenes, but not specifically to the alloantigenic determinants, were first obtained by immunizing guinea-pigs and rabbits with red blood cells of Macaccus rhesus monkeys. Hence the designation Rh. Rh alloimmunization to the D antigen is the most frequent cause of hemolytic disease of the newborn. The alloimmunization of mothers occurs when Rh positive red blood cells of the baby, which bear the D antigen, enter the circulation of a mother whose red blood cells are Rh negative (i.e., do not bear the D antigen). The mother makes alloantibody of the IgG class to antigenic determinants of the D antigen. During a subsequent pregnancy with an Rh-positive baby the alloantibodies, which cross the placenta, cause hemolysis of the baby's red blood cells. Alloimmunization can be prevented by administration of $Rh_o$(D) immune globulin in women whose red blood cells are Rh-negative and who have just given birth to a baby whose red blood cells are Rh-positive.

***Rhesus Factor*** (Rh Factor). Antigen carried on the erythrocytes of certain humans that is responsible for the problems of rhesus incompatibility involved in the rhesus system.

***Rhesus System.*** Isoantigens present on erythrocytes and important in erythroblastosis foetalis. According to the Fisher and Race theory followed in England the system consists of five antigenic determinants (D, C, E, c and e) which are the products of genes at three distinct, but closely linked chromosomal loci, with the D antigen being important clinically. A second theory by Wiener and followed in the USA holds that one locus is responsible for production of several antigenic determinants leading to the notation RH rh′, rh″, hr′ and hr″ and corresponding respectively to D, C, E, c and e.

***Rheumatoid Arthritis.*** Common disease of humans affecting about one in 50 of western populations. There is a weak hereditary element and some association with specific HLA antigens.

***Rheumatoid Arthritis (RA).*** Chronic disease presumed to have an immunological cause and characterized by symmetrical multiple joint swellings, particularly of the fingers and writsts. The disease tends to wax and wane in severity. The synovial membranes are infiltrated with neutrophils, macrophages, lymphocytes and plasma cells. Eventually, vascular graulation tissue, called a pannus, forms and erodes the cartilage of the joint, causing deformities. The disease is two to three times more common in women than in men. Rheumatoid factor occurs in approximately 70 percent of patients. The cause of rheumatoid arthritis is not known.

***Rheumatoid Factor.*** Autoantibody to IgG or IgA, usually of the IgM class, found most frequently in serum of patients with rheumatoid arthritis. These autoantibodies may be monoclonal or polyclonal. To detect rheumatoid factors, particles, usually of latex, are coated with IgG or IgA and their agglutination by test serum in measured. The different reactivities of various individual rheumatoid factors define human allotypic determinants (e.g., Gm, Am and Km allotypic determinants).

***Rheumatoid Nodule.*** Subcutaneous nodule in a patient with rheumatoid arthritis that usually forms at pressure points such as the elbow. Microscopically, the nodule has a central area of necrosis surrounded by palisading connective tissue cells and an outer mantle of infiltrates of lymphocytes.

***Rhizobium.*** Genus of symbiotic bacteria that live in root nodules of leguminous plants and facilitate the fixation of atmospheric nitrogen.

***Rhizopoda.*** Phylum to which the protozoan such as Amoeba belong.

***Rhodamine.*** Red fluorescent dye often employed as a fluoresent marker when conjugated to protein.

***Rhodoplast.*** Red plastid found in the red algae, the Rhodopyta.

***Rhodopsin (Visual Purple).*** The light-sensitive pigment of vertebrate rod cells, composed of retinal, the aldehyde of vitamin A, attached to a protein, opsin. Light initiates a series of reactions leading to separation of retinal from opsin, which initiates nervous activity in the rod. The bleached pigment is reconstituted in the dark. Adaptation to low levels of illumination is aided by increase in the amount of pigment.

***$Rh_o$(D) Immune Globulin.*** Preparation of human immune serum globulin from donors who have been hyperimmunized to the $Rh_o$(D) antigen. It contains sufficient antibodies to suppress an immune response to 15 ml of packed $Rh_o$(D)-kpositive erythrocytes. It is given within 72 hours after delivery to prevent alloimmunization of Rh-negative women by Rh-positive red blood cells from the baby.

***Rho Factor*** (ρ factor). Hexameric protein (monomer $M_r$ = 55000) involved in transcription termination in prokaryotes. It binds tightly to RNA (but not to DNA or to RNA polymerase), and when bound hydrolyses nucleoside triphophates (NTPs) to nucleoside diphosphates. A model for rho action supposes it to move along the RNA transcript (using the energy provided by hydrolysis of NTPs) until it meets and releases RNA polymerase stopped at a terminator site on the DNA template.

***Rhyzoid.*** Cellular filament found in some algae and bryophytes, and used to secure the plant to the substratum.

***Riboflavin (vitamin $B_2$).*** An essential nutritional factor for mammals that forms part of the vitamin B complex. It is obtained from green vegetables, yeast, milk, liver, etc. Riboflavin was first detected in 1879 by Blyth and its structure was determined by synthesis in 1935 by Kuhn,

Karrer, and others. Riboflavin is essential for carbohydrate metabolism, functioning as a precursor of the coenzymes FMN and FAD. See Figure R.8.

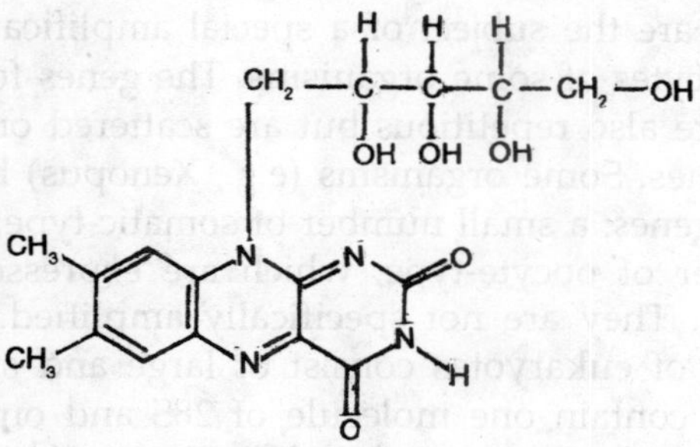


Figure R.8. Riboflavin.

***Ribonucleoprotein (RNP).*** Complex of RNA and protein. Particles of RNA occur in both nuclei and cytoplasm of eukaryotic cells, and are formed in order to protect RNA from degradation and probably also to assist in its transport and localization within the cell.

***Ribonucleotide.*** Compound consisting of a purine or pyrimidine base bound to a ribose sugar, which is itself bound to a phosphate group. RNA is a polymer of such units.

***Ribose.*** Five-carbon sugar ($C_5H_{10}O_5$), the dextrorotatory form of which (D-ribose) is used in the formation of ribonucleotides and RNA.

***Ribosomal Cistron.*** Gene coding for ribosomal RNA.

***Ribosomal Protein.*** Protein used in the formation of ribosomes in which each molecule of RNA is associated with up to 30 molecules of small protein molecules, most of which are distinct proteins.

***Ribosomal RNA*** (rRNA). RNA that is used in the composition of ribosomes. Such RNA consists of four distinct classes in eukaryotic cells, designated as 28S, 18S, 5.8S and 5S according to their sedimentation coefficients. The genes for the first three occur as tandem repeats in the nucleolar-organizing centre of the genome, the numbers of such repeats being as high as 450 in Xenopus and 250 in Homo. Initial transcription products from these repeats consists of a 45S precursor RNA which is processed to yield three distinct RNA molecules. The 5.8S RNA molecule is later hydrogen bonded with the 28S. These genes for the large ribosomal RNAs are the subject of a special amplification process in the oocytes of some organisms. The genes for the 5S molecule are also repetitious but are scattered on various chromosomes. Some organisms (e.g., Xenopus) have two types of 5S genes: a small number of somatic-type; a much larger number of oocyte-type, which are expressed only in the oocyte. They are not specifically amplified. The 80S ribosomes of eukaryotes consist of large and small sub-units, which contain one molecule of 28S and one of 18S RNA, respectively. Bacterial cells have large ribosomal RNAs of 23S and 16S, plus a 5S, and have only seven copies of each gene coding for these molecules. Mitochondria have ribosomal RNAs of 23S and 19S and some plants have 25S and 16S RNAs.

rRNA is synthesized from the ribosomal genes by the action of RNA polymerase, the type I enzyme being responsible for synthesis of the larger molecules and the type III enzyme for the 5S molecules.

***Ribosome.*** A particle consisting of roughly equal amounts of RNA and protein (i.e. a ribonucleoprotein particle), many of which (up to several million) occur in virtually all living cells and are the sites of protein synthesis. Two types of ribosome are recognized, according to their S values (rate of sedimentation in a centrifuge). Both types consist of two subunits. The prokaryote type is 70S (with 50S and 30S subunits) and about 18 nm in diameter. This type is also found in chloroplasts and mitochondria of eukaryotes. The eukaryote type is 80S (60S and 40S subunits) and about 22 nm in diameter. It is found in the cytoplasm, though its RNA is made in the nucleolus. The RNA molecules of ribosomes have characteristic sizes and base composotions and are called ribosomal RNA (rRNA). During protein synthesis ribosomes associate with messenger RNA (mRNA), usually forming polysomes (polyribosomes). Each polysome is a single mRNA molecule in the process of translation by a variable number of ribosomes arranged along its length like beads on a string. Polysomes occur either free in the cytoplasm or bound to the surface of the endoplasmic reticulum (ER) or outer membrane of the nucleus (usually adopting spiral forms in the latter case). Proteins from free ribosomes are released into the hyaloplasm but those from membrane-bound ribosomes are usually passed into the ER cisternae to be later secreted or otherwise transported.

***Rickettsiae.*** A group of obligate interacellular prokaryotic parasites of fleas, lice, ticks, and mites. They are similar in structure to bacteria (for example, their cell walls contain mucopeptide, a substance characteristic of bacterial cell walls), but they can multiply only within their arthropod hosts and aree therefore considered to be intermediate between bacteria and viruses. In arthropods they produce no ill effects; however, if they are transmitted to mammals, including man, by a bite of the artthropod host they cause severe, sometimes fatal, disease,Rickettsial diseases of man include typhus, Rocky Mountain spotted fever, and Q fever.

The group takes its name from the principal genus, Rickeettsia, which was named after H. T.Ricketts (1871-1910), an American pathologist who died of typhus while investigating the cause of the disease.

***Ricin.*** Highly potent toxin from the seeds of Ricinus communis plants. It is a heterodimer, in which each chain- A and B - has an $M_r$ of 30,000. The B chain is responsible for binding to cells and the A chain is responsible for cytotoxicity. The B chain binds to galactosyl residues on the cell surface, enabling the molecule to enter the cell in endocytic vesicles. The A chain then dissociates from the B chain, reaches the cytosol, binds to ribosomes and inhibits protein synthesis. Ricin or its A chain, coupled to an antibody, can be used in immunotoxins.

***Rifampicin*** (rifampin). Antibiotic that inhibits RNA synthesis. Rifampicin, a derivative of rifamycin SV, specifically inhibits DNA-dependent bacierial and chloroplast, but not mamalian RNA polymerase. It is also reported to inhibit the assembly of DNA and protein into mature virus particles.

***Rifamycin.*** Antibiotic that inhibits RNA synthesis by binding to RNA polymerase and blocking the initiation of RNA chains. The activity is limited to prokaryote RNA polymerase.

***Right Bivalent.*** Chromosomal configuration resudlting from terminal chiasma in both arms of a meiotic chromosome.

***Ring Chromosome.*** (1) Abnormal chromosome where both arms are joined to form a ring structure. (2) Association of metacentric tetrads of chromosomes which forms a temporary ring structure.

***Ringer's Solution.*** An aqueous solution of calcium, sodium, and potassium chlorides, used as a medium for living cells or tissues undergoing in vitro investigations. It is named after the 19th-century physiologist Sidney Ringer. Sometimes other salts are added, in order to mimic closely the natural surroundings of the cells in vivo. The solution must be isotonic with the cells and at the correct pH. To achieve this it must be buffered with bicarbonate or phosphate. The resulting solution is often also known as physiological saline. It is now known that virtually all tissues can be kept alive at least for a time in such a solution.

***Ring-porous.*** Designating wood with most of the vessels aggregated in the early wood.

***Ring Species.*** Two or more species that do not interbreed where their ranges overlap but are connected by a ring of subspecies between which breeding can occur. For example, Larus argentatus (herring gull) and L.fuscus (lesser black-backed gull) behave as good species in western Europe where their ranges overlap. However there are subspecies of L.argentatus in North America and of L.fuscus in Siberia that interbreed with each other as well as with members of their own species. They thus form a circumpolar chain linking the two good species.

***Ring Test.*** Qualitative test for detecting, by precipitation, the presence of antigens or antibodies. A solution containing antibodies (or antigen) is layered on top of a solution containing antigen (or antibodies) without mixing the two solutions. If the complementary reactants are present, a precipitate forms at the interface. The test, which can be carried out in test tubes or capillary tubes, is a simple way to establish the presence of a precipitating antigen-antibody system.

***Ritualization.*** The process, in the course of the evolution of animal behaviour, in which activities of one individual (often displacement activities) come to cause a certain response in another individual of the same species. It is particularly evident in courtship displays; for example, the courtship of the great crested grebe shows elements of nest-building behaviour, which have evolved by ritualization.

***R-loop.*** A region in a DNA double helix where one DNA strand has become displaced and paired with a complementary RNA strand instread of its DNA partner. See Figure R.9.

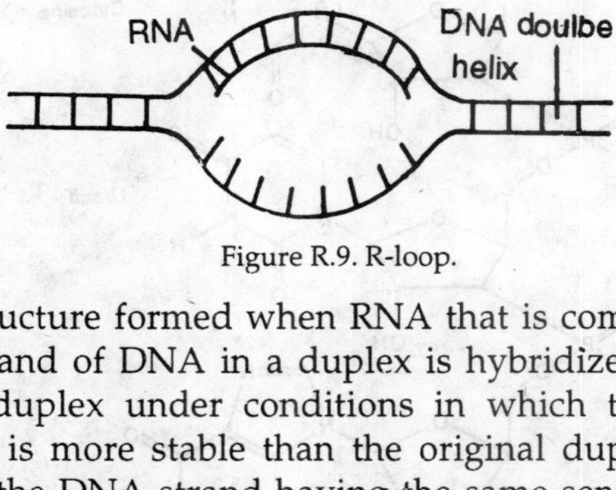


Figure R.9. R-loop.

***R-loop.*** Structure formed when RNA that is complementary to one strand of DNA in a duplex is hybridized to the denatured duplex under conditions in which the RNA-DNA hybrid is more stable than the original duplex. RNA displaces the DNA strand having the same sense and forms a double-stranded hybrid with the complementary DNA strand. This structure: an RNA-DNA hybrid and a displaced DNA strand form a loop (the R-loop), which can be detected by electron microscopy. When a gene containing an intron is hybridized with the corresponding mRNA, the DNA of the intron is not complementary to any part of the mRNA and is extruded as a double-stranded loop between two adjacent R-loops. This technique has been used to show that the coding sequences of many eukaryotic (e.g., immunoglobulin) genes are interrupted by introns.

***RNA (Ribonucleic Acid).*** A nucleic acid that serves as the genetic material of some viruses and has many important roles as an intermediate molecule in protein synthesis. An RNA molecule normally consists of a single strand of nucleotides, each consisting of the sugar ribose (which replaces the deoxyribose of DNA) and phosphoric acid with one of four nitrogenous bases: adenine, guanine, cytosine, or uracil. Uracil is the only base that occurs in RNA, but not in DNA: in the sequence arrangement of RNA it is analogous to the thymine of DNA.

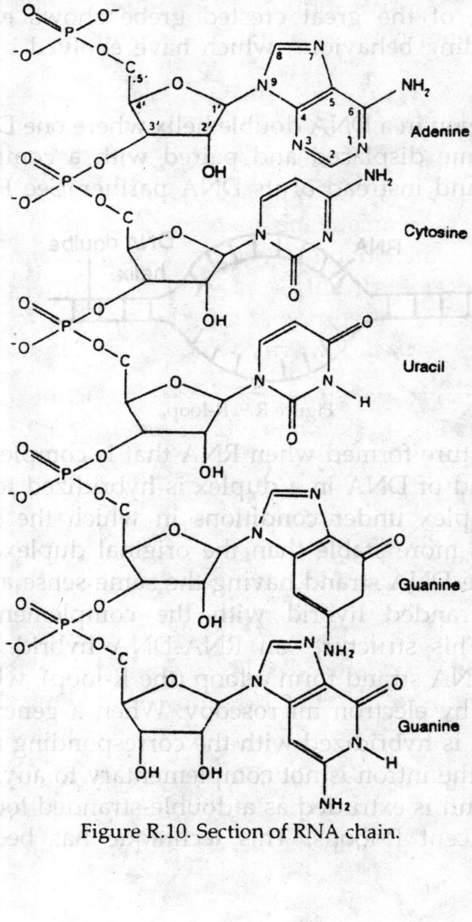


Figure R.10. Section of RNA chain.

Some forms of RNA can fold into double-stranded regions of complementary base pairs, but more RNA molecules are substantially single-stranded and are not base paired. The chief types of RNA found in cells are the heterogenous nuclear RNA (HnRNA), which is the immediate transcription product of the structural genes; messenger RNA, which is produced from HnRNA; ribosomal RNA (rRNA), which, together with ribosomal protein, forms the ribosomes; and transfer RNA, which is responsible for carrying specific amino acid molecules to the messenger RNA on the ribosome during protein synthesis.

Although RNA is normally the product of transcription from the template molecule DNA, in some viruses DNA can be synthesized from an RNA template by the action of reverse transcriptase. See Figure R.10.

***RNA-directed DNA Polymerase*** (reverse transcriptase; EC 2.1.7.7.49). DNA polymerase found in retroviruses (e.g., Rous sarcoma virus, avian myeloblastosis virus (AMV), human immunodeficiency virus (HIV) that can synthesize DNA from an RNA template. It requires a primer with a free 3'-hydroxyl group, which is base-paired with the template. The product of the reaction is a DNA-RNA hybrid. Despite its name, the enzyme also catalyses DNA synthesis from a DNA template. The reverse transcriptase molecule also carries a ribonuclease H activity, which selectively degrades the RNA strands in DNA-RNA hybrids (therefore lthe designation H) in either the 5'—>3' or 3'—>5' direction.

The polymerase (pol) from AMV is derived from a larger precursor polyprotein (gag-pol); it consists of two subunits, alpha ($M_r$ 60,000) and beta ($M_r$ 92,000). The alpha subunit is generated by proteolytic cleavage of some of the beta subunits. The alpha subunit carries the polymerase as well as the ribonuclease H activity, the latter activity being associated with a $M_r$ 24,000 domain that is probably derived from the carboxy-terminal portion of the chain. The remaining $M_r$ 32,000 fragment of the beta subunit is a DNA endonuclease.

Reverse transcriptase is an important enzyme in recombinant DNA procedures as it is used for first-strand synthesis of cDNA. That from AMV is used most commonly. The enzyme can also be used in a 'filling reaction' to label the ends of DNA fragments having protruding 5'ends.

***RNase (ribonuclease).*** Any of various enzymes that degrade RNA by hydrolysing the phosphodiester bonds in the sugar-phosphate backbone. Many attack only specific structures (e.g. RNase T attacks only the ends of hairpin loops, such as those in transfer RNA molecules) and so yield specific RNA fragments that can be used for fingerprinting.

***RNA Splicing.*** Excision of specific segments from a primary RNA transcript and subsequent ligation of the resulting non-contiguous segments to form a mature RNA molecule (tRNA, rRNA or mRNA). Splicing reactions occur in the cell nucleus (or mitochondrion or chloroplast) and are extremely precise. In the formation of mRNA of higher eukaryotes, the introns that are spliced out most always begin with the dinucleotide GU and end with the dinudeotide AG. An additional sequence, located 20-50 base pairs upstream of the 3' splice site also appears to play a role in the splicing reaction. Typically, before splicing, the RNA is capped (addition of 7-methylguanylate and, usually, methylation of one or two terminal riboses) at the 5' end and polyadenylated at the 3' end. Small nuclear ribonucleoprotein particles (snRNPs) appear to be required for the splicing of mRNA precursors. (Antibodies to these particles are found in some patients with autoimmune disease such as systemic lupus erythematosus). Sometimes, a primary transcript can be processed in more than one way to yield two or more different mature mRNAs (alternative splicing). This can occur by choice of different splice sites (e.g. as in synthesis of related forms of class I histocompatibility molecules, fibronectin and some viral proteins) or by completition between polyadenylation and splicing (as in the processing of immunoglobulin heavy chain transcripts that give rise to secreted and membrane forms of the protein).

***RNA-coding Triplets.*** Triplets found on mRNA that code for the amino acids, the code being recognized by the anti-codon present on the molecule of tRNA changed with the specific amino acid.

***RNA-coding Triplets.*** Triplets reverse transcriptase.

***RNA-driven Hybridization.*** Competition hybridization in which a small amount of single-stranded DNA competes with a large excess of RNA for the complementary sequences.

***RNA Ligase.*** Enzyme that joints RNA molecules by the formation of phospodiester bonds between 5'-phosphate and 3'-hydroxyl ends.

***RNA Phages.*** Series of bacteriophages that have RNA as genomic material (e.g., Qb and MS2).

***RNA Polymerases*** (DNA-dependent RNA polymerases, transcriptases). Group of enzymes for catalysing the synthesis of RNA from a DNA template (sense strand). Bacteria possess only a single type of RNA polymerase, but eukaryotic cells possess at least four. They are designated: type I (pol I), which is responsible for synthesis of ribosomal RNA (except 5S RNA); type II (pol II), which is responsible for synthesis of messenger RNA (and its precursor, heterogeneous nuclear RNA); type III (pol III), which is responsible for synthesis of transfer RNA and the small ribosomal 5S RNA; type IV, which is the RNA polymerase of the mitochondria. RNA polymerases are sensitive to various antibiotics: for example, pol II is sensitive to α-amanitin and pol I to actinomycin D. Since a single species of RNA polymerase is responsible for synthesis of all messenger RNA, the specificity of gene expression is clearly not determined by the polymerase enzyme, but since the promoter sequence upstream of the initiation site of the coding sequence is recognized by the enzyme, differences in the sequence of the promoter between different genes will affect transcription rates.

RNA polymerases are complex proteins. The bacterial enzyme consists of a core enzyme comprising α-, β– and β'-

subunits, and a sigma factor, which recognizes the pribnow box.

***RNA Primase.*** Enzyme that synthesizes the short primer RNA of about 10 nucleotides that is elongated by DNA polymerase to form an okazaki fragment of DNA during DNA replication. The leading strand of DNA is presumed also to be initiated by such a primer.

***RNA Replicase*** (RNA-dependent RNA polymerase). Enzyme found in certain RNA phages (e.g., MS2).

***RNases*** (Ribonucleases). Enzymes that degrade RNA. Distinct forms which are extensively used or analysied include RNase A, which attacks the phosphate linkages of pyrimidines internally located in an RNA, RNase P which cleaves bacterial tRNA precursor to yield mature tRNA, and RNase T1 which specifically cleaves the phosphate groups of internal guanosine residues.

***RNA Splicing.*** In vivo phenomenon by which exon sequences are joined following intron removal. Although snRNA molecules are believed to be involved, the mechanism of RNA splicing remains unclear.

***Rod Cell.*** Cell forming a rod of the vertebrate eye. Rod cells are capable of producing a measurable electrical signal in response to even a single photon of light.

***Rocket Immunoelectrophoresis.*** Quantitative test to determine the concentration of an antigen in a test sample (usually serum). One of the reactants (usually antiserum) is incorporated into an agarose gel; wells cut into the gel are filled with the second reactant (usually antigen). An electric current is applied so that the antigen migrates into the gel. The area of the resulting rocket-shaped zone of precipitation is proportional to the concentration of antigen. By comparison with a set of antigen strandards, the concentration of antigen added to the well can be determined. Provided that the antiserum is specific, the antigen need not be pure. The major advantage of this technique, compared to single radial immunodiffusion, is speed; the migration of antigen into the gel is completed in hours instead of days.

*Roentgen.* Amount of ionizing radiation that release 2.083 x $10^9$ ion pairs per millilitre of air at a pressure of 760 mmHg and 0°C. If one gram of tissue is exposed to one roentgen of gamma-radiation it absorbed 93 ergs.

*Rogue* (sport). Deviant specimen occurring in a population of relatively standardized individuals. The term is most often used in relation to crop plants where a few plants may show phenotypic characteristics with involve expression of undesirable recessive genes.

*Rolling Circle.* Method by which some types of circular DNA molecules (e.g. fX174) are replicated. One of the two strands of native DNA is nicked and the free 5'-end attached to a stable support such as an internal cell membrane. DNA polymerase uses the free 3'-end as a primer and then copies the second (unnicked) strand, during the course of which the nicked strand unravels and the intact one rolls along it away from the fixed attachment point.

*Root Hair.* Outgrowth from an epidermal cell in the root, thereby increasing the surface area of the root. Root hairs occur in a part of the root behind the region of root extension, known as the piliferous layer. Root hairs make close contact with the soil particles and are responsible for the absorprtion of water and solutes.

*Root Nodule.* Growth that develops on the roots of certain plants in response to infection by symbiotic microorganisms. Root nodules on leguminous plants result from infection with Rhizobium and in these nodules nitrogen fixation occurs. Nitrogen-fixing nodules also occur on the roots of a few species from other families, but these develop in response to other microorganisms.

*Rosette.* Cluster resembling a rose, such as is formed by erythrocytes (E) adhering to CD2 on T lymphocytes (i.e., E-rosette) or by sensitized erythrocytes to Fc receptors or complement receptors of neutrophils.

***Rot.*** The product of RNA concentration ($R_o$) and incubation time (t) in an RNA-driven hybridization reaction. When a small amount of single-stranded DNA is hybridized with a large amount of RNA, the Rot value is a measure of the amount of RNA complementary to the DNA probe.

***Rot.*** Expression representing the hybridization of RNA at a given concentration following a specific incubation time, in an RNA-driven hybridization reaction. It is the analogue of the cot value in DNA-driven hybridization reactions.

***Rough Endoplasmic Reticulum (RER).*** Rough-surfaced endoplasmic reticulum found in most eykaryotic cells, and especially concentrated in highly secretory cells of pancreas and other tissues. It consists of membranes of endoplasmic reticulum densely studded with ribosomes and is the main site of protein synthetic activity in the cell. See Figure R.11.

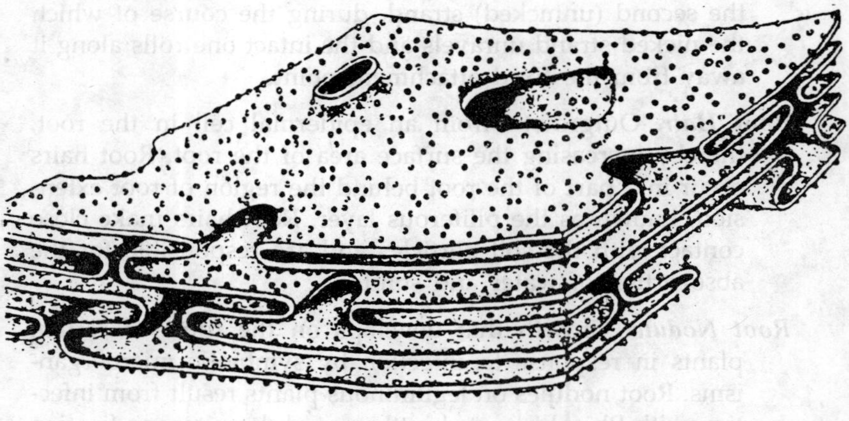

Figure R.11. Rough endoplasmic reticulum. Three-dimensional representation of the rough endoplasmic reticulum.

***Rous Sarcoma Virus (RSV).*** Retrovirus discovered by Peyton Rous in the chicken. The oncogene of this virus is the src gene.

***Royal Jelly.*** Secretion produced from salivary glands by nurse worker honey bees, and used to feed larvae destined to be queens. It contains 40 percent dry matter including lipoproteins, free fatty acids, glycerides, sugar, amino acids and all B vitamins. High contents of acetylcholine (1mg/g), pantothenic acid, folic acid and biopterine are found in royal jelly. Larvae destined to be workers receive much less royal jelly and are fed mainly with pollen and honey. The nature of the queen-determining factor is not known, although the relatively high amounts of protein in royal jelly (compared with mainly carbohydrate worker larvae food) has been suggested.

***rpm*** (revolutions per minute). Indication of the speed of a centrifuge rotor. The more useful expression is that of g (i.e., the number of times the gravitational force), since this can be precisely repeated experimentally in centrifuges of different size or manufacture.

***Rubella*** (German measles). Human disease that is caused by a virus and involves relatively slight illness in affected patients. However, it results in serious teratogenic effects in pregnant women especially it encountered in the first four weeks of pregnancy.

***Ruffing.*** Throwing of the 'dorsal' or uppermost cell surface into a series of undulations (i.e. ruffles) during tissue cell locomotion in culture. They are initially formed at motile areas of the cell margin (lamellipodia) and appear to move backwards over the cell. Such ruffles are not a causal component in cell locomotion in vitro, but simply a consequence of the typically flattened phenotype presented by cultured cells.

***Runting Disease.*** Condition in which young experimental animals fail to thrive following injection of cells that cause a graftversus-host reaction.

***Russell Body.*** Globular mass in the endoplasmicreticulum of normal plasma cells or myeloma cells. Russell bodies are composed of immunoglobulins and stain with eosin.

***Rusts.*** A group of parasitic basidiomycete fungi belonging to the order Uredinales, many of which attack plants of agricultural importance, including the Gramineae (grasses). The life cycle is typically as follows. A basidiospore infects the secondary host, such as Berberis vulgaris (barberry) for

Puccinia graminis, to produce a mycelium with one nucleus per cell. This produces spermogonia, which results in the formation of a dikaryotic mycelium. This then produces aecidiospores which infect the primary host, such as a grain crop, and form a dikaryotic mycelium in it. This mycelium produces uredospores (or brand spores), in the early part of the season, for dissemination, and later two-celled teleutospores. The latter act as the resting stage of the life cycle, germinating the following season to produce basidiospores.

***Ruthenium Red.*** Compound that inhibits calcium ion transport into mitochondria.

# S

***4S RNA.*** Transfer RNA (tRNA) which sediments as a 4S particle.

***5S RNA.*** Species of small ribosomal RNA, of 120 nucleotides, one molecule of which is included in the larger of the two ribosomal subunits. Transcription of the 5S genes is quite independent of the nucleolar group of 28S, 18S and 5.8S genes. They are present as multiple copies and are located near to the ends of chromosome arms. These genes are not specifically amplified, as are the 28S and 18S genes. Two distinct species of 5S occur in many vertebrates: oocyte-species 5S and somatic 5S. The former are active only in the oocyte, the latter in the oocyte and all stages of development.

***5.8S RNA.*** Small 120 nucleotide molecule that is part of the initial transcript from the large ribosomal genes located in tandem array in the nucleolar chromatin. The 5.8S molecule, following transcription and processing, is hydrogen-bonded to the 28S rRNA.

**$^{35}$*S.*** Radioactive isotope of sulphur with a half-life of 81 days and decaying with the emission of a beta-particle. It is commonly used to label proteins by using the sulphur-containing amino acids methionine and cysteine.

***S*˙** (1) Svedberg unit. (2) Symbol for sulphur. (3) Phase of the cell cycle in which DNA replication occurs.

***S.*** (1) Sedimentation coefficient. (2) Standard deviation. (3) selection coefficient.

***$S_1$, $S_2$, $S_3$, etc.*** Indicating successive generations of self-fertilized plants, each subsequent generation being again self-fertilized.

***S1 nuclease.*** Endonuclease from Aspergillus that attacks single-stranded RNA or DNA to yield mononucleotides. This enzyme is different from an S1 exonuclease that also exists.

***S1 Nuclease*** EC 3.1.31.1). Endonuclease, from Aspergilus oryzae, that degrades single-stranded DNA or RNA to 5'-phosphomononucleotides or oligonucleotides. S1 nuclease ($M_r$ 32,000) requires $Zn^{2+}$ and is active at pH 4.0-4.5. It is used in S1 nuclease mapping, in the removal of cohesive ends from restriction fragments, and to open the hairpin loop generated during the synthesis of double-stranded cDNA. S1 nuclease has been found to cleave active genes in the region of the promoter.

***S1 Nuclease Mapping.*** Procedure for mapping the ends and splice points of RNA transcripts in relation to specific sites (e.g., positions of restriction endonuclease cleavage) in their template DNAs. Conditions are established that favor the formation of RNA-DNA hybrids) (relative to DNA-DNA hybrids). The resulting structures are treated with S1 nuclease, which degrades single-stranded RNA and DNA tails; the remaining RNA-DNA hybrid, which is resistant to digestion, is analysed by gel electrophoresis. If the DNA was first labeled with $^{32}P$, it can be detected by autoradiography of the gel. If the DNA is unlabeled, it can be detected with an appropriate $^{32}P$-labeled DNA or RNA probe after transfer to nitrocellulose (i.e., by Southern blotting).

***Sabin-Feldman Dye Test.*** Serological test for toxoplasmosis. Dilutions of heat-inactivated human test serum are mixed with Toxoplasma organisms in the presence of complement. If antibodies to the Toxoplasma are present in the serum, the Toxoplasma organisms are killed, as indicated by uptake of methylene blue. The titer refers to the serum dilution at which 50 percent of the test organisms are killed.

***Saccharomyces Cerevisiae.*** Brewer's or bakers' yeast; a budding yeast widely used in genetics and cell biology. Mitochondrial mutation which app;ear as slow-growing petite mutants have been much studied in this organsm, as have the genes controlling mating type.

***Sacculus Rotundus.*** Terminal portion of rabbit ileum, which is rich in lymphoid tissue. At one time it was thought to be the mammalian equivalent of the bursa of fabricius.

***Safranin.*** Stain used to indicate the presence of various structures in plant cell sections, especially those containing suberin. It iis commonly used in alcoholic solution.

***Saliva.*** The secreton of the salivary glands, basically consistiing of mucus, which moistens and lubriicates food. In some tetrapods and insects the saliva contains amylases, e.g. ptyalin in mammals, which initiate the digestion of strarch. The saliva of blood-sucking animals, e.g. leeches, mosquitoes, contains an anticoagulant.

***Salivary Glands.*** Ectodermal glands that are derived from the buccal cavity (vertebrates) or the foregut (invertebrates) and secrete saliva. The salivary glands may be specialized to produce poisons (some carnivores, e.g. lizards) or adhesive substances (birds, for building nests).

***Salivary Gland Squash.*** Procedure for preparing salivary gland tissue from larvae of Drosophila and related insects for studies on their polytene chromosomes. The cells are squashed in a drop of aceto-orcein and examined directly without prior fixation or sectioning.

***Salmo.*** Genus containing fish species such as S.salar, the Atlantic salmon, and S.gairdneri, the rainbow trout, which are not only of economic importance, but are now being investigated genetically in detail in terms of strains, races, hybrids, triploids and gynogenetic individuals. Gene libraries are available in clone for both species.

***Salmonella Typhimurium.*** Facultative, gram-negative, rod-shaped (0.5 x 1.0—3.0 μm), motile, non-spore-forming bacterium found in warm-blooded animals, including man (where it causes food poisoning). It differs from the colkiform bacteria (e.g., E.coli) in not utilizing lactose as a fermentable carbon source. S.typhimurium is readily cultivated in standard nutrient medium, but has not been as widely adopted as E.coli as an experimental organism for biochemistry and genetics.

***Saltatory Replication.*** Increase in the number of gene copies of a specific DNA sequence by laying down numerous strands of DNA in parallel without nuclear division. Such specific increase in the number of copies of ribosomal cistrons occurs in some strains of Drosophila and is evident in the polytene chromosomes where these genes are over-represented (or in other cases, under-represented).

***Salting out.*** Procedure for bringing molecules such as nucleic acids out of solution by gradually increasing the ionic concentration of one salt, often sodium chloride.

***Sandhoff Disease.*** Autosomal recessive gene in the human causing invariably lethal disease. A gene on chromosome 5 coding for a hexosaminidase subunit is defective and mental deterioration results. Similar symptoms occur in tay-sachs disease.

***Saponication.*** Production of soap plus glycerol by alkaline hydrolysis of glycerides.

***Saprophyte.*** An organism that obtains its nourishment from dead or decaying organic matter. Enzymes produced by the saprophyte are secreted onto the organic matter, which is digested externally, absorbed, and assimilated. Many fungi and bacteria are saprophytes: they play an important part in the recycling of nutrients.

***Saprozoic.*** Designating organisms that feed on solutions of organic material rather than on solid organic matter. Saprozoic organisms include the flagellate protozoan Polytoma uvella and many gut parasites.

***Sarcoidosis.*** Disease characterized by the occurrence of granulomas, with little or no necrosis. Sarcoidosis occurs most frequently in young adults and may affect any organ of the body, but most commonly the lymphnodes of the lungs. The disease is characterized by mild polyclonal hypergammaglobulinemia and anergy to skin test materials that elicit delayed-type hypersensitivity. Sarcoidosis is usually mild and approximately 60 percent of patients recover spontaneously or after treatment with corticosteroids. The cause is not known.

***Sarcoma.*** Any tumour arising in connective tissue and normally constituting a solid mass of cells. Sarcomas are often highly malignant and represent one of the commonest forms of cancer.

***Sarcomere.*** Functional unit of striated muscle bounded by the Z lines. The sarcomeres lie parallel and in register, and so give the muscle its characteristic striped appearance. Within each sarcomere are the thick (myosin) and thin (actin) myofilaments. Active sliding of these fiilaments across one another shortens the individual sarcomeres and results in contraction of the muscle cell.

***Sarcoplasmic Reticulum.*** The form of the endoplasmic reticulum found in muscle cells, specialized for the transmiission of nervous excitation to the contractile filaments.

***Sarcosome.*** Large mitochondrion found in the flight muscles of many insects.

***Satellite Chromosome.*** Piece of chromosome that is connected to the distal end of a chromosome arm only by a thin filament of chromatin termed a secondary constriction. Under low magnification the thin filament may be invisible, and the small piece looks superficially like a supernumerary chromosome.

***Satellite DNA.*** A fraction of DNA that separates from the bulk of the genomic DNA of an organism during centrifugation. DNA of mitochondrial, chloroplast, centromeric, and ribosomal types may all be recovered from centrifuged samples as distinct satellites, especially when the DNA is run through gradients of sucrose or caesium chloride.

***Satuaration Hybridization.*** Hybridization of nucleic acids in which one of the components is in great excess, thus ensuring that all complementary sequences in the other sample are hybridized. If the DNA is the molecule in excess and RNA the scarce component, the reaction would be said to be DNA-driven and the DNA referred to as driver DNA.

***Scanning Electron Microscope.*** Electron microscope that usues back-scattered electrons to provide information on the surface topography of solid specimens. The advent of high-resolution scanning electron microscopy, coupled with freeze-etching techniques can reveal the three-dimensional ultrastructure of cells and tissues in a new and unique way.

***Scarce mRNA.*** Refers to the may mRNA species that exist as very few copies per cell.

***Scatchard Equation.*** Equation used to describe the binding of a univalent ligand to a multivalent macromolecule (e.g., antibody): r/c = Kn—Kr. At equilibrium, r is the molar concentration of bound ligand divided by the molar concentration of antibody (i.e., the average number of ligand molecules bound per antibody molecule), c is the molar concentration of free ligand, n is the valence of the antibody molecule, and K is the association constant.

***Scatchard Plot.*** Plot of experimental binding data in which r/c is plotted against r. If all the binding sites are identical and independent, the plot should be a straight line with slope of -K (negative value of the association constant) and intercept on r axis of n (maximum value of r or number of sites per molecule). If the binding sites are not identical or not independent, the plot is not linear, the slope (-K) varying with the extent of site occupancy. For the binding of ligands to heterogeneous antibodies, an average association constant is often defined as the reciprocal of the free ligand concentration required for half-saturation of the antibody sites.

***Scattering.*** Random reflection of light rays or electrons due to collisions or interactions. Light scattering may cause aberrations in spectrophotometry, whereas electron scattering by the specimen is used to provide the image in the electron microscope.

***Schick Test.*** Skin test for circulating antibodies to diptheria toxin. Diptheria toxin (0.2 ml) is diluted so as to contain about 1 ng and is injected into the skin. At another site, 0.2 ml of diluted toxin heated at 70ºC for 5 minutes is injected as a control. A red, raised circular area (1-2 cm in diameter), appearing in four to seven days, indicates a lack of antibodies to diphtheria (i.e., susceptibility to diptheria). A reaction occurring within 24 hours is called a 'pseudo reaction' and does not indicate whether the test subject is immune kor susceptible.]

***Schiff's Reagent.*** Reagent used in the feulgen stain and periodic acid schiff's reagent and which colours compounds containing aldehyde pink.

***Schizogony.*** Production of schizont spores by rapid mitosis within a cell but without increase or division of the cell membrane or wall.

***Schizomycetes.*** Now obsolete classification for some bacteria.

***Schizont.*** Sporozoan spore that results from schizogony.

***Schizophrenia.*** Mental disease with a large hereditary component, however the gene, or genes,that is responsible for the syndrome remains unknown. It affects up to 5 percent of the human population, depending on race and culture, and is characterized by a so-called split mind, often involving severe delusion, paranoia and other types of mental disturbance, but usually interspersed with periods of remission.

***Schizosaccharomyces Pombe.*** Fission yeast that grows by simple fission following the formation of a central cell plate rather than by budding as in baker's yeast. The organism has been much used for studies on the cell cycle.

***Schlepper.*** Synonym for carrier.

***Schultz-Dale Reaction.*** Contraction of isolated uterine or intestinal strips in a water bath upon addition of antigen. The tissue strips are either taken from a primed donor or from an unprimed donor followed by sensitization of the tissue by antiserum in vitro. The contraction is due to release of histamine and other mediators of anaphylaxis.

***Schwann Cell.*** Cell that surrounds an axon during its early stages of outgrowth in an embryo and generates the myelin sheath.

***Sciara.*** Genus of small flies, which, like Drosophila, have polytene chromosomes in the larval salivary glands. Certain puffs of these chromosomes have been extensively studied.

***Scion.*** Graft from the shoot of one plant that is grafted onto the stock of another.

***SCID Mouse.*** Mouse of a mutant strain derived from BALB/C17 (CB-17/SCID) characterized by severe combined immunodeficiency (SCID). The trait is autosomal recessive. SCID mice have no B lymphocytes or T lymphocytes because of a selective defect in hematopoietic stem cells that generate lymphoctes. They have normal lymphoid storma in lymph nodes and spleen, which can be repopulated by bone marrow stem cells from normal CB-17 mice. Bone marrow stem cells from CB-17/SCID mice will not generate lymphocytes after transplantation into X-irradiated CB-17 mice. SCID mice have normal numbers of mononuclear phagocytes, natural killer cells and granulocytes. Serum of SCID mice lacks immunoglobulins and they do not manifest cell-mediated immunity. About 15 percent of SCID mice develop serum immunoglobulin late in life. SCID mice appear to lack a lymphocyte-specific DNA recombinase so that effective rearrangement of the T cell receptor genes and immunoglobulin genes does not occur.

***Scission.*** Breaking or separation of a long molecule or a pair of cells, or the breakage of one piece of tissue from another as in the abscission of leaves (i.e. leaf fall) in decidous trees.

***Sclereids.*** Plant cells, varied in shape but characteriistically having a thick secondary wall which is typically lignifieid. Sclereids form a component of sclerenchyma and have been classified into a number of types based on their shape and form. Brachysclereids (stone cells) are shaped like parencyma cells and occur iin the flesh of fruiits such as pear. Macrosclereids are elongated and columnar, and are found in seed coats of peas and beans. Osteosclereids are bone-shaped and occur in seed coats and leaves. Asterosclereids are highly elongated and hair-like and sometimes branched.

***Sclerenchyma.*** Plant tissue made up of thick-walled cells, often lignified, whose principal function is to provide mechanical support. At matuarity, the cells are frequently devoid of living contents. Sclerenchyma can be subdivided into fubres which are elongated cells with tapering ends and sclereids which are variously shaped.

***Scleroproteins.*** Group of proteins, including collagen, keratin and elastin, that contribute to connective and skeletal tissues of animals and are insoluble in most common solvents.

***Scrapie.*** Transmissible disease of the sheep and goat, involving degeneration of the nervous system following infection wiith a prion particle.

***Scratch Test.*** Skin test to ascertain the presence of IgE antibodies to particular allergenes. A small abrasion is made in the skin with a needle. A drop of an aqueous solution of an allergen is placed on the abrasion and the site is observed for an immediate wheal and flare reaction (urticaria), which occurs when IgE antibodies to the allergen are present on mast cells of the test subject.

***Scurvy.*** Disease caused by lack of ascorbic acid. Symptoms include superficial haemorrhages from skin and gums.

***SDS-PAGE.*** Sodium dodecyl sulphate polyacrylamide gel electrophoresis.

***SDS-polyacrylamide Gel.*** Modification of polyacrylamide gel electrophoresis in whiich the solution of proteins to be analysed is dialysed against a solution of the detergent sodium dodecyl sulphate (SDS). The proteins bind to the SDS and all become negatively charged, having similar weight-to-charge ratios. In an electric field, electophoretic separation will occur dependent on the proteins' size and shape. Use of differing concentrations of polyacrylamide gel permits different molecular weight ranges to be analysed. It is usual to reduce the disulphide bonds in the protein by treatment with 2-mercaptoehanol: this results in the reduced proteins having similar shapes, so separation will be by size alone. It should be noted, however, that a SDS binds less to heavily glycosylated proteins than to unglycosylated proteins of similar molecular weight.

***Searle Translocation.*** X chromosome autosomal reciprocal translocation n the mouse which has the effect to preferential inactivatiion of the paternal X in female heterozygotes.

***Secondary Disease.*** Chronic graft-versus-host disease in mice.

***Secondary Granule.*** Cytoplasmic organelle of polymorphonuclear leukocytes. In neutrophils, secondary granules contain lactoferrin, vitamin B12-binding protein and lysozyme. In eosinophils, secondary granules contain cationic peptides. In basophils, secondary granules contain heparin, histamine and platelet activating factor.

***Secondary Growth*** (secondary thickening). Growth from cambium that gives rise to the secondary plant body.

***Secodary Immune Response.*** Accelerated, enhanced immune response that develops upon encouter with an antigen for the second time. The secondary immune response can be detected within a few hours after antigen is introduced, whereas in the primay immune response there is usually a lag period of several days after antigen administration. The secondary response is characterized by strong cell-mediated immunity and high titers of IgG antibodies often of high affinity. Antigens that induce a secondary immune response are proteins or glycoproteins that stimulate T cell reactivity. Immunological memory denotes the capacity to develop a secondary immune response. The term secondary immune response is also used to describe the third, fourth, fifth or $n^{th}$ response to an antigen; such responses are similar to the second response. Synonym for anamnestic reaction.

***Secondary Immunodeficiency.*** Any faiure or compromise of specific immunity that is not due to an intrinsic defect in B or T lymphocytes. Secondary immunodeficiency results from loss of immunoglobulins or T lymphocytes, as occurs in inflammatory bowel disease; from destruction of B or T lymphocytes by cytotoxic drugs or ionizing radiation; from displacement of normal B or T lymphocytes by malignant cells as in multiple myeloma or chronic lymphocytic leukemia; from infection of B or T lymphocytes, as in acquired immunodeficiency syndrome.

***Secondary Lymphoid Organ.*** Lymphoid organ where mature T and B lymphocytes encounter antigen to initiate an immune response. The secondary lymphoid organs include lymph nodes, spleen, tonsils and gut-associated lymphoid tissue. The structure of all these organs is such as to maximize interaction between lymphocytes and antigen-charged accessory cells.

***Secondary Lysosome.*** Vesicle in cell cytoplasm that results from fusion of a primary lysosome with an endosome (i.e. membrane-bound endocytotic vesicle). Degradation of ingested material occurs in the secondary lysosome.

***Secondary non-disjunction.*** Non-disjuction affected the sex chromosomes of an XXY individual, so that gametes may have an XX, XY, X or Y complement of sex chromosomes.

***Secondary Ray.*** Radial line of parenchyma cells in the secondary xylem and phloem arising from a ray initial in the vascular cambium. Rays may be uniseriate (one cell wde) or multiseriate (composed of several cells) when viewed in tangential longitudinal section.

***Secondary Sexual Characteristic.*** A characteristic of an adult animal that is restricted to one sex but does not include the gonads or their associated ducts and glands. Most secondary sexual characteristics develop under the influence of steroid hormones produced by the gonads (e.g. androgens and oestrogens). Examples include antlers in stags, the bright plumage of male birds, the mane of lions, and in humans enlargement of the breasts (women) and growth of beard (men).

***Secondary Structure.*** That aspect of macromolecular structure dependent on hydrogen bonds, e.g. the helical arrangement of a polynucleotide chain and the alpha-helix and beta-pleated sheet structure in protein.

***Secondary Structure.*** Organization of the peptide backbone of a polypeptide or protein chain due to formation of hydrogen bonds between carbonyl oxygen and amide nitrogen atoms. The alpha helix, beta-pleated sheet and collagen helix are examples of secondary structures.

***Secondary Wall.*** Inner layer of cell wall laid down by some plant cells. The microfibriils run in different directions in each layer, so increasing the strength of the compound structure. Secondary cell walls lack pectic substances.

***Second Messenger.*** Molecule that carries the stimulus from cell surface to cytoplasm and nucleus followiing attachment of a polypeptide hormone to the outer surface of the plasma membrane of a cell. Many such hormones do not enter the cell, but transmit their effective stimulus to the cell cytoplasm and nucleus via the second messenger. molecule. This molecule is, in most cases, cyclic amp.

***Second-set Rejection.*** Accelerated rejection of a graft because of prior immunization of the recipient (e.g., by previous grafting).

***Secreted Immunoglobulin.*** Immunoglobulin that is secreted by a plasma cell. The secreted immunoglobulin is the form that accumulates in serum and other body fluids.

***Secretin.*** A straight-chain polypeptide hormone of 27 amino acid residues synthesized and secreted by the duodenal mucosa when acidified food leaves the stomach. It stimulates the release of relatively enzyme-free pancreatic juice (further enzyme release occurs with stimulation of the vagus nerve). Secretin was the first substance shown to be a hormone, by the classic studies of Bayliss and Starling in the early 1900s, but it was not until the mid 1960s, that it was characterized and synthesized and found to resemble glucagon.

***Secretion.*** The discharge or extrusion of intracellular molecules into the surrounding medium. The term is also applied to the molecules that are secreted, which include ions, enzymes, hormones, glycoproteins, fluids, inorganic molecules, etc. There are three principal mechanisms of secretion. Exocytosis (merocriine or eccrine secretion) is the most common type and involves the release of small membrane-bound granules of the secreted substance by a complex process in which the granule membrane fuses with the plasma membrane. Neurotransmitter is released from nerve endings by exocytosis. Apocrine secretion involves the loss of the apical plasma membrane, resulting in the release of the secretory product and some cytoplasmic constituents. It occurs in the glands around the anus. Holocriine secretion involves the loss of the entire cell in releasing its secretory product; it occurs in the sebaceous glands. The secretion of fluids such as sweat and small ions, often against osmotic or electrochemical gradients, is complex and requires energy, usually in the form of nucleotides.

***Secretor.*** Person whose secretions (e.g., gastric, juice, saliva, tears, ovarian cyst mucin) contain ABO blood group substances. Secretors are homozygous (Se/Se) or heterozygous (Se/Se) for the gene Se; they constitute approximately 80 percent of the population.

***Secretor Genē.*** Dominant autosomal gene in the human that allows secretion of A and B type blood group antigen into saliva and other body fluids.

***Secretory Cell.*** Cell involved in secretion, as are, for example, many epithelial cells in the pancreas. Secretory cells have abundant endoplasmic reticulum and numerous secretory vesicles, which release their contents at the cell surface through exocytosis.

***Secretory Component (SC).*** Polypeptide chain ($M_r$ 75,000) that is found in a variety of external secretions (e.g., tears, bile, colostrum) usually complexed to secreted polymeric immunoglobulins (IgA or, less frequently, IgM), but sometimes also found in free form. It is derived, by proteolytic cleavage, from the polyimmunoglobulin receptor on the surfaces of epithelial cells or hepatocytes.

Human SC contains kabout 550 amino acid residues and seven N-linked oligosaccharides. The polypeptide can be divided into five domains; these are the five amino-terminal (extracellular) domains of the poly-immunoglobulin receptor. As in immunoglobulin domains, each domain contains a disulfide bridge spanning 60-70 amino acid residues. The cysteine residues forming these disulfide bridges are in homologous positions to cysteines in the five extracellular immunoglobulin-like domains of the rabbit polyimmunoglobulin receptor. In addition, four of the domains of human SC have a smaller disulfide loop. In free secretory component, the fifth domain contains yet another intrachain disulfide bridge, which is labile to reduction and which may rearrange to form two interchain disulfide bridges to the alpha chain when SC becomes covalently bound to IgA. In humans, SC appears to be joined, by two disulfide bridges, to only one of the two monomer units of secretory IgA. In some varieties of IgA, Sc may not be covalently bound to the immunoglobulin. Human SC is similar in amino acid sequence (55 percent identity) to the amino-terminal five domains of rabbit polyimmunoglobulin receptor and is a member of the immunoglobulin superfamily.

For transport of polymeric immunoglobulins into external secretions, the immunoglobulin, secreted by a plasma cell, binds to the polyimmunoglobulin receptor on the basolateral surface of an epithelial cell. During or after transcitosis of the resulting complex, proteolytic cleavage of the receptor occurs; most of the exrtracellular portion (called the secretory component) of the receptor remains bound to the immunoglobulin and this complex is released into the secretions. The carboxy-terminus of human SC is uneven, presumably due to variable proteolytic cleavage from the intact receptor. It is thought that binding of SC to IgA increases the resistance of IgA to cleavage by proteolytic enzymes found in external secretions.

***Secretory Component Deficiency.*** Very rare disorder in which no IgA is found in secretions due to the failure of secretory component synthesis by epithelial cells. The few reported cases have had prolonged diarrhea following infection of the gastrointestinal tract. It is not known if the polyimmunoglobulin receptor is absent or defective.

***Secretory Granule*** (Zymogen granule). Specialized secretory vesicle in the pancreas and some other tissues.

***Secretory Protein.*** Protein such as enzyme amylase or trypsinogen or the polypeptide hormone insulin or growth homone, that is secreted by cells by means of exocytosis.

***Sectioning.*** Technique in cell biology and histology in which thin sections are cut from tissues or organisms prior to microscopy. Sectioning may be carried out crudely on live plant material, and more precisely using a microtome on fixed material following its embedding in way or resin. Sections for electron microscopy must be ultra-thin and are cut with a special microtome using a glass or diamond knife.

***Sedimentation Coefficient*** (Sedimentation costant). Constnat s for a macromolecule (protein, nucleic acid, nucleoprotein, etc.) sedimenting in a strong centifugal field as provided by the ultracentrifuge.

$$s = \frac{dx/dt}{\omega^x}$$

where dx/dt is tthe rate at whiich the particle travels at a distance x from the centre of rotation, and ω is the angular velocity of the rotor in radians per second. The sedimentation coefficient is usually expressed in Svedberg units (S) (after the inventor of the ultracentrifuge), where 1S = $10^{-13}$ seconds. The sedimentation coefficient can be used to calculate molecular weight.

***Segmentation Gene.*** Gene in insects and other segmented animals that regulates the number or polarity of the body segments.

***Segregation.*** The separation of a pair of alleles on homologous chromosomes during meiosis, so that only one member of each pair is present in the gametes. For example, in the allelic pair Aa, segregation results in equal numbers of gametes containing A and a.

***Segregational Petition.*** Type of petite mutant in yeast in which the mutation is located not in the mitochondrial genome (as it is in normal petite mutants). but in a nuclear gene that produces mitochondrial defects. Thus segregational petites may show a mixture of petite and wild-type cells among progeny.

***Selection.*** Process of the greatest importance in evolution, in which individuals with certain genotypes makes a greater or lesser contribution to the population pool of progeny than do other individuals. When the contribution to the pool of progeny is greater, the parental individuals are said to have a selective advantage or 'to be selected for' whereas if such contribution is lesser, the individuals are said to have a selective disadvantage or 'to be selected against'. The selective effect of a given gene is determined by the probabiliity that the individuals carrying that gene will reproduce and produce viable offspring. Selection pressure may be applied artifically by modifying the culture conditions. An extreme example of cell selection in vitro is forced amplification involving one specific gene sequence. Selection is based on the phenotype of an organism, but what is effectively selected is the genotype and its contribution to the future gene pool.

***Selection Coefficient*** (s). Expression that indicates the relative selection against a particular genotype. It is the proportional reduction in the contribution to the gene pool of the next generation made by individuals with one particular genotype, as compared to the contribution made to this pool by some other genotype, usually the one of greatest fitness. If a genotype is not selected aganst the s=0. If individuals with a particular genotype, leaves only 50% as many viable progeny in a population as do the most fit, then the selection coefficient of such indiviiduals is 0.2 or 20 percent.

***Selection Differential.*** Difference between the value of a particular character in terms of selectiive advantage, taken for the whole population, and the value of that character in the individuals which, through selection, become parents of the next generation.

***Selection Pressure.*** Effectiveness of natural or artificial selection is changing the average genotype of a population over a series of generations.

***Selective Advantage.*** Increased fitness of one or a series of individuals expressing a particular phenotypic character, as compared with other individuals in the same population not expressing the character in precisely that form.

***Selective Neutrality.*** Situation in which the fitness of individulas in a population carrying a mutant allele is no different from that of the other individuals in the population carrying the wild-type allele.

***Selective Plating.*** Technique for the isolation of recombinant colonies of bacteria by placing two auxotrophic mutants in mixture together on agarplate of minimal medium. Under such conditions, only colonies representing chance recombinants will grow.

***Selective Theory.*** Theory that explains the specificity of the immune response by antigen selection of pre-existing antibodies or antibody-like cell receptors. Selective theories differ from instructive theories, which state that antigen is required to induce specificity of the antibody. An early form of selective theory was proposed by Paul Ehrlich. The current, widely accepted selective theory is the clonal selection theory.

***Self.*** (1) In an immunological sense, the cells and molecules specific to one unique individual, recognized by the immune mechanisms as self rather than non-self. (2) To undergo or to use a procedure involving self-fertilization or self-pollination, and in this sense often used as a verb.

***Self-assembly.*** Spontaneous aggregation of performed macromolecules into supramolecular structures such as multienzyme complexes, protein filaments, ribosomes, membranes and viruses in which the components are non-covalently linked. Examples of self-assembly are the formation of actin filaments, the aggregation of the protein cylinder around the helical RNA core of tobacco mosaic virus, and the maturation of simple bacteriophages.

***Self-fertilization.*** Fusion of genetically similar gametes and ones usually derived from the same individual.

***Self-replicating*** (of plasmids and other extrachromosomal DNA and RNA molecules). Able to control the timing and rate of their own synthesis rather than being under the same control as chromosomal DNA.

***Self-sterility.*** The condition in hermaphorodite plants and animals in which male gametes cannot fertilize female gametes of the same organism. It occurs in flowering plants in which an incompatibility mechanism operates.

***Self-sterility Gene.*** Gene that operates against self-fertilization in monoecious plants, usually by control of the rate of pollen tube growth down the style.

***SEM.*** Scanning electron microscope.

***Semen.*** A fluid, produced by the male of animals with internal fertilization, consisting of spermatozoa and secretions from various accessory sex glands (in mammals, these include the prostate gland and seminal vesicles). Semen is transferred from the male to the female during coitus.

***Semiconservative Replication.*** Manner of DNA repliication. Each new DNA duplex contains one original parental strand and one newly synthesized strand.

***Semidiscontinuous Replication.*** Manner of DNA replication in which one strand—the leading strand— is synthesized continuously, whereas the other strand—the lagging strand—is synthesized disicontinuously iin small sections termed okazaki fragments.

***Semipermeable Membrane.*** Membrane that allows some, but not all molecules to pass. Biological membranes (e.g., plasma membranes, nuclear membranes and vesicle membranes) are semipermeable, allowiing some small molecules such as water iin and out relatively freely, but impeding the passage of other molecules such as proteins.

***Semispecies.*** Distinct population of organisms that, although not recognized as being a separate species, appear to be destined to become one in time.

***Semisyngeneic Graft.*** Graft from a member of one strain into an $F_1$ hybrid produced by mating any member of that strain with a member of another strain (e.g., A into A x B). Such a graft is usually accepted.

***Semliki Forest Virus.*** Well-studied example of a single-stranded RNA virus which has an enveloped icosahedral capsid. It is a member of the Toga viridae.

***Sendai Virus.*** Enveloped myxovirus with a single-stranded RNA genome. The virus caused a widespread infection in laboratory mice, but is now used, in an attenutated form after ultraviolet irradiation, to promote cell fusion experimentally.

***Senescence.*** Deletrious changes that occur as an organism ages, and result in a loss of vitality (i.e. the ability of the organism to sustain life in the face of its internal and external environments). All organisms senesce, and the pattern of senescence seems to be characteristic for each species. The causes of senescence are probably many, but are not fully understood.

***Sensitive Developmental Period.*** Period during development in which an embryo or larva is particularly sensitive to genetic malfunction (e.g., amphibian gastrulation).

***Sensitization.*** Procedure, natural or artificial, that increases the reactivity of cells or organisms to an antigen or hapten, radiation or inflammatory agent. The process happens naturally in many animals when a prior exposure to antigen dramatically increases the response on a subsequent encounter.

***Sensitization.*** Administering antigen (i.e., priming) so that a heightened response (i.e., secondary immune response) is obtained upon subsequent challenge with that antigen.

***Sensitized Cell.*** (1) Cell that has been coated with antibodies and/or complement components. (2) Cell from a primed donor.

***Sensitizing Agent.*** Agent that, in a biological system, increases the damage incurred on exposure to radiation, potentiates a subsequent immune response, or protentiates an inflammatory response in subsequent encounter with an irritant. Thus an eczematous response to, for example, a detergent, is often dramatically increased by prior contact with nickel.

***Sensory Neurone.*** Neurone responsible for detecting a specific stimulating factor such as light or touch.

***Sephadex.*** Trade name for a group of absorbent resins used in chromatography.

***Septate Junction.*** Cell junction found in the cells of invertebrates and replacing tight junctions in such cells. Sepate junctions differ from tight junctions in the more orderly arrangement of the junctional proteins and in that the proteins rather than the membranes themselves from the seal. Like tight junctions they serve to hold cells together and form complete septal ribbons around cells.

***Sequenator.*** Machine that automatically determines amino acid sequences of peptide fragments, and can thus be used to determine such sequences in complete proteins.

***Sequence Analysis.*** Determination and study of the sequence of bases in DNA or of amino acids in proteins. Although both are related, the former cannot be accurately deduced from the latter because of the degeneracy of the genetic code.

***Sequential Determinant.*** Antigenic determinant that is dependent on the sequence of a few contiguous residues in a macro-molecule. The amino acid residues comprising the sequential determinant of a protein are clustered within a relatively small (about six residues) peptide segment. Such a determinant is not expected to be affected by denaturation of the protein. The binding of antibodies to a sequential determinant of a protein can often be inhibited by an appropriate peptide derived from the protein.

***Sericin.*** Minor gummy protein of silk that forms a covering for the twin filaments of fibroin in each silk fibre. There are a number of different molecular forms of sericin, but each is composed of more than 30 percent serine.

***Serine*** (Ser). One of the 20 common amino acids found in proteins and a precursor of sphingosine.

***Serine Proteases.*** Family of enzymes including the digestive enzymes chymotrypsin, trypsin, elastase and proteases such as thrombin. All contain an activated serine residue in their active site.

***Seroconversion.*** Conversion from negative to positive reactivity in a test for serum antibodies.

***Serology.*** The study of in vitro reactions between antigens and antibodies. The three main serological tests are agglutination reactions, the complement fixation test, and precipitation reactions such as the precipitin reaction.

***Serotherapy.*** Treatment of an infectious disease by the administrative of antiserum in order to achieve passive immunity. Serotherapy was frequently practised for the treatment of pneumococcal infections before the introduction of antibiotics.

***Serotonin*** (5-hydroxytryptamine). Potent vasoconstrictor of large blood vessels, vasodilator that enhances permeability of small blood vessels, and constrictor of bronchi. Serotonin is widely distributed in animals and plants. In humans 90 percent of serotonin is in the enterochromaffin cells of the gastrointestinal tract; the remainder is in platelets and the brain where it is a neurotransmitter. In rodents (e.g., rats, mice and Bovidae (e.g., cows) serotonin is present in mast cells and is a mediator of anaphylaxis. In humans, platelet activating factor, released from mast cells during anaphylaxis, induces release of serotonin from platelets. However, serotonin is not thought to play a role in human anaphylaxis. Serotonin is synthesized from the amino acid tryptophan in two enzymatic reactions involving hydroxylation and decarboxylation. The activity of serotonin is inhibited by ergot alkaloids, such as lysergic acid diethylamide (LSD) and reserpine.

***Serotonin (5-hydroxytryptamine).*** A compound with neurotransmitter properties that is released from certain neurones and is associated with the control of mood. Serotonin is concentrated in the hypothalamus region of the brain, where it is localized in granular synaptic vesicles in the nerve endings. Serotonin nerve terminals are also found in nuclei of the parasympathetic and sympathetic nervous system and in the pineal body. Serotonin is synthesized in the brain from the amino acid tryptophan.

***Serotype.*** Antigenic properties and characteristics of a cell as determined by serology.

***Serotype.*** Antigenic variant within a bacterial species identified with antibodies to surface antigenic determinants of the variants. Serotyping is used to classify Salmonella, Shigella and streptococci.

***Serpin.*** Acronym for serine protease inhibitor(e.g.,C1 inhibitor).

***Sertoli Cell.*** Specialized cell found in the epithelial wall of the seminiferous tubules of the vertebrate testis. Sertoli cells provide an important supportive/nutritional role in the maturation of the spermatozoa (in this respect these cells are sometimes considered homologous to the follicle cell in the ovary).

***Serum.*** Fluid remaining in blood after clotting. Serum is plasma from which fibrinogen and clotting factors have been removed. The major protein components in serum are: serum albumin (35-55 mg/ml), immunoglobulins of all isotypes (~20 mg/ml in total), α1-antitrypsin (~3 mg/ml), transferrin (~3 mg/ml), α2-macroglobulin (~2.5 mg/ml), haptoglobin (~2 mg/ml).

***Serum Albumin.*** The major protein component of serum or plasma. Its concentration ranges from 35 to 55 mg/ml. Human serum albumin is a single chain of 585 amino acid residues crosslinked by 17 disulfide bridges. It is synthesized in the adult liver in a precursor form with a signal sequence of 18 amino acid residues and an additional basic precursor (i.e., 'propeptide') sequence of six residues, which is cleaved from proalbumin in the Golgi apparatus, thereby generating mature serum albumin. Serum albumin is important in maintaining the osmolarity of the blood and it binds a great many blood constituents including fatty acids, hormones, bilirubin and drugs. It is the most anionic (negatively charged) of the serum proteins.

***Serum Amyloid A Component*** (SAA). Serum protein ($M_r$ 20,000) that is the precursor of the major component of amyloid deposits in secondary amyloidosis. SAA is a single polypeptide chain of 114 amino acid residues. After peptides are cleaved from the amino- and carboxy-terminal ends of SAA the residual protein ($M_r$ 8,000) forms fibrillar amyloid deposits. In inflammation, the serum level of SAA may rise 1000-fold to 1 mg/ml.

***Serum Amyloid P Component (SAP).*** Serum protein of unknown function that is a minor component (10-15 percent) of amyloid deposits in secondary amyloidosis. SAP is composed of two disk-like structures; each disk is a pentamer of identical subunits of 204 amino acid residues. Serum concentration of SAP is 30 μg/ml; the level does not rise during inflammation. The gene for SAP has been mapped to chromosome 1q2.1 and is linked to the gene for C-reactive protein.

***Serum Sickness.*** Immune complex disease that may develop several days after the introduction of a large amount of foreign protein into the circulation. The usual signs and symptoms of serum sickness include fever, joint pains, skin rash and red blood cells and protein in the urine. These are the consequences of the deposition of antigen-antibody complexes that fix complement and attract neutrophils, which cause tissue injury upon degranulation. Serum sickness occurred frequently during serotherapy for infectious diseases.

***Severe Combined Immunodeficiency (SCID).*** Syndrome of infants that is caused by a profound deficiency of T lymphocytes and a variable deficiency of B lymphocytes. Infants with SCID are extremely susceptible to opportunistic infections (e.g., with Pneumocystis carini, adenovirus, Candida albicans) and die of these infections in infancy or early childhood. SCID may be inherited as an X-linked recessive or autosomal recessive. Of the latter group, half of the affected infants have adenosine deaminase deficiency or purine nucleoside phosphorylase deficiency. In all cases of SCID, regardless of the cause, the thymus has few or no lymphocytes and Hassell's corpuscles. SCID is treated with transplants of bone marrow cells.

***Sex.*** (1) Reproduction dependent on fusion of haploid gametes produced by meiotic division. (2) Distinction between organisms depending on the type of gametes produced. If gametes are morphologically indistinguishable they are termed isogametes, and the sexes may be termed simply plus and minus, as in mating type in yeast. Individuals producing both male and female gametes are termed hermaphrodite, if animal, and monoecious, if plant.

***Sex Chromatin.*** Strictly speaking chromatin of the sex chromosome, but in common usage chromatin of the inactivated X chromosome, say in the human female.

***Sex Chromosome.*** Any chromosome that is associated in some way with sex determination. There are two types: the X chromosome and the Y chromosome. X chromosomes are similar in appearance to the other chromosomes, whereas the Y chromosome is usually much smaller. In diploid organisms, sex chromosomes are represented as XX in the homogametic sex and XY in the heterogametic sex. In some cases the Y chromosome is missing and the heterogametic sex is XO. The determination of sex by these chromosomes is somewhat variable. In some cases, as in man and many other mammals, XX is the female sex and XY is the male and the Y chromsome is important in sex determination. In Drosophila, however, although XX is female and XY is male, the loss of the Y chromosome does not result in an abnormal male. In this case the dosage of X is more important in sex determination and the Y chromosome is practically inert; thus XX is female and X is male. In some organisms the Y chromosome has been lost in the course of evolution; the female of certain grasshoppers is XX and the male is XO, while in caddis flies the female is XO and the male is XX. in lepidopterans, birds, and some fishes the homogametic (XX) sex is male and the heterogametic (XY) sex is female. Most plants are hermaphrodite. Of the few unisexual groups, Melandrium dioicum (campion) and Salix (willows) have an XX/XY mechanism of sex determination. In all methods of sex determination involving sex chromosomes, equal numbers of males and females are produced.

The sex chromosomes also contain genes concerned with processes oher than sex determination, which results in the phenomenon of sex linkage.

***Sex-conditioned Character.*** Phenotypic character that, although determined by an autosomal gene, is conditioned by the sex of the individual. Thus human baldness is dominant in males but recessive in females; even when females are homozygous, the gene is expressed only to a minor degree.

***Sex Determination.*** Mechanism by which sex is determined within any given species. Sex chromosomes represent the commonest method of sex determination, in which one sex is homogametic and one heterogametic. Sometimes, as in mosquitoes, a single gene with two alleles is responsible, and one sex is homozygous recessive (female) and the other the heterozygous (male).

Many insects of the order Hymenoptera have a haploid/diploid sex-determining system, fertilized eggs producing females and non-fertilized eggs producing males. Workers and queens differ only in their diet, the latter being fed on large quantities of royal jelly.

Many marine worms and fishes use environmental cues to determine sex, and adults may change sex depending on water temperature, or even, as in the snail Crepidula, depending on whether a male is found. Egg incubation temperature is also used to determine sex in reptiles. It is said that the female alligator can alter the sex of her progeny by regulating the temperature of the nest.

***Sex Hormones.*** Hormones (e.g., oestrogens, progestogens, androgens and gonadotrophins) that are secreted by or influence the developement of the gonads. Many secondary sexual characteristics result from the activity of sex hormones.

***Sex Index.*** Indication of the number of X chromosomes per set of autosomes; used chiefly in relation to genetics to Drosophila.

***Sex-limited Gene (Sex-limited Character).*** A gene, or the character produced by it, that has its effect in only one sex. The gene may be on any chromosome, but because of the influence of certain sex hormones or other sex-determining factors, it is expressed in only one sex. The genes for secondary sexual characteristics, such as breast development and milk production in women and deep voice and growth of beard in men, are sex limited.

***Sex Linkage.*** The presence of one or more genes on a sex chromosome, usually the X chromosome, resulting in certain characteristics appearing in only one sex. In those species in which there is no crossing over between X and Y chromosomes, the genes on the X chromosome are permanently linked there. When there is crossing over, or when the Y chromosome is not inert, only the unpaired part of the X chromosome contains sex-linked genes. These genes are present in duplicate only in the homogametic sex (XX); in the homorogametic sex (XY), sex-linked genes are present singly. If a gene is recessive, and therefore usually deleterious, it is more likely to show up in the heterogametic sex. In man, several sex-linked diseases are due to sex-linked recessive genes, such as haemophilia and red-green colour blindness. A woman is more likely to be heterozygous for the recessive and therefore will not show the disease, although she will carry it and pass it on to her sons. A man with the disease cannot pass it on to his sons but his daughters will become carriers. Women with sex-linked diseases are rare, since the recessive must be present on both sex chromosomes. Sex-linked genes in other organisms include the gene for ginger coat colour in cats (it is more usual for ginger cats to be toms) and that of white eye colour in Drosophila.

***Sex Ratio.*** The proportion of males to females in a population, often expressed as the number of males per 100 females.

***Sexual Reproduction.*** Any form of reproduction in which two haploid cells (gametes) or nuclei fuse to produce a diploid cell that develops into a new organism. The gametes (or nuclei) are typically of two kinds, male and female, and may be derived from one individual or from separate male and female organisms. Sexual reproduction permits genetic recombination and therefore results in greater variation in the offspring, on which natural selection can act, than is possible in asexual reproduction.

Certain types of reproduction, notably parthenogenesis and apomixis, involve the development of individuals from female gametes without fusion taking place. These are usually regarded as special types of sexual reproduction.

***Sex Linkage.*** Type of genetic linkage in which the gene responsible for determining the character concerned is carried on a sex chromosome. In humans this is always the X chromosome, but it varies in other species depending on the mechanism of sex determination and the types of sex chromosomes present. This may mean that the particular phenotypic trait is almost exclusively expressed in the heterogametic sex (e.g., haemophilia in humans). Differences between reciprocal crosses may also arise with sex-linked genes.

***Sex Ratio.*** Proportion of males to females in a population. Usually the figure is corrected for age, since individuals of one sex may live longer than another. Although ratios close to 1:1 are common, they are by no means the rule. In some species, one sex, often the male, is less viable in embryonic life; in other species, males may be scarce or unknown.

***Sex Reversal.*** Change from one sex to another during the lifetime of an organism. In some species,such as the marine fishes—the wrasses—where sex is dependent on environmental factors, sex reversal is common. In mammals it normally only results from pathology or artificial interference, the latter sometimes being practised for psychological reasons.

***Sexual Dimorphism.*** Existence of morphological distinctions in colour, size or other features between sexes of one species, so that the population consists of two distinct types differing by sex. Thus sexual dimorphism is pronounced in species like the lion and the pheasant, but scarcely apparent in leopard or the partridge.

***Sexual Isolation.*** Inability of closely related species or subspecies to produce progeny because of differences in courtships or mating behaviour, or physical inability to mate.

***Sexual Reproduction.*** Production of offspring dependent on fusion of haploid gametes produced by meiotic division. This contrasts with non-sexual reproduction in some lower eukaryotes, such as vegetative growth of yeast, and vegetative propagation in plants.

***Sexual Selection.*** A subsidiary mechanism bringing about some aspects of evolution according to Darwinism. Sexual selection is thought to be the cause of exaggerated secondary sexual characteristics in one sex, typically the male. Females of the species are assumed to prefer to mate with such males, whose characteristics are therefore inherited by their male progeny. Sexual selection is said to have accounted for the evolution of brilliant plumage of male birds, courtship behaviour, large antlers in stags, etc. The importance of sexual selection in evolution is probably less than Darwin supposed, as the less brilliantly marked males of many species usually do find a mate.

*S Gene Complex.* Group of genes in certain plant families (e.g.,Cruciferae) that combine to prevent self-fertilization. Thus pollen tubes are inhibited from growth by ovules carrying identical alleles of such genes.

*Shine-Dalgarno Sequence.* A short sequence in bacterial mRNA, lying 4-9 bases 5'to the initiater triplet AUG, which is complementary to a sequence in 16 S ribosomal RNA. It promotes binding of the mRNA to the ribosome and the initiation of translation. The consensus shine-Dalgarno sequence is 5' UAAGGAGGU 3'.

*Shine-Delgano Sequence* (SD Sequence). Sequence forming a leader in the mRNA molecules upstream from the AUG initiation codon. The sequence is AGGAGG and is precisely complementary to a sequence at the 3'-end of 16S rRNA (in bacteria) and so acts as a binding site on the small ribosomal subunit for an mRNA molecule.

*Shope Papilloma Virus.* Virus that causes papilloma in rabbits, it is a double-stranded DNA virus with an icosahedral capsid some 50 nm in diameter.

*Short-period Interspersion.* Pattern of gene sequence arrangement in the genome of an organism in which non-repetitious coding sequences of some 1000 base pairs in length alternate with short repetitious DNA sequences of about 300 base pairs.

*Shotgun Cloning.* Procedure in which a number of different restriction endonucleases are used to cut up purified genomic DNA prior to cloning of the fragments in bacterial or phage vectors to form a genomic library.

*Shuttle Vector.* Plasmid vector that replicates in more than one host, for example in both E.coli and Agrobacterium tumefaciens, or in both E.coli and Neurospora crassa, allowing transfer of genes spliced into such plasmids from one cell to another in gene-cloning techniques.

***Shwartzman Reaction.*** Hemorrhagic lesions induced by lipopolysaccharides (LPS). In the local Shwartzman reaction, LPS is injected intradermally, followed by a second injection intravenously; hemorrhage occurs at the site of the first injection. In the systemic or generalized Shwartzman reaction, both injections are given intravenously, resulting in acute tubular necrosis of the kidney and hemorrhagic lesions in lung, liver and other viscera. Contrary to earlier opinion, the Shwartzman reaction has no immunological basis.

***Sialic Acid*** (N-acetylneuraminic acid). Amino sugar derived from neuraminic acid. Sialic acid is found in glycoproteins and glycolipids, and is abundant on the outer surface of many animal cell plasma membranes.

***Sialophorin*** (CD43). Major cell surface glycoprotein on all T lymphocytes, thymocytes, some B lymphocytes, platelets, monocytes and neutrophils, detected by monoclonal antibodies. Sialophorin from lymphocytes and monocytes ($M_r$ 115,000), or from neutrophils and platelets ($M_r$ 135,000) is a single polypeptide chain; the two forms differ only in carbohydrate content. Twenty-seven percent of the amino acid residues are threonine or serine, to almost all of which are attached O-linked saccharides, containing galactose β1-3 galactosamine. In mature T lymphocytes and medullary thymocytes sialic acid is attached to the galactose and galactosamine; the cortical thymocytes are only partially sialylated. The adherence of cortical thymocytes, but not of medullary thymocytes or T lymphocytes, to peanut lectin is due to this incomplete sialylation. Completely sialyated O-linked saccharide structures do not adhere to peanut lectin.

Human sialophorin consists of 400 amino acid residues, incuding a signal sequence of 19 residues, an extracellular domain of 235 residues, a putative transmembrane segment of 23 residues and a cytoplasmic domain of 123 residues. Sialophorin contains one site for N-linked oligosaccharides. The gene encoding sialophorin is on chromosome 16.

Antibody to sialophorin activates T lymphocytes; during activation of T lymphocytes, the cytoplasmic domain is phosphorylated. This glycoprotein is defective in the membrane of T lymphocytes from males with the Wiskott-Aldrich syndrome. The equivalent protein in the rat is called leukosialin.

***Sibling*** (sib). Offspring of the same parents, whether brothers or sisters.

***Sibling Species.*** Species that are reproductively isolated, but nearly identical morphologically.

***Sickle-cell Anaemia.*** A human disease affecting Black Africans in which the red blood cells have a tendency to assume spiked or sickle-like shape when the blood is deprived of oxygen. The disease results from the inheritance of a defective allele coding for β-globin, which results in the production of an abnormal type of haemoglobin, sickle haemoglobin (HbS). Affected blood cells are removed from the circulation, leading to anaemia.

***Sickle Cell Trait.*** Condition in which sufferers are heterozygous for the codominant sickle cell gene and so possess both sickle cell haemoglobin (HbS) and normal adult haemoglobin (HbA) in their erythrocytes. Such persons are mildly debilitated. It seems that possession of HbS in the erythrocytes confers a greater resistance to malaria, probably due to the increased viscosity of the cytosol, as well as the tendency of parasitized cells to sickle and be ingested by phagocytes. Thus the sickle cell gene survives in the population because heterozygotes are more 'fit' with respect to survival in the face of malaria.

***Side-chain Theory.*** Form of selective theory proposed by Paul Ehrlich in 1900 to explain the presence of antitoxin in serum after immunization with bacterial toxins. Ehrlich postulated that cells contained surface extensions of their protoplasm (haptophores) that bind to the antigenic determinants of the toxin (toxophores); after the cell is stimulated, the haptophores are shed into the circulation and become the antitoxin. Proposed at a time when there was no understanding of the cellular basis of immunity, this theory was a remarkably prescient (explanation of cellular recognition of antigen).

***Sieve Area.*** Depression in the primary wall of sieve tube elements with clusters of pores through which the protoplasts of adjacent sieve elements are connected by cytoplasmic strands. These strands are encased in a cylinder of callose.

***Sieve Plate.*** Area, usually on the end walls of sieve tube elements, perforated by relatively large pores. These pores are larger than those found in sieve areas, but like them are linked with callose and are penetrated by cytoplasmic strands.

***Sieve Tube Element.*** Characteristic cell of the phloem that is responsible for translocation of dissolved nutrients. Sieve elements are of two kinds; less specialized sieve cells found in pteridophytes and gymnosperms; sieve tube elements (or sieve tube members). Sieve cells are commonly elongated and have tapering ends or steeply inclined end walls. Distributed on the walls are sieve areas through which the protoplasts of adjacent cells are interconnected. In sieve tube elements, some of the sieve areas are more highly specialized than others, having larger pores and being localized on or near an end wall, and form a sieve plate. A vertical series of sieve tube elements arranged end to end with the sieve plate on their common walls constitutes a sieve tube. At matuarity, sieve elements usually have no nucleus, ribosomes or dicytosomes and lack a large central vacuole. In angiosperms the sieve elements are associated with companion cells, and frequently the cytoplasm contains a characteristic proteinaceous material, P protein.

***Sigma Factor.*** A protein molecule that is one of the five distinct subunits of RNA polymerase in prokaryotes. Sigma factor plays a crucial role in enhancing the preference of the enzyme for promoter regions at the initiation end of gene sequences. RNA polymerase without sigma is referred to as core enzyme; that with sigma is holoenzyme.

***Sigma Virus.*** Virus that infects Drosophila melanogaster, resulting in increased sensitivity to carbon dioxide.

***Signal Sequence.*** Sequence of 16 to 30 amino acid residues that is thought to initiate transport of secreted proteins across the membrane of the endoplasmic reticulum. Signal sequences typically contain a core of 4 to 12 hydrophobic residues, which may facilitate interaction with the membrane. Transmembrane proteins may also have signal sequences; these proteins usually also contain a 'stop-transfer' sequence of about 20 hydrophobic residues, which stops translocation of the growing polypeptide and anchors it in the phospholipid bilayer. The signal sequence of most secreted and many transmembrane proteins is at the amino-terminus and is removed by enzymatic cleavage of the nascent chain in the endoplasmic reticulum. Some membrane proteins and a few secreted proteins (e.g., ovalbumin) have uncleaved internal signal sequences that facilitate membrane insertion. The interaction of secreted and some integral membrane proteins with the endoplasmic reticulum is mediated by a signal recognition particle (6 distinct polypeptides and a 300-base RNA) and is receptor, known as 'docking protein', which is an integral membrane protein (single chain of $M_r \sim 72{,}000$) of the rough endoplasmic reticulum. Synonym for signal peptide, leader sequence, leader peptide.

***Silent Allele.*** Allele whose product can not be detected at a phenotypic level. Such alleles should not be assumed to be untranscribed. Often the protein product is defective as an enzyme or structural molecule, and thus goes unnoticed.

***Silect Mutation.*** Mutation with no phenotypic effect in that the protein product is just as effective as that of the wild-type allele.

***Silk.*** Fibre produced by both insects and spiders, but nest known as the product of the larva of the silk moth, Bombyx mori, being used to form the cocoon in which the larva pupates. Fibroin is the chief protein constitutent of silk, the other being sericin.

***Silurian.*** The third period of the Palaeozoic era, extending from 440 to 400 million years ago. It was named after a Celtic tribe that lived in the region of Wales where rocks of the period were first recognized. Silurian·fossils consist of many marine invertebrates, including bryozoans, trilobites, crinoids, and corals. In some Silurian rocks scales and spines of ostracoderms (jawless fish) have been found.

***Simple Allotype.*** Allotype that varies from another allotype in amino acid sequence at only one or a few positions. Simple allotypes (e.g., Km) are usually products of alleles at a single genetic locus.

***Simple Pit.*** Pit lacking a surrounding border. Simple pits are found in certain parenchyma cells, sclereids and some fibres.

***Single-coil Protein.*** A protein produced by fermenting microorganisms with petrolkeum hydrocarbons. Some microorganisms, such as the yeast Candida and the bacteria Nocardia and Pseudomonas, are able to convert petroleum hydrocarbons to protein in the presence of air and suitable aqueous nutrients. The protein is nutritionally acceptable and a potential food source if large-scale production were to be undertaken.

***Single-copy DNA.*** DNA that hybridizes extremely slowly or not at all in a cot plot experiment and therefore is made up of sequences that occur only once, or very few times, in the genome.

***Single-copy Gene.*** Gene sequence that, like that coding for fibroin, is present once only in the haploid genome. Other genes, such as those coding for globins, occur as small families of similar, but non-identical sequences, or as repetitious copies or identical sequences, as with some histone genes.

***Single-copy Plasmid.*** Plasmid present in bacterial cells at a frequence of only one copy per cell.

***Single Immunodiffusion.*** Type of immunodiffusion in which one reactant (e.g., antiserum) is incorporated into a gel and the second reactant (e.g., antigen) is introduced onto the surface of a gel-filled tube (method of Oudin), or into a well of an agar plate (method of Mancini). The antigen diffuses into the gel and forms a precipitate when the antigen concentration reaches equivalence with the antibodies, forming a line or ring of precipitation. Single immunodiffusion can be used to quantitate either the mobile or stationary reactant.

***Single Radial Immunodiffusion.*** Quantitative immunodiffusion test (method of Mancini). One of the reactants (usually antiserum) is incorporated into a gel (e.g., agarose) before it solidifies. The other reactant (usually antigen) is placed into a well made in the gel. When the antigen diffuses from the well into the gel, it precipitates with the antiserum. As antigen continues to diffuse from the well, the precipitate comes into anigen excess, dissolves and reforms further from the well. At the equivalence ratio of antigen and antibody, a ring or halo of precipitate is finally formed; the area within this ring is proportional to the antigen concentration. By comparison with a set of antigen standards, the concentration of antigen added to the well can be determined. Provided that the antiserum is specific, the antigen need not be pure.

***Single-hit Theory.*** Theory that complement-mediated hemolysis is brought about by a single lesion produced in the erythrocyte membrane as a result of the activation of complement.

***Sinusoid.*** Small blood-filled space in liver surrounded by flattened epithelial cells with hepatocytes behind them. This arrangement allows the rapid transport of metabolites and products of metabolism to be exchanged between blood and hepatocytes.

***Sips Distribution.*** Distribution, originally used to describe the adsorption of gases to (heterogeneous) catalyst surfaces, that has been applied to the distribution of association constants in a heterogeneous population of antibody sites.

The Sips distribution resembles closely the normal (Gaussian) distribution. As applied to antibody sites, the logarithms of the association constants (log K) are distributed about a mean, which is denoted log $K_o$; the dispersion about this mean is described by a parameter, a, that varies from 0 to 1 and that is inversely related to the width of the distribution (i.e., the smaller a, the greater width). The explicit function for the distribution is log r/(n-r) = a log c + a log $K_o$, where r is the molar concentration of the bound ligand divided by the molar concentration of antibodies, n is the valence of the antibodies and c is the molar concentration of free ligand. The values of a and log $K_o$ are estimated from the linear plot of log r/(n-r) against log c. By convention , $K_o$ (the antilog of the mean of the distribution, log $K_o$) is called the 'average association constant'. However, this is a misnomer because, although log $K_o$ is the mean of all the log K, $K_o$ is not the mean of all the K. Nevertheless, for symmetrical distributions, such as the Sips and normal distributions, $K_o$ will be the median association constant.

When the antibody sites are half-saturated with ligand, r = n-r, log $K_o$ = -log c, and $K_o$ = 1/c. Again, by convention, the 'average association constant' has been taken to be the reciprocal of the free ligand concentration resulting in half-saturation of the sites. However, as discussed above, this value is not actually the mean of the association constants and, only in an ideal symmetrical distribution, will it be the median value of these constants.

If the population of antibody sites is homogeneous, a =1 and the Sips equation reduces to the Scatchard equation r/(n—r) = Kc.

***Sips Plot.*** Plot of data obtained in measuring the binding of ligand to a population of antibodies, in which log r/n-r is plotted against log c. If the plot is a straight line (i.e., the data conform to the Sips equation), the slope, a, is a meausre of the heterogeneity of the antibodies with respect to affinity.

***Sister Chromatid Exchange.*** Exchange of pieces of DNA molecules between sister chromatids prior to mitosis. Unlike crossing over in meiotic chromosomes, no genetic recombination is involved; sisten chromatid exchange is revealed simply as a phenomenon appearing in autoradiography of chromosomes following DNA radio-labelling during the S phase of the cell cycle.

***Site.*** Location of a mutation in a coding sequence of DNA, or the location of DNA cutting or integration. Thus some phage integrate in a 'site-specific' manner, implying that they can integrate only at certain locations on the DNA.

***Site-specific Recombination.*** Recombination of short, specific nucleotide sequences. It does not depend on DNA homology.

***Sjogren's Syndrome.*** Autoimmune disease characterized by keratoconjunctivitis sicca (dry eyes) and xerostomia (dry mouth), and usually accompanied by connective tissue disease such as rheumatoid arthritis. The salivary glands are enlarged and heavily infiltrated with lymphocytes. There are numerous autoantibodies, both organ non-specific (e.g., rheumatoid factor and a variety of antibodies to uridine-rich nuclear RNA) and organ-specific (e.g., to ductal epithelium of the lacrymal and salivary glands). Sjogren's syndrome has been observed in recipients of bone marrow transplants who have graft-versus-host disease. Pathology similar to Sjogren's syndrome has been observed in NZB x NZW $F_1$ mice.

***Skin*** (cutis). Cellular layer that covers almost the entire body of vertebrates, consisting of epithelial cells, connective tissue and associated structures. It consists of both epidermis and dermis, the former being the outer layer of epithelial cells, and the latter the inner connective tissue layer. Skin contains numerous glands, hairs, and is also modified to form spines, nails, claws and beaks of different vertebrate groups. Skin is important in temperature regulation, due to sweat glands, blood vessel dilation or construction, and insulation by fur. Skin cells are constantly being sloughed off and replaced by rapid cell division of stem cells in the underlying dermis.

***Skin-sensitizing Antibody.*** Antibody that binds to mast cells in skin and thus prepares a skin site for an immediate hypersensitivity reaction.

***Skin-specific Histocompatibility Antigen.*** Minor histocompatibility antigen found in the skin of mice. The existence of this antigen is demonstrated by the following experiment. Spleen cells from an $F_1$ offspring of two inbred strains are transplanted into a heavily irradiated parent. Sunsequently (three months later) various tissues are transplanted from the opposite parent onto the chimera. Skin grafts are rejected, albeit at a low and inconsistent rate. However, tissues other than skin are not rejected. The spleen cells of the $F_1$ mouse are initially tolerant to the tissues of both parents but eventually lose tolerance to the skin of one parental strain when residing in the other parent. The putative gene encoding the sensitizing antigen has been named Sk.

***Skin Test.*** Any test carried out by injecting or applying substances to the skin to ascertain the state of immunity of the host.

***Skin Window.*** Technique for observing the evolution of inflammation. Skin is injured by scraping. Cover slips are successively placed on the abrasion and stained upon removal to ascertain the types of cells responding to the injury. For the first four hours, neutrophils are mainly found on the cover slips; subsequently, increasing numbers of monocytes and decreasing numbers of neutrophils are found. Skin window is also called Rebuck window after the physician who developed the technique.

***Sliding Filament Model.*** Mechanism that is widely accepted as the model for muscular contraction. It involves sliding of actin and myosin filaments relative to one another by making and breaking of cross-bridges between them. Microtubular contraction, as in the mitotic spindle, may involve a somewhat similar mechanism.

***Sliding Growth.*** Growth of plant cells in which new cell slide over previously formed cells without disturbing the underlying organization.

***Slime mould*** (slime fungus). Term applied to two distinct and probably unrelated types of organisms: the Acrasiomycota, which includes the organism Dictyostelium; the Myxomycota, which includes the organism Physarum. The former are referred to as cellular slime molds and the latter as acellular slime moulds (since for most of their life history they exist as syncitial plasmodia.)

***Slow Reacting Substance of Anaphylaxis (SRS-A).*** Leukotrienes C4, D4 and E4, thought to be responsible for many of the symptoms of anaphylaxis. SRS-A was first identified as a biological activity in extracts of guinea-pig lung following anaphylaxis induced by cobra venom. The activity contracted guinea-pig ileum, but at a slower rate than histamine and was not inhibited by antihistamines.

***Slow Stop.*** Mutants of bacterial cells that are able to complete a round of cell division after being raised to 42°C.

***Slp.*** Sex-limited proteins of mice (found normally only in males and inducible in females by androgens). It is the product of the complement locus, C4A, and is not hemolytically active.

***Small Nuclear RNA*** (snRNA). Species of RNA of between 100 and 300 base pairs, found in the nucleic of eukaryotic cells at a frequency of $10^5$-$10^6$ for each individual species. They exist chiefly in small ribonuleoprotein particles, and also include some species—the UsnRNA— which has a role in splicing of some intron sequences.

***Smooth Endoplasmic Reticulum (SER).*** Regions of the endoplasmic reticulum devoid of ribosomes as observed by electron microscopy and indicative of little if any, protein synthesis.

***Smooth Muscle.*** Tissue consisting of long, tapering cells with single nuclei and with both thick and thin filaments running along the long axis of the cell. These filaments do not adopt the ordered array characteristic of striated muscle cells.

***Snake Venom.*** Source of important biochemical compounds. The toxins of venomous snakes operate in quite diverse ways. For example, corbratoxin from venomous cobra species and α-bungarotoxin from a Formosan snake are neurotoxins that bind acetylcholine receptors at the neuromuscular junction. Other snake venoms are enzymes that cleave phosphodiesterase bonds. Venoms with important enzymic properties are also produced by spiders.

***Snell-Bagg Mouse.*** Mouse belonging to a mutant strain (dw/dw), characterized by pituitary dwarfing. The dw mutation is an autosomal recessive trait. These mice have a small thymus and depressed cell-mediated immunity.

***Sodium Dodycyl Sulphate*** (SDS, sodium lauryl sulphate). Anionic detergent much used to deproteinize cell homogenates and in SDS-PAGE electrophoresis for protein fractionation on gels.

***Sodium Pump.*** Mechanism whereby sodium ions are actively pumped out of cells across the plasma membrane. The mechanism of this biochemical pumping action is part of a combined sodium and potassium pump, the sodium being pumped out and potassium in. A specific pump ATPase is implicated, using ATP to provide energy for the movement. Indeed at least one-third of all the ATP used by a resting animal is employed in the activity of this pump. The movement of the sodium and potassium ions helps to control cell volume, drives the active transport of sugars and animo acids, and renders nerve and muscle cells electrically excitable.

***Solenoid Model.*** Model proposed for compaction of nucleosomes into the 30-nm diameter thread which is basic to the chromatin structure of most chromosomes. The string of nucleosomes along a length of DNA is believed to condense by an alteration in the binding of histone H1, and the nucleosomes then form a tight spiral stack in the form of solenoid. Such solenoids must themselves be further folded or coiled to acieve the tight packing of chromatin in chromosomes.

***Solid-phase Immunoassay.*** Any immunoassay in which antigens or antibodies are attached to an insoluble matrix. For example, in a typical assay for antibodies, an antigen is attached to the matrix and a test sample, containing antibodies to the immobilized antigen, is added. There should be an excess of antigen relative to the antibodies. After a suitable interval, the matrix is washed and radiolabeled antibodies directed to constant region determinants of the bound antibodies (e.g., anti-Fc) are then added in excess. Unbound radiolabeled antibodies are washed away and the residual radioactivity adhering to the matrix is determined. The assay can be standardized by adding known amounts of antibodies to the antigen. The insoluble matrix may be beads (e.g., Sepharose) or wells in a polystyrene or polyvinyl chloride tissue culture plate to which proteins (e.g., antigens) adhere non-specifically. Care must be taken so that excess sites on the plate (i.e., sites not containing the immobilized antigen) are saturated with unrelated protein before addition of the test antibody.

***Soluble Complex.*** Antigen-antibody complex that is soluble (i.e., not precipitated). Such complexes usually contain excess antigen.

***Soluble RNA.*** Low-molecular-weight RNA of ill-defined composition, but mainly consisting of transfer RNA. the term is something of a misnomer since all RNA, including high-molecular-weight species, are readily soluble in aqueous media.

***Somatic cell.*** Generally body cell. The majority of tissues in the adult organism are composed of somatic cells. The somatic cells divide by mitosis, and most contain he diploid number of chromosomes.

***Somatic Cell Hybrid.*** Cell resulting from the fusion of two somatic cells or substantial parts of such cells.

***Somatic Hybridization.*** The fusion of diploid cells from different species in tissue culture; for example, a mouse cell an a human cell. The technique can be used to map human genes, since a hybrid cell that immediately after fusion contains a full complement of (for example) human and mouse chromosomes progressively loses the human chromosomes. Thus, loss of particular traits can often be ascribed to loss of a particular chromosome.

***Somatic Mutation.*** Mutation that has occurred in a cell other than a germ cell. Most somatic mutations will have no phenotypic effects since the gene affected may not be expressed in the tissue of which the cell forms a part. Some somatic mutations can be detected as a distinct line of cells in the tissue arising from the cell in which the mutation originally occurred. Some types of variegation in plants result from somatic mutations, as do certain changes in leaf form or branching pattern.

***Somatic Mutation.*** Mutation in a somatic cell, which is inherited only by its descendants. Accelerated somatic mutation (called somatic hypermutation) is thought to be important in generating diversity in the variable regions of the light and heavy chains of antibodies. Evidence for the occurrence of somatic mutations can be obtained by comparing sequences of expressed variable regions with germline V,J (and D) gene segments. Somatic mutations are found more frequently in IgG and IgA antibodies than in IgM antibodies.

***Somatic Pairing.*** Association of homologous chromosomes in somatic cells. This is a rare phenomenon, but occurs in cells of Drosophila larvae in which polytene chromosomes occur. It is the side-to-side alignment of homologous chromosomes (each chromosome replicates many times to form the ribbon-like polytene formation) which permits visualization of deletions or inversions in one of the two homologous chromosomes as a loop in the ribbon of the other homologue.

***Somatomedin (Plasma Growth Factor).*** A polypeptide (molecular weight about 4000) in mammalian plasma that is released from the liver (and possibly the kidneys) by growth hormone, most of whose actions it is thought to mediate.

***Somatostain.*** Peptide hormone, released by the hypothalamus, that inhibits the production of growth hormone (somatotrophin) by the anterior lobe of the pituitary gland. It also inhibits insulin and glucagon production by the pancreas. The somatostatin gene has been isolated from the human and cloned in E.coli, active somatostatin being recovered from the clone.

***Somite.*** Segmentally arranged series of blocks of mesoderm that lie on either side of the neural tube in vertebrate embryos. Each somite consists of three regions: myotomes, which develop into striated muscle: sclerotome, which develops into the vertebral column and proximal parts of the ribs; dermatome, which develops into the dermis.

***Sonication.*** Technique in which ultrasound is used to homogenize tissue. The procedure has fallen out of favour in moecular biology because it tends to damage large, long molecules by shearing, but it may be used intentionally to reduce drastically the molecular weight of a nucleic acid solution.

***Sordaria Fimicola.*** Ascomycete fungus used widely for genetic studies. Separate strains produce black or white ascospores, and hybridization between the strains results in hybrid asci which have been much used for studies on gene conversion.

***Sorting Out.*** Phenomenon in cell and developmental biology, in which cells with distinct surface properties will separate, selectively from one another by dint of the differential adhesion of the cell surfaces. Such differential adhesion can be demonstrated to be tissue-specific, so that a mixed aggregate of cells from differing tissues will eventually sort out into separate aggregates of only one cell type, or aggregates in which one cell type is internal and the other is external in the cell mass.

***SOS.*** DNA sequence of the operator gene that is recognized by the hex A repressor protein.

***SOS Repair.*** Process of DNA repair, involving a number of different enzymes. It is highly important because it is error-prone and thus generates mutations. Regulation of SOS repair in E.coli is known to depend on the fact that the repair enzymes are coded by genes which have common SOS boxes in their regulatory regions. These boxes are specifically repressed by a protein called hex A. However, this protein is specifically cleaved and inactivated by a rec A protease, which is, in turn, activated by damaged DNA. So damaged DNA is able to induce its own repair.

***Southern Blotting.*** Technique, described by and subsequently named after E.M. Southern, for detecting particular sequences in a mixture of DNA fragments, usually obtained by digestion with one or more restriction endonucleases, that have been separated, according to size, by gel electrophoresis. The resulting fragments are denatured (by soaking the gel in sodium hydroxide) and 'blotted' onto a sheet of nitrocellulose or nylon that is laid on top of the gel. The relative positions of the DNA fragments are preserved during the transfer. The DNA in the filter is then hybridized with an appropriate labeled probe (e.g., radiolabeled DNA or RNA) which hybridizes to complementary sequences in the fragments. Unbound probe is washed away, and the location of the hybridized probe is revelaed by autoradiography. The technique can be used both to detect specific sequences in cloned DNA and in digests of genomic DNA. It is sufficiently sensitive to detect single-copy genes in the total mammalian genome. Strictly speaking, 'blotting' refers to the method for transferring DNA from the agarose gel to the nitrocellulose, but the term is often used to describe the entire procedure; electrophoresis, transfer and hybridization.

***Southern Blotting Technique.*** A widely used method in gene manipulation invented by Ed Southern in 1975. An agarose gel containing denatured DNA fragments is placed between buffer-saturated filter paper and a cellulose nitrate filter. The DNA is eluted from the gel onto the cellulose nitrate filter, to which it blinds strongly. This filter can then be used for complementary nucleic acid hybridization, which reveals the identity of the sequences in the blotted filter and thus in the original agarose gel. Other similar techniques, which have been given the jargon names of 'Northern' blots and 'Western' blots, are used for elution of RNA fragments from gels. See Figure S.1.

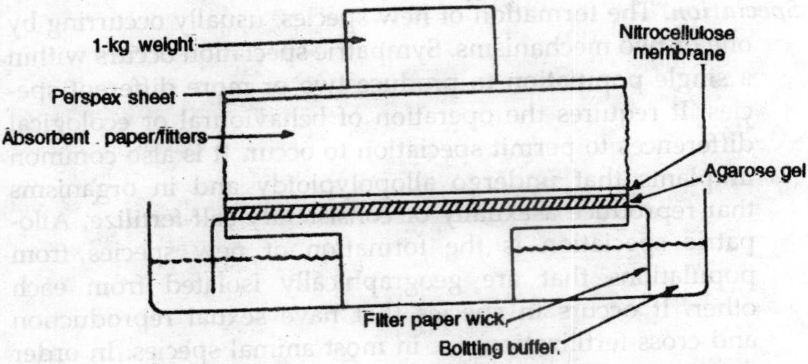


**Figure S.1. Southern Blotting. Diagrammtic representation of southern blotting apparatus showing capillary transfer of DNA from a gel to a solid supporting matrix (nitrocellulose membrane).**

***Spacer DNA.*** DNA that is located between genes and may or may not be transcribed by RNA polymerase. Spacer DNA is found, for example, between the cistrons coding for 18S and 28S ribosomal RNA is most eukaryotic organisms.

***Special Creation.*** Hypothesis of the origin of life that presupposes the existence of a divine power responsible for the creation of life. Various different forms of the hypothesis exist. It may be conceived as a process in which the first cell was created and all other organisims were derived from that cell by natural evolution. Alternafives are that many different, diverse organisms were created all at once or that it is a continuing process. The degree to which the divine power might use natural selection, and evolution in the creation process is also a matter for speculation. No scientific evidence exists to confirm the idea of special creation.

***Specialization.*** The evolution of a special adaptation to suit an organism to a particular environment. An organism with such an adaptation is less capable of evolving in other directions, and this could result in extinction of the species in the environment were to change considerably.

***Specialized.*** Descriptive of organisms that will tolerate only a narrow range of environmnental conditions, or have a restricted capacity for future evolutionary change.

***Speciation.*** The formation of new species, usually occurring by one of two mechanisms. Sympatric speciation occurs within a single population to produce two or more different species. It requires the operation of behavioural or ecological differences to permit speciation to occur. It is also common in plants that undergo allopolyploidy and in organisms that reproduce asexually or consistently self-fertilize. Allopatric speciation is the formation of new species from populations that are geographically isolated from each other. It occurs in species that have sexual reproduction and cross-fertilization, i.e. in most animal species. In order that two separate species may develop, the two populations must evolve some sort of sexual and/or genetic isolating mechanism so that they do not interbreed if they come into contact again.

***Species.*** A unit used in the classification of plants and animals. Ideally a species is defined as a group of organisms that interbreed with each other to produce fertile offspring. Members of different animal species do not normally interbreed; if they do, the progeny are sterile. Hybrids of two plant species are usually sterile but may occasionally be made fertile by allopolyploidy. Members of the same species usually resemble each other closely, but when species are subdivided into subspecies, clines, or cultivated varieties, the members of these subgroups often differ from one another in appearance. Not all species have been tested for the breeding definition, and this definition cannot be applied to specimens studied from dead or preserved material only or to species that habitually self-fertilize or have only asexual reproduction. Such species can be defined only in terms of observable similarities between their members. Each species has a holotype, which was used in the original naming and description of the species, and two names.

Species can be designated according to the criteria used in defining them. The taxonomic species, the unit in general use, satisfies all possible criteria and meets the requirements of the International Rules of Nomenclature. The morphospecies is a species named only on morphological evidence, for example from herbarium or preserved specimens. These species must often be modified if live material becomes available. The palaeospecies, an exinct group, is named from fossil material only; such species often have to be modified as more fossil material becomes available. A biospecies is a species that fulfils the breeding requirements of the definition. The term can therefore be applied only to species with sexual reproduction and cross-fertilization and in practice only to species that mature quickly and breed fairly frequently. The agamospecies consists of a group of organisms that reproduce only asexually and must therefore be treated as morphospecies since the breeding definition cannot be applied.

***Species Transformation.*** Gradual evolution of one species into another with time. Since both species do not coexist at the same time, no increase in the number of species is involved.

***Specific Activity.*** Ratio of radioactive atoms or molecules to non-radioactive ones in the same sample. It may sometimes be expressed as the number of radioactive atoms per million atoms of the non-radioactive compounds, or as curies per mole or millimole.

***Specific Granule.*** Synonym for secondary granule.

***Specific Ionization.*** Number of pairs of ions per unit mass of tissue, or per unit path length of the ionizing radiation in the medium.

***Specificity.*** Selective requirement on the part of one reactant molecule or cell for its substrate, receptor or macromolecular complex. Thus antibody is specific for antigene, and an enzyme and its substrate share specificity.

***Specificity.*** Ability of antibodies or lymphocytes to discriminate among different ligands.

***Spectrin.*** Most abundant protein of the erythrocyte plasma membrane. It is a long, fibrous molecule comprising two large polypeptides ($M_r$= 240,000 and 220,000). The molecules form a filamentous network on the cytoplasmic side of the membrane, and some 3 x $10^5$ molecules of spectrin exist in each human erythocyte.

***Spectrotype.*** Pattern of bands on an isoelectric focusing gel. The spectrotype can serve as a marker for a single protein (that may appear as a cluster of bands because of post-translational modifications) or a group of proteins. A spectrotype of secreted antibody can be used as a marker for a clone of antibody-producing cells.

***Spermatheca (Seminal Receptacle).*** A cavity or sac in the body of some female and hermaphrodite animals in which spermatozoa received from the male (or hermaphrodite partner) during copulation are stored until required for fertilizing the ova.

***Spermatid.*** A haploid cell of the animal testis produced by the second meiotic division of a spermatocyte (one spermatocyte produces four spermatids). The spermatid then matures and changes shape to form a spermatozoon.

***Spermatium.*** A minute spherical non-motile male gamete produced by the red algae and by certain fungi, including some Pyrenomycetes (a subdivision of the Ascomycetes) and the Uredinates (rusts).

***Spermatocyte.*** A cell within the seminiferous tubules of the testis that undergoes meiosis to form a spermatid with a haploid nucleus. Typically a primary spermatocyte undergoes the first division to form two secondary spermatocyts, which each undergo a second division to form two spermatids.

***Spermatogenesis.*** Process of production of sperm cells (spermatozoon) involving both haploid division of the spermatocytes and spermiogenesis.

***Spermatogonia.*** Cells in the testis of the male which divide mitotically and are the progenitors of the primary spermatocytes.

***Spermatophore.*** Mass of sperm held together by mucus, which may be deposited within the body of the female during copulation (as in some insects) or deposited into water or onto a surface by the male, to be later taken up by the female into her cloaca (as in salamanders).

***Spermatozoon (sperm).*** The small motile male gamete formed in the animal testis and released in large numbers to fertilize the female gamete during the process of sexual reproduction. It generally comprises a head region (acrosome) containing a compact haploid nucleus, a middle region containing mitochondria, and a tail region (often a flagellum).

***Sperm Bank.*** Store of sperm, normally in semen with additives such as glycerol, derived from many individuals, and maintained in liquid nitrogen at -196°C for many years. Such sperm may be used in artificial insemination. Sperm banks permit storage of gene pools which might otherwise be lost for ever.

***Spermidine.*** Highly basic polyamine, somewhat smaller than spermine, but with a similar biological distribution and presumed function.

***Spermine.*** Small, highly basic polyamine, found in both prokaryotes and eukaryotes and probably responsible for stabilizing the DNA double helix.

***Spermiogenesis.*** That part of spermatogenesis which involves development of spermatozoon (sperm) from spermatid.

***S Phase*** (synthetic phage). Phase in the cell cycle after the G1 phase and before the G2 phase and during which the DNA is replicated.

***Spheroplast.*** Protoplast to which remnants of bacterial cell wall remain attached. Spheroplasts are able to regenerate cell walls.

***Spheroplast.*** Type of protoplast prepared from Gram-negative bacteria and hence retaining remnants of the outer membrane.

***Spherosome.*** An organelle of eukaryote cells, bounded by a single membrane, that store and synthesizes lipids (fats and oils). Derived from the endoplasmic reticulum, it measures up to 1 μm in diameter and is usually spherical.

***Sphingosine.*** A lipid alcohol consisting of a long hydrocarbon tail and a polar head. It is a component of the sphingomyelins, gangliosides, and cerebrosides.

***Spina Bifida.*** Result in the human of incomplete closure of the neural tube in the non-cephalic region. Its cause remains obscure, although there is a distinct hereditary aspect. The condition may be detected in pregnancy by a raised maternal serum alpha-foetoprotein.

***Spindle.*** A structure formed within the cytoplasm during mitosis and meiosis. It is shaped like two cones joined at their bases and is made of longitudinally arranged contractile protein microtubules or fibres. Chromosomes come to be orientated on the equatorial plate of the spindle by their centromeres. The spindle microtubules are of different types: some are continuous between the poles (interpolar microtubules); some are discontinuous and involved in attaching to the centromeres (kinetochores) of the chromosomes (kinetochore microtubules). The precise mechanism by which the spindle microtubules accomplish movement of the chromosomes to the spindle poles during anaphase

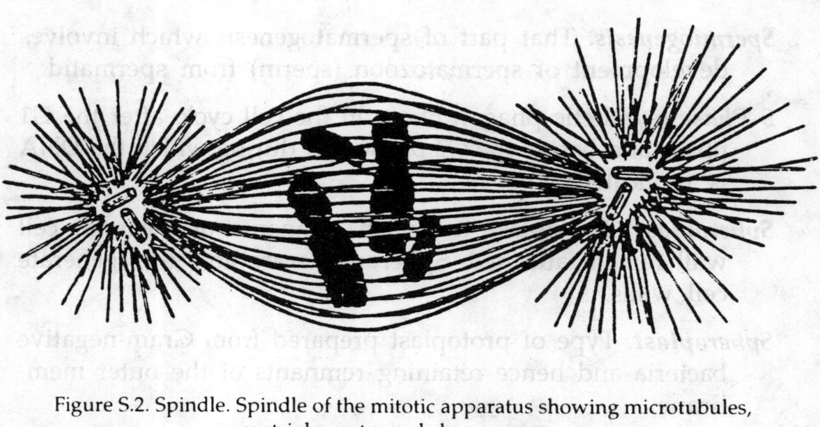

Figure S.2. Spindle. Spindle of the mitotic apparatus showing microtubules, centrioles, aster and chromosomes.

remains unclear. Organization of the spindle is associated with activity of the centrioles in the cells of animals and some lower plants. Higher plant cells lack centrioles but still generate spindles, and there is no envidence that the presence of centrioles is essnetial for spindle formation even in higher animal cells. See Figure S.2.

***Spiral Cleavage.*** Type of embryonic development found in molluscs and annelids in which the horizontal cell divisions in the blastula result in quartets of cells that are slightly out of line with the quartet above or below, so giving the embryo a spiral appearance. Complex genetic influences, including strictly maternal influences, determine the direction of the spiral.

***Spiral Thickening.*** Pattern of wall formation in tracheids and xylem vessels in which the thickening is laid down in spiral bands. Such thiickenng is usually secondary to other forms of thckening in these cell walls.

***Spirochaetes.*** Unicellular bacteria whose cells are flexible, elongated and arranged in a helix around an axial fibrillar fiilament. The cells are enclosed within an outer flexible, close-fittng envelope. Some spirochaetes are free-livng, whereas others are parasitic or pathogenc. Syphylis in humans is caused by the spirochaete Treponema pallidum.

***Splanchnopleur.*** Lower layer of lateral mesoderm whch in the development of vertebrates becomes applied to endoderm to form the alimentary canal; derived from the Greek pleura meaning siide. In reptiles, birds and mammals iit also forms the yolk sac and allantois.

***Spleen.*** Major secondary lymphoid organ located in the upper abdomen in direct communication with the main arterial circulation. In contrast to lymph nodes, which filter lymph, the spleen filters blood. The spleen consists of lymphoid tissue around arterioles (white pulp) surrounded by lakes of blood (red pulp). The periarteriolar lymphoid sheath consists of small masses of B lymphocytes (follicles) interskpersed among T lymphocytes. The arterioles terminate in specialized venules that lie between the white pulp and the red pulp - the so-called marginal sinus. B and T lymkphocytes traverse the marginal sinus, circulate through the white pulp for about six hours, and return to the venous circulation via the red pulp. The spleen traps blood-borne antigens and immune responses to them are initiated there. The red pulp scavenges old red blood cells and is a reserve site for hemopoiesis. Individuals lacking a spleen are very susceptible to some blood-borne bacterial infections (e.g., with pneumococci and Hemophilus influenzae). See Figure S.3.

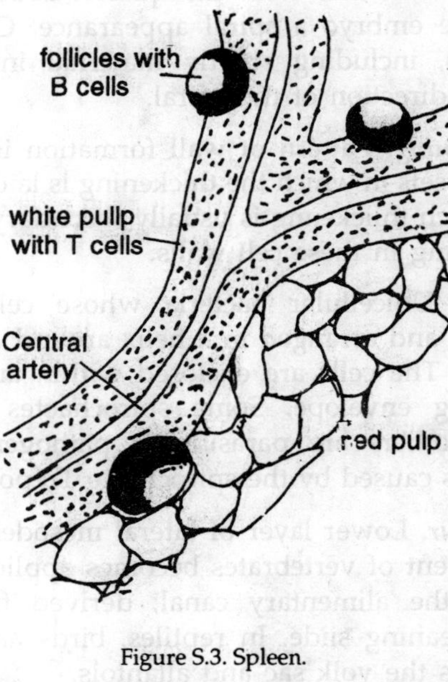


Figure S.3. Spleen.

***Spleen Colony-forming Cell.*** Bone marrow cell injected into the circulation of a mouse followiing its irradiation. Injected cells 'rescue' the mouse by replacing its own killed bone marrow cells, many growing to form colonies in the spleen. Analysis of such colonies has been used to shed light on the proliferative cells of the marrow and how they differentiate into lymphocytes, red cells and macrophages.

***Splice Junction.*** Short sequence that resides at the end of an intron and facilitates intron excision and exon splicing. The sequences at either end of an introl are termed donor junctions and acceptor junctions, being at the 5'-end and 3'-end, respectively, and UsnRNA contains a sequence complementary to both.

***Splicing.*** The enzyme-catalysed joiniing of conserved sections of messenger RNA, following excision of the intron sequences. The term is also used for the joining of fragments of DNA in genetic engineering. The enzymes effecting both types of splicing are known as splicing enzymes.

***Split Gene.*** Gene that consists of both exon coding sequences and intron non-coding sequences interspersed. Most eukaryotic genes are split, as are the genes of some animal viruses. The genes of prokaryotes lack introns, as do all but a few mitrochondrial genes.

***Split Tolerance.*** Form of partial tolerance in which there is tolerance to some antigenic determinants and an immune response to other antigenic determinants of allogeneic cells.

***Spontaneous Generation (Abiogenesis).*** The doctrine that living organisms arise from nonliving material. Until the middle of the 17th century it was widely believed that microorganisms arose in this way, from rotting meat, infusions of hay, etc. However, the work of bacteriologists, especially Pasteur (1822-95), proved that microorganisms are always present in the air and merely undergo rapid growth and reproduction when they come into contact with a suitable substrate.

***Spontaneous Mutation.*** Mutation that occurs without any added agent such as a mutagen, and therefore results most commonly from the mutagenic effects of cosmic rays.

***Sporangium.*** Structure in which spores are formed. Sporangia found in the algae and fungi are usually simple in structure, whereas those of the bryophytes and the vascular plants are more complex in form.

***Spore.*** Reproduction until normally microscopic in size. Spores are produced by bacteria, protozoa, fungi and plants, and are adapted for different functions. Spores may act as a means of asexual reproduction for rapid vegetative spread.

Others may function as a resistant, resting stage in the life cycle. In plants, spores are produced by the sporophyte after meiosis and are then haploid. They germinate to produce the gametophyte. The term spore is often prefixed to give an indication of its function (e.g., endospore, megaspore, microspore, zoospore, zygospore).

***Spore Mother Cell*** (Sporocyte). Diploid cell that give rise to four haploid spores by meiosis.

***Sporophyll.*** Leaf-bearing sporangia on the sporophyte phase of a vascular plant.

***Sporophyte.*** Diploid generation in the life cycle of organisms that exhibit an alternation of generations. It arises from the fusion of gametes derived from the haploid gametophyte generation. Meiosis occurs in the sporophyte, producing asexual spores which develop into the gametophyte.

***Sporopollenin.*** Compound found in the walls of fungal spores and polen grains, which is a long, polymerized cyclic alcohol somewhat similar to cutin and suberin. The stability of the compound allows the persistance of the outer layers of spores and pollen grans for thousands of years.

***Sporozoa.*** Class of parasitic Protozoa, containing the malarial parasite Plasmodium. They have complex life cycles and alternating sexual and asexual reproduction, with spore production. No locomotory phase is present.

***Sport (Rogue).*** An organism produced by a naturally ocurring mutation.

***Spot Desmosome.*** Type of adhereing intercellular junction in which epithelial cells are held together by button-like points of contact. Desmosomes also act as anchoring sites for keratin filaments.

***Spreading Position Effect.*** Phenomenon in which the effect of an inversion or translocation in inactivatiing adjacent gene sequences affects more than one such sequence.

***S Protein.*** Protein in human serum that inhibits the formation of the membrane attack complex of complement. S protein is a single polypeptide chain of 478 amino acid residues, including a signal sequence of 19 residues; it contains three sites for attachment of N-linked oligosaccharides. Three molecules of S protein bind to each nascent complex of C5b, C6 and C7, and prevent the insertion of the complex into cell membranes. S protein also prevents the polymerization of C9 on complexes of C5b, C6, C7 and C8.

S protein is identical to vitronectin (serum spreading factor), which is functinally similar to fibronectin. Vitronectin, so called because of its affinity for glass surfaces, binds to certain cell membranes and to complexed of thrombin and antithrombin III.

***Squarmes.*** Flattened, scale-like dead cells, filled with keratin filaments, which form the outermost layer of the mammalian epidermis.

***src Gene.*** Oncogene of the Rous sarcoma virus, a retrovirus, which induces sarcoma-type tumours in chickens.

***S region.*** Segment of the mouse major histocompatibility complex (MHC) in which the genes for complement components C2, Factor B, C4A (Slip) and C4B (Ss) are encoded. The term is also used to describe the homologous region of the human MHC, between HLA-B and HLA-D, where the genes for the four similar components are located. The products of the S region are called class III molecules.

***SSC.*** (1) Sister stand cross-over. (2) Solution of 'saline citrate', comprising a mixture of sodium chloride and sodium citrate.

***ssDNA.*** Single-stranded DNA.

***Ss Protein.*** Product of the complement locus, C4B in mice. Unlike the product of the C4A locus, slp, Ss is hemolytically active.

***Stab Culture.*** Culture of bacteria made by stabbing a long needle, carrying some of the bacteria from another culture, deep into an elongated test-tube containing a solid nutrient agar. It represents an easy way of culturing relatively non-fastidious anaerobic bacteria, since the oxygen concentration deep in the agar is low.

***Stabilizing Selection.*** Selection which involves removal of alleles that cause deviation from the mean population phenotype. Such selection reduces genetic variance in future generations.

***Stacking.*** Arrangement of adjacent nitrogenous bases in a DNA molecule.

***Stacking Gel.*** Technique employed in gel electrophoresis in which a gel of differing concentration is placed above the normal gel in order to help concentrate the molecules into distinct bands.

***Stage Micrometer.*** Etched glass slide bearing a sclae in 10 μm units; used for calibration of eyepiece micrometers in light microscopy.

***Staggered Cuts.*** Cuts in a DNA duplex which, although affecting both strands, are distant from one another by one or more bases. Most restriction endonucleases introduce such cuts in DNA.

***Staining.*** A process used in the preparation of temporary or permanent microscope slides of organisms or tissues. In light microscopy the specimens are coloured by adding solutions of dyes, so that they become visible under the microscope. The different dyes used for temporary and permanent preparations are shown in the table. The stain solvent is usually either water or alcohol, and it is necessary to know which has been used if dehydration is to follow, in the making of permanent preparations. Some stains are general and colour any nucleus or cytoplasm, while others are specific and are taken up by certain tissues only. Several specific stains can be used in sequence, a process known as counterstaining or double (or triple) staining. For example in animal tissues, haematoxylin or haemalum can be counterstained with Van Geison stain; in plant tissues safranin can be counterstrained with light green. Strains are described as acidic, basic, or neutral; this refers to the coloured radicals of he molecules, not to the pH of the solution. In acidic stains the actively staining part is an anion, which is usually combined with a metal; in basic stains the actively staining part is a cation, which is usually combined with an inorganic acid. Acidic stains colour the cytoplasm and collagen while basic stains colour the nucleus (and also the cytoplasm to some extent) because they are taken up by nucleic acids. Materials that stain strongly with basic dyes are known as basiphilic (or basophilic); those that stain strongly with acid dyes are termed acidophilic. Metachromatic stains produce colours in certain tissues or cells that are different from the colour of the stain solution. For example, methyl violet (violet-blue) becomes purple or reddish.

***Standard Deviation*** ***(s).*** In satistics, the square root of the variance

$$\text{standard deviation} = s = \sqrt{\text{variance}}.$$

s is a measure of the variation in individual observations from the mean in a normally distribution population.

***Standard Error (of the mean)*** (SE). If several sample observations from a population are made, and the mean value is calculated, the standard error (SE) of the mean will give an idea about the true mean value for the whole population. This estimate of how accurately the sample mean approximates to the true mean is measured by the standard deviation of the distribution of sample means or SE of the mean.

$$SE = \frac{s}{\sqrt{n}}$$

where s = standard deviation, and n = number of samples observed.

***Staphylococcus.*** A genus of spherical nonmotile Gram-positive bacteria. Streptococci form short chains of clusters and do not produce spores. They cause a variety of suppurative infections in man, including abscesses, wound infections, and meaningitis. Some strains produce a toxin and can cause food poisoning.

***Starch.*** Polysaccharide used as a storage compound in plants; an α-D-glucose polymer. Amylopectin, which comprises

75 precent of starch, is based on 1,4-linked glucose molecules with numerous 1,6-links. Amylose, comprising 25 precent of starch, is based on 1,4-linked glucose molecules without the 1,6-links.

***Starch Gel Electrophoresis.*** Zone electrophoresis method in which the support medium is a starch gel. As components of the mixture migrate through the gel under the influence of the electric current the pore structure of the gel acts as a molecular sieve. As a result, proteins of the same charge to mass ratios separate if their molecular sizes are suffiiciently different.

***Stasipatric Speciation.*** Speciation that results in development of individuals which have increased fitness within one part of the geographical range of the population as a result of a novel chromosomal rearrangement.

***Stasis.*** (1) Persistance of a species without significant evolutional change, over a long geological time span. (2) Stoppage of blood flow or of the circulation of some other body fluid.

***Stationary Phase.*** Phase of cell growth when tissue cells or microorganisms are cultured in vitro. It follows the exponential growth phase and is a period of slowing growth, terminating in complete cessation of growth and frequently in cell death. Such growth cessation results either from depletion of essential nutrients in the medium of from the accumulation of toxic waste products, or both. Note, however, that growth of explanted tissue cells may also slow as a result of the hayflick phenomenon.

***Statolith.*** Large starch grain or group of such strains found on the inner side of the lower plasma membrane of some plant cells. Since such cells are known to be gravity-sensitive, the statoliths are though to play a part in the geotropic mechanism.

***Steady-state System.*** Biological system in which the rate of molecules and other components leaving the system exactly balances the rate of those entering.

***Stem Cell.*** Progenitor cell of any lineage or differentiation pathway, but in a more specialized sense usually applied to those progenitor cells of a 'self-renewing' stem cell population (i.e., ones in which after each successive mitosis, one daughter will become differentiated and non-mitotic whereas the other remains undifferentiated and mitotic, thereby maintaining the stem cell line). Examples include plant cambium, haemopoietic stem cells, the malpighian layer of the vertebrate epidermis.

***Stereoisomer.*** Molecules that differ in the spatial arrangement of side groups bonded to a common atom, but having the same structural formula.

***Steric.*** Referring to stereochemical structure, the three-dimensional arrangement of atoms in molecules.

***Sterile.*** Free from all living organisms.

***Sterlization.*** Process applied to objects or environments that renders them sterile. Sterilization is irreversible and eliminates all viable organisms. Both physical and chemical methods of sterilization are available.

Physical agents include: dry heat (1-2 hours at 160ºC), used for clean glassware, etc.; moist heat (steam), more rapidly lethal than dry heat and used for heat-stable liquids and solid objects that cannot withstand dry heat; ultraviolet irradiation (260nm) has limited ability to penetrate liquids and is mainly used to sterilize air and exposed surfaces in enclosed spaces; ionizing radiation (x-radiation, gamma-radiation) has higher energy than ultraviolet light and greater penetration, used for surgical equipment and prepacked plastic laboratory ware; filtration, for heat-labile liquids. Physical methods, apart from filtration, rely on the destruction of proteins and/or nucleic acids.

Chemical agents include gases and volatile liquids (e.g., ethylene oxide, glutaraldehyde, β-propiolactone) used to sterilize heat-sensitive objects.

***Steroid Hormones.*** Hormones, such as oestrogens and androgen, which are steroids. These are comparatively small molecules and are to be contrasted with the large polypeptide hormones (e.g., insulin, growth hormones). Steroids are able to pass through the gut and can also enter the cytoplasm by traversing the plasma membrane, and so the levels of steroid in food should be carefully monitored. By contrast the large polypeptide hormones do not normally enter cells, but act by stimulating a second messenger system at the cell surface; they are also broken down in the gut and so the growth hormone content of ingested food has no effects on the metabolism of the animal eating the food.

***Steroids.*** Group of complex lipid molecules with a 17-carbon nucleus. Included in this group are many biologically important molecules, such as vitamin D, sex hormones (e.g., oestrogens, progesterone and androgens), corticosteroid and sterols (e.g., cholesterol).

***Sterols.*** A group of steroid alcohols that includes cholesterol, the most abundant animal steroid, and ergosterol.

***Sticky Ends.*** Self-complementary single-stranded ends of double-stranded DNA molecules produced by a restirction endonuclease cutting the DNA at specific points in its recognition sequence.

***Stochastic Process.*** Process consisting of one or more steps each of which involves a random choice or random movement. Thus the onset of cell commitment is regarded as a stochastic . process.

***Stoichiometric.*** Relating to proportions of compounds in a reaction or of elements in a compound; usually a simple ratio.

***Stoma.*** Small aperture in the epidermal surface of a plant leaf, stem or flower through which gaseous exchange and water transpiration occur. Each stoma is provided with a pair of guard cells, which control the opening and closing of the aperture through alternation in their shape when turgid.

***Stomium.*** A weak area for dehiscence in the walls of certain plant structures. A stomium is present in anthers and in fern sporangia (where it may be associated with an annulus).

***Stomodaeum.*** An anterior invagination of the ectoderm of the embryo that opens into the archenteron. It gives rise to the regions of the alimentary canal specialized for the reception of food, e.g. the buccal cavity of vertebrates and the foregut of arthropods.

***Strain.*** Alternative term for variety, but used where differences between the describe groups are somewhat less. Both words are used to indicate intraspecific subpopulations maintained artificially within crop plants or domesticated animals. Many strains are genetically fairly homozygous and will breed true.

***Strand Displacement.*** Method of replication in some viral genomes in which the newly synthesized strand physically displaces one of the previous homologous strand of the DNA duplex.

***Streak Plating.*** Technique for isolating single colonies of bacteria (and other microorganisms) and thereby obtaining pure cultures (clones). A small amount of the bacterial specimen is drawn over the surface of a solid medium (e.g., nutrient medium solidified with agar) in a petri dish using a sterile wire. The agar surface is thoroughly covered in a criss-cross fashion so that the bacteria are well distributed and will produce isolated colonies after a period of incubation.

***Streptococcus.*** A genus of spherical non-motile Gram-positive bacteria that form long chains. Streptococci do not form spores. Many are haemolytic (i.e. they destroy red blood cells) and are responsibe for a variety of diseases, including throat infections, puerperal fever, scarlet fever, and rheumatic fever.

***Streptomyces.*** Gram-positive prokaryotic organisms, growing slowly as branching filaments (1 μm, or less in diameter), and ubiquitous in soil where they decompose organic materials. Their filamentous growth leads to mycelium formation, and they were long regarded as fungi, but their cells lack a nuclear envelope, their walls contain mucopeptide and lack chitin and glucans, and their mebranes do not contain sterols. Aerial portions of the mycelium form asexual spores. Streptomyces, together with other actinomycetes, are important as the main source of antibiotics including streptomycin, neomycin, tetracycline and chloramphenicol.

***Streptomycin.*** Aminoglycoside antibiotic, produced by certain species of Streptomyces, discovered by S. Waksman in 1944. It has a broad spectrum of action (active against both gram-positive and gram-negative bacteria) and was the first really effective drig against tuberculosis, but its use is limited by the development of resistant strains and by toxic side-effects. The bactericidal action of streptomycin, as with other aminoglycoside antibiotics (e.g., neomycin) is through selective inhibition of protein synthesis on 70S ribosomes; it is inactive against 80S ribosomes. Streptomycin allows initiation of translation but, through an interac-

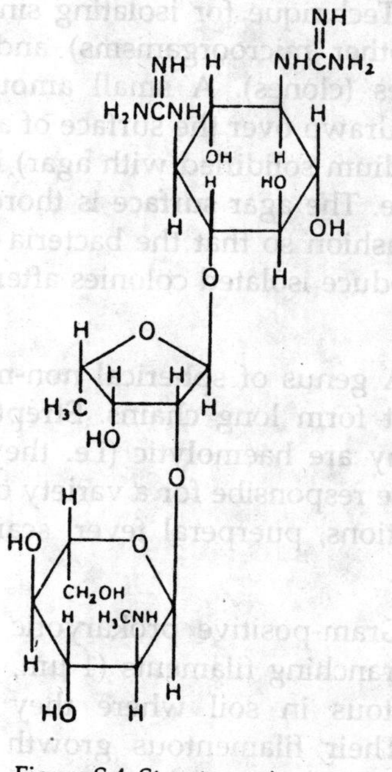

Figure S.4. Streptomycin.

tion with the 30S ribosomal subunit, prevents the initiating complex from becoming a chain-elongating ribosome. See Figure S.4.

***Stress Fibres.*** Bundles of microfilaments that lie in parallel array beneath the plasma membrane of many eukaryotic cells. They contain actin, myosin, and tropomyosin and are involved in cell motility and anchorage. They are particularly noticeable in tissue culture cells such as fibroblasts.

***Striated Muscle*** (skeletal muscle, striped muscle). One of the three major types of muscle tissue. Viewed by light microscopy, the cells or fibres of striated muscle show dark transverse bands. Striated muscle fibres are large, multinucleate cells packed with myofibrils in parallel arrays. Contraction is effected by the active sliding of two types of filaments—thick filaments composed of myosin and thin filaments composed of actin—across one another. This process utilizes ATP. See Figure S.4.

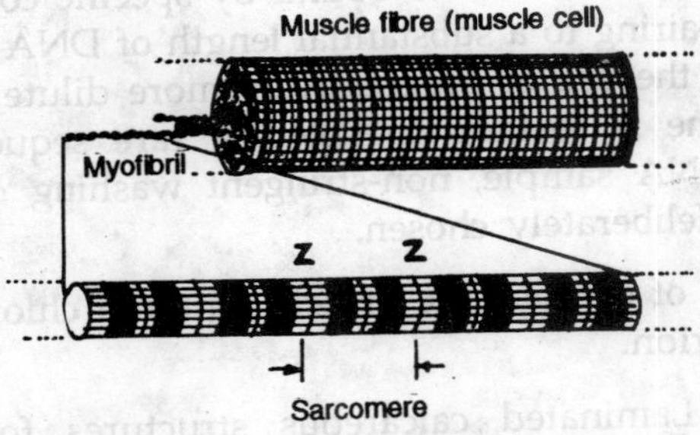


Figure S.5. Striated Muscle. Relationship between muscle fibres, myofibrils and sarcomeres.

***Striated Muscle Cell.*** Multinucleate cell, resulting from fusion of numerous myoblasts. The cells are packed with myofibrils, so forcing the nuclei to locations on the surface of cell cylinder. The multinucleate cells are also referred to as muscle fibres.

***Stridulation.*** The production of sound by an insect, usually by rubbing one part of the body, modified as a hard ridge or knob (the scraper), against another part, modified as a series of ridges or projections (the file). For example, crick-ets stridulate by rubbing together modified veins on their forewings but other insects use elytra, legs, the abdomen, etc. Cicadas stridulate by vibrating a membrane at the base of the abdomen, which produces a series of clicks. The majority of insect sounds are used in sexual behaviour but they may also be used in the maintenance of territory, for warning, etc.

***Stringent Control.*** Situation in which the numbers of any one type of plasmid in a bacterial cell are strictly regulated and do not normally number more than 10.

***Stringent Mutant.*** Bacterial mutant that shuts down RNA synthesis abruptly in a depleted growth medium.

***Stringent Washing.*** Procedure that follows hybridization of probe DNA, usually radioactively tagged, to a southern blot containing DNA fragments separated by gel electrophoresis. Stringent washing is used to remove all probe DNA except that which is bound by specific complementary base pairing to a substantial length of DNA sequence. It involves the use of progressively more dilute salt solutions. If one is seeking to detect a rare sequence in a genomic DNA sample, non-stringent washing conditions might be deliberately chosen.

***Stroma.*** Matrix of cytoplasmic protein within a chloroplast or mitochondrion.

***Stromatolites.*** Laminated calcareous structures formed by blue-green algae in intertidal zones of warm waters, such as those of the Bahamas. In the last two decades interest in stromatolites has been aroused by the discovery of similar structures in Pre-Cambrian rocks nearly $3.0 \times 10^9$ years old.

***Structural Change.*** Chromosomal mutation or aberration that involves a gross change in chromosome structure.

***Structural Gene.*** DNA sequence that codes for a protein or an RNA (e.g., transfer RNA, ribosomal RNA), although in some terminology structural genes code only for protein and do not include sequences where the sole final product is RNA. The term is used to contrast with spacer sequences, or regulatory regions which are not transcribed.

***Structural Protein.*** Protein that has, as its chief function, a contribution to the shape and structure of cells and tissues (e.g., collagen, actin, myosin). The term is slightly misleading since many enzymes have structural roles, and many structural proteins also have enzymic fuctions.

***Struggle for Existence.*** Phrase used by Darwin in the context of evolution to describe the competitive nature of an organisms's attempts to find food, shelter and a suitable mate.

***Stud.*** Animal kept for breeding, or the place where such breeding stock is housed.

***Subculture.*** Culture established by inoculation of fresh sterile medium with a sample from a previous culture.

***Suberin.*** A fatty substance similar to cutin. It occurs in the Casparian strip in young roots and certain stems and also forms a protective layer on the primary cellulose walls of cork cells.

***Subhymenium.*** The tisue layer between the hymenjum and the trama in certain fungal fruiting bodies.

***Submetacentric.*** Describing a chromosome in which the centromere is nearer one end than the other, rather than being centrally or terminally placed.

***Subsidiary Cell (Accessory Cell).*** One of the epidermal plant cells that surround the guard cells. They can be distinguished structurally from guard cells and unspecialized epidermal cells and their function is to aid the guard cells when the stoma is opening and closing.

***Subspecies.*** Subdivision of the species that may be geographically isolated and have distinct distinguishing characteristics, but is not reproductively isolated. Subspecies are normally indicated by a third Latin name following the Latin binomial of the species. Although there is no hard and fast distinction between a subspecies and a race, the latter term is normally used for populations which are less marked or consistent than those found in subspecies.

***Substitution.*** Single alteratiion at a defined state iin the primary structure of a protein or nucleic acid chain. One monomeric unit (amino acid, base pair or nucleotide) is removed and replaced by a different monomer. Substitution in a protein follows from a point mutation in the corresponding structural gene for the protein.

***Substrate.*** Specific compound or molecule that is acted on by an enzyme. There is therefore specificity between an enzyme and is substrate.

***Substratum.*** Surface on which an organism moves, or by which it is supported.

***Subunit.*** Single unit of a compound molecule or molecular aggregate; thus proteins with quaternary structure such as haemoglobins are composed of subunits, as are molecular aggregates such as ribosomes.

***Succession.*** The establishment of a sequence of different communities in a particular area over a period of time. Primary succession occurs during the colonization of an uninhabited area, such as a recent lava flow or a sand dune. Algae and lichens are usually the first plants to be established and they constitute the pioneer community. They are followed by mosses and, as the soil develops, higher plants, eventually resulting in a completed succession of plants and animals—the sere. Secondary succession is the establishment of communities on sites previously occupied by well-developed communities, such as a clear forest or a burnt patch of soil.

***Succinate.*** Important intermediate in the citric acid cycle.

***Suicide.*** In immunology, the death of cells that have specifically taken up highly radiolabeled antigen.

***Sucrose.*** Disaccharide composed of glucose and fructose. It is a major storage molecule of many plants and is the sugar of commerce.

***Sucrose Gradient Centrifugation.*** Method of separating biological components from cellular homegenates, in which the centrifugal separation is aided by the presence of a gradient of sucrose, set up in the centrifuge tube prior to the run. Although such gradients are referred to as density gradients, they act chiefly as viscosity gradients. They are widely used for the isolation of membrane, mitochondrial or ribosomal fractions.

***Sudan Black B.*** Dye widely used for the staining of lipids.

***Sugars.*** Small carbohydrates; commonly present in plants as short-term or long-term storage molecules.

***Sulphanilamide.*** Antimetabolite used to control bacterial growth.

***Sulphatide.*** Cerebroside which contains a sulphur group esterfied to the C-3 atom of the galactose molecule. Sulphatides are abundant in the white matter of the brain.

***Sulphatide Lipidosis.*** Human autosomal recessive disease due to defective production of lysosomal arylsulphatase A. Clinical symptoms include paralysis, blindness and premature death.

***Sulphonamides.*** Drugs derived from the dye sulphanilamide that inhibit bacterial growth. Some bacteria that do not require folic acid synthetic reactions are not affected by this group of drugs.

***Supercoiling.*** Coiling of a covalenty closed circle of DNA upon itself, or the further coiling of a long length of double helix with fixed ends, thus forming a superhelix. Further coiling in the same direction as the helix, for example, right-handed coiling of B from DNA is referred to as positive supercoiling, whereas twisting in the opposite direction is termed negative supercoiling.

***Superfemale*** (metafemale). Female mammal with more than two X chromosomes. Such females often lack normal female secondary sex characteristics.

***Supergene.*** DNA sequence that is protected from crossing-over and is thus transmitted intact from generation to generation.

***Supernatant.*** Fluid layer overlaying the precipitate following centrifugation.

***Supernumerary Chromosome.*** Chromosome that is additional to the normal chromosome complement of a species. In some species these are referred to as B chromosomes, and are particularly common in some species of grasshoppers and certain other insects.

***Superovulation.*** Release of more than the normal number of eggs from the ovary, more or less simultaneously. Such an event can be induced hormonally and is used to provide eggs for in vitro fertilization prior to transfer to surrogate mothers or to the donor mother.

***Superoxide Dismutase (SOD).*** Enzyme, coded by a nuclear gene. The gene sequence in higher organisms coding for the mitochondrial enzyme (but not the cytoplasmic one) resembles the sequence in prokaryotes, especially at the amino-terminus, a fact that suggests that mitochondria may be derived from prokaryotes.

***Superspecies.*** Complex made up of a number of allopatric species, all with certain morphological similarities.

***Supersuppressor.*** Mutation that itself suppresses the expression of other mutant alleles at different chromosomal loci.

***Suppression.*** (1) In immunology, a state of immune non-responsiveness that is specially induced. (2) Recovery or restoration of normal genetic function due to the silencing of some aberrant or deleterious gene activity.

***Suppressor Cell.*** Population of T lymphocytes that has the function of suppressing the antigenic response of other lymphocytes.

***Suppressor Macrophage.*** Highly activated macrophage from infected or tumor-bearing animals that inhibits in vitro immune reactions by releasing products of arachidonic acid metabolism (e.g., prostaglandins and/or oxygen radicals.

***Suppressor Mutation.*** Mutation which, if intragenic, restores the original reading frame after an earlier frameshift mutation, or, if intergenic, may act by coding for an aberrant tRNA species which reads an aberrant codon as if it were a normal codon, so restoring the original protein sequence.

***Suppressor T Lymphocyte.*** T lymphocyte involved in the inhibition and/or termination of an immune response and perhaps in the induction and maintenance of immunological tolerance. It is though that the outcome of an immune response is the result of the opposing effects of helper T lymphocytes and suppressor T lympholcytes. It is also though that the activity of suppressor T lymphocytes predominates in situations where some molecules of antigen are not processed. Suppressor T lymphocytes bear CD8 molecules on their surface. The identity of suppressor T cells as a separate subset is seriously questioned.

***Suramin*** (Antrypol, 8,8'- (carbonylbis (imino-3,1-phenylenecarbonylimino)m bis-1,3,5-naph thalene trisulfonic acid). Drug used in the treatment of trypanosomiasis (African sleeping sickness). Suramin is of interest to immunologists because it binds to C3b thereby preventing the binding of factor H and factor I. Suramin also inhibits complement-mediated lysis by inhibiting the binding of the membrane attack complex to cell membranes. See Figure S.6.

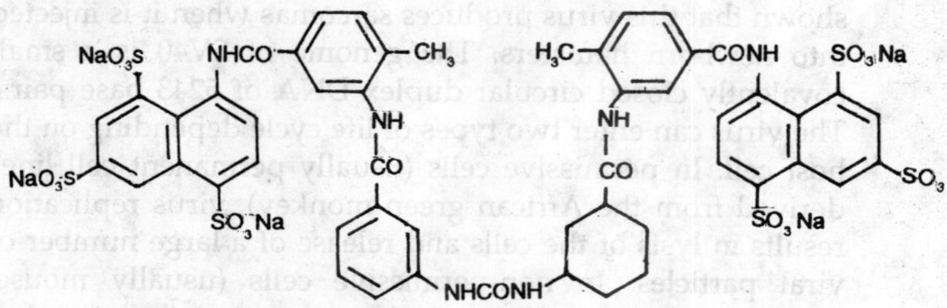


Figure S.6. Suramin sodium.

***Surrogate Genetics.*** Genetic experiments in which vertebrate oocytes (especially those of Xenopus) are injected with molecules of novel DNA, RNA or protein as a means of studying mechanisms of gene regulation and molecular processing.

***Surrogate Mother.*** Female mammal that has received an embryo transplant, the egg having been derived from a separate female donor, often as a result of superovulation.

***Suspension Culture.*** A tissue-culture system in which single cells and small cell clumps are grown in suspension in an agitated liquid medium. Suspension cultures are used to study cell division, cell differentiation, and the regulation of cell metabolism both in microorganisms and in isolated plant cells. Plant suspension cultures are obtained by adding fragments of friable callus tissue to the medium. Under appropriate conditions single plant cells may develop into embryos and subsequently into complete plants.

***Suspensor.*** Embryonic structure in plants that develops from one of the cells derived from the first division of the zygote: the suspensor elongates to push the embryo into the parental gametophyte tissue and so ensure development.

***SV40.*** Oncogenic animal virus, member of the polyoma family. SV40 was discovered as an agent that multiplied in rhesus monkey kidney cultures (used for propagating polio virus) and was subsequently found to produce cytopathic changes in cell cultures from African green monkeys. It was then shown that this virus produces sarcomas when it is injected into newborn hamsters. The genome of SV40 is a small covalently closed circular duplex DNA of 5243 base pairs. The virus can enter two types of life cycle depending on the host cell. In permissive cells (usually permanent cell lines derived from the African green monkey), virus replication results in lysis of the cells and release of a large number of viral particles. In non-permissive cells (usually mouse, hamster or human cell lines), there is no lytic infection but oncogenic transformation of the cells can occur. In such cells, DNA sequences of the SV40 genome are integrated into the host genome. Transformed cells have distinctive morphology and growth characteristics (e.g., ability to grow in suspension in soft agar).

SV40 was the first animal virus to be developed as a cloning vector. Requirements for assembly of SV40 virions impose a strict limitation on the amount of foreign DNA that can be packaged. Therefore, strategies to circumvent this size limitation have had to be developed. In one such strategy, a region of the viral genome is removed and replaced with an equivalent amount of foreign DNA; the recombinant can replicate and be packaged into virions in permissive cells. A helper virus must be supplied to provide the genetic functions lost by removal of native virus sequences. In a second strategy, recombinants are consturcted but are not packaged into virions and produce no lytic infection. They are maintained in host cells transiently as high copy number plasmid-like DNA molecules, which are not integrated into the host chromosome.

***SV40 Antigen.*** Gene regulatory protein coded on the genome of SV40 virus. It represses transcription of specific viral genes and is essential for DNA replication to be initiated at a nearby site. Thus this protein shuts down gene transcription in order to permit DNA replication.

***SV40 Virus*** (Simian virus 40). Small, double-stranded DNA virus that infects animal cells; a papovavirus. The virus was originally isolated from cells of the green monkey. It has been widely used in research and, although it will grow freely and induce cell lysis in cultured monkey cells, in mouse cells it does not freely replicate, such cells being non-permissive. However, occasional mouse cells undergo transformation following SV40 infection. The genome of SV40, which consists of 5227 bases of DNA, has been entirely sequenced and consists of a minichromosome of DNA complexed with histone. Some genes of SV40 are overlapping and some have intron sequences.

***Svedberg Unit (Svedberg, S value).*** Symbol: S. The rate of sedimentation of a particle in an ultracentrifuge is expressed as the sedimentation coefficient (s) and is a function of its weight and shape. A Svedberg unit is a sedimentation coefficient of 1 x $10^{-13}$ seconds. Since sedimentation depends also on the solvent properties, it is usual to express S values for the solvent water at 20°C (S20/W). S values are quoted as indicators of size or molecular weight when comparing cellular particles and macromolecules. For example 70S ribosomes have 30S and 50S subunits, containing 23S, 16S, and 5S RNAs.

***SV40 Virus.*** A small animal virus, belonging lto the papovavirus group of double-stranded DNA viruses. The name is short for Simian Virus 40: the virus was originally isolated from cell cultures derived from an African green monkey. The virus has been widely used in research and is noted both for its ability to induce cellular transformation and for the fact that its genome consists of a minichromosome of chromatin. The entire genome of SV40 virus has been sequenced and is now known to consist of only six genes.

***Svedlberg Unit.*** Unit for expressing sedimentation coefficients; one Svedberg unit (S) equals $10^{-13}$ second. IgG antibodies sediment at 7S, IgM antibodies at 19 S.

***Switch (S) Region.*** Region of DNA that meditates the recombination events that lead to class switching. Switch regions are approximately one to six kilobases in length and lie about one to four kilobases upstream (5') to each heavy chain C gene segment, except $C_\delta$. These regions are composed of tandem repetitions of short (<80 base pairs) DNA sequences. $S_\mu$ contains tandemly repeated blocks of two pentameric sequences; GAGCT and GGGGT, which are contained in other switch regions, although not in the form of precise tandem repeats as in $S_\mu$. In the other switch regions, the pentamers are embedded in larger repeat units. The four $S_\gamma$ are homologous to each other and are based on an approximately 50 base pair repeat; their similarity to $S_\mu$ diminishes with distance, i.e., $S_{\gamma 3}$ is most similar and $S_{\gamma 2a}$ least similar to $S_\gamma$. However, $S_\varepsilon$ and $S_{\alpha'}$,.the 3'-most switch regions, are most similar to $S_\mu$. Sequences unique to a particular switch region may be important for meditating isotype-specific switching.

***Symbiont.*** Organism that lives together with an organism of a different species, both gaining benefit from such a close relationship.

***Symbiosis.*** Interaction between two species of organisms living together, including parasitism. The term is sometimes used to denote mutant benefit, such as in mutualism.

***Sympathetic Neurone.*** Peripheral nerve cell, either sensory or motor, that innervates a gland or smooth muscle, forming part of the autonomic nervous system. Sympathetic neurones are highly dependent on supplies of nerve growth factor.

***Sympathin.*** Archaic alternative name for adrenaline and noradrenaline when they function as neurotransmitters.

***Sympatric Speciation.*** Situation in which two populations become reproductively isolated although sharing the same geographical range, or having overlapping ranges.

***Sympatric Species.*** Species whose geographical ranges overlap or coincide.

***Symplast.*** Interconnecting system of plant cell protoplasts, bounded by the cell wall/apoplast complex, but, through the medium of the interconnecting plasmodesmata which link adjoining protoplasts through the cell wall, forming a cytoplasmic continuum.

***Symplastic Growth.*** Growth in plants in which adjacent cell walls grow in unison, rather than sliding over one another or growing intrusively.

***Symport.*** Transport protein system within a cell mebrane in which transfer of one solute depends on the simultaneous or sequential transport of a second solute in the same direction.

***Synapse.*** Area of contact between two neurones or between one neurone and an effector cell, throughout which information is transferred by chemical neurotransmitters. The commonest synapses are between the axon of one neurone and termini of dendrites of another. Synapses involve close juxtaposition of the two cell membranes, the space between being termed the synaptic cleft. Synaptic vesicles in the presynaptic cell are stimulated by an electrical impulse to discharge neurotransmitter molecules into the synaptic cleft, whence they are absorbed by the postsynaptic cell via specific receptor molecules. Their attachment induces specific changes in ion permeability in the plasma membrane of the receptor cell.

***Synaptonemal Complex.*** An organelle or molecular structure that can be observed by electron microscopy between homologous chromatids of meiotic chromosomes. It is presumed to play an important role in mediating movement of DNA and its fissure and rejoining during meiotic chiasma formation. See Figure S.7.

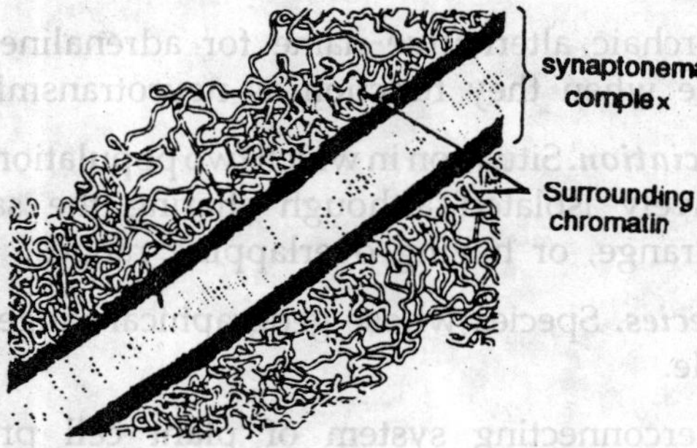


Figure S.7. Synaptonemal complex. Paired chrmosomes of a grasshopper. The narrow space between the chromosomes contains the synaptonemal complex.

***Synchronous Culture.*** Cells that pass through the stages in their cell cycles in synchrony. If mammalian cells are grown in a tissue culture dish, those in the M phase of the cell cycle adhere very weakly to the dish surface and can be removed by gentle agitation. The removed cells, which almost immediately enter the G1 phase of the cell cycle, can in turn be cultured and form a synchronous culture.

***Syncytium.*** An animal tissue consisting of a mass of protoplasm containing many nuclei and bounded by a plasma membrane. Syncytia occur in many animal groups; for example they form the epidermis of nematodes, the body wall of rotifers, and the fibres of striated muscle.

***Syndesis.*** Synapsis of meiotic chromosomes.

***Syndrome.*** Series of symptoms that, taken together, characterize a particular disease state.

***Synergid.*** Haploid cell, one of two that occur in plant embryos lying beside the embryo sac and responsible for its nourishment.

***Synergism.*** The interaction of two or more substances (e.g. drugs, hormones, plant growth substances) having a similar effect in a given system to produce an effect that is greater than the sum of the effects of the substances acting in isolation. This interaction is also termed potentiation to distinguish it from summation, the synergistic action of two substances to produce an effect greater than either is capable of in isolation.

***Syngen.*** Group of identical organisms carrying the same surface antigens. The term is widely used in relation to the ciliate Paramecium aurelia which contains a number of distinct syngens, each of which is geneticaly isolated and biochemically unique.

***Syngeneic.*** Of the same genetic constitution. Synonomous with isogeneic and used to describe tissue transplants in animals.

***Syngeneic.*** Possessing almost identical genotypes (e.g., individual mice of an inbred strain).

***Synkaryon.*** Cell in which the nucleus consists of a combination of two or more different genotypes. A synkaryon arises when the nuclei of a heterokaryon combine to form a monoculeate hybrid cell. The term hybrid cell has become more or less synonymous with the synkaryotic condition.

***Syntenic Genes.*** Genes that are believed to be linked (i.e. reside on the same chromosome) because of their concurrent loss along with a specific marker gene known to be located on a particular chromosome.

***Synthetase*** (synthase). Enzyme that catalyses molecular synthesis by the coupled breakdown of a nucleotide triphosphate (e.g.,ATP).

***Synthetic Polynucleotides.*** Molecules of DNA or RNA synthesized in vitro without a nucleic acid template by enzymic or other chemical means.

***Synthetic Antigen.*** Molecule synthesized in the laboratory and used for immunization. Synthetic polypeptides have been used to study the molecular basis of immunogenicity. Immunogenicity of synthetic polypeptides is enhanced by the presence of a variety of amino acid residues and, in particular, by aromatic and charged amino acid residues.

***Systemic Lupus Erythematosus (SEL).*** Common autoimmune disease in which there are inflammatory destructive changes in many organ systems and many antinuclear antibodies. A combination of signs and symptoms and laboratory findings are characteristic of SLE; a rash of fixed erythema forming a butterfly pattern on the face and exacerbated by exposure to sunlight, oral ulcers, pain in the joints, inflammation of the pleural and/or pericardial sacs, seizures or psychosis, antinuclear antibodies, protein in the urine, leukopenia, thrombocytopenia and hemolytic anemia. SLE is ten times more common in wormen than in men. The symptoms tend to wax and wane in severity. The immunological basis of SLE appears to be an uncontrolled differentiation of B lymphocyte clones, many of which produce autoreactive antibodies. The most characteristic antibodies in SLE are to double-and single-stranded DNA and to soluble ribonucleoproteins (Sm). Deposits of immune complexed containing DNA have been found in the kidney and in other organs. Serum complement is decreased. The use of corticosteroids and immunosuppresive drugs (e.g., cyclophosphamide) has markedly improved the survival of patients with SLE, which was almost invariably fatal in the past. SLE also occurs in NZB x NZW $F_1$ mice and other inbred strains of mice, as well as in dogs. SLE can be induced by drugs (e.g., hydralazine). The serum of patients with drug-induced SLE contains antibodies to histones, which are usually not found in other forms of SLE A mild form in which the only symptom is the butterfly rash of the face, is called 'discoid lupus'.

***Systematics.*** The study of the diversity of plants and animals and of the relationships between them, including their identification, classification, and nomenclature. It is sometimes used as a synonym for taxonomy.

***Systemic.*** Describing a process that affects the whole organism or of a factor that is distributed throughout a whole organism.

***Systemic Sclerosis.*** Disorder of connective tissue, characterized by induration and thickening of the skin (scleroderma), that may affect only the fingers and face or that may be extensive and involve the viscera, notably the gastrointestinal tract, heart, lungs and kidneys. When it affects only the skin it is called 'scleroderma'. Patients have hypergammaglobulinemia, cryoglobulinemia, rheumatoid factor, antinuclear antibodies and antinucleolar antibodies. Antinucleolar antibodies react with a degradation product ($M_r$ 70,000) of DNA topoisomerase I, which is found in the nucleolus. The disease is presumed to have an immunologic cause; the systemic form is usually fatal.

# T

**2,4,5-T.** 2,4,5-trichlorophenoxyacetic acid: a synthetic auxin widely used as a herbicide.

***T.*** Symbol for thymine or thymidine in molecular biology.

***t.*** Indicating a translocation in cytogenetics.

***$T_4$*.** Tetraiodothyronine.

***Tac (CD25).*** Antigenic determinant of the interleukin-2 (IL-2) receptor of human T lymphocytes. It is defined by a mouse monoclonal antibody, anti-Tac, which blocks the binding of IL-2 to the receptor and inhibits the proliferation of T lymphocytes.

***Tactoid*.** Aggregate with some crystalline characteristics or form.

***Takayasu's Arteritis.*** Severe, usually fatal, disease involving the aortic arch and its branches. All layers of the walls of involved arteries are inflammed and infiltrated with mononuclear cells. Immunoglobulin deposition in the arteries can be detected by immunofluorescence. Intimal proliferation results in stenosis (marked narrowing) of the arterial lumen. Aneurysms (local dilatation of artery) may form and rupture. This rare disease occurs predominantly in young women. It is presumed to have an immunological cause.

***Tailing.*** The modification of some nuclear RNA molecules after transcription by the addition of 10-20 adenosine residues to the 3' end of the RNA. Most messenger RNA. (mRNA) is tailed, the adenosine residues being added to the HnRNA precursor and surviving the removal of any intron sequences in the processing of the HnRNA to form mRNA.

***Tandem Duplication.*** Situation in which a segment of a chromosome is duplicated and the extra copy or copies inserted in line in the chromosome. Thus the genes for large ribosomal RNAs are tandemly duplicated in eukaryotes.

***Tandem Genes.*** Genes that are arranged tandemly in the chrosome, especially multiple copy genes where the copies are tandemly duplicated.

***Tannin.*** Plant phenol derivative that is used commercially because of its attachment to animal hide to form leather. Tannins are widely distributed in plans, giving an astringent taste and pigmented colour of orange, brown and yellow. They are abundant in leaves, seed coats and bark, and often occupy specialized enlarged cells termed tannin cells.

***T Antigen.*** Antigen found on normal human erythrocytes but which is only exposed by treating them with neuraminidase. A normal component of serum is anti-T anti-body which can cause agglutination of erythrocytes infected with bacteria, since the latter produce small quantities of neuraminidase.

***Target Cell.*** Cell that is killed by cytotoxic T lymphocytes, by antibody and complement, or by lymphokines, such as lymphotoxin.

***Targeted Mutagenesis.*** Use of a mutagen, such as ultraviolet light or nitrogen mustard, which is specific for a particular target within the cellular DNA.

***Target Organ.*** Organ in which the effect of a hormone is evident or in which a particular drug is selectively effective.

***Target Theory.*** Hypothesis developed to account for the mutagenic effects of ionizing radiation on cells. It is postulated that only a small target exists in the cell and that one or more ionizing events or 'hits' are necessary within the target area for radiation to produce effectively a mutation. This target is now accepted as being the DNA in the chromosomes.

***Target Tissue.*** Tissue that respnds specifically to a molecule or factor such as a hormone, antibody or specific dye.

***Taste Blindness.*** Inability to taste phenylthiocarbamide (PTC) in humans. Affected individuals are homozygous for a recessive gene carried on an autosome. Those carrying the dominant allele detect a bitter taste to PTC.

***TATA Box (Hogness Box).*** A sequence of homology found some 20-40 bases from the initiation site of many gene sequence in DNA. The TATA box is so called because the homologous sequence is TATAA (T=thymine; A =adenine). This sequence has the property of binding RNA polymerase and so seems to function as a promoter region. A similar sequence of homology is prokaryotes is known as the Pribnow box.

***Taurine.*** Rare amino acid containing a sulphonic acid group that occurs in the bile salt taurocholate and has an effect on some neurones of the nervous system.

***Tautomerism.*** Phenomenon in which an equilibrium exists between two isomeric forms of a molecule.

***Taxis*** (Tactic Movement). Locomotory movement of a cell or organism in response to an external directional stimulus.

***Taxol.*** Drug that increases the polymerization of tubulin in vitro.

***Taxon.*** Unit of taxonomic rank at any level of the hierarchial scale.

***Taxonomy.*** Study of the principles and procedures for classification of the variation and diversity of living organisms. The term is often used synonymously with the term systematics, although strictly the latter is concerned with the description of living organisms and the relationships that exist between them.

***Tay-Sachs Disease.*** Inherited disease, resulting from homozygous inheritance of a recessive gene carried on chromosome 15, a gene which codes for the allpha-subunit of hexosaminidase A. In affected individuals, gangliosides accumulate in the brain, and mental retardation and paralysis are followed by early death. The disease is found most frequently among Askhenazki jews, of whom some 3 percent are heterozygous for the allele.

***T-B Cell Collaboration.*** Interaction between B lymphocytes and helper T lymphocytes that results in the growth and differentiation of B lymphocytes into antibody-secreting cells (plasma cells). In T-B cell collaboration, membrane immunoglobulin on B lymphocytes interacts with protein antigen, which, after endocytosis, is processed and presented to helper T cells. The T cell receptor recognizes the processed antigen plus class II histocompatibility molecules on the surface of the B lymphocyte; this results in the secretion by helper T cells of lymphokines that are essential for the growth and differentiation of the B lymphocytes into antibody-secreting cells. T-B cell collaboration is required for immunoglobulin class switching. The antigens recognized by B and T lymphocytes are usually different. Ordinarily, B lymphocytes recognize native protein antigens, but they can also recognize denatured proteins or peptide fragments. However, T lymphocytes have an absolute requirement that the antigen (usually a peptide) be presented in association with class I or class II histocompatibility molecules.

The collaboration between B and T lymphocytes has been demonstrated with model antigens consisting of hapten-protein complexed. After an animal has been immunized initially (i.e., 'primed') with a hapten (e.g., the dinitrophenyl (DNP) group) coupled to a 'carrier' protein (e.g., bovine serum albumin (BSA) a second injection of the same hapten-carrier complex elicits a strong secondary response.

However, if the second injection consists of the same hapten attached to a different protein carrier (e.g., ovalbumin (OVA), there is a much weaker response, unless the animal had also been primed with the second carrier (OVA). This requirement for recognition of the original carrier is known as the 'carrier effect'. It can be shown that B lymphocytes in the primed animal recognize the hapten and T lymphocytes the carrier (after processing). The hapten and carrier must be physically linked to elicit the maximum response.

***TCA.*** (1) Tricarboxylic acid.

***T Cell Growth Factor-1.*** Synonym for interleukin-2.

***T Cell Growth Factor-2.*** Synonym for interleukin-4.

***T Cell Receptor (TcR).*** Protein on the surface of T lymphocytes that specifically recognizes molecules of the major histocompatibility complex (MHC), either alone or in association with foreign antigens. The nature of the T cell receptor remained elusive for many years; it was eventually identified by highly specific antibodies to individual T cell clones and also by examination of unique gene rearrangements in T lymphocytes. Since different T cell clones express TcR that vary in binding specificity and idiotype, the receptors are also sometimes called Ti, i denoting idiotype. In the cell membrane, the TcR is closely associated with the CD3 complex. The CD3 chains are believed to mediate signal transduction when the T cell receptor is engaged.

There are two types of TcR; both consist of two distinct membrane-embedded polypeptide chains, either alpha and beta (αβ TcR) or gamma and delta (γδ TcR). The first TcR to be described was the αβ receptor. This receptor is widely distributed on mature T lymphocytes, usually on CD4+ or CD8+ T cells, but it has also been reported to occur on a subpopulation of thymocytes that lack CD4 and CD8. Another TcR, the γδ receptor, is found on a small fraction of thymocytes and peripheral T cells (~0.2 percent of adult thymus and 0.2-1 percent of peripheral blood cells). Most cells bearing the γδ TcR are CD4-, CD8-. Dendritic epidermal cells in mouse skin and cells in mouse and chicken intestinal epithelium also bear γδTcR. Like immunoglobulins, the TcR polypeptide chains are encoded by gene segments that are assembled by somatic rearrangements. However, unlike immunoglobulins, the αβ TcR recognize antigens only when these are presented in association with major histocompatibility molecules, usually on the surface of a cell (e.g., macrophage, B lymphocyte, target cell). The αβTcR on CD4+ cells recognize class II MHC molecules (non-self (allogeneic) class II or self class II + antigen); the αβTcR on CD8+ cells recognizes class I MHC molecules (non-self (allogenic) class I or self class I+antigen). The specificity of the γδ TcR is not yet clear.

The γδ TcR appears in the mouse thymus at about 14 days of gestation, at least three days before the appearance of the αβ TcR. It has not been established whether T lymphocytes that express the γδ receptor, are precursors of those expressing the γβ receptor or whether the two cell types represent distinct lineages but the weight of evidence favors the latter possibility.

Most information about the TcR polypeptide chains has been derived from the analysis of cDNA and genomic clones. These chains resemble immunoglobulin heavy and light chains in overall structural features. The $M_r$ of the primary translation product (before glycosylation and cleavage of the signal peptide) is approximately 30,000; the $M_r$ of the mature chain varies from 32,000 to 55,000. Each chain consists of a signal sequence, a variable domain and a constant domain that are each similar in size to an immunoglobulin domain and that also contain a centrally-placed disulfide bridge spanning about 50-60 amino acid residues, a short connecting peptide, a hydrophobic transmembrane region, and a short hydrophilic cytoplasmic tail. (Each of the poutative transmembrane segments contains a conserved lysine residue that has been proposed to form a salt bridge with an acidic residues (aspartic or glutamic acid) in the transmembrane segments of the CD3 gamma, delta and epsilon chains). With the exception of one isotype of mouse gamma chain, the TcR chains contain one or more acceptor sites for attachment of N-linked oligosaccharides. The chains of αβ receptors in both mouse and humans are cross-linked by disulfide bridges (between the connecting peptides); the chains of mouse, but of only some human, γδ receptors are also cross-linked by disulfide bonds. The TcR are members of the immunoglobulin superfamily. The constant domains of the beta and gamma chains are substantially similar in amono acid sequence to immunoglobulins; those of the alpha and delta chains show less similarity to immunoglobulin chains. See Figure T.1.

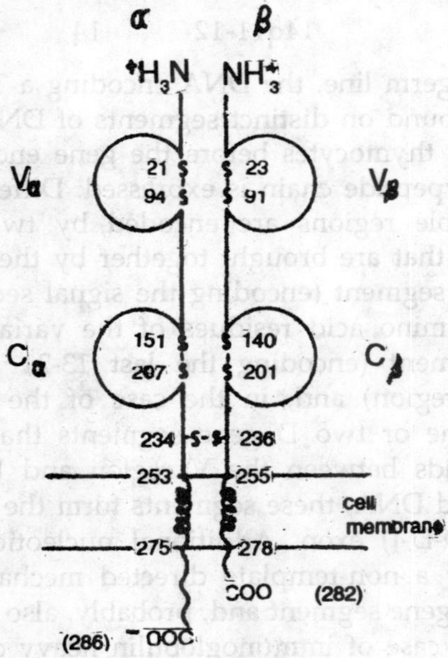


Figure T.1. T cell receptor.

***T Cell Receptor Genes.*** Genes that encode the variable regions and the constant regions of the polypeptide chains of the T cell receptor (TcR). In the mouse, the genes for the alpha, beta and gamma chains are on separate chromosomes. In both mice and humans, genes encoding the delta chain have recently been located within the alpha gene complex. The human beta and gamma chains are on the long and short arms, respectively, of chromosome 7. There are many similarities between the structure, organization, and rearrangements of genes encoding T cell receptors and those encoding immunoglobulins. Both families of genes exist in two configurations, germ line and rearranged.

Chromosome map locations of T cell receptor genes

| *Gene* | *Human* | *Mouse* |
|---|---|---|
| α | 14q11-12 | 14 |
| β | 7q32-35 | 6 |
| γ | 7p15 | 13 |
| δ | 14q11-12 | 14 |

In the germ line, the DNA encoding a TcR polypeptide chain is found on distinct segments of DNA that are rearranged in thymocytes before the gene encoding the complete polypeptide chain is expressed. Different portions of the variable regions are encoded by two to four gene segments that are brought together by the rearrangement; a V gene segment (encoding the signal sequence and first ~95-100 amino acid residues of the variable region), a J gene segment (encoding the last 13-21 residues of the variable region) and, in the case of the beta and delta chains, one or two D gene segments that encode a few amino acids between the V region and J region. In the rearranged DNA, these segments form the V-J or the V-D-J (or V-D-D-J) exon. Additional nucleotides may be inserted, by a non-template directed mechanism, on either side of D gene segment and, probably, also at V-J junctions. As in the case of immunoglobulin heavy chain gene rearrangements, a $D_\beta$ may rearrange to a $J_\beta$ without rearrangement of a $V_\beta$; such a rearranged gene may be transcribed, but corresponding tranlated polypeptides have not been identified.

The structure of the V gene segment of the TcR genes resembles that of the immunoglobulin genes. Most of the signal sequence and an untranslated region are encoded in a exon at the 5' end of the segment; the rest of the signal sequence as well as the bulk of the variable region are encoded at the 3' end of the segment. The two coding regions in the V gene segment are separated by an intron of

100-400 base pairs. The constant region of each TcR chain is usually encoded by three or four exons, which are located downstream (3') from one or more J gene segments. In contrast to the immunoglobulin C gene segments, these exons do not correspond exactly to the presumed functional domains of the constant regions of the TcR (e.g., the connecting peptide of the beta chain in both mice and humans is encoded on three separate exons).

Two $C_\beta$ gene segments in both mice and humans, separated by about 6 and 8 kilobases, respctively, have been described; each of these gene segments containfour exons. The amino acid sequence of the two constant regions differ by four (mouse) or five (human) amio acid residues. In mice, there are two clusters of seven $J_\beta$ gene segments, each located 2-3 kilobases 5' to one of the $C_\beta$ gene segments; the $J_\beta$ in each cluster, six of which are functional, are separated by 36-421 base pairs. (An additional exon of 72 base pairs, $C_\beta 0$, is located between the $J_\beta 1$ cluster and $C_\beta 1$; this sequence is found in some beta chain transcripts.) About 500-600 base pairs 5' to each $J_\beta$ cluster, there is a single $D_\beta$ segment either 12 or 14 base kpairs in length. The number and organization of $J_\beta$ and $D_\beta$ in humans is very similar to that in mice. The number of $V_\beta$ gene segments in mice is probably relatively small (less than 30); 20 of these gene segments have recently been localized within a span of 250 kilobases of DNA 5' to the two $D_\beta J_\beta C_\beta$ clusters. The distance from the 3' end of this cluster to the $D_\beta J_\beta C_\beta$ is about 320 kilobase. One $V_\beta$ segment ($V_\beta 14$) is located 10 kilobases 3' to the $D_\beta J_\beta B_\beta$ clusters; although it is in reverse transcriptional orientation, it is known to be utilized by a functional T cell clone. The $V_\beta$ have been divided into different families, the members of each family being at least 75 percent identical in DNA sequence. In the $V_\beta$ of mice most families seem to have only one member. Humans appear to have a similar number of families of $V_\beta$ but fewer have only one member; accordingly, the total number of $V_\beta$ is greater than in mice. In mice, the complete T cell receptor beta locus has been estimated to span 700 to 800 kilobases.

There is only a single $C_\alpha$ gene segment, containing four exons, in both mice and humans. An unusual aspect of the alpha gene family is the presence of many J gene segments spread over a large region of the chromosome. In the mouse, there are probably 50 or more $J_\alpha$ located 3-63 kilobase 5' to the single $C_\alpha$; the different $J_\alpha$ are separated from one another by at least 500 base pairs. Presumably, when a $V_\alpha$ rearranges to one of the more 5' $J_\alpha$, the resulting primary transcript is very long, including an intron of up to 63 kilobases. No D elements have been identified in the alpha gene complex. There seem to be 75-100 $V_\alpha$; their location is not known but they are thought to be 5' to the $J_\alpha$. The $V_\alpha$ have also been grouped into families and most of these contain more than one member. Therefore, the potential exists for many $V_\alpha$-$J_\alpha$ combinations. The organization of the alpha-chain genes in human seems to be similar to that in mice.

There are four $C_\gamma$ gene segments in mice; one of these is a pseudogene in some strains and delted in others. There are two $C_\gamma$ in humans, separated by about 10 kilobases. Three of the mouse $C_\gamma$ contain three exons (the detailed structure of the fourth is not yet determined); one of the human $C_\gamma$ has three exons and the other has four or five exons. Two of the functional mouse $C_\gamma$ and both human $C_\gamma$ contain sites for N-linked oligosaccharides. One of the human $C_\gamma$ does not encode a cysteine residue that ordinarily participates in interchain disulfide bridging, presumably accounting for the non-covalent association of some gamma-containing TcR beterodimers. In mice, one J segment has been found upstream to each of the four $C_\gamma$. In humans, one of the two $C_\gamma$ has two upstream $J_\gamma$ segments and the other $C_\gamma$ has three such segments. No D segments have been identified in the mouse or human gamma locus. The number of $V_\gamma$ gene segments appears to be relatively limited. Seven $V_\gamma$ have been identified in mice, and they have been grouped into five families: four single-member families and one three-member family. Six of the $V_\gamma$ have been linked in pairs; one of these pairs is in head-to-head orientation. In humans, fourteen $V_\gamma$ have been found, but not all are functional. The $V_\gamma$ and $C_\gamma$ are interspersed in mice but not in humans. An unusual feature of the gamma gene family is that gene rearrangement and expression of mRNA frequently occurs without expression of the protein product on the cell surface. The TcR gamma locus in humans appears to span about 150 kilobases and that in mice at least 200 kilobases.

Recently, gene segments encoding the delta chain have been identified nested within the alpha chain locus. In mice, a single $C_\delta$ gene segment is located about 10 kilobases 5' to the $J_\alpha$ cluster. Two $J_\delta$ and two $D_\delta$ gene segments have been identified upstream of the $C_\delta$. The V gene segments used for alpha and delta chains are largely distinct, but there is some overlap. Some rearranged delta genes seem to contain both $D_\delta$ segments. The arrangement of alpha and delta genes is consistent wth other evidence that the delta chan s expressed before the alpha chain since $V_\alpha$ to $J_\alpha$ rearrangement results in deleton of the D, J and C segments of the delta gene complex.

The ways in which diversity is generated by the TcR genes resemble the generation of diversity by the immunoglobulin genes, but there are some differences. The relative contribution of germline diversification may be relatively less than that due to gene rearrangements. Different variable-region sequences are generated, from a relatively limited repertoire of gene segments in the germ line, by combinatorial joining (utilization of different combinations of V, J and D segments), junctional diversity (variation in the position of the recombnation point between two gene segments) and the addition of N nucleotides, which occurs in all four T cell receptor polypeptides (but only in the heavy chains of immunoglobulins. Thus, much of the potential variability, especially of gamma and delta chains, is concentrated near the V-(D)-J junctions. Somatic hypermutation does not appear to occur in the TcR (in contrast to the immunoglobulins).

***T Cell Subset.*** Subpopulation of T lymphocytes usually defined by a reaction with monoclonal antibodies (e.g., CD4 subset).

***T Cell-conditioned Medium.*** Medium from cultures of T lymphocytes that were stimulated with lectins, antigens or allo-antigens in a mixed lymphocyte reaction. The medium contains a variety of lymphokines.

***T-DNA.*** Part of the genome of the Ti plasmid that integrates into the host cell genome in crown gall disease of plants.

***Teichoic Acid.*** One of a group of linear polymers of either glycerol phosphate or ribitol phosphate. Ribitol teichoic acids are one of the two characteristic constituents of the cell wall of Gram-positive bacteria (the other being mucopeptide); glycerol teichoic acids are associated with the bacterial cell membrane. See Figure T.2.

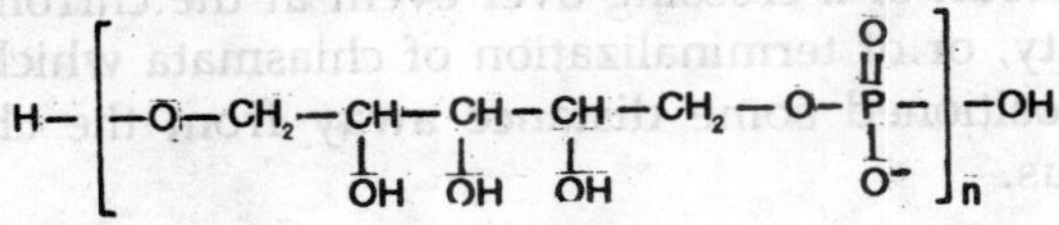

Figure T.2. Teichoic acids.

***Telegony.*** Hypothesis that the offspring of one mating can be influenced by the genes of a male that had previously mated with their mother. The idea is no longer accepted except in species where multiple matings with different males may result in litters of truly mixed parentage.

***Telology.*** The theory that all organisms or their parts have evolved for a particular purpose.

***Teleonomy.*** Proposal that the presence of a structure or function in an organism can be assumed to imply earlier evolutionary advantage in the possession of such a structure or function.

***Telocentric.*** Chromosome in which the centromere is located terminally.

***Telomere.*** The end of a chromosome. The molecular structure of telomeres has recently been studied and it has been shown that the chromosomal DNA molecule forms a loop (i.e.the sugar-phosphate backbone is continuous, as in the hairpin loops in transfer RNA molecules).

***Telome Theory.*** The theory, expanded by Zimmerman from a suggestion made by Lignier (1903), that the megaphyll originated from a stem structure, i.e. that it is fundamentally a cladode. Zimmerman suggested that primitive plants consisted of a system of dichotomizing axes whose ultimate divisions he termed telomes, which either bore sporangia (fertile telomes) or were sterile (phyloids). The megaphyll evolved from the phylloid-bearing axes.

***Telophase.*** Final stage of mitosis and meiosis.

***TEM.*** Transmission electron microscope.

***Temperate Phage.*** Bacteriophage (e.g., lambda phage) which can either enter, as a prophage, into a stable and quiescent relationship (lysogeny) with its host bacterium or can undergo lytic growth.

***Temperature-sensitive Mutation.*** A mutation giving a normal phenotype at one temperature but a mutant phenotype at another. This effect is usually due to a heat-labile mutant gene product.

***Template.*** Molecular structure that is effective in dictating the structure of another molecule copied from it. This other molecule will often be an antti-template, and can in turn dictate the structure of a new template molecule. Thus a single strand of DNA or RNA acts as a template strand for the elaboration of the complementary antitemplate strand.

***Teratocarcinoma.*** Malignant and transplantable form of a teratoma. It may contain a bizarre range of tissue types without morphogenesis or organization, but importantly contains stem 8cells, the embryonal carcinoma cells, which may be isolated and grown as a cell line. Such cells can be used to study differentiation in vitro and, interestingly, will contribute to normal development if transplanted back to a normal blastocyst.

***Teratogen.*** Agent that give ise to contgential malformation, especially to terratomas. Thalidomide acts as a teratogen in the human.

***Teratology.*** Study of plant or animal congenital abnormalities and monstrosities.

***Teratoma.*** Tumour that typically contains derivatives of the three embryonic germ layers (ectoderm, endoderm and mesoderm) (e.g., skin, muscle, gut, and also embryonal carcinoma cells). It is believed to originate both from primordial germ cells and disorganized growth of early embryos. Derives from the Greek root teraton meaning monster.

***Terminal Cell.*** Cell at the top or tip of an embryo.

***Terminal Chiasmata.*** Association of homologous chromosomes at meiosis, involving only the chromosome ends. This may be the result of a crossing-over event at the chrromosomal extremity, or of terminalization of chiasmata which earlier were positioned some distance away from the chrosome terminus.

***Terminal Differentiation.*** Differentiation that cannot progress further, as in the production of non-dividing end cells (e.g.,neurones, erythrocytes).

***Terminalization.*** Process in which chiasmata tend to move towards the ends of chromosomes during meiosis. At one time it was assumed that terminalization permitted chromosomes to disengage from one another and complete segregation, but it is now clear that such terminalization does not normally go to completion. Instead the DNA is cut and rejoined to permit the separate chromosomes to move apart.

***Terminal Redundancy.*** Repetiton of the same DNA sequence at either end of a long DNA molecule. Some bacteriophages have DNA that is terminally redundant and can be circularized by removal of a few bases from each end.

***Terminal Transferase.*** Enzyme that will synthesize homopolymer single-stranded tails at the 3'-ends of DNA molecules. It is used in gene manipulation technology, most frequently to add poly A tails to one DNA duplex and poly T tails to another, thus permitting the formation of a hybrid molecule of cloned circular DNA. Recombinant plasmids for cloning in E.coli are frequently constructed by such homopolymer tailing.

***Terminal Web.*** Perpendicular network of actin filaments at the base of a microvillus.

***Terpenes.*** Lipids made up of multiples of the unsaturated hydrocarbon isoprene. Many trepenes are found in plants, where they are responsible for characteristic odours and flavours. In the strict sense terpenes have the empirical formula $C_{10}H_{16}$ and are volatile aromatic hydrocarbons. In a broader sense the term includes sesquiterpenes ($C_{15}H_{24}$),diterpenes ($C_{20}H_{32}$) and higher polymers. The term can also be extended to cover various oxygen-containing compounds derived from the terpene hydrocarbons. The term terpenoid is sometimes used to cover all of these compounds.

***Tertiary.*** The first period of the Cenozoic era, extending from 70 to 1 million years ago. It is the first period in which mammals are the dominant fauna and modern families of angiosperms are the dominant flora. The Tertiary is subdivided into the following epochs: Palaeocene, Eocene, Oligocene, Miocene, and Pliocene. The mammal fossil of these epochs show a gradation from primitive to advanced forms, and the angiosperms show increasing specialization.

The Palaeocene extended from 70 to 60 million years ago. Placental mammals appeared in such primitive forms as the creodonts (primitive carnivores) and condylarths (primitive herbivores).

The Eocene, extending from 60 to 40 million years ago, saw the appearance of the true ungulates and the first ttype of horse, eohippus (Hyracotherium), which was a small browser.

The Oligocene extended from 40 to 25 million years ago. The fossil fauna of this epoch is much more modern and archaic groups have disappeared. In many groups of mammals there is a trend to increased size and complexity. In the evolution of the horse, eohippus had evolved to the larger Mesohippus and Miohippus.

The Miocene extended from 25 to 11 million years ago and is characterized by a general drying of the climate, which is reflected in the fossil fauna in many groups. For example the horses, such as Merychippus, were faster moving larger grazers compared with their small broad-footed ancestors. Many groups tthat could not adapt to the drier environment died out.

The Pliocene extended from 11 and 1 million years ago and ended with the onset of the Pleistocene Ice Age. Pliocene fossils are similar to modern types.

***Tertiary Granule.*** Cytoplasmic organelle of neutrophils that contains acid hydrolases, gelatinase and the precursor of complement receptor 3. Tertiary granules are poorly characterized.

***Tertiary Structure.*** Folding of a protein chain by virtue of interactions among the side-chains of its constituent amino acid residues. The tertiary structure may be stabilized by disulfide bridges.

***Tertiary Structure.*** The three-dimensional folding of a protein molecule.

***Test Cross.*** Mating between two individuals, one of known and one of unknown genotype, in order to ascertain the genotype of the tested parent. Normally the tester parent is selected to carry only recessive genes, so that any dominant alleles carried by the tested parent will be revealed.

***Tester Strain.*** Strain of multiple recessive individuals used to test the genotyes of the other individuals in a test cross.

***Testicular Feminization.*** Genetic males lacking cellular receptors for testosterone. Despite the presence of testosterone-secreting testes, such individuals appear to be females since all mammals develop as females unless exposed, as embryos, to testosterone, and response to testosterone (in different ways by different body cells) is dependent on the presence of testosterone receptors. Testicular feminization has been describe in humans, mice, rats and cows.

***Testis.*** The main reproductive organ of male animals. In vertebrates there is a pair of testes, which produce both spermatozoa and steroid hormones under the control of the pituitary gonadotrophins.

In mammals and most other vertebrates the testis is composed of seminiferous tubules, which are lined with a germinal epithelium containing cells (spermatogonia) that produce haploid spermatozoa by meiosis. The seminiferous tubules also contain larger Sertoli cells, which are thought to facilitate the development of the spermatozoa. Between the tubules lie interstitial cells of Leydig, which are the major androgen-producing cells of the testis. The endocrine function of the testis was first demonstrated in 1849, when Berthold showed that a capon (castrated cock) with a testis transplanted into its abdomen redeveloped male characteristics and behaviour. In most mammals the testes are found within a pouch of skin (scrotum) outside the abdominal cavity. This helps to maintain them at the optimal temperature (lower than body temperature) for their development.

***Testosterone.*** Principal and most potent androgen secreted mainly by the leydig cells. In the circulation almost all of the testosterone is bound either to a protein that also binds other steroids, sex hormone-binding globulin (SHBG), or albumin. Testosterone is responsible for the development, both during embryogenesis and at puberty, and for maintenance of the male secondary sexual characteristics. Androgens, including testosterone, alsc have an anabolic effect, resulting in the increased rate of growth in males at puberty. The level of circulating testosterone is controlled

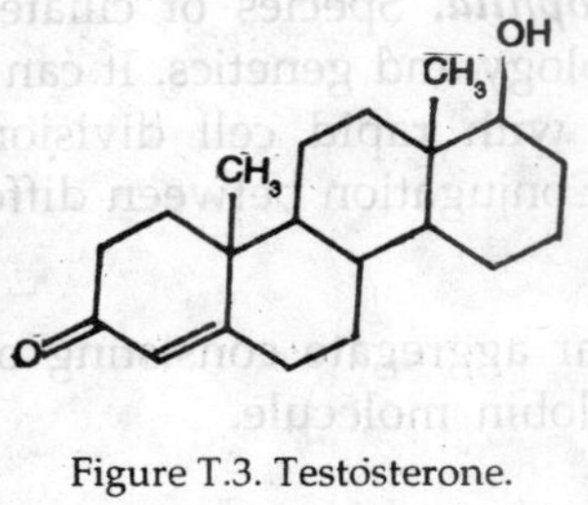


Figure T.3. Testosterone.

by a feedback mechanism. Luteinizing hormone, secreted by the anterior pituitary gland, stimulates androgen productions; testosterone inhibits the secretion of luteinizing hormone. See Figure T.3.

***Test-tube Baby.*** Production of a child following in vitro fertilization, after which the embryo is transplanted into the uterus of its biological mother or a surrogate mother to permit implantation and normal gestation.

***Tetra-allelic.*** Situation in which four distinct alleles occur at a particular gene locus in a polyploid organization.

***Tetracyclines.*** Group of broad-spectrum antibiotics obtained from various species of the mould Streptomyces. They bind to the 30S subunit of tthe bacterial ribosome, preventing attachment of tthe aminoacyl-tRNA.

***Tetrad.*** Group of four homologous chromatids, synapsed together during meiotic prohase. The term is also used to indicate the four haploid products of a single meiotic division.

***Tetrad.*** The group of four haploid cells that is formed by meiosis of a diploid cell.

***Tetrad Analysis.*** Analysis of the products of meiotic division, especially in haploid phases of such fungi as Neurospora and Sordaria. Such fungi produce an ordered sequence of spores witthin a long capsule, the position of the spores in a group of four representing the arrangement of chromosomes at the earlier meiotic division. Thus analysis of the genetic characteristics of the ordered spores can be used to reveal information about crossing over during meiosis.

***Tetrahymenathermophila.*** Species of ciliate protozoan widely used in cell biology and genetics. It can be grown easily in axenic culture with rapid cell division in its vegetative growth cycle. Conjugation between different strains is also common.

***Tetramer.*** Molecular aggregate consisting of four subunits, as in the haemoglobin molecule.

***Tetraparental Mice*** (allophenic mice). Mice produced by artificial fusion of cells from two different blastulas in vitro, followed by reintroduction of the hybrid embryo into a pregnant mouse for development. The resulting progeny have therefore four parents rather than two and contain cells of distinct genetic origins.

***Tetraparental Mouse.*** Synonym for allophenic mouse.

***Tetraploid.*** Descriptive of a cell or organism in which four genome equivalents are present in each nucleus (i.e. four times the haploid amount of DNA).

***Tetrasomic.*** Describing a cell or organism in which one chromosome in the set is present as four copies in an otherwise diploid nucleus.

***Tetroses.*** Group of monosaccharides with four carbon atoms.

***Thalassaemias.*** Group of related human anaemias of greater or lesser severity, showing themselves by the existence of abnormal haemoglobin profiles. Most types of thalassaemias are caused by mutations of the beta-globin genes, resulting in an inability to make beta-globin. Many such patients compensate by making foetal haemoglobin (HbF) with two alpha-globin chains and two gamma-globin chains and/or by increasing the proportion of delta-haemoglobin. Thalassaemias that are characterized by an inability to make alpha-globin chains are also known: some patients synthesize haemoglobin Barts ($\gamma_4$) or compensate with haemoglobin H($\beta^A{}_4$).

***Thalidomide.*** Compound used as a tranquillizer in the early 1960s. Although no undesirable side-effects were apparent in adults, it proved to be a teratogen, including phocomelia in some babies born to women who had taken the drug during pregnancy.

***Thallus.*** Form of plant body, found in many lower plants and in the gametophyte stage of higher plants, consisting only of parenchyma tissue with no vascular bundles and no differentiation into leaves, stems or roots.

***T Haplotype.*** Variant of the proximal region (~20 centiMorgans) of chromosome 17 of mice. These variants are defined by the occurrence of : (1) chromosomal inversions. Two such inversiions have been identified; the major histocompatibility complex is included in the distal inversion. (2) Suppression of recombination between t haplotypes and wild-type chromosomes; presumably, recombination is suppressed as a result of the chromosoal inversion. (3) male transmission distortion. Up to 99 percent of the offspring of a male heterozygote inherit the t haplotype. Most t haplotypes contain at least one recessive lethal mutation. These mutations affect embryonic development at different stages. Different t haplotypes, containing different mutations, can complement each other. Thus, heterozygotes $t^x/t^y$ are viable although both homozygotes $t^x/t^x$ and $t^y/t^y$ are not; ($t^x/t^y$ males are sterile, but females of this genotype are completely fertile). At least 16 complementation groups have been identified. The t haplotypes were originally identified because they carry a mutation that enhances the effect of the T mutation, i.e., a mouse carrying T/t has no tail; a mouse carrying T/+ has a short tail. The male transmission distortion is believed to be responsible for maintaining the t haplotype at high levels in natural populations, despite it deleterious features.

***Thelytoky.*** Type of parthenogenesis in which unfertilized eggs yield females; males are absent. It occurs in some insects (e.g., stick insects).

***Theophylline*** (1,3 dimethylxanthine). Drug used in the treatment of asthma; it dilates bronchi because it is a potent relaxant of bronchial and other smooth muscle. Theophylline is rendered more soluble by complexing it with ethylenediamine; the complex is called aminophylline.

***Thermal Denaturation.*** Loss of structural conformation of a molecule induced by heating. Proteins and nucleic acids can be readily denatured by heating (as, for example, when the white of an egg hardens on boiling). Thermal denaturation of nucleic acids is used in technology involving hybridization and also in determining Cot values.

***Thermodynamics.*** Study of energy and energy flow. The laws of thermodynamics are as follows.

*First law of thermodynamics.* Energy cannot be created or destroyed, but may be transformed from one from to another.

*Second law of thermodynamics.* When energy is transformed from one form to another, some remains as the heat energy of the molecules at the end of the reaction, so only some is available for useful work.

*Third law of thermodynamics.* At absolute zero temperature all molecules are motionless and their entropy is zero.

***Thermogenesis.*** Production of internal heat; especially applied to processes in hibernating mammals and other coldadapted mammals (including the newborn) by which the mitochondria of brown fat serve as ATP generators for production of heat energy.

***Thermophilic.*** Designating microorganisms that require an optimum temperature of 55-75°C for growth, with a minimum of 35-40°C.

***Thiamine (vitamin $B_1$).*** A water soluble vitamin, part of the vitamin B complex, that serves as a precursorr of the coenzyme thiamine pyrophosphate, which is involved in decarboxylation in carbohydrate metabolism. Most vertebrates and many microorganisms are unable to synthesize thiamine and it therefore has to be supplied from an external source. A deficiency of this vitamin in the diet of man leads to the disease beriberi. See Figure T.4.

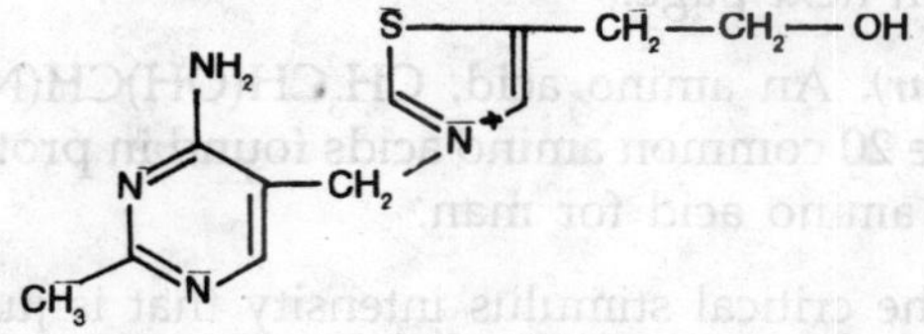


Figure T.4. Thiamine.

***Thick Filaments.*** Filament of the striated muscle that extends over the A band but not the I band, and is overlapped in the A band by thin filaments.

***Thin Filament.*** Filament of striated muscle that overlaps thick filaments in the A band and also continues into the I band, running from the Z disc which lies at the centre of the I band.

***Thin-layer Chromatography.*** Type of chromatography in which the stationary phase, through which molecular migration occurs, is a thin layer of silica gel or alumina spread on a glass plate and acting as an absorbent layer.

***Thoracic Duct.*** Duct that returns lymph to the blood. It leads from the cisterna chyli to the left subclavian vein. The cisterna chyli is a dilated chamber at the origin of the thoracic duct in the lumbar region. Lymph from the abdomen, chest and retroperitoneum collects in the cisterna chyli.

***Thoracic Duct Drainage.*** Prolonged drainage of lymph from the thoracic duct. This technique is used to deplete lymphocytes from an animal or patient.

***Three-point Cross.*** Cross carried out to determine, on the basis of recombination frequency, the order in which three non-allele-linked genes are located on the chromosome. The orientation of markers b and c carried by two strains is determined relative to a marker a (introduced into the strain carrying marker b). If the order is abc then, using each strain in turn as donor, the yield of wild-type ($a^+b^+c^+$) recombinants will be approximately the same for the two crosses. If, however, the order is acb then one cross (that requiring four cross-over events) will give many fewer wild-type recombinants than the reciprocal cross. See Figure T.5 on next page.

***Threonine (thr).*** An amino acid, $CH_3CH(OH)CH(NH_2)COOH$, one of the 20 common amino acids found in proteins and an essential amino acid for man.

***Threshold.*** The critical stimulus intensity that is just sufficient to initiate a response in an irritable tissue.

***Thrombin.*** A proteolytic enzyme, present only in blood removed from the circulation, that catalyses the conversion of fibrinogen to fibrin during blood clotting. It is formed from an inactive precursor, prothrombin, which is present in normal plasma; the conversion is highly complex and requires many cofactors, the most important of which are calcium ions, thromboplastin, and platelets. The absence of thrombin in normal blood appears to be the means by which its fluidity is preserved, as intravenous injection of thrombin results in immediate clotting.

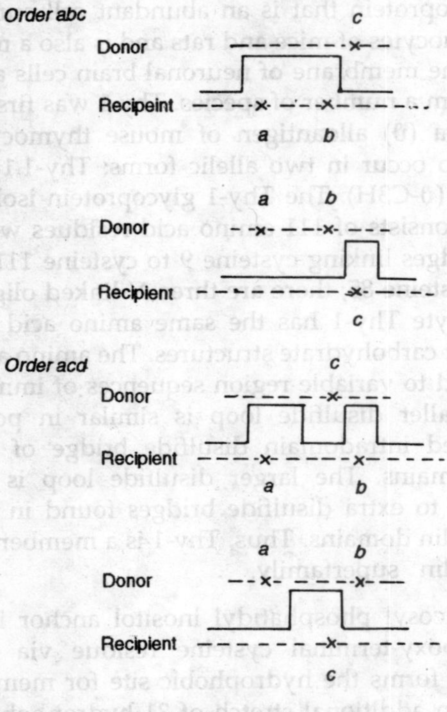


Figure T.5. Three-point cross.

***Thrombocyte.*** The former name for a platelet, which was originally incorrectly thought to be a true cell.

***Thrombocyte.*** Synonym for platelet.

***Thrombocytopenia.*** Decrease in the number of platelets in the blood to less than 100,000/mm$^3$ (normal: 150,000-300,000/mm$^3$).

***Thrombocytosis.*** Condition in which the number of blood plasteles is drastically reduced.

***Thromboplastin.*** Protein required, along with other factors, for the conversion of prothrombin to thrombin during blood clotting. Tthese proteins are found in blood that has been exposed to injured tissue and can be recovered from intact lung, placenta, brain and other tissues.

***Thy-1.*** Clycoprotein that is an abundant cell surface molecule on thymocytes of mice and rats and is also a major constituent of the membrane of neuronal brain cells and of fiibroblasts from a number of species. Thy-1 was first identified as the theta (ϑ) alloantigen of mouse thymocytes and was found to occur in two allelic forms: Thy-1.1 (ϑ-AKR) and Thy-1.2 (ϑ-C3H). The Thy-1 glycoprotein isolated from rat brains consists of 111 amino acid residues with two disulfide bridges linking cysteine 9 to cysteine 111 and cysteine 19 to cysteine 85; there are three N-linked oligosaccharides. Thymocyte Thy-1 has the same amino acid sequence but different carbohydrate structures. The amino acid sequences is related to variable region sequences of immunoglobulns. The smaller disulfide loop is similar in position to the conserved intradomain disulfide bridge of immunoglobulin domains. The larger disulfide loop is is similar in position to extra disulfide bridges found in a few immunoglobulin domains. Thus, Thy-1 is a member of the immunoglobulin superfamily.

A glycosyl phosphatidyl inositol anchor is attached to the carboxy-terminal cysteine residue via ethanolamine and this forms the hydrophobic site for membrane attachment. An additional stretch of 31 hydrophobic amino acid residues, predicted from the cDNA sequence, is not present in the mature protein. Mouse Thy-1 is very similar in structure to rat Thy-1, except it has one additional amino acid residue. A single amino acid substitution, arginine or glutamine at position 89, distinguishes Thy-1.1 from Thy-1.2. In the mouse, but not in the rat, Thy-1 is present on mature T lymphocytes as well as on thymocytes. It has been widely used as marker for mouse T lymphocytes. Treatment of lymphocytes with antibodies to Thy-1, in the presence of complement, leads to selective lysis of T lymphocytes and abrogation of T-dependent reactions. Thy-1 has been mapped to mouse chromosome 9.

Human Thy-1 is expressed on only a very small percentage of lymphocytes but is a major surface component of neurons and fibroblasts. The function of Thy-1 is not known. Mouse T lymphocytes cultured with phorbol myristic acid can be triggered to divide by cross-linking of Thy-1 with antibodies.

***Thylakoid.*** Flattened sac bounded by membrane that forms the lamellar grana of photosynthetic mebrane in chloroplasts. Thylakoids also form the photosynthetic systems of photosynthetic bacteria. Chlorophylis and other pigments of the photosynthetic pathway are located in the thylakoid mebranes.

***Thymectomy.*** Surgical removal of the thymus. Clinically, thymectomy is used to treat myasthenia gravis. In newborn mice, this procedure is used to deprive the animal of T lymphocytes and therefore cell-mediated immunity and antibody responses to thymus-dependent antigens. Neonatally thymectomized mice do not gain weight and have atrophy of their lymphoid tissue. This is called runt disease or wasting disease.

***Thymic Epithelial Cell.*** Cell derived from the endoderm of the third and fourth pharyngeal pouches and having the characteristic of an epithelial cell. These cells express class I histocompatibility and class II histocompatibility molecules and are though to influence thymocyte differentiation. Fewer epithelial cells are found in the thymic medulla than in the cortex. Large thymic epithelial cells in close contact with thymocytes are called thyumus nurse cells.

***Thymic Hormone.*** Peptide (e.g., thymopoietin, thymosin) extracted from the thumus that has been proposed to regulate T cell differentiation. Thymic hormones have been assayed by diverse methods such as incubation of hormone with spleen cells from nude mice to induce expression of Thy-1 antigen.

***Thymidine.*** Deoxyriboside of the pyrimidine base thymine.

***Thymidine Kinase.*** Enzyme that catalyses the conversion of thymidine to thymidine monophosphate by phosphorylation.

***5'-thymidylic acid.*** Nucleotide, the 5'-phosphate ester of thymidine, and one of the monomeric units in DNA. See Figure T.6.

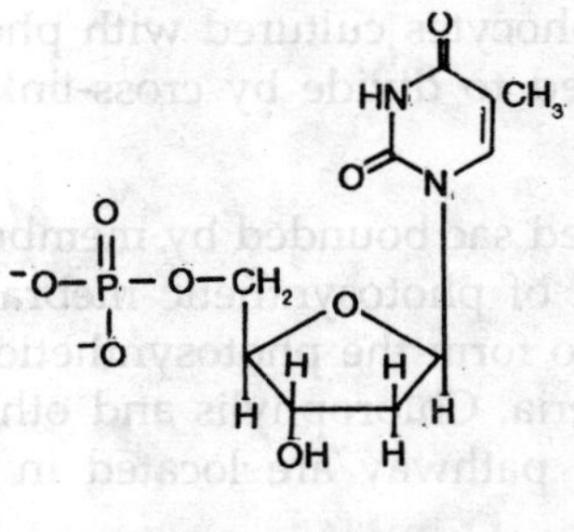


Figure T.6. 5'-thymidylic acid.

***Thymine.*** One of the two pyrimidine bases found in DNA. It is not represented in RNA, where it is replaced by uracil.

***Thymocyte.*** T lymphocyte derived from or processed by the thumus gland.

***Thymocyte.*** Lymphocyte in the thumus.

***Thymoma.*** Tumor of thymocytes. Thymomas, which usually grow slowly, are found in the mediastinum and may be associated with myasthenia gravis or immunodeficiency.

***Thumus.*** Primary lymphoid organ for T lymphocyte development. The thymus is located in most mammals in the superior anterior mediastinum (chest). It consists of epithelial cells derived during embryogenesis from cells of the third and fourth branchial (or pharyngeal) pouches, thymocytes (T lymphocytes in various stages of differentiation), macrophages and dendritic cells. The thymus is divided into a cortex rich in immature T lymphocytes tightly packed between the epithelial cells and a medulla containing mature T lymphocytes and macrophages. At birth the weight of the thymus, relative to body weight, is maximal and the cortex is the site of intense mitotic activity. However only 5 percent of thymocytes emigrate from the thymus into the circulation. The thymus increases in absolute size until puberty; it then begins to decrease in size and may atrophy in later life.

***Thymus Cell Differentiation.*** Proceess of maturation of stem cells into mature T lymphocytes that occurs in the thymus. The differentiation of stem cells involves the sequential acquisition and loss of cell surface markers that demarcate various stages of maturation. In humans, stem cells bearing CD38 become early thymocytes when they express CD2 and CD7 and then the transferrin receptor. Early thymocytes subsequently express CD1, which is the marker of common thymocytes at mid-stage of differentiation. During this stage, the genes for the gamma and delta, and subsequently those for alpha and beta chains of the T cell receptor rearrange. The thymocytes then express CD3, CD4 and CD8; the CD1 marker is progressively lost at this stage. Finally two distinctive subsets of mature T lymphocytes appear: the helper/inducer subset that is CD3+4+8- and the cytoxic/suppressor subset that is CD3+4-8+.

In mice, a similar maturation process occurs. The stem cells can be identified by antibodies to Ly5. Mouse thymocytes express TL molecules that, like CD1 in humans, are lost in the late stages of differentiation. Thy-1 is expressed by mouse thymocytes in all stages of differentiation and by mature T lymphocytes.

During differentiation, thymocytes are in intimate contact with epithelial cells, which bear both class I and class II histocompatibility molecules. With bone marrow transplants into irradiated mice, it has been possible to show that the alleles of class I and class II molecules in the stromal cells influence T cell recognition. For example, marrow stem cells from a mouse of haplotype AxB transplanted into an A recipient will develop helper T lymphocytes that recognize antigen in the context of antigen-presenting cells of haplotype A; when AxB cells are transplanted into a B recipient, the helper T lymphocytes will recognize antigen + B. How this process of acquisition of receptors restricted by the major histocompatibility complex allele develops is not yet understood. Overall, thymus cell differentiation is an inefficient process since about 90 percent of thymocytes die in the thymus.

***Thymus-dependent Antigen.*** Antigen that requires interaction with helper T lymphocytes in order to stimulate B lymphocytes to produce antibodies. Thymus-dependent antigens must be presented to T lymphocytes by cells bearing class II histocompatability molecules. All proteins and polypeptides are thymus-dependent antigens.

***Thymus Gland.*** An irregular two-lobed gland that develops ventrally in the lower neck region of vertebrates from the third gill pouch. In mammals it consists primarily of epithelial cells, large numbers of rapidly dividing lymphocytes, and cells of suspected endocrine function. The thymus specifically controls cell-mediated immunity, homograft rejection, and hypersensitivity (or allergic) aspects of the immune response of the animal. Such effectts were first clearly demonstrated in the early 1960s using mice that had been thymectomized at birth. Certain lymphocytes are either derived initially from the thymus or require its mediation (possibly via a hormone) before they are immunologically competent. Following sexual maturity the gland atrophies and is active only if the established lymphocyte pool is depleted.

***Thymus-independent Antigen.*** Antigen that does not require interaction with T lymphocytes in order to stimulate B lymphocytes to produce antibodies. T-independent antigens include polysaccharides with repeating antigenic determinants and lipopolysaccharides from Gram-negative bacteria. Such antigens induce production of IgM and lead to little, if any, immunological memory. Whether or not any antigen is completely thymus-independent is not clear.

***Thyroglobulin.*** Glycoprotein ($M_r$—650,000) that binds to throxine during its synthesis and storage in the thyroid gland. When thyroxine is secreted into the circulation, it is separated from thyroglobulin. In the serum, the free thyroxine becomes bound to a thyroxine-binding globulin (TBG).

***Thyroid Gland.*** A paired endocrine gland of vertebrates that is formed in the embryo from ventral endoderm of the pharynx and is concerned primarily with regulation of the metabolic rate by the secretion of thyroid hormone. It probably evolved from the endostyle of protochordates and occurs as diffusely scattered tissue in some lower vertebrates (e.g. teleost fish). In mammals it consists of two lobes on either side of the trachea, joined anteriorly by an isthmus of tissue. Histologically it is composed of follicles of variable size that are lined with secretory epithelium, contain a colloidal substance, and are embedded in vascular connective tissue. The mammalian thyroid also contains C-cells, which secrete calcitonin. Normal growth of the gland and secretion of thyroid hormone requires trace amounts of iodine in the diet and stimulation by thyrotrophin.

***Thyroid Hormone.*** Either (or both) of two iodine-containing amino acid hormones secreted by the follicles of the vertebrate thyroid gland. Thyroid hormones are synthesized from a large precursor protein, thyroglobulin, in the colloidal substance of the follicles. Thyroglobulin is hydrolysed into various iodotyrosines, some of which are coupled together by specific enzymes to form iodothyronines, which are secreted. Of these, only thyroxine (tetraiodothyronine) and 3,5,3'-triiodothyronine have biological activity. Evidence suggests that triiodothyronine is the active form and thyroxine is metabolized to this form in the target tissues. Both hormones produce a large number of metabolic effects on many tissues; in particular they increase oxygen consumption and energy production (they probably interact synergistically with growth hormone, adrenal corticosteroids, and adrenaline in producing these effects). Thyroid hormone also stimulates developmental changes, such as moulting and metamorphosis; its effect on precocious metamorphosis in the amphibian tadpole has been known since 1912. Thyroid hormone effects involve RNA and protein or enzyme synthesis.

***Thyrotrophin (Thyroid-stimulating Hormone, TSH).*** A glycoprotein hormone, secreted by the pars distalis of the mammalian pituitary gland and homologous tissue of other vertebrates, that stimulates the growth of the thyroid gland, its uptake of iodine, and the secretion of its hormones. It consists of two large peptide subunits, one of which is similar to those of the glycoprotein pituitary gonadotrophins (LH and FSH).

***Thyroxine*** (Tetraiodothyronine, $T_4$). Principal hormone secreted by the thyroid gland in mammals. Thyroxine is an iodine rich derivative of tyrosine. Thyroxine release is controlled by thyrotrophin. In the circulation thyroxine is bound to thyroxine-binding globulin (TBG). Some thyroxine is converted to triiodothyronine ($T_3$). Thyroxine controls the level of metabolism throughout the body and is essential for normal growth. Excess thyroxine secretation, leading to hyperthyroidism, increase metabolism and results in body-wasting. A deficiency of thyroxine (hypothyroidism) in childrren causes dwarfism and mental retardation. Thyroxine is also required for metamorphosis in amphibians; tadpoles in which the thyroid has been removed or chemically ablated by treatment with thiourea fail to metamorphose.

***Tight Junction*** (Zonula Occludens). Continuous, band-like, intercellular junction around the lateral surface of epithelian cells that serves to seal epithelia against leakage. The outer leaflets of the plasma membrane of adjacent cells appears to have fused, thereby excluding completely any intercellular space. Tight junctions are rarely seen in tissues other than epithelium.

***Time-lapse Photography.*** Technique used in the production of films of moving cells using a photomicroscope and a camera which takes exposures at set intervals of, say, one frame per minute. By projecting the film at a more rapid speed, gains of over 1000 times the lapse of real time are readily obtained, allowing detailed study of the mechanisms of cell movement.

***Ti Plasmid.*** Large (150-230 kilobases) Plasmid possessed by strains of Agrobacterium tumefaciens, which incite crown gall in plants. A small part of this plasmid, the T-DNA, is transferred to and stably integrated into the host plant nuclear genome and is responsible for the oncogenic transformation of the plant cells. One of the characteristic features of the crown gall tumour cells is the production of opines. The genetic information for the synthesis of opines resides on the Ti plasmid and is transferred to the plant cell genome as part of the T-DNA. In relation to opine synthesis, there are two families of Ti plasmids: those that specify the synthesis of octopine and related opines; those that specify nopaline and related compounds. Using restriction mapping and insertional mutagenis, it has been established that the octopine group have extensive homology, whereas the nopaline family are less closely related. Between the two groups there is only some 30 percent homology. Apart from inciting tumour formation and opine production, the Ti plasmid encodes a number of other functions, and these are located outside of the T-DNA region. These include the information for the catabolism for the specific opine produced by the plant tumour cell and for the catabolism of arginine and ornithine, agrocin sensitivity, transfer functions and host range specificity. Since the Ti plasmid leads to the trransfer of genetic information from a prokaryote to a eukaryote, it has attracted considerable interest as a possible vector for genetic engineering in plants. Unfortunately, the size and complexity of the Ti plasmids presents problems for their direct manipulation in vitro. Various strategies are being developed to solve this problem, one of which is the development of binary vector systems. One plasmid contains the T-DNA region, whereas the other possesses the virulence features. Individually they do not lead to gene transfer, but when both are present oncogenicity occurs. The T region plasmid is able to replicate in E.coli as well as in Agrobacterium. Manipulation of the plasmid can ttake place in E.coli and the plasmid returned to Agrobacterium for transfer of the required genetic information to the host plant.

***Tissue.*** Aggregation of cells, together with associated extracellular matrices, specialized to perform differentiated functions. Some tissues may be made up substantially of one cell type, or of many different cell types.

***Tissue Culture (Explanation).*** The gorwth in a suitable medium of piece of tissue removed from a living animal or plant. The medium is often Ringer's solution supplied with oxygen and nutrients and kept free of microorganisms. A similar medium is used for the culture of organs.

***Tissue Typing.*** Use of serological tests to determine the major histocompatibility complex antigens of potential transplant donors or recipients.

***Titer.*** Estimate of amount of antibody activity. The antibody-containing fluid (e.g., serum) is diluted raidly unto an end-point (e.g., failure to agglutinate red blood cells) is reached. The titer is often expressed as the reciprocal of the end-point dilution.

***Titre.*** An assessment of the amount of anibody present in serum. It is estimated from the highest dilution of the serum at which agglutination by antigen-antibody reaction will still occur to a detectable extent and is expressed as the reciprocal of this dilution.

***Tla Complex.*** A segment of DNA, about 1.5 centiMorgans in length, on the telomeric side of the H-2 complex, and consisting of two regions called Qa and Tla.

The Qa region (220 kilobases) encodes the alpha chains of certain tissue-restricted class I histocompatibility molecules; these chains associate noncovalently with beta-2 microglobulin. The eight to ten genes in the Qa region of various inbred strains are designated Q1, Q2, Q3, Q4, Q5, Q6, Q7, Q8, Q9 and Q10. Three molecules, encoded in the Qa region, have been characterized: Qa-1, Qa-2 and Q10. Qa-1 and Qa-2 are expressed on lymphoid cells; Q10 is expressed on liver cells. The genes in the Qa region exhibit very little polymorphism.

The Tla region (155 kilobases) encodes the alpha chains of other class I histocompatibility molecules; these chains also associate noncovalently with beta-2 microglobulin. Therre are 13 to 18 genes (depending on the inbred strain). The molecules encoded in the Tla region are called TL and are found on thymocytes of certain inbred strains and on some leukemia cells, the origin of the designation TL. TL+ leukemias may occur in mice that do not express TL on their thymocytes. The Tla region molecules also exhibit very little polymorphism. The function of Qa and TL molecules is not known.

***T Locus.*** Locus near the centromere of chromosome 17 of mice. The dominant mutation, T, was the first gene to be identified in the T/t complex. Heterozygotes for T and wild-type (T/+) have a short tail. Homozygotes (T/T) die as embryos hecause the notochord is not formed. Heterozygotes for T and a t haplotype (T/t) are tailless. The T locus is also known as the brachyury locus.

***T lymphocyte.*** Lymphocyte that matures in the thymus and is responsible for cell-mediated immunity and the regulation of the growth and differentiation of other immunologically competent cells (e.g., B lymphocytes, mononuclear phagocytes). Mature T cells leave the thymus and recirculate in blood, lymph and secondary lymphoid organs. In lymph nodes, the T lymphocytes are localized to the deep cortex. T lymphocytes circulating in blood bind to specialized endothelial cells in the post-capillary venules of lymph nodes or the marginal sinus of the spleen. They then traverse the venules into the deep cortex of the lymph node or white pulp of the spleen where they remain for about 12-24 hours and leave by the efferent lymphatics to reach the major lymphatic circulation and the blood.

Mature T lymphocytes can be divided into two subsets that differ in function on the basis of surface antigenic determinats- CD4 and CD8. CD4+ cells recognize antigen associated with class II histocompatibility molecules, and CD8+ cells recognize antigen associated with class I histocompatibility molecules. Most CD4+ cells are helper T lymphocytes or responsible for delayed-type hypersensitivity reactions. Most CD8+ cells are cytotoxic and/or suppressor cells. Mature T lymphocytes in humans and mice bear CD3 and a transferrin receptor. All human and many mouse T cells also have CD2, which is the E-rosette receptor. T lymphocytes also bear an antigen-specific receptor.

***T Lymphocyte.*** Vertebrate white blood cell involved in cell-mediated immunity. Precursor T lymphocytes undergo an antigen-independent phase of differentiation within the thymus to become immunocompetent virgin T lymphocytes. These have membrane-bound receptors for antigens on their surfaces with properties similar to the antibody receptors of B lymphocytes, as well as characteristic differentiation antigens. T lymphocytes are classed into several different types of effector cells depending upon their function in the immune response, (i.e. $T_c$, cytotoxic T cells; $T_D$, responsible for delayed hypersensitivity; $T_H$, help B lymphocytes to differentiate; $T_S$, suppress immune responses).

***T lymphocyte Clone.*** Progeny of a single T lymphocyte. T lymphocytes from human blood or mouse spleen are suspended in medium and stimulated with antigen. T lymphocytes that have responded to antigen by blast transformation are separated on density gradients from resting T lymphocytes. The activated T lymphocytes are appropriately diluted and aliquots are added to the wells of a tissue culture plate, and then stimulated with antigen and interleukin-2. The dilution is such that usually, no more than a single T lymphocyte is added to each well. Therefore, single clones are obtained.

***T Lymphocyte Hybridoma.*** Clone resulting from the fusion of a mouse spleen T lymphocyte and a thymoma cell, BW 5147, derived from the AKR strain of mice. The cells are fused by polyethylene glycol. The hybrid cells proliferate continuously and produce interleukin-2 when stimulated with the appropriate antigen on an antigen-presenting cell. Unlike a T lymphocyte clone, T lymphocyte hybridomas grow in the absence of growth factors (e.g., interleukin-2).

***$T_m$***. Melting temperature for a sample of double-stranded nucleic acid. The more accurate figure is $T_{12m}$ being the temperature at which half the sample has become dissociated or melted into single strands.

***Tobacco Mosaic Virus (TMV).*** First plant virus to be isolated. TMV is a long filamentous virus consisting of a helical array of 2130 protein capsomeres, within which a coil of single-stranded RNA of 6500 nucleotides is located. The virus causes a mottling pattern on the leaves of plants and greatly reduces the strength of the plant.

***Tolerance.*** State of specific, immunological non-reactivity to a given antigen which in other circumstances would elicit an immune response. Tolerance to an antigen may be acquired if the animal is exposed to it early in foetal life or, as an adult, is exposed to very high or very low doses of the antigen.

***Tolerance.*** Immunological phenomenon consisting of the acquired incapacity of an individual to respond to a particular antigen. Tolerance can be induced by introducing an antigen into an individual at a very early stage in life, either during fetal or early postnatal life. Such as individual will not respond when challenged with the same antigen during adulthood. In contrast, the response to unrelated antigens is normal (i.e., there is selective loss of the response to the antigen that had been introduced in eary life, tolerogen).

Tolerance was discovered in non-identical twin cattle in which there had been exchange of blood in utero that resulted in a chimeric state (i.e., each twin has hemopoietic cells from the other). In adulthood, each cow can accept grafts from its twin. Tolerance can be induced in fetal/neonatal mice by injections of foreign cells or purified proteins. Immunological tolerance can also be induced in adult individuals by giving weak protein antigens either in repeated small doses or in larger amounts (i.e., low-zone tolerance or high-zone tolerance, respectively).

The mechanisms involved in tolerance are complex. Three possibilities have been proposed: (1) inactivation or deletion of B lymphocytes (which apparently occurs if B lymphocytes are exposed to antigen in the absence of interactions with T lymphocytes); (2) inactivation or deletion of helper T lymphocytes; and (3) induction of suppressor T lymphocytes. The lack of immunological response to autologous proteins is self-tolerance.

***Tolerogen.*** Substance that is capable of inducing tolerance. In general, tolerogens are also immunogens. Whether tolerance or immunity follows antigen administration depends on a number of factor: dose, route of administration, immunological status of the recipient. For example, foreign cells are strong immunogens when given to an adult, but may be tolerogens when given to a fetus. Heterologous immunoglobulins are usually strong immunogens when aggregated, but are often tolerogens in the monomeric form.

***Tolerogenic.*** Capable of inducing tolerance.

***Toluene.*** Organic solvent widely used as a base for cocktails used in liquid scintillation counters.

***Toluidine Blue.*** Dye widely used in cytochemistry.

***Tolmetin.*** (1-methyl-5-p-toluoylpyrrole-2-acetic acid). Drug used in the treatment of rheumatoid arthritis, juvenile rheumatoid arthritis and ankylosing spondylitis because of its anti-inflammatory effects. See Figure T.7.

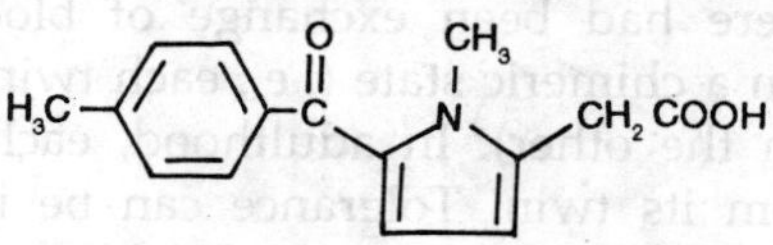


Figure T.7. Tolmetin.

***Tonofilament.*** Pre-keratin filaments, which are anchoured on the cytoplasmic side of spot demosomes and which extend as a network through the cytoplasm of epithelial cells. Tonofilament networks in adjacent cells are thus indirectly connected via the spot desmosomes and constitute a tonofilament array running throughout an epithelium. Such arrays can have a critical role in any folding morphogenesis displayed by the epithelium.

***Tonoplast.*** Membrane that bounds the vacuoles of plant cells. It consists of a single unit membrane with little mechanical strength and so bulges in response to hydrostatic pressure form inside or outside, thus helping to maintain turgor pressure within the cell.

***Tonsil.*** Mass of lymphoid tissue in the oropharynx. The palatine tonsils lie between the palatoglossal and palatopharyngeal arches; the lingual tonsils are at the base of the tongue; the pharyngeal tonsils, also called adenoids, are at the back of the pharynx. Tonsils are secondary lymphoid organs and are composed mostly of B lymphocytes.

***Topoisomerases.*** Group of enzymes that alter the topological form of DNA—previously termed swivelase, DNA-relaxing enzyme or nicking-closing enzyme. Two distinct types of topoisomerases are known: type I enzymes, which introduce transient nicks in single strands of DNA; type II enzymes, which introduce transient nicks in double-stranded DNA. These enzymes are capable of interconverting normal linear double-helical DNA, supercoiled DNA and DNA forming knots or concatenates.

***Topological Isomers.*** Molecules of DNA that are identical to one another except for their linking numbers (i.e. they vary in the degree of coiling or supercoiling of the DNA molecule).

***Tortoiseshell Cat*** (Calico Cat). Female cat in which black and orange patches of fur make a mosaic pattern in the coat. This mottled colour results from random inactivation of one or other X chromsome. Each group of cells of one pigment colour represents a cell clone in which a particular allele of the pigment gene, carried on the X chromosome is expressed.

***Totipotent.*** Describing a cell (or nucleus) that retains complete potential, so that it is able to differentiate into all the cell types represented in an adult organism (or cell), or to give rise to cells of all types on transplantation into appropriate cytoplasm (or a nucleus). Although the zygote is totipotent, almost all differentiated cells are not. Many nuclei remain totipotent, as proved by their insertion into enucleated egg cells of the same species, when normal development into adult may follow. See Figure T.8.

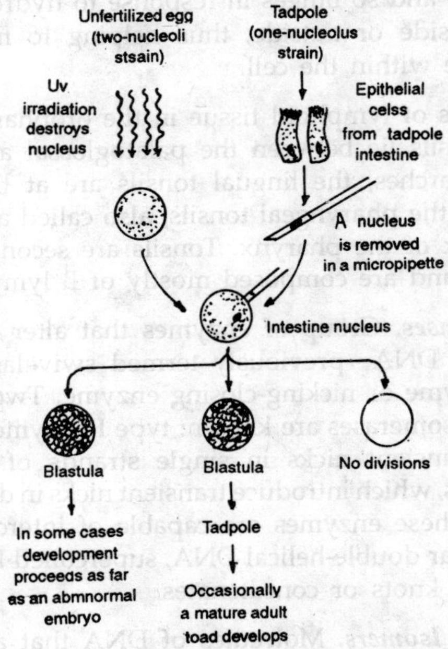


Figure T.8. Totipotent. Procedure employed to demonstrate the totipotency of the nucleus from a differentiated cell.

***Toxin.*** Substance that is poisonous to cells or organisms and is the product of another organism. Microorganisms, fungi, and certain plant tissues and animal secretions are toxins.

***Toxin.*** Poison, usually of high molecular weight, that is produced by a living organism and that is usually immunogenic.

***Toxoid.*** Toxin treated (e.g., with formalin) so that it retains its immunogenicity, but loses its toxicity. Diphtheria and tetanus toxoids are routinely used to immunize infants.

***Toxoid.*** Protein toxin that has lost its toxic properties, but retains its antigenic potential. Toxoids are thus useful as vaccines in the production of antitoxins by animals.

***Tp44*** (CD28). Membrane glycoprotein of T lymphocytes identified by a mouse monoclonal antibody. Tp44 is a homodimer, $M_r$ 74,000-92,000 (depending on cell source and probably due to variations in glycosylation); under reducing conditions the $M_r$ is 39,000-50,000. In the presence of phorbol esters, anti-Tp44 causes T lymphocytes to proliferate. The function of Tp44 is not known. Tp44 is composed of 220 amino acid residues, including a signal sequence of 18 residues, an extracellular domain of 134 residues, a transmembrane segment of 27 residues and a cytoplasmic domain of 41 residues; there are five sites for attachment of N-linked oligosaccharides. Tp44 is a member of the immunoglobulin superfamily. The amino-terminal 119 residues of the mature protein are homologous to variable region-like domains.

***T Phages.*** Group of bacteriophages of somewhat diverse form, but all having double-stranded DNAa genomes, an icosahedral head, and a hollow tail section. Notable T phages include the very large $T_2$ and $T_4$ bacteriophages.

***TPN.*** Triphosphopyridine nucleotide.

***Trace Element.*** Element required in minute amounts for growth, development or healthy survival of an organism. Copper, zinc and boron are trace elements for most animal species.

***Tracheary Elements.*** Certain lignified cells in the xylem. Strictly the term refers only to the tracheids and vessels (from the type of secondary wall thickening they show), but now it is commonly used to include fibres, fibre-tracheids, tracheids, and vessel elements. Because of the gradation in form between fibres, fibre-tracheids, and tracheids, these are sometimes grouped together as imperforate tracheary elements.

***Tracheid.*** An elongated empty lignified tracheary element with somewhat tapered ends and bordered pits that forms part of the vertical system of the xylem and is concerned with water conduction and mechanical support. It is regarded as the fundamental cell of the xylem from which fibres, fibre-tracheids, and vessel elements have evolved, and in more primitive ttacheophytes it forms the only type of water-conducting and mechanical cell in the wood. Cells termed ray tracheids, which have very thick lignified walls but are otherwise similar tto the ray parenchyma cells, occur in the medullary rays os some plants.

***Trailer.*** Any sequence that is downstream of the termination signal of a messenger RNA molecule and is therefore untranslated. It does not include the poly A tail.

***Trait.*** Particular phenotypic property of an individual, especially if expressed only to a slight degree. Thus individuals heterozygous for the sickel cell haemoglobin allele are said to have sickle cell trait.

***Trans.*** Situation in genetics when mutants of two nonallelic genes are carried on separate homologous chromosomes.

***Trans-acting Locus.*** Gene locus that affects another gene locus on another chromosome, generally though the production of a regulatory protein.

***Transamination.*** Biochemical transfer of an amino group from an amino acid to a keto acid, resulting in the production of novel amino acid and keto acid molecules. Pyridoxal phosphate is a coenzyme for all transaminases.

***Transcobalamin 2 Deficiency*** (TC2 deficiency). Deficiency of the principal vitamin B12 transport protein, transcobalamin 2. Affected infants have megaloblasic anemia and agammaglobulinemia. Vitamin B12 is required for terminal differentiation of B lymphocytes. The anemia and agammaglolbulinemia are corrected by administration of large doses of vitamin B12. TC2 deficiency is inherited as an autosomal recessive.

***Transcribed Spacer.*** Spacer sequence lying between the tandem repeats of the rRNA genes of certain eukaryotes, which is transcribed but of which the transcript is subsequently discarded.

***Transcriptase.*** Alernative term for an RNA polymerase.

***Transcription.*** The transfer of information in the form of nucleotide sequences from DNA to RNA. A single strand of a DNA acts as a template for the synthesis of a complementary RNA sequence, the synthesis being catalysed by DNA dependent RNA polymerase. Genes coding for ribosomal RNA or transfer RNA are transcribed into a precursor RNA, which is modified to yield the final RNA. DNA sequences coding for protein, i.e. structural genes (or cistrons) are transcribed initially into haterogeneous nuclear RNA (HnRNA), which is processed after transcription by removal of introns to yield the final product, messenger RNA. Transcription involves no elementary change to the coding language, i.e. the sequence of bases is the coding information. This contrasts with the process of translation, which involves conversion of the nucleotide code to a radically different amino acid code. See Figure T.9.

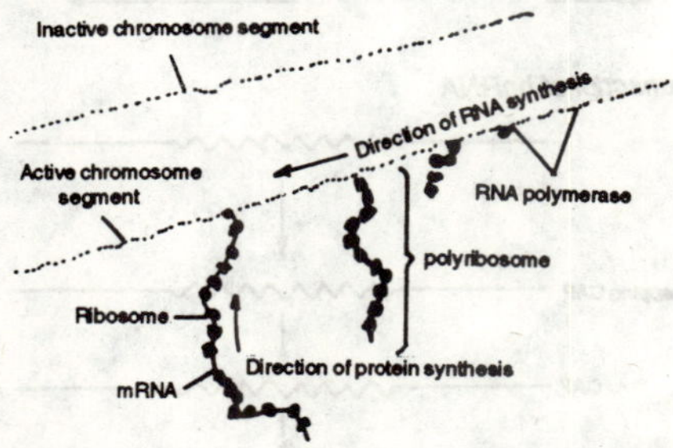


Figure T.9. Transcription. Transcription and trnaslation processes in bacteria. Two stretches of DNA, one naked, the other with nascent mRNA arranged at right angles, are observed.

***Transcription Control.*** Conttrol of gene expression at the level of transcription, as distinct from post-transcriptional or post-translational regulation. Transcriptional control of gene activity may be positive or negattive. The lac operon of E.coli is negatively controlled and must be depressed by inducer for transcription to occur. Many other genes in prokaryotes and eukaryotes are known to be positively controlled.

***Transcription Factor.*** Protein important in effecting transcription of a specific gene sequence. One such factor, known as TFIIIA (transcription factor/RNA polymerase III.A), has been found to bind to the central position of the 5S RNA coding sequence in Xenopus, and to facilitate greatly transcription of the sequence by the type III RNA polymerase. No doubt many other transcription factors exist. CAP acts as a transcription factor in E.coli. See Figure T.10.

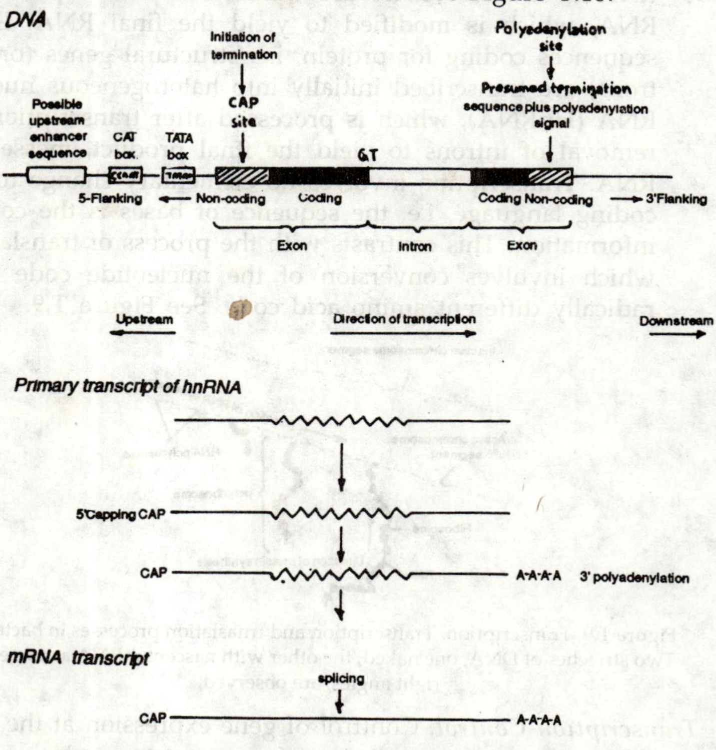


Figure T.10. Transcription. Transcription of class II gene.

***Transcytosis.*** Process whereby ligands, which have been internalized by receptor-mediated endocytosis, are directed to the surface of the cell opposite to that at which they entered. The best-characterized examples of transcytosis involve transport of immunoglobulins across epithelia. The polyimmunoglobulin receptor on the basolateral surface of epithelial cells bind IgA or IgM; the complex is internalized (receptor-mediated endocytosis), transported across the cell, and released at the apical surface by exocytosis, In transcytosis of IgA or IgM, the receptor is cleaved, and the ligand-binding portion, known as secretory component, remains bound to the polymeric immunoglobulin, which is released into secretions. Other epithelial cells transport monomeric IgG via Fc receptors (e.g., maternal IgG is transported from the small intestine of suckling rats into the circulation, in the direction opposite to that of IgA in adult intestine).

***Transdetermination.*** Change in the state of determination of a cell or tissue. The best known example of the phenomenon is found with imaginal discs of Drosophila larvae. With a frequency that is rare butt considerably greater than the basic rate of mutation, a disc, or more frequently, part of a disc will alter its state of determination so that, in the pupa, it develops and differentiates into an organ or organ part quite distinct from that dictated by its original state of determination.

***Transdifferentiation.*** Change in the state of differentiation of a cell or tissue. It is a phenomenon of relatively infrequent occurrence, but is known to occur in Hydra, and at least in experimental situations in plants. A well-authenticated example involves the transdifferentiation of pigmented iris cells into non-pigmented lens cells in the eyes of salamanders following earlier lens removal.

***Transduced Element.*** Fragment of DNA transferred from one cell to another in the process of transduction.

***Transduction.*** Transfer of genetic material from one bacterium to another by a bacteriophage. It was discovered in 1951 for Salmonella typhimurium and its temperate bacteriophage P22. Transduction has since been observed for E.coli and phage P1 (and under special conditions phages T1 and T4), and for species of Shigella, Proteus, Pseudomonas, Bacillus and Staphylococcus. Transduction is used for gene mapping and analysis in bacteria, and for strain construction. There are two kinds of transduction--generalized and specialized—each with a different underlying mechanism.

During generalized transduction any donor gene (chromosomal or plasmid) can be transferred with a probability of $10^{-4}$ — $10^{-8}$ per phage particle. Random fragments of bacterial DNA are encapsulated in phage heads, by error, during lytic growth of the phage in tthe donor culture. About 0.3 percent of the phage population (transducting phage) carry bacterial rather than phage DNA, the amount incorporated being limited by the size of the phage head (1 and 2.3 percent of the donor genome for P22 and P1, repectively). The lysate, containing transducing phage particles, is then used to infect recipient bacteria. At a multiplicity of infection (MOI) of less than one, lysis of transduced recipient bacteria by non-defective phage is avoided. The role of the phage vector ends with injection of the donor DNA. The injected DNA (the exogenote), within the partially diploid merozygote, can be degraded by host nucleases or can replace recipient genes by recmediated homologous recombination with the host chromosome (the endogenote).

Generalized transduction is ideal for detailed mapping of small bacterial chromosome segments. The method may entail measuring cotransduction frequency, or deletion mapping, or the two-point cross and three-point cross. If two or more genes are cotransduced, they are assumed to be carried by the same fragment of donor DNA, and are thus closely linked.

Deletion mapping allows the rapid positioning of single-site mutations. Using transduction, a small number of pairwise crosses are performed involving a set of strains carrying overlapping deletions with known end-points.

A two-factor transductional cross can give an estimate of genetic distance from recombination frequency. Transduction can also be used to order mutations by reciprocal three-point crosses.

In generalized transduction the majority of donor DNA fragments are stably inherited as non-replicating structures within recipient bacteria; this gives rise to abortive transduction.

Specialized (restricted) transduction occurs following induction of a lysogen. Only those bacterial genes immediately adjacent to the ends of the integrated prophage can be transduced. Thus specialized transduction is non random. On induction of a lysogen a small proporttion of virions (about one in 100 000) have genomes that contain some bacterial genes. These genomes are produced by illegitimate (rec-independent) recombination between the prophage and the bacterial chromosome during excision (compare formation of F plasmids in bacterial conjugation). For example, lamda (λ) heads cannot package DNA that is more than 110 percent of the length of the normal λ chromosome. A transducing phage lacks genes from one end of its genome and carries instead, at the opposite end, bacterial genes depending on the position of the illegitimate excision cross-over.

A lysate from a normal lysogen promotes low-frequency transduction (LFT) because it contains only a small proportion of phages capable of transducing bacterial genes. High-frequency transduction (HFT) lysates, considerably enriched in transducing phages of one type, can be produced by induction of cultures of transduced bacteria.

Specialized transducing phages have several important uses apart from mapping genes and creating recombinants. Transduced genes in an HFT preparation are enriched from one per bacterial genome (about 0.02 percent of the genome) to one per phage genome (about 2.5 percent of the genome). DNA from transducing phages can be readily obtained pure in large quantities, and can then be used in vitro for analysing gene transcription and translation, or the binding of specific regulatory proteins. Transducing phages are also a useful source of bacterial DNA for gene cloning in vitro. Genes carried by transducing phages are presented as multiple copies during vegetative replicattion of the phage DNA. The increased gene dosage may amplify expression of specific bacterial genes and serve to enrich cells for the protein products of these genes. This is particularly useful for genes which have an inherent low-level of expression (e.g., genes for repressor molecules).

***Transduction.*** Transfer of genetic information by a virus. Originally, the term described the transfer of genes from one bacterium to another by bacteriophage. Transduction is now also used to describe the transfer or genes by other viruses. For example, transducing retroviruses acquire proto-oncogenes (c-onc) from normal cells and transfer these genes (as oncogenes or v-onc) to other cells.

***Transfection.*** Uptake of foreign DNA by eukaryotic cells and its subsequent incorporation into the cellular genome.

***Transfection.*** Hybrid of transformation and infection, originally used to describe the introduction of phage DNA into bacteria. Subsequently, its use was broadened to include the introduction of viral (i.e., infectious) DNA into any cell, bacterial or eukaryotic. Presently, the term transfection is used quite loosely. In the context of eukaryotic cell biology, the transfer of any type of DNA (viral, cellular or plasmid) into an animal cell is often called transfection. This terminology was developed because the term transformation also has another meaning (i.e., malignant transformation). Some workers use the term transfection to describe the process whereby DNA is introduced into a cell, transformation being the relatively rare event of stable incorporation of DNA into the genome such that the cell is permanently altered. Several methods are used for the transfection of DNA into a variety of cells including lymphoid cells (e.g., coprecipitation of DNA with calcium phosphate, treatment with DEAE-dextran, protoplast fusion, electroporation).

***Transfectoma.*** Stable line of antibody-producing cells created by the transfer of genetically engineered antibody genes into myeloma cell lines. Usually, genomic DNA (rather than cDNA) is used in order to facilitate expression by virtue of inclusion of unique regulatory sequences (e.g., promoters, enhancers). The immunoglobulin heavy and light chain genes may be introduced one at a time in separate vectors or they may be cloned into the same vector.

***Transferases.*** Enzymes responsible for catalysing the transfer of functional groups such as phosphate or amino groups from one molecule to another.

***Transfer Cell.*** Plant cell with numerous mitochondria, abundant endoplasmic reticulum, and highly involuted plasma membrane. Transfer cells are abundant in situations where high rates of solute flow occur, as in xylem and phloem loading and unloading. They may also be involved in glandular and secretory plant tissues.

***Transfer Factor.*** Extract of T lymphocytes that is able to transfer cell-mediated immunity from one individual to another.

***Transfer Factor.*** Substance in dialysates of lysates of human peripheral blood leukocytes that may be capable of transferring delayed-type hypersensitivity from one individual to another.

***Transferrin Receptor (T9).*** Cell membrane receptor for transferrin, a serum protein ($M_r$76,000) that transports $Fe^{3+}$. The transferrin receptor is detected in humans with a mouse monoclonal antibody, anti-T9. Although the transferrin receptor is found on many cell types, it is most prominently expressed on the surface of activated T lymphocytes (about 250,000 molecules per cell). It is absent or barely detectable on resting T lymphocytes. The transferrin receptor is also expressed by early thymocytes. It is a glycoprotein, composed of two identical polypeptide chains ($M_r$ 100,000) which are linked by disulfide bonds. When T lymphocytes are stimulated with mitogens or antigens, the transferrin receptor is expressed before the onset of DNA synthesis. Monoclonal antibodies to T9 inhibit DNA synthesis in activated T lymphocytes. The gene encoding the transferrin receptor has been mapped to chromosome 3p12-ter in humans.

***Transferrins.*** Serum glycoproteins that bind iron and transport it from the intestine, where it is absorbed, and liver, where it is stored, to the other tissues of the body. Receptors on the surfaces of cells bind ferrotransferrin (transferrin with iron) and the complex is then taken into the cell by endocytosis.

***Transfer RNA*** (tRNA, adaptor RNA, soluble RNA, sRNA, 4S RNA). Species of RNA responsible for the transfer of specific amino acids to the growing end of a polypeptide chain during translation. The appropriate amino acid is positioned in the polypeptide chain since the tRNA molecule also bears an anticodon sequence which pairs up with the appropriate coding triplet on the mRNA molecule. There are thus at least 20 different species of tRNA (i.e. one for each amino acid) and many amino acids have more than one form of tRNA. The clover-leaf shape of the molecule is explained by the partial hydrogen bonding where regions of the RNA strand folds back on itself. The 3'-end of all tRNA molecules has an ACC terminus which acts as the amino acid binding site, whereas the anti-codon occupies bases 36-38 out of the 70-80 base length of the RNA. A ribosome binding site is also present. tRNA molecules sediment at 4S, and contain certain rate bases such as

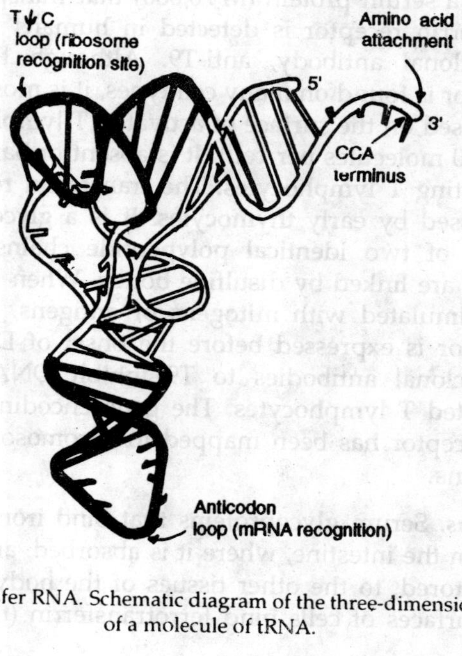


Figure T.11. Transfer RNA. Schematic diagram of the three-dimensional structure of a molecule of tRNA.

ribothymidylic acid and pseudouridylic acid which arise by post-transcriptional modification of existing bases. See Figure T.11.

***Transfilter Induction.*** Induction experiment in which a filter of precise pore size is interposed between two cell layers growing in vitro. The ability of one cell type to induce differentiation in another can thus be shown to be dependent or independent of cell contact between inducing and induced tissue.

***Transformant.*** Cell or organism that has been transformed by exposure to foreign DNA.

***Transformation.*** 1. A permanent genetic change in a cell following its acquisition of new DNA. The process was originally observed in bacteria: the classic experiment of Griffith in 1928, in which living nonvirulent bacteria acquired the property of virulence from dead bacteria in the same culture, was the first recognized example of transformation. In 1944 Avery, MacLeod, and McCarty demonstrated that the 'transforming principle' was DNA. Cells other than bacteria can also be transformed, but less easily than bacteria.

2. A permanent inherited change in a cell or cells in tissue culture. It is seen as a change in properties of growth and adhesiveness to neighbouring cell in culture and it involves changes similar to those associated with tumour formation. Some transformed cells are clearly malignant. Transformation is often associated with the growth of viruses in the tissue culture cells but may also result from the action of another agents.

***Transformation.*** Inherited change in a cell as the result of some experiental treatment. The term is used in three different contexts. (1) Transformation by DNA (genetic transformation): acquisition of a heritable altered phenotype as a result of the incorporation of exogenous DNA into a bacterial or eukaryotic cell. (2) Neoplastic (cellular) transformation: conversion of cultured animal cells to a state of unrestrained growth such that these cells come to resemble malignant cells. (3) Lymphocyte transformation: activation of a resting lymphocyte so that it grows, divides and differentiates, i.e., becomes a blast cell. The degree of blast transformation can be quantitated by measuring the incorporation of [$^3$H] thymidine into the cell's DNA. Blast transformation can be induced by stimulation with lectins, lymphokines, alloantigens (e.g., in the mixed lymphocyte reaction) and, in the case of cell from immune individuals, by antigen.

Genetic transformation was discovered in bacteria when it was shown that living non-virulent pneumococci could acquire the property of virulence from dead bacteria in the same culture. Subsequently, the material responsible for the 'transformation' was shown to be DNA.

***Transfusion Reaction.*** Untoward immunological reactions observed in the recipient of a transfusion of blood or blood products. Such reactions are usually due to allo-antibodies that cause hemolysis of donor red blood cells. The reaction is characterized by pain in the extremities and back, shortness of breath and falling blood pressure, which may lead to shock. The patient sustains a brief period of hypothermia followed by fever. Hemoglobin appears in the urine.

***Transgenic Organism.*** Organism carrying an exogenous gene in its genome. For example, in mice, the gene is usually introduced by microinjection into one of the two pronuclei of a recently fertilized egg. To allow the egg to develop, it is placed into the oviduct of a pseudopregnant female. The gene may become integrated into a chromosome; this occurs at a random position. If the DNA is integrated, it is transmitted through the germ line to subsequent generations and will be present in every cell; all tissues, at any developmental stage, can be analysed for expression of the inserted gene. Retroviruses may also be used to introduce foreign DNA into a mouse; in this case, infection is usually initiated at a later developmental stage (i.e., four to eight cell stage) and the resulting transgenic animal will be a mosaic; if germ line cells are infected, the exogenous DNA will be transmitted to progeny.

***Transgenesis.*** Transfer of new genetic material to a cell or organism, or between organisms.

***Transgenic Organism.*** Organism that has become transformed following the introduction of novel DNA into its genome. Such introduction is most frrequently achieved by integration of cloned DNA sequences following their injection into the fertilized egg. Transgenic animals produced by this technology include mice, Drosophila, Xenopus and some fish species.

***Transient Hypogammaglobulinemia of Infancy.*** Self-limited disease of infants, characterized by a delay in the capacity to synthesize antibodies normally until 30-36 months of age. Although affected infants have normal numbers of B lymphocytes, their helper T lymphocyte function appears to be defective.

***Transient Polymorphism.*** Temporary polymorphism in a population which occurs while one particular allele is in process of being replaced by an allele that confers increased fitness.

***Transition.*** Mutant in which a purine is substituted by a different purine, or a pyrimidine by a different pyrimidine. Such a change infers a base pair change between a G-C pair and an A-T pair in the DNA.

***Translation.*** The conversion of the sequence of nucleotides in a molecule of messenger RNA (mRNA) into a corresponding sequence of amino acids in a polypeptide chain, a stage in protein synthesis. The process occurs on the ribosomes, several to many of which are usually attached to a single molecule of mRNA, forming a polysome. Each triplet of nucleotides (codon) in the mRNA determines a single amino acid. Each amino acid is bonded to a specific molecule of transfer RNA (tRNA); base pairing occurs between the appropriate codon of the mRNA and the anticodon of the tRNA, during which the amino acid is added to the growing polypeptide chain on the ribosome. See Figure T.12.

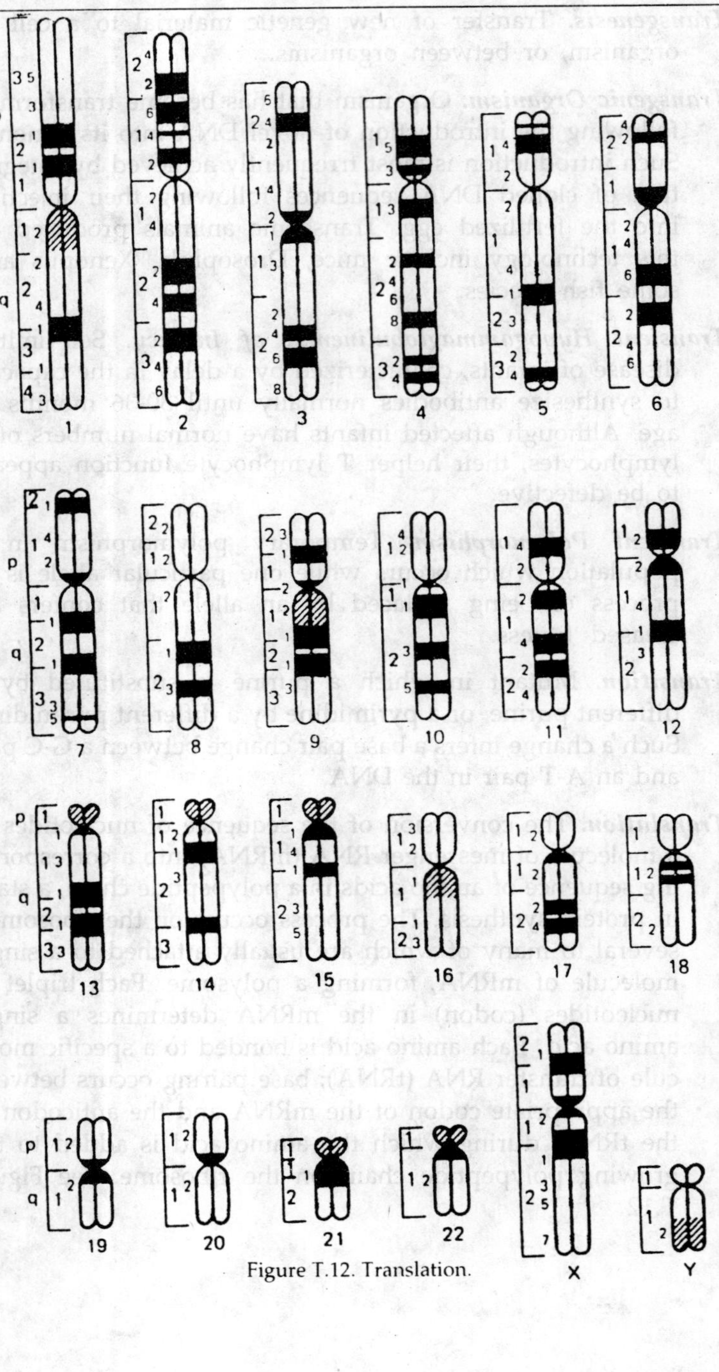


Figure T.12. Translation.

***Translational Amplification.*** Use of the same mRNA molecule many times, allowing the synthesis of large amounts of polypeptide from a single mRNA and therefore from a single gene product.

***Translational Control.*** Regulation of gene expression at the level of translation. Such control is chiefly a matter of modulating the rate of translation rather than modifying the message itself, but the timing of gene expression may also be modulated at this level by sequestering of mRNA for translation long after its initial transcription.

***Translocase.*** Protein that helps in the movement of tRNA molecules between different ribosomal sites during translation. The protein forms a complex with GTP and the ribosome and hydrolysis of GTP is coupled with the tRNA movement.

***Translocation.*** Movement of a DNA sequence or a substantial segment of a chromosome from one chromosomal location to another. It may be inter- or intrachromosomal and often involves an exchange between two segments of chromosome (i.e. reciprocal translocation).

***Translocation Down's Syndrome.*** Condition in which familial down's syndrome results from trisomy 21, one copy of chromosome 21 being translocated to another chromosome (most often chromosome 14).

***Translocation Heterozygote.*** Cell or organism in which non-homologous segments of two chromosomes are exchanged, but one copy of each of these chromosomes remains normal. Such an event induces the formation of a quadrivalent association between chromosomes at meiosis.

***Transmembrane Protein.*** Protein that traverses the cell plasma membrane.

***Transmission Genetics.*** Aspect of genetics that is concerned with transmission of genes from parents to progeny.

***Transmutation.*** Change of one element into a different element due to loss of some subatomic structure in radioactive decay.

***Transplantation.*** Grafting of tissue from a donor to a recipient organism or the transfer of organelles from one cell to another as in nuclear transplantation.

***Transposable Element.*** Element that function as a transposon.

***Transposition.*** Movement of a transposable element from one site to another in the genome.

***Transposon.*** A DNA element that has the ability to insert itself into other DNA sequences; plasmids and the genomes of bacteria and some eukaryotic cells are known to harbour transposons. Most transposons possess special insertion sequences, which facilitate entry into another DNA sequence. Transposons often carry genes that are involved in the insertion process, but their most significant effect is that of disturbing the expression of the genes with which they become associated.

***Transversion.*** Mutation in which a purine is converted to a pyrimidine or a pyrimidine to a purine.

***Triallelic.*** Describing a polyploid organism in which three different alleles occur at any one locus.

***Triassic (Trias).*** The first period of the Mesozoic era, extending from 225 to 180 million years ago. It was named after the German strata of this period, which are divided into thrree groups. In many places the Triassic system grades into the Permian and the two can be considered as a single system: the Permo-Triassic (or Permo-Trias).

***Tribe.*** A unit used in the classification of plants as a subdivision of the subfamily. It is used only in very large families. The name of the tribe ends in -eae and is derived from one member of the tribe. In the Compositae, for example, the subfamily Carduoideae consists of ten tribes; one of these is the Astereae, which contains the genera Aster, Bellis (daisy), Erigeron (midsummer daisy), etc.

***Trichloracetic Acid (TCA).*** Acid widely used for protein precipitation, especially during nucleic acid preparation. Its use has largely replaced that of the potentially explosive perchloric acid (PCA).

***Trichome.*** Hair-like outgrowth from the epidermis of vascular plants. Such outgrowths are entirely epidermal in origin and include glands and papillae as well as true hairs.

***Trichocyst.*** Small, spindle-shaped organelle that lies beneath the pellicle of many ciliated protozoa, forming a protrusible sac.

***Trichogen Cell.*** Cell that gives rise to the hair-like process which forms an insect bristle.

***Trichogyne.*** Specialized hypha that extends from the fruiting body of some fungi and forms a receptive organ for the male gamete.

***Triglycerides*** (triacylglycerols). Major component of animal and plant fat; fatty acid esters of glycerol.

***Triodothyronine*** ($T_3$). Hormone synthesized by the thyroid gland in response to thyrotrophin.

***Trilobita.*** A class of extinct marine bottom-dwelling Arthropoda, abundant from the Cambrian to the Silurian. The oval flattened body was divided longitudinally into three lobes and transversely into a head, thorax, and abdomen. The head bore a pair of compound eyes, a pair of antennae, and four pairs of jointed forked appendages with a inner projection used as an aid in feeding. There were numerous similar paired appendages on the body. Trilobites are thought to have been closely related to the ancestors of other arthropods, particularly the Crustacea.

***Trioses.*** Group of monosaccharides with three carbon atoms.

***Triparental Recombinant.*** Recombinant bacteriophage (phage) that can be recovered from phage-injected bacteria which contain marker genes derived from three different original infecting phages. Such triple recombinant phage emphasize the frequency of recombinational events during the replication of the phage DNA in the infected cell.

***Triploblastic.*** Designating animals with three embryonic cells layers: ectoderm, endoderm, and mesoderm. All the Metazoa are triploblastic with the exception of the Coelenterata, which are diploblastic.

***Triploid.*** Describing a cell or organism in which three haploid sets of chromosomes are present, rather than the usual diploid condition with only two sets.

***Tris*** (Tris (hydroxymethyl) aminomethane). Compound widely used as a buffering agent in biological media and solutions.

***Triskelion.*** 'Three-legged' protein complex of clathrin and another small protein which forms the polyhedral coat on the surface of coated vesicle.

***Trisomic.*** Describing an organism in which one chromosome is present in triplicate in an otherwise diploid set.

***Trisomy.*** The condition in which one or more chromosomes are represented three times in a nucleus, cell, or organism, so that the diploid chromosome complement is 2n + 1, where n is the haploid number. Down's syndrome in man is caused by chromosome 21 being present three times, resulting in a chromosome number of 47 rather than 46.

***Tritanopia.*** State of being colour blind for the colour blue. Unlike red/green colour blindness, blue colour blindness is determined by an autosomal rather than an X-linked gene.

***Tritium*** ($^3$H). Radioactive isotope of hydrogen; an emitter of beta-particles. Tritiated precursor are used to study the synthesis of macromolecules such as DNA ([$^3$H]thymidine), RNA ([$^3$H)uridine) or protein ([$^3$H]amino acids) or to mark cells by incorporating [$^3$H]thymidine into their nuclei and identifying the cells within histological sections of tissue by autoradiography.

***Triton Detergent.*** Uncharged (non-ionic) detergent widely used in cell biology for solubilizing the proteins of cell membranes. The commonest is Triton X100.

***Triturus Cristatus.*** Great crested or warty newt; a urodele (tailed amphibian) native to most of Europe including the UK. Crested newts have been much used in cytogenetics due to the occurrence of large, readily visible lampbrush chromosomes in their oocytes. This species has also been shown to carry an unusual genetic load; viability requires heterozygosity of chromosome 1, with the result that 50 percent of fertilized eggs are unable to develop beyond the early embryo stage because they are homozygous for this chromosome.

***Trivalent.*** Arrangement in meiosis in which three copies of a homologous chromosome are associated.

***Trivial Equilibrium.*** Situation of supposed genetic equilibrium in a population, relative to one locus in which the equilibrium is explained by the fact that only one type of allele is present at the locus.

***tRNA Gene.*** Gene that codes for transfer RNA. The total number of these genes in the genome varies from 360 in yeast to over 1000 in humans. Each of the 20 common amino acids have specific tRNA genes coding for molecules with specificity of binding to their coding triplet on the message and to their own structure. Because of degeneracy in the code, different species of tRNA will bind the same amino acid but have variant anticodon triplets (e.g.,UCA and UCG for serine). In addition, some species of tRNA are coded by highly repetitious genes; thus Xenopus carries 240 copies of the gene coding for valine tRNA. Within the genomes of eukaryotes, the tRNA genes are widely scattered among the chromosomes, but many copies may be clustered at any one of the numerous chromosomal loci.

***tRNA Isoacceptors.*** Differing species of tRNA that bind the same amino acid but, because of coding degeneracy, have differing anticodon triplets. Such isoacceptors are coded by separate genes.

***Trophectoderm.*** Rim of cells that surrounds the blastocoelic cavity (containing fluid) and inner cell mass of the early mammal embryo at the blastocyst stage. Trophectoderm is an extraembryonic tissue, some of whose cells give rise to the trophoblast.

***Trophoblast.*** Layer of extraembryonic epithelium that forms around the mammalian blastocyst. It forms the outer layer of the chorion and attaches the early embryo to the uterus wall, absorbing nutrients from the mother and which derives from the trophectoderm.

***Trophocyte.*** Nurse cell of the insect ovary that provides nutrient for the developing oocytes.

***Tropism*** (Tropic Movement). Directional growth movement by part of a plant, or movement of part of a sedentary animal in a particular direction in response to light (phototropism), chemicals (chemotropism) or other stimuli. Movement in the direction of the stimulus is called positive tropism, and movement away negative tropism.

***Tropocollagen.*** Large molecule consisting of a rope of three alpha-collagen molecule wrapped around to give a trriple helical rod.

***Tropomyosin.*** One of the constituents of skeletal muscle. It is a rod-shaped protein that lies in the long grooves formed by the actin aggregates in the muscle filaments.

***Troponin.*** Protein found in skeletal muscle filaments. It is a complex of three polypeptides and helps to position tropomyosin along the filaments of actin molecules. It helps mediate the calcium ion regulation of muscle contraction.

***trp Gene.*** Gene concerned with tryptophan biosynthesis in E.coli. A number of such genes are located together in the genome, forming the tryptophan operon (trp operon).

***trp Promoter.*** Promoter of the tryptophan operon in E.coli.

***True Breeding.*** Production of a progeny which, like their parents, express a particular genotype in their phenotype. The term may be applied to a single gene, but more often to a particular pattern of gene expression in the individuals concerned, so that animals of a particular breed are expected to 'breed true' and produce progeny resembling themselves.

***Trypsin.*** Proteolyic enzyme secreted by the pancreas. Its initial form is trypsinogen, which is inactive, and is converted to the active form by enterokinase in the intestine. In cleaves proteins by cutting off the carboxyl arginine and lysine residues.

***Trypsinogen.*** Relatively inert form of trypsin. It is synthesized in the pancreas, and is converted to trypsin in the gut by enzymic removal of some terminal amino acids.

***Tryptophan*** (trp). One of the 20 common amino acids; a precursor of serotonin and indole compounds (e.g., indoleacetic acid). Tryptophan carries a non-polar sidechain.

***Tryptophan Synthetase.*** Enzyme that catalyses the formation of tryptophan from serine and indole.

***TSH.*** Thyroid-stimulating hormone.

***T/t Complex.*** Proximal region of chromosome 17 of mice in which recombination is suppressed between t haplotypes and the wild-type chromosome. The region of recombination suppression spans about 20 cM and includes the T locus and the major histocompatibility complex. There is about 5-11 cM of normal chromosome between the centromere and the beginning of the recombination-suppressed region. The T/t complex contains genes involved in early embyronic development.

***t Test.*** Statistical method used to determine the significance of differences between means.

***Tube Nucleus.*** Vegetative nucleus found in the pollen tube of the germinating plant pollen grain.

***Tuberculin.*** Mixture of proteins from culture filtrates of Mycobacterium tuberculosis. It is employed in skin tests for delayed-type hypersensitivity to this organism. The term includes old tuberculin and purified protein derivative.

***Tuberculin Test.*** Intradermal test for delayed-type hypersensitivity to tuberculin. Positive reactions are presumptive evidence of cell-mediated immunity to Mycobacterium tuberculosis.

***Tumor-associated Antigen.*** Membrane or nuclear antigen of tumor cells that is not found - or found in lesser amounts - in normal cells of the type from which the tumor was derived. Tumor-specific transplantation antigens (TSTA) have been found in methylcholanthrene-induced skin tumors of mice. When such tumors are transplanted to a syngeneic mouse, the recipient becomes immune to the tumor and rejects it and is resistant to the successful engraftment of a second tumor from the same source. Each tumor appears to have a distinct antigen. Oncogenic viruses can also induce expression of tumor-associated antigens. For each virus, the same antigen is expressed regardless of the tissue of origin of the tumor or the animal species in which the tumor is induced. These tumor-associated antigens are actually host antigens whose expression is induced by the virus. Oncofetal antigens are also considered to be tomor-associated antigens.

***Tumour (Neoplasm).*** A swelling in an organism resulting from the abnormal or uncontrolled proliferation of cells. Tumours that do not invade and destroy other parts of the body are described as benign; those that do are termed malignant.

***Tumour Cell.*** Neoplastic cell. Tumour cells are likely to show properties of rapid growth and can often be established as cell lines in tissue culture.

***Tumor Enhancement.*** Prevention, by antibodies, of cell-mediated destruction of tumors. Two mechanisms that have been invoked to account for this phenomenon are: (1) antibody molecules cover tumor-associated antigens and block the induction of cell-mediated immunity; (2) antibodies cover tumor-associatd antigens, thereby preventing their destruction by cytotoxic T lymphocytes.

***Tumour-inducing Principle*** (tip). Putative genetic element transferred from bacterium to plant cell in crown gall disease. The element has now been identified as the Ti pasmid.

***Tumor Necrosis Factor (TNF).*** Monokine that induces leukocytosis, fever, weight loss, the acute phase reaction and necrosis of some tumors (e.g., methylcholanthrene-induced sarcomas in mice). TNF was first found in serum of animals primed with Bacille Calmete-Guerin (BCG) and then challenged with lipopolysaccharide. A molecule identical to TNF, and named cachectin, was isolated from serum of animals with heavy parasitic infestations. Cachectin was found to have profound effects on general cellular metabolism and to be responsible for weight loss during infection or from neoplasia. Synthesis of TNF can be induced in mononuclear phagocytes by a variety of agents including lipopolysaccharides and phorbol esters; secretion of TNF is maximal 8 to 24 hours later.

TNF (also called TNF-$\alpha$) is a single polypeptide chain of 157 amino acid residues; it is not glycosylated. The gene for TNF has been mapped to the H-2 region of mouse chromosome 17 and the HLA region of human chromosome 6. The gene encoding TNF is closely linked to the gene encoding lymphotoxin (LT), a lymphokine that is also called TNF-$\beta$. TNF and LT are homologous proteins having approximately 30 percent amino acid sequence identity. They bind to the same receptor and have common biological activities: (1) inducing differentiation of myeloid cells; (2) activating neutrophils; (3) killing of RNA and DNA viruses by macrophages in synergy with interferon-gamma. Both TNF and LT are assayed by their capacity to kill a mouse fibroblast line (L-929). In contrast to the other major monokine, interleukin-1, TNF does not induce synthesis of interleukin-2.

***Tunica-Corpus Theory.*** The theory of Schmidt (1924) proposing that the apical meristem of vascular plants consists of two parts, each with its own separate initials: an outer tunica of one or more layers, characterized by anticlinal cell divisions, and an inner corpus, in which cell division occurs in various planes. Since Schmidt first put the theory forward it has been modified a number of times, and as more plants are studied it has become more difficult to define and delimit the two parts. However, the terms are still used in describing apex growth patterns.

***Tunicamycin.*** Antibiotic that inhibits glycosylation of membrane glycoproteins.

***Turbidimetry.*** Estimation of numbers of bacterial cells in a culture by determination of turbidity using a spectrophotometer.

***Turbid Plaque.*** Plaque formed by growth of a lytic phage in a bacterial lawn, but in which cloudiness persists due to some phage becoming lysogenic and failing to lyse the bacterial cells.

***Turgor.*** State of cellular and tissue turgidity in a prokaryotic or plant cell, resulting from exertion of turgor pressure (itself a result on entry of water in the cell or cells by osmosist against a rigid cell wall. The plant cell vacuoles also help to maintain and control turgor pressure. Such pressure is essential for the maintenance of form and for mechanical support of flowers, stems and leaves, especially in succulent plants. Turgor pressure is also involved in plant movements, flower opening, stomatal movement and phloem translocation.

***Turner's Syndrome.*** A syndrome involving reduced stature, webbing of the neck, infertility, and some degree of mental retardation in the human female, resulting from a sex chromosome anomaly. Affected individuals have a sex chromosome constitution of XO, ratther than the normal XX, and lack a Barr body. This would seem to indicate that the Barr body of normal females must play a role in normal development and is probably not heterochromatic.

***Turnover.*** Replacement of atoms or molecules in a living system by synthesis, usually in a steady state where synthesis precisely equals degradation. For example, prokaryotic mRNA is said to turn over rapidly.

***Tween 80*** (Polyoxyethylenesorbitan monooleate). Non-ionic detergent. It is sometimes used as an emulsifying agent in the preparation of microbiological tissue culture media (such as thioglycolate broth).

***Twins.*** Paired progeny. Such pairs may consist of identical twins, (monozygotic twins), or non-identical twinns (dizygotic twins).

***Twisting Number.*** Number of base pairs in a DNA duplex sequence, divided by the number of base pairs for every helical turn.

***Two-dimensional Electrophoresis.*** Method for enhancing the separation of proteins and other macromolecules that are of similar size and charge and not resolved by electrophoresis in one dimension. There are ·various ways of doing this, for example, by altering the pH of the supporting medium in the second dimension, by changing the nature of the medium itself (i.e. polyacrylamide gel as opposed to agar) or by carrying out combinations of pore gradient electrophoresis and isoelectric focusing.

***Two-point Cross.*** Genetic cross in which either one parent is a double mutant (— —) and the other is wild type (++) with respect to two markers being followed in the cross (an 'in-coupling' cross), or each parent carrries one of the two markers (+—x—+) being followed in the cross (an 'in-repulsion' cross).

***Ty Element.*** Tansposable element of yeast. About 30 transposable elements exist in each haploid genome.

***Tylose.*** Protursion of part of a parenchyma cell into the lumen of an adjacent tracheary element tthrough the pit pairs connecting the two cells. It may remain thin-walled or develop a secondary wall with lignification. These tyloses are often sufficiently large and abundant as to block the lumen of the element. They develop when the element becomes inactive or damaged and are frequently found in elements in the abscission zones. Their presence may prevent the spread of fungal and other infections through the xylem.

***Type II Interferon.*** Synonym for interferon-gamma.

***Tyrosinaemia.*** Inherited disease of the human resulting from deficiency of p-hydroxyphenylpyruvic oxidase.

***Tyrosinase.*** Enzyme involved in the production of melanin from tyrosine. Tyrosine is first converted to DOPA, then DOPA is oxidized to form DOPA quinone, and these molecules polymerize spontaneously to form melanin.

***Tyrosine (try).*** An amino acid, $(OH)C_6H_4CH_2CH(NH_2)COOH$, one of the 20 common amino acids occurring in proteins. Tyrosine is important as a precursor of noradrenaline,

adrenaline, melanin, thyroid hormone, isoquinoline alkaloids (e.g. papaverine), and opium alkaloids (e.g. morphine).

***Tyrosine Aminotransferase*** (TAT). Enzyme that is inducible by steroids in mammalian tissue culture cells. The X chromosome is known to carry a gene for a factor capable of blocking TAT inducibility.

# U

***U.*** Symbol for uridine and uracil in molecular biology.

***Ubiquinone*** (coenzyme Q). Quinone with a long isoprenoid tail; the number of isoprene units depends on the species in which the quinone occurs. In mammals there are 10 such units (hence uniquinone-10 or coenzyme $Q_{10}$). Ubiquinone is a membrane-soluble component of electron transport chains which meditate hydrogen transfer between membrane-bound dehydrogenase which contain flavoprotein and iron-sulphur proteins, and membrane-bound cytochrome complexes containing b-type cytochrome. The coenzyme alternates between the quinone and quinol forms during hydrogen transfer and the free radical semiquinone is probably an intermediate in the reacttion.

***Ubiquitin.*** Acidic protein widely, and perhaps universally, distributed among eukaryotes. It binds strongly tto chromatin and may have a structural role in chromatin conformation. Binding specifically to histone H2A by a covalent linkage, the complex has come to be known as protein A24.

***Ubiquitin.*** Polypeptide of 76 amino acid residues that is present in all eukaryotes, but apparently not in prokaryotes. Ubiquitin is highly conserved, differing in only three amino acid residues from yeast to mammals. Ubiquitin exists their free or covalently bound to many cellular proteins, thereby marking them for selective degradation. Ubiquitin is also present in chromosomes, where it forms covalent complexes with histones; the functional role of ubiquitin in chromosomes is not known. Ubiquitin was originally found in extracts of thymus and was erroneously belived to be one of the 'thymic hormones'. It is found on the lymphocytes homing receptor (gp90MEL-14) and other cell surface receptor.

***UI RNA.*** Species of small nuclear RNA (snRNA), of 165 bases is length, that is complementary to the donor and acceptor splice junctions and is therefore believed to be involved in the excision of introns and splicing of exons, the UI RNA is associated with a specific protein which is involved in intron excision, and together they form the UI ribonucleoprotein particle called either the UI particle or snRNP.

***Ultracentrifuge.*** Instrument in which tissue homogenates or solutions are rotated at high speed and thereby subjected to intense centrifugal force, sometimes in the region of several hundred thousand times gravitational force. Subcellular particles (cell membranes, mitochondria, ribosomes) and macromolecules (mtRNA, rRNA, mtDNA) sediment rapidly according to their size, shape, densitty and molecular weight. There are basically two types of ultracentrifuge: preparative and analytical. Preparatie ultracentrifugation is used to purify components for further use, and the centrifuge is solely designed to generate large centrifugal forces for a set period of time. In analytical centrifugation the instrument is designed to allow the progress of the components during centrifugation to be monitored, allowing the sedimentation coefficients of various molecules and particles to be determined.

***Ultrasonography.*** Visualization of a foetus in utero by ultrasound in order to check on possible gross malformation or difficult presentation.

***Ultrastructure (fine structure).*** The structure of a cell or tissue at the molecular level or at the microscopic level using resoluttions unobtainable with the visual spectrum, e.g. as observed using an electron microscope.

***Ultraviolet Absorption Curve.*** Plot that shows the relationship between differing wavelengths of light in the ultraviolet rrange and the percentage absorbance by a solution of biological molecules. Such a curve helps to distinguish nucleic acids from proteins; the former absorb maximally at about 260 nm and the latter at about 280 nm.

***Ultraviolet Fluorescence Microscope.*** Ultraviolet microscope in which the ultraviolet light is directed on biological material which fluoresces in a particular colour when so irradiated. This may be because of natural fluorescence or because of staining with fluorescent dyes such as fluorescein or association with fluorescently tagged antibody.

***Ultraviolet Irradiation.*** Irradiation with ultraviolet light, which may induce melanin formation in low doses, but is also a mutagen and, in high doses, lethal to living cells. It is widely used for the maintenance of sterility in cabinetts used for tissue culture, but will not penetrate glass or plastic efficiently. Its mutagenic effect results from its induction o^f pyrimidine dimers in DNA.

***Ultraviolet Light.*** Lightt,actually invisible to the human eye and forming part of the electromagnetic spectrum between 100 and 400 nm.

***Ultraviolet Microscope.*** Microscope in which ultraviolet light is generated from the light source, usually a high-pressure mercury vapour lamp, and which is provided with excitation and barrier filters so that ultraviolet light can excite fluorescent molecules in the specimen, harmful ultraviolet light can be filtered out, and fluorescent light only allowed to pass through the eyepiece.

***Unbalanced Translocation.*** Chromosome translocation in which some loss of chromosomal material has resulted or in which a deleterious genetic effect is evident following the translocation.

***Uncoiling of Chromomeres.*** Situation most readily seen in the puffing of polytene chromosomes and the looping out of chromatin loops in lampbrush chromosomes.

***Uncondensed Chromatin.*** Chromatin that is not highly compacted and is therefore more likely to be transcriptionally active; there is a strong correlation between gene activity and chromatin decondensation. Both the puffs and interbands of polytene chromosomes are uncondensed and are sites of intense and moderate transcriptional activity, respectively.

***Uncoupling Agent.*** Weak acid that is, to some extent, lipid-soluble. It can therefore mediate the movement of protons across membranes, and so uncouple electron transport from phosphorylation of ADP.

***Underwinding.*** Negative supercoiling; coiling of normal B-form DNA in a left-handed direction, and therefore opposite to the direction of coiling of the double helix itself.

***Unequal Crossing-over.*** Imprecise pairing of deuplicated segments prior to crossing over, leading to chromatids with unequal copies or numbers of copies of the segments concerned.

***Unicellular.*** Designating organisms or parts that consist of one cell only. Unicellular organisms include the Protozoa and some algae.

***Unidentified Reading Frame (URF).*** Oopen reading frame (ORF) that does not correspond to a known protein.

***Unidirectional Replication.*** Movement of a single replicating fork from a replication origin.

***Unineme Hypothesis.*** Concept that an unduplicated chromosome, that is one prior to the S phase of DNA replication, has a single molecule of DNA duplex running from end to end. The concept is now generally accepted, although it is clear that the molecule is highly twisted upon itself both by reason of packing around nucleosomes, packing of nucleosomes in the 30-nm fibres of chromatin, and further packing of these fibres relative to the chromosome axis.

***Uniparental Inheritance.*** Type of inheritance in which all the offspring from one mating resemble only one of the two parents in one of a range of characteristics. Such a phenomenon is commonly an example of maternal inheritance and is explained by the presence of cytoplasmic determinants in the egg.

***Uniport.*** Protein responsible for ion transport from one side of a cell plasma membrane to the other.

***Unique DNA.*** Sequence of nucleotides present only once per haploid genome. The great majority of prokaryotic DNA and almost all protein-coding genes is eukaryotes are unique in this respect.

***Unisexual.*** (Designating) a plant or animal species that bears either male or female reproductive organs but not both.

***Unitarian Hypothesis.*** View that the multiple functions of antibodies (e.g., agglutination, complement fixation, lysis, precipitation) are all results of the same type of antibody molecule reacting with different ligands. The opposing view is that each activiy is associated with a distinct type of antibody molecule. Today, it is known that neither of these views is entirely correct, since different immunoglobulin classes and subclasses do vary in their activities, but a particular activity (e.g., precipitation) is usually manifested by more than one class.

***Unit Membrane.*** Single biological membrane, resolvable at the ultrastructural level into the characterisitc two electron-dense leaflets enclosing an electron-lucent layer.

***Univalent.*** Describing a chromosome that exists singly at meiosis, when other chromosomes are present as paired homologous chromsomes. Thus the X chromosome of an XO turner's syndrome individual is univalent.

***Univalent.*** Having one binding site.

***Universal Donor.*** Out-moded term used to describe human blood group O donors in the early days of blood transfusion. All blood is potentially incompatible due to the presence of a wide variety of erythrocyte antigens and isoagglutinins, and must be cross-matched with the patient's serum before transfusion. There is no universal donor.

***Universal Recipient.*** Out-moded term used to describe human blood group AB recipients in the early days of blood transfusion.

***Unscheduled DNA synthesis.*** Synthesis that occurs at times other than the S phase of the cell cycle. Most of such synthesis is DNA repair, although synthesis of mitochondrial DNA in the cytoplasm is also continuous.

***Untranscribed Spacer.*** DNA sequence that lies between two coding sequences and is not transcribed by RNA polymerase. Although such sequences do exist, some identified in the past (e.g., the spacers between the multiple copy of rRNA genes) are now known to be transcribed.

***Unwinding Protein.*** Protein that untwists the DNA double helix before the replicating fork reaches that region during DNA synthesis. Such a protein, discovered in phage T4, has been termed the gene 32 protein.

***Up.*** Describing a mutation in the promoter that increases the frequency of transcriptional initiation.

***Upstream.*** In the direction opposite to the direction of DNA transcription, and therefore going from 5' to 3' on the coding strand, or 3' to 5' on the mRNA.

***Uracil.*** Pyrimidine base found in RNA, but not DNA, and pairing with the adenine base.

***Uranyl Acetate.*** Electron-opaque compound used to stain ultra-thin sections of tissue for viewing by transmission electron microscopy.

***Urea.*** A nitrogen-containing water-soluble organic compound, $H_2NCONH_2$, that is the main nitrogenous excretory product of the catabolism of amino acids in ureotelic animals. Urea is produced in the liver via the urea (or ornithine) cycle.

***Urethane.*** Simple organic molecule that induces tumours when inhaled, especially in the lung.

***Uric Acid.*** Main product of amino acid catabolism in reptiles and birds; product of nucleic acid catabolism in mammals.

***Uridine.*** Riboside consisting of ribose linked to a uracil base.

***Uridine Diphosphate Galactose*** (UDP-Gal). Nucleoside diphosphate sugar, found as an intermediate in the metabolism of galactose, and formed in a reaction between uridine triphosphate (UTP) and galactose-1-phosphate catalysed by the enzyme UDP-Gal pyrophosphorylase: UTP + galactose-1-phosphate —> UDP-Gal + PPi. UDPG epimerase then catalyses an inversion of configuration converting UDP-Gal to uridine diphosphate glucose.

***Uridine Diphosphate Glucose*** (UDPG). Nucleoside diphosphate sugar formed in a reaction between uridine triphosphate (UTP) and glucose-1-phosphate catalysed by UDPG pyrophosphorylase: UTP + glucose-1-phosphate—UDPG+PPi. UDPG donates the activated monomers in the biosynthesis of glycogen: $(\text{glucose})_n$ + UDPG —> $(\text{glucose})_{n+1}$ + UDP. UDPG is also an intermediate in the metabolism of galactose. See Figure U.1.

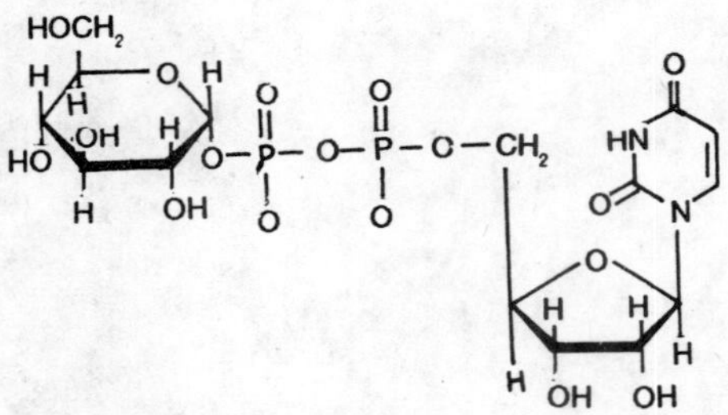


Figure U.1. Uridine diphosphate glucose.

***5'-Uridylic Acid.*** Nucleotide, the 5'-phosphate ester of uridine, and one of the monomeric units of RNA. See Figure U.2 on next page.

***Urticaria.*** Intensely itchy, patchy rash consisting of a raised, irregularly shaped wheal with a blanched center surrounded by a red flare. Urticaria is caused by histamine released from mast cells due to immunological reactions or to chemical or physical agents. Among the immunological reactions causing histamine release are interactions between antigens and IgE antibodies bound to mast cells or generation of anaphylotoxins by activation of complement.

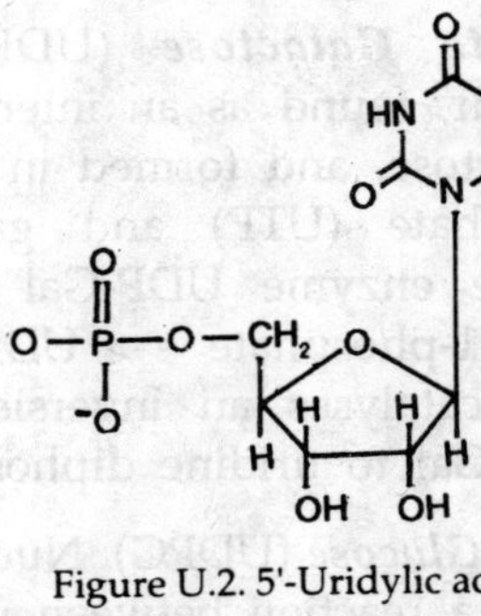

Figure U.2. 5'-Uridylic acid.

***Uveitis.*** Inflammation of the uveal tract (uvea, iris, ciliary body and choroid) of the eye. Uveitis is found in several immunological diseases, such as sarcoidosis, Behcet's disease and juvenile rheumatoid arthritis.

# V

***$V_k$*.** Variable region of an immunoglobulin kappa chain; sometimes used to denote only that portion of the variable region encoded by the $V_k$ gene segment.

***$V_\gamma$*.** Variable region of an immunoglobulin lambda chain; sometimes used to denote only that porton of the variable region encoded by the $V_\gamma$ gene segment.

***Vaccination.*** The administration of antigenes for the purpose of inducing active immunity, by establishing adequate levels of antibody and lymphocytes carrying cell-bound antibcdy. Antigens are injected or ingested in the form of vaccines. These may be toxins derived from pathogenic bacilli, dead pathogenic bacteria or viruses, or attenuated organisms.

***Vaccinaton.*** Production of actve iimmuniity by administration of a vacciine. Vaccinatiion was introduced by Edward Jenner. Jenner showed that immunity aganst small-pox could be induced by inoculating with cowpox, a virus that is not pathogenic for humans but that shares antigenic determinants wiith smallpox viirus.

***Vaccine.*** Pathogenic microorganisms or materials derived from such organisms that contain antigens in an inocuous form. When inoculated into a non-immune individual, the vaccine will provoke active immunity to the microorganisms, but will not cause disease.

***Vaccine.*** Suspension of dead or attenuated viruses or bacteria used to immunize against these pathogens.

***Vaccinia.*** Viirus, Pox virus officinale, originally derived from cowpox and used in vaccination to produce active immunity to smallpox.

***Vaccinia Gangrenosa.*** Synonym for progressive vaccinnia.

***Vaccinia Virus.*** Cowpox virus, which used for vaccination against smallpox. It is a poxvirus with a double-stranded DNA genome.

***Vacuole.*** A fluid-filled often spherical membrane-bound compartment within a cell. Mature parenchyma cells of plants commonly have a large central vacuole bounded by a membrane, the tonoplast. The vacuolar solution (or cell sap) may contain salts, sugars, organic acids, oxygen, carbon dioxide, pigments (e.g. anthocyans), and waste products such as calcium oxalate in the form of single crystals or raphides, tannin in tannin cells, latex in laticifers. The vacuoles control turgor of plant cells by osmotic exchange of water. Plant vacuoles probably also have a lysosomal function; there is a growing tendency to describe all lysosomes as types of vacuole, with all vacuoles having similar origins. Vacuoles are also formed during endocytosis, particularly in animal cells, as in the formation of food vacuoles in Protozoa. Many freshwater unicellular organisms and sponges possess contractile vacuoles, which function in osmoregulation.

***Valence.*** Number of binding sites on an antibody or antigen molecule. The antibody valence corresponds to the maximum number of antigen molecules that can bind to one antibody molecule (barring steric hindrance). Antigen valence is more difficult to define. An antigen typically has a number of distinct determinants, each of which may bind a different population of antibody molecules; these determinants may be overlapping.

***Valine*** (Val). One of the 20 common amino acids found in proteins. It has a non-polar side-chain.

***Vanadate.*** Ion containing vanadium and oxygen, used in cell biology to block cross-bridge formation of dynein, and to block ATpase activity.

***Van der Waals forces.*** Weak, short-range attractive forces between atoms or molecules, chiefly between non-polar molecules and therefore of a hydrophobic nature. These forces result from interactions between varying dipoles.

***Variable Region.*** Portion of an immunoglobulin molecule that interacts with anigen.

***Variable (V) Region.*** In a set of equivalent proteins, that portion of each protein (or constituent polypeptiide chain) that varies in sequence from one molecule to the next. In the immunoglobulins, the variable region is the segment of a heavy or light chain that varies in sequence in chains of the same isotype and allotype: the amino-terminal domain of light chains (~110 amino acid residues) or of heavy chains (115-120 residues). The variable regions of heavy and light chains combine to form the binding site for antigen and, therefore, determine the specificity of the antibody molecule. The portion of the chain encoded by the V gene segment is sometimes also referred to as the variable or V region. By this definition, the V region would include the signal peptide, but not the portions of the variable region encoded by the J gene segment and, in the case of the heavy chain, the D gene segment. Thus the term 'V region' is sometimes ambiguous. Variable regions encoded by the V,J and sometimes D gene segments are also found in T cell receptors.

The term variable region is also used to refer to those domains of class I or class I major histocompatibility molecules that are most variable when equivalent molecules obtained from different members of the same species are compared the $\alpha_1$ and $\alpha_2$ domains of class II molecules and the $\alpha_1$ and $\beta_1$ domains of class II molecules.

***Variance.*** Mean of squared deviations from a mean value in a population or a set of observations.

***Variation.*** The differences in characteristics between members of a population or of a species. Variations are due to environmental influences, the genetic constitution of the individual (genotype), or to interactions between the two. Genetic variations are due to recombination of the genes during sexual reproduction or to mutations. These inherited variations are the raw material on which natural selection acts and are the basic cause of the evolution of species. Continuous variation (quantitative inheritance) is brought about by the action of many genes (polygenes), each having a small effect and causing a gradual change in a characteristic of the species. Examples are the height and weight variations in man.

Discontinuous variation (qualitative inheritance) is brought about by one or a few major genes, which may be present in the population in two or more allelic forms. These alleles give rise to alternative characteristics in the phenotype that differ sharply from each other, with no intermediates between them. Examples are the different blood groups in man, normal and vestigial wings in Drosophila, and round and wrinkled seed coats in peas.

***Variegation.*** Irregularity of pigmentation, usually resulting in plants due to differential chloroplast distribution in a chimaera or to viral infection, and in animals due to such factors as local physiological conditions or X chromosome inactivation.

***Variety.*** A unit of classification that is a subdivision of a species. The term is usually applied loosely to a number of a groups within the species. It is most often used for a cultivated form of a plant, usually produced vegetatively, but is sometimes applied to a new breed of animal. The name of a variety is usually added after the name of the species in the style Salix repens var, fusca (a variety of creeping willow), or simply as Salix repens fusca. Cultivated varieties produced in horticulture are known as cultivars. Cultivars have English names, rather than Latin ones, and the specific epithet is often omitted from the name (as in Gypsophila 'Briston Fairy').

***Variolation.*** Inoculation of pustular materiial from smallpox lesions into the skin of non-immune recipients with the aim of inducing immunity to smallpox. Variolation was difficult to control and frequently produced severe smallpox infection. Variolation was superseded by vaccination.

***Varve Dating (Geochronology).*** A dating technique that gives the absolute age of a sediment and therefore of the fossils it contains. Varves are finely stratified clays, formed especially in Scandinavia during the retreat of ice in the Pleistocene. Each varve is thought to be seasonal and to represent the yearly melting of the ice. In some places, varve formation has continued until the present day; by counting varves it has been possible to establish an absolute chronology for northern glaciated Europe that goes back to the end of the Pleistocene (i.e. to 20 000 years ago).

***Vascular Tissue.*** (1) In animals, all tissues involved in the circulation of blood, including the heart, arteries, veins and capillary networks. (2) In plants, the transporting tissues of the vascular bundles (i.e. phloem, xylem and associated cambium).

***Vasculitis.*** Inflammation and necrosis of blood vessels, as may ocur in immune complex disease.

***Vasopressin (Antidiuretic Hormone, ADH).*** A peptide hormone secreted by the pars nervosa of the mammalian pituitary gland. In 1895, Oliver and Schafer first showed that pituitary extract caused vasoconstriction and increased blood pressure in the dog. The mammalian vasopressins were characterized and synthesized by du Vigneaud in the 1950s. The main effects of vasopressin are: (1) the stimulation of water re-uptake by the epithelial cells of the kidney distal tubules in higher vertebrates (antidiuretic effect), (2) stimulation of the permeability of skin and bladder cells in amphibians, (3) contraction of the smooth muscle in the walls of blood vessels (vasopressor effect), and (4) the regulation of the release of hormones from the adenohypophysis. These effects are all mediated by cyclic AMP. The secretion of vasopressin is stimulated by most emotional, systemic, or reflex stimuli and by osmotic and electrolyte factors in the blood. Purified posterior pituitary extracts containing vasopressin are known as pitressin.

***Vasotocin.*** A peptide hormone secreted by the posterior pituitary of most lower vertebrates and by the mammalian foetus and pineal gland. It was first identified in the chicken in 1958, but subsequent work has shown that the amphibian water balance principle described by Heller in 1941 was vasotocin. Its wide distribution has led to the hypothesis that vasotocin was a stem hormone in the evolution of the neurohypophysial hormones. Vasotocin structurally resembles and exhibits similar properties to vasopressin and oxytocin but its most characteristic action is to increase permeability in the skin and bladder of amphibians.

***Vasotocin.*** Peptide hormone secreted by the posterior pituitary gland of lower invertebrates and by the pineal body in mammals. It increases skin permeability in amphibians and regulates bladder function and is structurally similar to vasopressin.

***Vector.*** (1) Organism responsible for parasite transfer one host to another. (2) Plasmid or other self-replicating DNA molecule that transfers DNA between cells in nature or in recombinant DNA technology. In the latter connection it may be called a cloning vector or cloning vehicle.

***Vector.*** DNA element used as a vehicle for cloning a fragment of foreign DNA. A vector should have the following properties: (1) capacity for autonomous replication in a host cell (i.e., it should contain an origin of replication); (2) presence of one or more selectable markers (e.g., antibiotic resistance); (3) presence of sites for restriction endonucleases in non-essential regions, allowing foreign DNA to be inserted into the vector or to replace a segment of the vector. Major types of cloning vectors are plasmids (e.g., pBR322), bacteriophages (e.g., lambda or M13 bacteriophage), cosmids, animal viruses (e.g., SV40, retroviruses).

***Vegetal Hemisphere.*** Part of the amphibian egg that is distant from the nucleus and contains most of the yolk.

***Vegetative Cell.*** Cell not directly involved in sexual reproduction.

***Vegetative Nucleus.*** (1) Tube nucleus of a pollen grain. (2) Macronucleus of a ciliate protozoan that carries both macronucleus (the vegetative nucleus) and micronucleus.

***Vegetative Petite.*** Petite mutant of yeast cells in which the genetic lesion is in the mitochondrial genome. When such a mutant results from a nuclear lesion, it forms a segregational petition.

***Vegetative Pole*** (Vegetal Pole). Region of the eggs of certain organisms. The eggs of most animals are spherical, but many have an asymmetrical distribution of pigment, cell organelles, etc. The lower most pole of the egg is the vegetative pole. In some animals the cells that form at these regions give rise to specific germ layers or embryonic tissues. Certain conditions or chemicals cause an overproduction of the embryonic tissues normally produced at the vegetative pole; such abnormal embryos are said to be 'vegetalized'. Other chemicals or conditions can produce 'animalized' embryos.

***Vegetative Propagation.*** Production of new organisms without a sexual process as in budding in Hydra, simple fission in bacteria or yeast cells, and propagation by cuttings, bulbs, corms, etc. in green plants.

***Vegetative State.*** Replication of viral particles within a bacterium or eukaryotic cell as an alternative to integration.

***Venom.*** Poison secreted by some animals (e.g., snakes, arthropods), delivered in bites and stings, and used for taking prey.

***Ventral.*** Relating to the side of an animal which faces downwards, or forwards in bipedal animals such as the human.

***Vermilion.*** Sex-linked recessive mutation of eye colour in Drosophila melanogaster.

***Vernalization.*** The exposure of certain plants to a period of cold, which in these plants is either required before flowering will occur or induces earlier flowering than usual. Flowering is usually subsequently controlled by photoperiodism. Winter varieties of rye, oats, and wheat, unlike spring varieties, require vernalization before flowering within one year. Therefore they are usually sown in autumn for vernalization during winter. Alternatively, the partially germinated seed is vernalized in cold storage, a technique perfected in Russia where severe winters would kill seedlings. Many biennials, which require a winter before flowering, can be induced to flower in the first year by vernalizing the young plants. Treatment with gibberellins can sometimes substitute for the cold period. Some perennials, e.g. wallflower, require annual periods of low temperature before flowering. The low-temperature stimulus is perceived by the apical bud, or sometimes by the leaves, and transmitted to the floral apex. The bud-perceived stimulus can also be transmitted across a graft to a second plant. A hormone, vernalin, has been postulated as being responsible, but has not been isolated.

***Veronal Buffer.*** Buffer prepared from sodium barbitone and used to maintain the pH of fixative such as glutaraldehyde used in the preparation of tissues for transmission or scanning electron microscopy.

***Vertical Transmission.*** Transmission of genetic material (or integrated viruses) via conventional hereditary processes.

***Vesicle.*** Membrane-bound cellular compartment, but especially applied to endocytotic vesicles, exocytotic vesicles and lysosomes.

***Vesicular Stomatitis Virus.*** Rhabdovirus, having a single-stranded RNA genome, and bullet-shaped virion covered in an envelope with many protroding microspikes.

***Vessel Element.*** Xylem cell witth specialized lignin thickening in the form of perforation plates. Vessels occur only in angiosperms and are water-conducting in plants that possess them.

***Vestigial.*** Descriptive of an organ that persists only as a vestige (i.e. in a reduced form) since the organism in which it occurs has so evolved that the organ is redundant. Human gill slits are vestigal organs.

***Vestigial Organ.*** An organ that has become reduced because the organism possessing it evolved in such a way that it was no longer required. Vestigial organs are important in that they show evolutionary relationships. For example, the skeleton of a snake shows that it possesses vestigial limbs, which cannot be seen in the external form but indicate that snakes evolved from limbed lizard-like ancestors.

***V Gene.*** Gene coding for the variable region (V region) of an immunoglobulin chain.

***V Gene Segment.*** Segment of DNA encoding most (i.e. the first ~95-100) amino acid residues of the variable regions of immunoglobulin and T cell receptor polypeptide chains. The V gene segment contains two coding regions, separated by an nitron of 100-400 base pairs. The first (5') of these coding regions is an exon that encodes a short untranslated region of mRNA as well as the first approximately 15-18 residues of the sgnal peptide. The second coding region, at the 3' end of the segment, is part of an exon; it usually encodes the last four residues of the signal peptide and 95-100 residues of the variable region. The remainder of the variable region is encoded by a J gene segment, and, in the case of immunoglobulin heavy chains and T cell receptor beta and delta chains, a D gene segment. Before transcription, the V gene segment is juxtaposed to the 5' end of a J or a D-J gene segment. (in preB-cells an unrearranged V gene may be transcribed.) As a result of this rearrangement, an exon is formed, which encodes the end of the signal peptide and the entire variable region.

***$V_H$.*** Variable region of an immunoglobulin heavy chain; sometimes used to denote that portion of the variable region encoded by the $V_H$ gene segment.

***Viability.*** Number of individuals surviving, especially in comparing the survival of two different groups within a species or population.

***Viable Count.*** Proportion of cells in a sample of tissue culture or bacterial cells that are able to grow and replicate.

***Vicariad.*** A group of species produced by allopatric speciation from one common ancestor.

***Vicia faba.*** Species name for broad bean or horse bean.

***Villin.*** Calcium-dependent, actin-fragmenting protein, also capable of nucleating actin assembly. It is abundant in intestinal brush border microvilli.

***Villus.*** Finger-like projection from an epithelial surface. Examples include the intestinal villi, which greatly increase the absorptive surface of the gut, and chorionic villi, which provide extensive contact between the placenta and the uterus. Note that villi consist of very many cells, and shound not be confused with microvilli, which are subcellular, and from a brush border on many absorptive cells.

***Vimentin*** (decamin). Cytoskeletal protein that is a major component of intermediate filaments in many cells.

***Vinblastine.*** Alkaloid from the plant Vinca that inhibits spindle formation in dividing cells and, for this reason, is used in the treatment of cancer. Vincristine is a similar, but distinct compound.

***Vinca Alkaloids.*** Toxins (e.g., vincristine, vinblastine) from plants of the genus Vinca, which includes the common periwinkle, that act as mitotic poisons.

***Vinculin.*** Fibrous protein responsible for the attachment of actin filaments to the inner surface of the plasma membrane. It is distributed in patches known as adhesion plaques, and these are believed to be involved in intercellular adhesion.

***Viral-specific Enzyme.*** Enzyme that is found in virus-infected cells, but is coded on the viral and not the cellular genome.

***Virion.*** Complete virus or bacteriophage particle, consisting of nucleic acid genome associated with a capsid protein coat.

***Viroid.*** A factor similar to a virus but with an even simpler organization, since it exists simply as a closed circle of single-stranded RNA (partially base-paired). Some viroids are believed to be pathogenic agents in higher plants, e.g. potato spindle tuber viroid.

***Virulence.*** Capacity of a pathogenic organism to produce a disease. Virulence is a function of invasiveness (the ability to colonize a host) and toxigenicity (the production of toxic substnaces such as exotoxins and endotoxins).

***Virulent Phage.*** Bacteriophage (e.g., the T phages of E.coli) which on infecting host bacteria enters a cycle of lytic growth terminating in lysis of the bacterial cell and the liberation of phage progeny.

***Virus.*** One of a group of minute infectious agents, formerly defined as unique obligate intracellular parasites. Since this is also a property of certain bacteria and the rickettsiae, viruses are now distinguished by their simple organization and structure and mechanism of replication. Many viruses cause disease in their hosts; they are metabolically inert outside the host cell and are no more alive than the pieces of nucleic acid used in transformation. A mature virus, known as a virion; is much smaller than a bacterium, with a diameter ranging between 20 and 400 nm. It consists basically of a shell or tube of protein subunits (capsomeres), the capsid, around a centrally located nucleic acid. Any particular virus contains only a single type of nucleic acid, RNA or DNA, as its genetic material. Some virus capsids resembly an icosahedron (a polyhedron of 20 triangular faces with 12 corners) and are called icosahedral virions; others have a cylindrical form with a helical structure and are called helical virions. Virus particles lack ribosomes, transfer RNA, ATP-generating systems, and biosynthetic enzymes. The virus genome contains no information for synthesizing ATP-generating systems. The virus shows a specificity for its host not shown by naked viral nucleic acid.

After the virus attaches to its specific host cell, the viral nucleic acid enters the cell, directs the synthesis of virus-specific proteins, and undergoes replication. The protein subunits of the virus coat are then assembled around the new copies of the viral genome to give complete virions. These are released by the dissolution of the infected cell either as naked virions or as enveloped virions, which acquire additional coats from the host cell envelope during release. Some viruses show other types of growth and development that do not necessarily cause dissolution of the host cell.

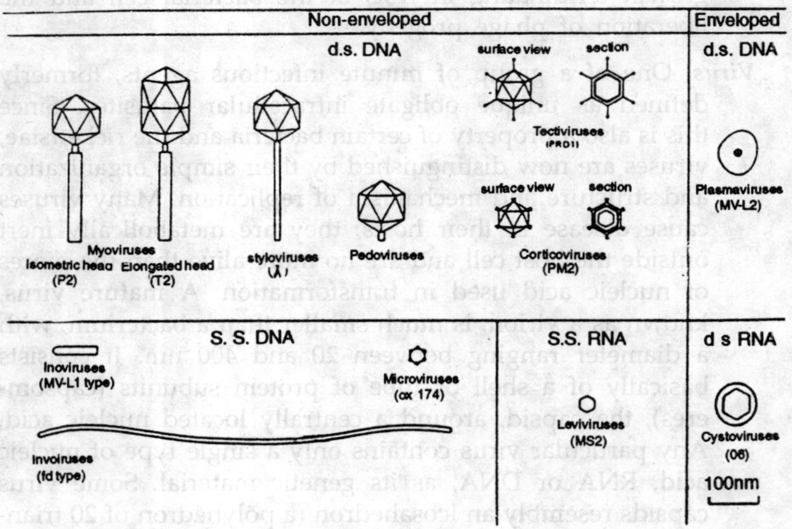


Figure V.1. Virus. Family of viruses infecting bacteria. Reproduced, with permission, from Matthews. R.E.F., Intervirology, 1982, 17 (1-2).

Viruses can be divided into four groups according to the types of organism they infect, i.e. animals, plants, insects, and bacteria. The host range depends both on the capsid and the specific receptors it interacts with on the host cell surface. Viruses can also be grouped into highly specific morphological types but the number of these is too small for adequate classification. The type of nucleic acid of the viruses can also be used for classification. Some important animal viruses are classified below :

Viruses containing double-stranded DNA. 1. Papovaviruses: naked icosahedral viruses causing tumours. There are two types: papillomaviruses, about 550 A in diameter, which include the viruses causing warts; and the smaller polyomaviruses, about 450 A in diameter, which include SV40 virus.

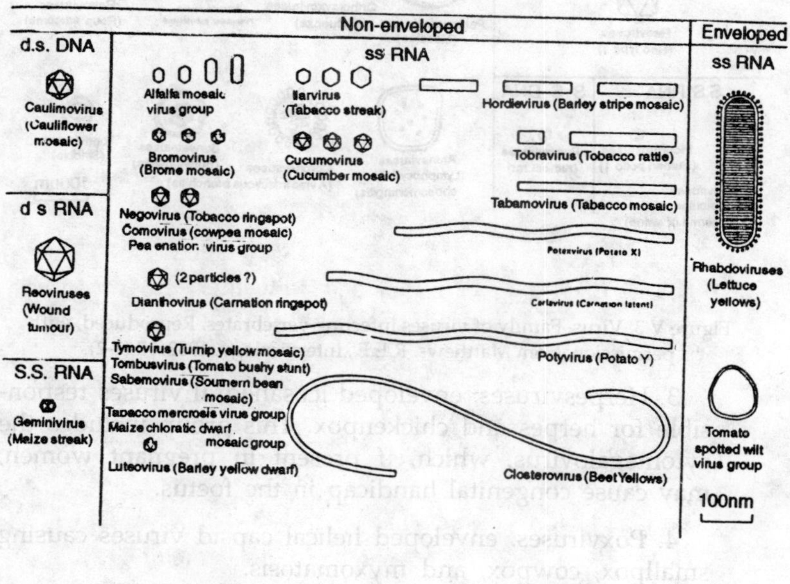


Figure V.2. Virus. Family of viruses infecting plants. Reproduced, with permission, from Matthews, R.E.F., Intervirology, 1982, 17 (1-2).

2. Adenoviruses: naked icosahedral viruses causing acute respiratory diseases in man. Adenoviruses possess a small genome of double-strand DNA associated with up to 12 different kinds of protein molecule. Like some other types of eukaryotic virus, adenoviruses have messenger RNA molecules that are mosaics of exon sequences spliced together after transcription.

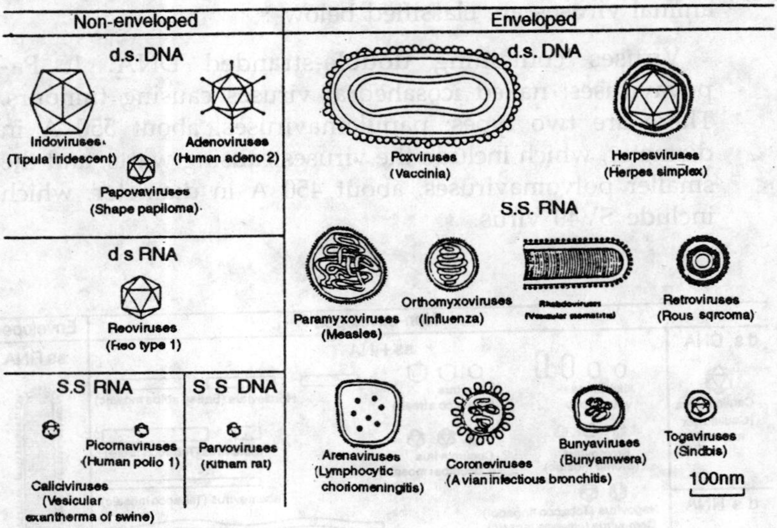


Figure V.3. Virus. Family of viruses infecting vertebrates. Reproduced, with permission, from Matthews. R.E.F., Intervirology, 1982, 17 (1-2).

3. Herpesviruses: enveloped icosahedral viruses responsible for herpes and chickenpox. This group includes the cytomegalovirus, which, if present in pregnant women, may cause congenital handicap in the foetus.

4. Poxviruses: enveloped helical capsid viruses causing smallpox, cowpox, and myxomatosis.

Viruses containing single-stranded RNA

1. Picornaviruses: naked icosahedral viruses, including the enteroviruses of man (such as those causing poliomyelitis), the rhinoviruses (responsible for colds), and the agents of foot-and-mouth disease in cattle.

2. Arboviruses: enveloped viruses causing such diseases as yellow fever and encephalitis.

3. Myxoviruses: enveloped helical capsid viruses responsible for influenza, mumps, measles, rubella, and rabies. See Figures V.1., V.2, V.3 and V.4.

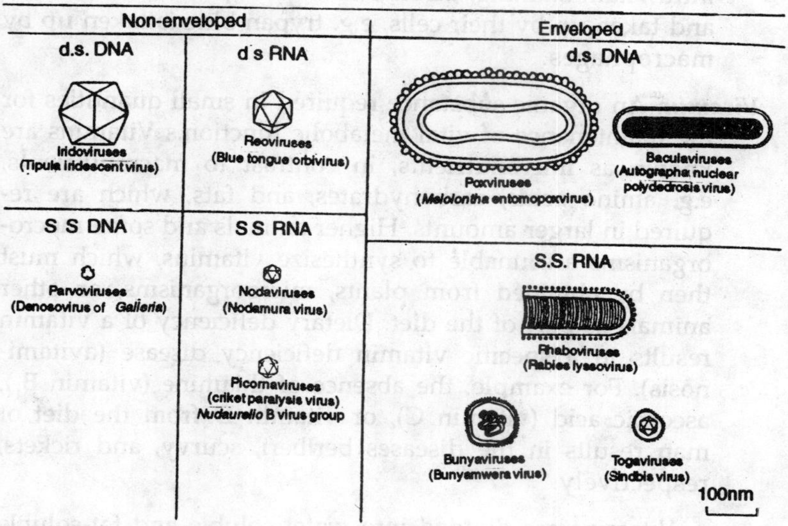


Figure V.4. Virus. Family of viruses infecting invertebrates. Reproduced, with permission, from Matthews. R.E.F., Intervirology, 1982, 17 (1-2).

***Virus Neutralization Test.*** Test to determine the titer of antibodies to a virus. The infectivity of the test virus (e.g, for tissue culture cells or susceptible animals) is neutralized by antibodies.

***Virus Receptor.*** Specific protein, glycoprotein or polysaccharide molecule on the surfaces of eukaryotic or bacterial cells that is the specific site to which viruses absorb.

***Visceral Endoderm.*** Inner layer of endoderm.

***Visible Mutation.*** Observable mutation.

***Vitalism.*** Concept or philosophy which holds that living systems possess and display characteristics that are not understandable in terms of chemistry and physics.

***Vital Staining.*** The process of staining cells while they are still alive. Some vital stains are specific, e.g. Janus green stains mitochondria. Supravital staining involves the immersion of cells in basic stains, e.g. methylene blue stains axons. In intra-vitam staining, acidic stains are injected into animals and taken up by their cells, e.g. trypan blue is taken up by macrophages.

***Vitamin.*** An organic substance required in small quantities for the maintenance of vital metabolic function.s Vitamins are known as micronutrients, in contrast to macronutrients, e.g. amino acids, carbohydrates, and fats, which are required in larger amounts. Higher animals and some mocro-organisms are unable to synthesize vitamins, which must then by obtained from plants, microorganisms, or other animals as part of the diet. Dietary deficiency of a vitamin results in a specific vitamin deficiency disease (avitaminosis). For example, the absence of thiamine (vitamin $B_1$), ascorbic acid (vitamin C), or vitamin D from the diet of man results in the diseases beriberi, scurvy, and rickets, respectively.

Vitamins are divided into water-soluble and fat-soluble groups. The water-soluble vitamins include the vitamin B complex and ascorbic acid. The former function as coenzymes (or the precursors of coenzymes) and the latter as a cofactor in several enzyme reactions. All the other vitamins, i.e. vitamin A(retinol), vitamin D, vitamin E (tocopherol), and vitamin K, are fat-soluble and have less well established mechanism of action.

***Vitamin A*** (Retinol). Substance derived from plant carotenes; deficiency in the diet leads to night blindness and eventual growth impairment. It is stored in the liver, and fish liver oil is a rich source of the vitamin. The aldehyde of retinol (retinene) is involved with opsin in the production of rhodopsin.

***Vitamin B Compex.*** Group of water-soluble vitamins functioning as coenzymes or coenzyme precursors. Included in the grouping are $B_1$ (thiamin), $B_2$ (nicotinic acid and riboflavin), $B_6$ (pantothenic acid and pyridoxine) and $B_{12}$ (cyanocobalamin and folic acid).

***Vitamin D.*** Fat-soluble steroid vitamins which include $D_2$(calciferol) and $D_3$. Actions of vitamin D include the increased absorption of phosphate and calcium by the gut, and deficiency leads to bone calcification abnormalities including rickets. Precursors of the vitamins are converted to the active form in animal tissues in the presence of ultraviolet light. Plant-derived precursors of $D_2$ and $D_3$, respectively, are ergosterol and 7-dehydrocholesterol.

***Vitamin D-resistant Rickets.*** Sex-linked dominant hereditary disease in humans involving defective renal transport of phosphorus. The disease resembles rickets due to vitamin D deficiency, but persists in the presence of adequate dietary vitamin D.

***Vitamin E*** (Tocopherol). Fat-soluble vitamin grouping consisting of $\alpha$–, $\beta$– and $\gamma$–tocopherol, and related molecules. The vitamin complex is found in some vegetables and especially wheat germ, and is thought to act by membrane stabilization. Deficiency leads to reproductive impairment and sterility.

***Vitamin K.*** Fat-soluble vitamin which, if deficient in vertebrate diet, leads to blood-clotting impairment due to failure in the synthesis of prothrombin.

***Vitellogenesis.*** Formation of yolk during the maturation of an egg or oocyte.

***Vitellogenin.*** Lipophosphoprotein: precursor of the two major proteins— lipovitellin and phosphovitin— in the yolk of oocytes. In amphibians vitellogenin ($M_r$—2000 000) is synthesized in the liver of vitellogenic females, secreted into the serum, transported to the ovaries and is taken into the growing oocytes by selective pinocytosis into small intracellular vesicels. Within the oocyte the vesicles coalesce, vitellogenin is converted into lipovitellin and phosphovitin, and the yolk proteins are arranged to form yolk platelets.

***Vitellogenin Genes.*** Genes coding for vitellogenin. Three such genes exist in Drosophila, each with only one or two introns, whereas in Xenopus laevis at least four distinct genes exist. Two of the Xenopus genes—A1 and A2—have been studied in some detail. They are 21 and 16 kilobases in length, respectively, both having 33 introns interrupting the coding sequence and both yielding messenger RNA about 6.3 kilobases long.

***Viviparity.*** 1. A type of reproduction in animals in which the embryo(s) develop within the derive nourishment from the maternal organism. Viviparity is characteristic of all placental mammals; it also occurs in some snakes, lizards, sharks, and invertebrates.

2. The process by which certain plants bypass the shedding of spores or seeds, producing instead small plants similar to themselves. For example, in Selaginella apoda (a lycopsid) the spores germinate on the parent plant so that the gametophyte phase is passed in the sporangium and an embryonic sporophyte plant is released.

***Viviparous.*** Describing an organism able to reproduce by retaining the embryo within the mother who provides the embryo with nourishment via placental connections. All placental mammals are viviparous, as are some snakes, lizards, sharks and invertebrates.

***$V_L$.*** Variable region of an immunoglobulin light chain; sometimes used to denote the segment encoded by the $V_L$ gene.

***VLA*** (Very Late Appearing Antigents). Five distinct heterodiers of cell membranes that share a common beta chain ($M_r$130,000) but have different alpha chains ($M_r$ 130,000-210,000). VLAs were first found on membranes of lymphocyte that had been in culture for several days. Subsequently, one or more VLAs were found on all types of nucleated cells. VLAs may function as cell matrix adhesion receptors. For example, VLA-5 is the fibronectin receptor.

***$V_{max}$.*** Expression used to define maximal diffusion rates achieved by satuaration of carrier protein binding sites for the solute substrate.

***Vollmer Test.*** Skin patch test using tuberculin.

***Voltage Clamp.*** Situation in which microelectrodes are placed in a cell and adjusted so that the membrane potential is held steady at a set voltage.

***Voltage Gating.*** Process in which certain ion channels are operated only at certain voltages.

***Voltinism.*** Variation in the presence or absence of dispause (temporary cessation of growth) which is evident as a polymorphism in strains of certain insects such as the silk moth Bombyx mori.

***Volutin.*** Cytoplasmic granules of polymerized inorganic phosphate that appear in the cytoplasm of both prokaryotic and eukaryotic microorganisms during nutrient stravation.

***Volvox.*** Simple multicellular alga in which the component cells are held in a hollow sphere without apparent cell specialization.

***Von Gierke Disease.*** Autosomal recessive disease in humans, presenting as defective glycogen storage due to malformation of glucose-6-phosphatase. It has an incidence of one in 100 000.

***Von Hippel-Lindau Disease.*** Inherited disease caused by an autosomal dominant gene, characterized by retinal haemangioma and renal carcinoma.

***V region.*** Variable region of immunoglobin light chain and heavy chain and containing the antigen binding sites.

# W

***Waardenburg Syndrome.*** Inherited human disease with a frequency of about one in 42 000. It is inherited as an autosomal dominant and is characterized by severe deafness and other symptoms.

***Wallace Effect.*** Hypothesis, advanced by Alfred Russell Wallace, that populations of organisms tend to become reproductively isolated at a species level.

***Waltzer.*** Mutant strain of laboratory mice that carries a neurological defect. Homozygous animals tend to walk in circles and have a head-shaking behaviour.

***Warfarin.*** Compound used as a rat poison and in the treatment of venous thrombosis, because of its antagonism of blood clotting. It is also a tetratogen in humans if taken in the first trimester of pregnancy.

***Waring Blender.*** Homogenizer consisting of rotating steel blades within a stainless steel vessel; widely used to homogenize tissue samples and to detach conjugating bacteria.

***Watson-Crick Model.*** Double-helical, right-handed model for DNA structure, proposed by J.Watson and F.Crick in 1953. The model proposed that two polynucleotide chains were associated by specific hydrogen bonds between complementary base pairs, the sugar phosphate backbones forming a double helix and thus providing a rigid framework of the bases. Although alternative structures for DNA (e.g., left-handed Z-form) have been discovered subsequently, the model has proved correct and has provided enormous stimulus and insight in the field of molecular genetics.

***Waxes.*** Esters of fatty acids and long-chain alcohols, commonly found as outer protective layers in plants and animals. For example, many leaves have a waxy cuticle, and beeswax is used for honeycomb formation by bees.

***Weak Interactions.*** Bonds that are less strong than covalent bonds, and inlclude van der waals forces and hydrogen bonds.

***Wegener's Granulomatosis.*** Disease charracterized by granulomas and vasculitis with necrosis of the upper and lower respiratory tracts and glomerulonephritis. The disease is thought to have an immunological cause. The disease process responds favourably to cyclophosphamide treatment.

***Weismannism.*** Proposition, now generally accepted, that characteristics acquired during the life time of an organism are not inherited and that only genetic changes in the germ line cells (in animals) are passed on to progeny.

***Western Blotting.*** Method for identifying proteins in complex mixtures. The proteins as separated by electrophoresis through a slab gel and then blot transferred onto a sheet of nitrocellulose by electrophoresis at 90° to the gel surface. The proteins bound on the nitrocellulose membrane can then be identified by reaction with specific reagents such as radioactive or fluorescent-labelled antibodies.

***Wheat Germ Lectin.*** Substance that specifically binds to N-acetyglucosamine and is used in cell biology to release these molecules from membranes.

***White Graft.*** Skin graft that is rapidly rejected prior to vascularization and lymphocytic infiltration, possibly because of the presence of pre-existing antibodies to the graft. Presence of a white graft is a manifestation of so-called hyperacute graft rejection.

***White Locus.*** Complex locus in the Drosophila genome affecting eye colour. Many mutants have been identified in the locus, including some which involve regulatory rather than structural sequences.

***Whole-arm Fusion*** (Centric fusion, robertsonian translocation). Fusion of the long arm of two chromosomes following breakage and loss of the small arms of two acrocentric chromosomes.

***Wild Mouse.*** Unconfined mouse that has not been raised under laboratory or domestic conditions and whose reproduction is not controlled.

***Wild Type.*** The type of individual (or the genotype or phenotype it possesses) that is most common in wild populations. For example in Drosophila, the wild tuype has normal wings, a grey body, and red eyes. Each of these genes is dominant to any other allele for that gene. Wild-type alleles are often represened as + rather than by a letter. Thus an insect homozygous for wild-type wings would be represented as ++. If a recessive gene becomes, by natural selection, the wild type, its status is modified so that it becomes dominant.

***Wild-type Gene.*** Gene that is the commonest of any series of alleles at that locus and is therefore regarded as normal. Wild-type alleles are frequently represented as +, and an organism homozygous for such a gene would be represented as ++.

***Wilm's Tumour.*** Rental tumour in children, often bilateral, of which about one in three results from inheritance of an autosomal dominant.

***Wilson's disease.*** Autosomal recessive inherited disorder in humans in which copper excretion is defective, and liver and brain damage results from copper accumulation.

***Winn Test.*** Procedure to evaluatee whether or not lymphocyrtes are sensitized to allogeneic cells or tumors. The allogeneic or tumor cells, together with the test lymphocytes, are injected into the skin of X-irradiated mice and the growtth of the cell mass is evaluated. Sensitized T lymphocytes will diminish the multiplication of the allogeneic cells or tumors. The test is frequently used to study immunity to tumors.

***Wiskott-Aldrich Syndrome.*** Inherited disease of immunodeficiency resulting from an X-linked recessive gene.

***Wiskott-Aldrich Syndrome (WAS).*** X-linked immunodeficiency disease, characterized by a low number of small platelets in the blood (thrombocytopenia), eczema and defective cell-mediated immunity. Affected males have small platelets, which are less than 1.8 μm in diameter (normal: 2.8-3.5 μm), and which lack surface glycoprotein Ib. The serum concentrations of IgA and IgE are elevated, that of IgM is decreased, but serum IgG concentration is usually normal. Patients have a markedly diminished antibody response to polysaccharide antigens (e.g., pneumococcal polysaccharides). Cell-mediated immuniy declines progressively with age. T lymphocytes are abnormal when examined by scanning electron microscopy; they appear to have bald surfaces in contrast to the richly fimbriated appearance of normal T lymphocytes. The sialophorin of T lymphocytes is abnormal. The defect in WAS can be completely corrected by transplants of normal bone marrow cells.

***Wobble Hypothesis.*** Proposal made by F.Crick to explain the fact that more than one codon triplet can be recognized by tRNA molecule bearing a single anticodon triplet. Degeneracy in the code means that in the mRNA, some amino acids are specified by differing codons, yet the same aminoacyl-tRNA recognizes them. Almost all of the variation is in the last of the three letters in the codon, and the hypothesis proposes that wobble in the anticodon to codon binding allows some third-letter variation.

***Wolman's Disease.*** Inherited human disorder determined by a recessive autosomal gene on chromosome 4, which involved deficiency of lipase in the lysosomes.

***Wright's Inbreeding Coefficient*** (F). Proportion of loci at which an individual organism is homozygous.

***Writhing Number.*** Number of times a supercoiled molecule of DNA is crossed or folded upon itself.

***Wu-Kabat Plot.*** Bar graph to illustrate the degree of variability at each amino acid residue position in the variable regions of immunoglobulins and T cell receptors. An index of variability is defined as the number of different amino acids found at a given position divided by the frequency of the most common amino acid at the position. Since 20 amino acids are utilized in the polypeptide chains, the index ranges from 1 to 400. (Suppose that at a particular position, valine occurs in 50 out of 100 chains, leucine occurs in 25 chains, and isoleucine in the remaining 25 chains. In this case, there are three different amino acids and the frequency of the most common (valine) is 0.5; therefore, the variability at this position is 3/0.5 or 6.) To display the variability graphically, the index is plotted (in bar graph form) at each residue position. The resulting plot shows the degree of variability at each position and has been used to localize the hypervariable regions of the polypeptide chains of immunoglobulins and T cell receptors. See Figure W.1.

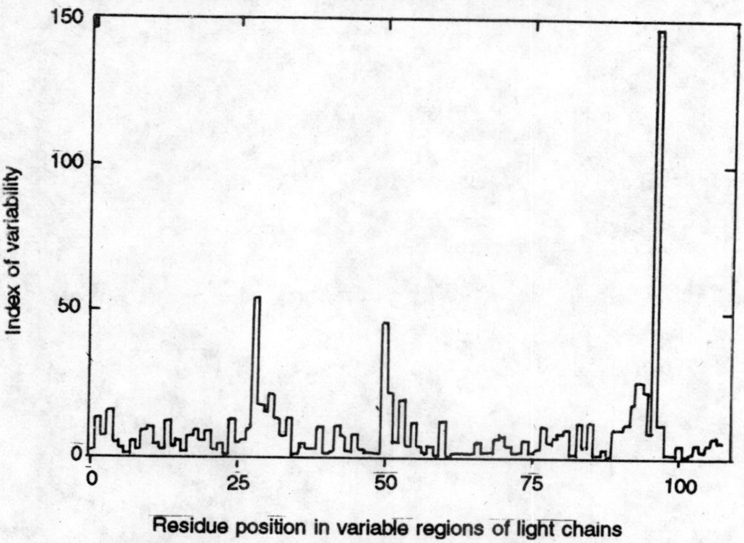


Figure W.1. Wu-Kabat plot. From Wu, T.T. and Kabat, E.A.J. Exper. Med. 132:210, 1970.

***W,Z chromosomes.*** Specification of sex chromosomes in some organisms (e.g., silk moth) in which the female is the heterogametic sex. Thus the male is ZZ and the female is WZ, and the W chromosome is female-determining.

# X

***Xanthinuria.*** Human disease in which the purine xanthine persists in the urine rather than being completely converted to uric acid.

***Xanthophylls.*** Class of oxygenated hydrocarbon compounds structurally related to carotene. Xanthophylls are yellow pigments, some of which function as photosynthetic acessory pigments in plants. However, in the brown algae the xanthophylls fucoxanthin and peridinin are the primary light-absorbing pigments.

***Xenogeneic Transplantation.*** Grafing of tissue between organisms of different species, or the transfer of organelles from a cell of one species to that of another.

***Xenograft.*** Graft to a member of a different species. Xenografts are usually rejected within a few days by antibodies and cytotoxic T lymphocytes to histocompatibility antigens. Synonym for heterograft.

***Xenoplastic.*** Pertaining to the grafting of parts between individuals of different species or genra.

***Xenopus Laevis.*** African clawed toad, a pipid anuran amphibian, which has been much used in experimental embryology, in studies of the control of gene expression and in developmental immunology where the existence of a free-living embryo (tadpole) and inbred, histocompatible strains of Xenopus laevis have been especially useful.

***Xeroderma Pigmentosum.*** Human metabolic disorder with a genetic basis, in which defects exist in the DNA repair mechanisms. One consequence is a high incidence of skin cancer due to the inability to repair damage caused by the ultraviolet irradiation from sunlight.

***X Inactivation.*** Repression by condensation of the transcriptional activity of one of the two copies of the X chromosome in all somatic cells of tthe female mammals. One of the two X chromosomes is randomly inactivated in early embryonic life, as a mechanism of dosage compensation. The condensed chromosome is visible in somatic cell nucleic as the barr body, although some genes at the distal end of the short arm of the X chromosome may escape inactivation. Tortoisehell cat coat colour results from the mosaic distribution of clones of epidermal cells in which either of the X chromosomes is inactivated, the pigment alleles being carried on this chromosome.

***X Linkage.*** Usual form of sex linkage in which a particular gene is located on the X chromosome.

***X-linked Agammaglobulinemia (XLA).*** Failure of immunoglobulin synthesis of all isotypes that results from an absence of B lymphocytes. Affected males have recurrent pyogenic infections. Their bone marrow contains a normal number of pre-B cells in which constant regions of immunoglobulin mu chains can be discerned in cytoplasm by immunofluorescence. There may be faulty $V_H$-D-$J_H$ gene rearrangement. The gene for X-linked agammaglobulinemia has been mapped to chromosome Xq 21.3-22.

***X-linked Hypogammaglobulinemia with Growth Hormone Deficiency.*** X-linked recessive form of hypogammaglobulinemia. Affected males have no B lymphocytes, and they are of short stature from 'failure of growth hormone synthesis. The gene for this deficiency does not map to Xq21.3-22, the location of the gene for X-linked agammaglobulinemia.

***XO.*** Situation in a heterogametic organism in which only a single X chromosome is present rather than an XX or XY. Human individuals with turner's syndrome are XO.

***X-radiation.*** Radiation of X-rays, which are produced when metal surfaces are bombarded with high-speed electrons. X-Rays are ionizing radiations and have wavelengths intermediatte between ultraviolet and gamma-radiation.

***X-ray Crystallography*** (X-ray diffraction analysis). Technique that makes a unique contribution to molecular biology because it provides the only method able to reveal the three-dimensional position of atoms in relation to each other in macromolecules such as proteins and nucleic acids. The technique depends on the fact that X-rays have a wavelength of 0.154 nm, which is similar to interatomic distances. X-Rays are passed through a crystal of the protein or other macromolecule, and those that are diffracted (scattered) by the atoms in the crystal are detected on photographic film. The detail in the structure deduced from the diffraction pattern depends on the resolution of the analysis, which for proteins has a limit of about 0.2 nm. It should be noted that to produce complete three-dimensional pictures of, say, enzyme molecules a great deal of conventional enzyme chemistry is necessary as well as the X-ray diffraction data.

***X-ray Diffraction Analysis (X-ray Crystallography).*** A technique for determining the arrangement of atoms in a crystalline substance by analysing the diffraction patterns produced when a narrow beam of X-rays is passed through the substance. The substance may be examined as a single crystal (used for detailed protein structure) or as a more-or-less randomly orientated mixture of crystals, as with powders and whole cell walls. X-ray diffraction has contributed to the elucidation of structure of many biological molecules, including some important macromolecules, e.g. DNA, haemoglobin, myoglobin. It is particularly useful for determining the tertiary and quaternary structure of proteins; the structure of myoglobin, for instance, has been determined at a resolution of less than 0.2 nm.

***Xylem*.** Complex cellular tissue, consisting of several cell types, that forms the principal water-conducting system in plants. The primary xylem is formed first and develops from the procambium of the primary meristem. It consists of protoxylem and metaxylem, the former differentiating while the tissue is still elongating. In those plants that undergo secondary thickening, the primary xylem is succeeded by secondary xylem which forms from the vascular cambium. The most characteristic cellular components are the tracheary elements, which conduct the water and also provide some mechanical support. Further support is provided by fibre tracheids and fibres. All these cell types have secondary wall thickening, which is usually lignified and at maturity they are devoid of living contents. Parenchyma cells are also present and constitute the living component and are important for the storage of food reserves. In secondary xylem some parenchyma, is present as radially arranged groups of cells, the rays, and some, the axial parenchyma, is more closely associated with the longitudinally aligned tracheary elements.

# Y

***Yeasts.*** Eukaryotic fungal cells that are widely used and studied in cell biology and genetics. Saccharomyces cerevisiae is the budding yeast used in baking and brewing, and Schizosaccharomyces pombe is a fission yeast. Yeast cells grow rapidly in culture and have been widely used in studying the cell cycle. Petite mutants of yeast, which have mitochondrial gene mutations, are also widely studied, and yeast cells are now used as expression systems for other eukaryotic gene sequences in recombinant DNA technology.

***Yeast Vectors.*** Yeast cells used as carriers of plasmids, in which novel genes may be replicated, or as transformed cells used to produce the products of integrated novel genes.

***Y Chromosomes.*** Chromosomes found in the heterogametic sex. In most mammals the male carries XY chromosomes and the female XX. The Y chromosome is male determining, as shown by the female phenotype of XO individuals (turner's syndrome). It is a small heterochromatic chromosome with few if any structural genes located on it.

***Y Linkage.*** Sex linkage, in which genes are located on the Y chromosome, and are therefore expressed only in males (holandric inheritance). In mammals the Y chromosome carries few, if any genes, but in some organisms (e.g., medaka fish) the Y chromosome does carry genes.

***Yolk.*** Inert, nutrient constituent of the ovum; consisting mainly of protein and fat. Ova of viviparous animals tend to have very little yolk.

***Y-suppressed Lethan Gene.*** Sex-linked recessive lethal gene that allows survival of XY males, but causes the death of XO individuals in Drosophila melanogaster.

# Z

***Zea Mays.*** Species name for maize, corn or Indian corn.

***Z Chromosome.*** Sex chromosome found in animal species in which the female is heterogametic and is therefore WZ; males are ZZ.

***Z DNA.*** Form of DNA in which the helix is screwed in a left-handed rather than a right-handed direction. Z DNA occurs in short stretches of DNA in nature.

***Zidovudine.*** (3'-azido-3'-deoxythymidine, AZT). Analogue of thymidine that inhibits reverse transcriptase. It has been used in the treatment of the acquired immunodeficiency syndrome. AZT is phosphorylated in vivo to 3'-azido-3'-deoxythymidine triphosphate, which binds to the reverse transcriptase of human immunodeficiency virus and other retroviruses, thereby terminating elongation of DNA.

***Zona Pellucida.*** Thin, non-cellular envelope that is secreted by follicle cells around the mammalian oocyte and which persists until the blastocyst stage just prior to implantation.

***Zone Electrophoresis.*** Type of electrophoresis in which the mobile ions or proteins move in a buffer through a support medium such as paper, cellulose acetate, starch gel, silica gel, polyurethane foam or acrylamide polymers. The sample is applied to the support in a narrow band approximately midway between the buffer reservoirs housing the electrodes. During electrophoresis, each component migrates towards the cathode or anode, depending on its charge, at a characteristic rate. Using this method charged species are separated into discrete zones. Sunsequently, the support can be divided into sections and individual components may be separately eluted.

***Zonula Adherens.*** Type of adhering cell junction; now known as a belt desmosome.

***Zoospore.*** Flagellated spore, produced from a zoosporangium of many algae and some fungi. It is often, but not invariablky functional as a gamete.

***Zoogeography.*** The study of the distribution of animals, especially in relation to the continents they occupy. There are three main areas of distinct fauna: Arctogea, Neogea, and Notogea, whose distributions can be explained by the theory of continental drift.

The diversity of marsupials found in Notogea is due to the fact that Australia has been a completely separate continent since Cretaceous times: thus its marsupial fauna has avoided unsuccessful competition with the more efficient placentals. Neogea, too, has a very distinct fauna. It was isolated for much of the period of mammalian evolution, and during the Tertiary period a great variety of marsupials and primitive placentals evolved there, cut off from the more advanced placentals of North America. In late Tertiary times a land bridge connecting the two continents was formed, and many advanced placentals invaded from the north and have now replaced most of the native marsupials. The continents comprising Arctogea have only recently drifted apart. During much of the Pleistocene they formed one continuous land mass over which the animals freely moved. Thus many families, and even genera, of animals are today present on several of the continents. Once the continents had separated, climatic and otther forces came into effect; the animals disappeared from some of the continents and evolved in different directions in others.

***Zwitterion.*** Ion bearing both a negative and a positive charge. All amino acids may exist as zwitterions.

***Zygonema.*** Little-used term for the zygotene sage of meiosis.

***Zygote*** (Zygospore). Diploid cell formed as the result of fusion between two gametes at fertilization.

***Zygotene.*** Meiotic stage during which synapsis of homologous chromosoms takes place.

***Zygotic Induction.*** Induction of bacteriophage proliferation and cell lysis in a nonlysogenic bacterial cell as a result of its conjugation with a lysogenic bacterium containing an integrated prophage. The transfer of DNA during the cojugation process results in the acquisition of the prophage gene by the recipient bacterium. However, the nonlysogenic characteristics of tthis cell lead to breakdown of the prophage state, induction of phage replication, and eventual lysis of the recipient cell. Zygotic induction is the technique normally used to map the incidence and location of prophage genes.

***Zygotic Lethal Gene.*** Gene that is lethal at some stage of development, but does not affect the function of gametes.

***Zygotic Meiosis.*** Meiosis that follows directly from zygote formation, as in protozoa and fungi.

***Zymogen.*** An inactive precursor of an enzyme. Large dense zymogen granules occur in the exocrine cells of the pancreas (i.e. those cells lining the branches of the pancreatic duct). They comprise a mixture of proteins (the precursors of the pancreatic juice enzymes carboxypeptidase, trypsin, and chymotrypsin), which are synthesized on the endoplasmic reticulum and concentrated in Golgi vesicles prior to release into the pancreatic duct.

***Zymogen Granules.*** Previously had a specific meaning in relation to zymogen, but currently used as an ultrastructural term for any cytoplasmic storage granule that is membrane-bound.

***Zymogram.*** Electrophoretic gels used to reveal and compare protein polymorphism, as of isoenzymes such as lactate dehydrogenase subunits.

***Zymosan.*** Dried cell walls of yeast. Zymosan is a complex polysaccharide that has been used to study the activation of the alternative pathway of complement.